MANUAL OF OBSTETRICS

Eighth Edition

Editors

Arthur T. Evans, MD
Professor and Chairman
Department of Obstetrics and Gynecology
University of Cincinnati College of Medicine
Cincinnati, Ohio

Emily DeFranco, DO, MS
Associate Professor
Department of Obstetrics and Gynecology
Division of Maternal-Fetal Medicine
University of Cincinnati College of Medicine
Cincinnati, Ohio

Donna Mc

http://inkling.com/read

password: donkeelbrivec

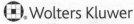

Wolters Kluwer
Health
Philadelphia • Baltimore • New York • London
Buenos Aires • Hong Kong • Sydney • Tokyo

Acquisitions Editor: Rebecca Gaertner, Jamie Elfrank
Product Development Editor: Morgan Hawk, Ashley Fischer
Production Product Manager: Priscilla Crater
Manufacturing Manager: Beth Welsh
Marketing Manager: Stephanie Manzo
Design Coordinator: Teresa Mallon
Production Services: SPi Global

8th Edition

Library of Congress Cataloging-in-Publication Data
Manual of obstetrics / [edited by] Arthur T. Evans, Emily DeFranco. — 8th edition.
    p. ; cm.
  Includes bibliographical references and index.
  ISBN 978-1-4511-8677-2
  I. Evans, Arthur T., editor of compilation. II. DeFranco, Emily, editor of compilation.
  [DNLM: 1. Obstetrics—Outlines. 2. Contraception—Outlines. 3. Perinatal Care—Outlines.
  4. Pregnancy Complications—Outlines.   WQ 18.2]
  RG531
  618.2—dc23   2013049597

Dedication

To my wife, Catherine, for her support and to our children and grandchildren for making it all worthwhile.

Arthur T. Evans, MD

To my mentor, colleague, and friend, Arthur Evans, for trusting me to carry on his work on the *Manual of Obstetrics*.

Emily DeFranco, DO, MS

Contributors

Alfred Abuhamad, MD
Professor and Chair
Department of Obstetrics and Gynecology
Eastern Virginia Medical School
Norfolk, Virginia

Albert Asante, MB, BCh
Fellow
Department of Obstetrics and Gynecology
Mayo College of Medicine
Fellow
Division of Reproductive Endocrinology and
*   Infertility*
Department of Obstetrics and Gynecology
Mayo Clinic
Rochester, Minnesota

Kristin L. Atkins, MD
Assistant Professor
Department of Obstetrics, Gynecology and
*   Reproductive Sciences*
University of Maryland School of Medicine
Medical Director of Labor and Delivery
Department of Obstetrics, Gynecology and
*   Reproductive Sciences*
University of Maryland Medical Center
Baltimore, Maryland

Bill Atkinson, MD
Clinical Associate Professor
Department of Obstetrics and Gynecology
Division of Maternal-Fetal Medicine
Texas Technical University Health Sciences
*   Center*
Medical Director, Women's Service
Department of Obstetrics and Gynecology
Division of Maternal-Fetal Medicine
Covenant Health
Lubbock, Texas

John R. Barton, MD
Associate Professor
Department of Obstetrics and Gynecology
University of Kentucky
Director, Maternal-Fetal Medicine
Perinatal Diagnostic Center
Baptist Health Lexington
Lexington, Kentucky

Cynthia Bean, MD
Assistant Professor
Department of Obstetrics and Gynecology
University of Cincinnati College of Medicine
General Obstetrician and Gynecologist
Department of Obstetrics and Gynecology
University of Cincinnati Medical Center
Cincinnati, Ohio

Eliza M. Berkley, MD
Assistant Professor
Department of Obstetrics and Gynecology—
*   Maternal-Fetal Medicine*
Eastern Virginia Medical School
Norfolk, Virginia

Kathleen M. Berkowitz, MD
Perinatologist
MemorialCare Center for Women
Miller Children's and Women's Hospital
Long Beach Medical Center
Long Beach, California

Brett Blake, MD
Procedural Dermatology Fellow
Department of Dermatology
VCU Medical Center
Richmond, Virginia

Jennifer Cavitt, MD
Associate Professor
Department of Neurology
University of Cincinnati Medical Center
Cincinnati, Ohio

Christian A. Chisholm, MD
Associate Professor and Vice-Chair for
*   Medical Education*
Department of Obstetrics and Gynecology
University of Virginia
Attending Physician
Department of Obstetrics and Gynecology
University of Virginia Health System
Charlottesville, Virginia

James T. Christmas, MD
Director, Maternal-Fetal Medicine
Commonwealth Perinatal Services
HCA Physician Services
Henrico Doctors Hospital
Richmond, Virginia

Charles C. Coddington, MD
Professor of Obstetrics and Gynecology
Mayo College of Medicine
Consultant
Division of Reproductive Endocrinology and
    Infertility
Department of Obstetrics and Gynecology
Mayo Clinic
Rochester, Minnesota

Alan M. Coleman, MD
Research Fellow
Division of Pediatric, General, Thoracic
    and Fetal Surgery
Cincinnati Children's Hospital Medical
    Center
Cincinnati, Ohio

Joseph Collea, MD
Professor
Department of Obstetrics and Gynecology
Division of Maternal-Fetal Medicine
Georgetown University
Washington, DC

David F. Colombo, MD
Assistant Professor
Department of Maternal-Fetal Medicine
Wexner Medical Center
The Ohio State University
Columbus, Ohio

Hope M. Cottrill, BM, MD
Volunteer Faculty
Department of Obstetrics and Gynecology
University of Kentucky
Physician
Medical Director of Robotic Surgery Program
Cancer Committee Chair of Quality
    Improvements
Member Institutional Review Board
Department of Gynecologic Oncology Services
Baptist Health Lexington
Lexington, Kentucky

Bonnie J. Dattel, MD, FACOG
Professor and Assistant Dean
Department of Obstetrics and Gynecology
Division of Maternal-Fetal Medicine
Eastern Virginia Medical School
Norfolk, Virginia
Director, Labor and Delivery
Women's Health
Sentara Norfolk General Hospital
Norfolk, Virginia

David D'Alessio, MD
Professor
Department of Internal Medicine
Division of Endocrinology
University of Cincinnati
Director of Endocrinology
University Hospital
Section Chief, Endocrinology
Cincinnati VA Medical Center
Cincinnati, Ohio

Emily DeFranco, DO, MS
Associate Professor
Department of Obstetrics and Gynecology
Division of Maternal Fetal Medicine
University of Cincinnati
Cincinnati, Ohio

Margarita deVeciana, MD
Professor
Department of Obstetrics and Gynecology
Eastern Virginia Medical School
Norfolk, Virginia

Arthur T. Evans, MD
Chair and Professor of Obstetrics and
    Gynecology
Division of Maternal-Fetal Medicine
University of Cincinnati College of Medicine
Cincinnati, Ohio

James E. Ferguson II, MD, MBA
William Norman Thornton Professor and
    Chair
Department of Obstetrics and Gynecology
University of Virginia
Obstetrician and Gynecologist-in-Chief
Department of Obstetrics and Gynecology
University of Virginia Health System
Charlottesville, Virginia

Kellie Flood-Shaffer, MD, FACOG
Associate Professor, Division Director-
  General Obstetrics and Gynecology
Department of Obstetrics and Gynecology
University of Cincinnati College of Medicine
Faculty Attending Physician
Department of Obstetrics and Gynecology
University of Cincinnati Medical Center
Cincinnati, Ohio

Todd Fontenot, MD
Director of Maternal-Fetal Medicine
Baton Rouge Medical Center
Baton Rouge, Louisiana

Regina Fragneto, MD
Professor
Department of Anesthesiology
University of Kentucky College of Medicine
Director of Obstetric Anesthesia
Department of Anesthesiology
UK Healthcare Chandler Medical Center
Lexington, Kentucky

Glen A. Green, MD
Associate Professor
Department of Pediatrics
Eastern Virginia Medical School
Neonatologist
Division of Neonatology
Children's Hospital of the King's Daughters
Norfolk, Virginia

R. Moss Hampton, MD
Chairman
Department of Obstetrics and Gynecology
Texas Tech University Health Sciences
  Center of the Permian Basin
Odessa, Texas

Wendy F. Hansen, MD
Department of Obstetrics and Gynecology
Division of Maternal-Fetal Medicine
University of Kentucky
John W. Greene Jr., MD Chair
Department of Obstetrics and Gynecology
University of Kentucky College of Medicine
Lexington, Kentucky

Kimberly W. Hickey, MD
Assistant Professor
Department of Obstetrics and Gynecology
Uniformed Services University
Chief, Maternal-Fetal Medicine
Department of Obstetrics and Gynecology
Walter Reed National Military Medical
  Center
Bethesda, Maryland

Nicolette P. Holliday, MD
Assistant Professor
Department of Obstetrics and Gynecology
University of South Alabama
Mobile, Alabama

Andra H. James, MD
John M. Nokes Professor and Vice-Chair for
  Research
Department of Obstetrics and Gynecology
University of Virginia
Attending Physician
Department of Obstetrics and Gynecology
University of Virginia Health System
Charlottesville, Virginia

Donna D. Johnson, MD
Professor and Chair
Department of Obstetrics and Gynecology
Medical University of South Carolina
Charleston, South Carolina

Elizabeth A. Kelly, MD
Associate Professor
Department of Obstetrics and Gynecology
University of Cincinnati
Medical Director
Division of Community Women's Health
University of Cincinnati Medical Center
Cincinnati, Ohio

Jamil H. Khan, MD
Associate Professor
Pediatrics
Eastern Virginia Medical School
Medical Director
Neonatal Intensive Care Unit
Children's Hospital of The King's Daughters
Norfolk, Virginia

David F. Lewis, MD, MBA
Professor and Chair
Division of Maternal-Fetal Medicine
Department of Obstetrics and Gynecology
University of South Alabama School of Medicine
Mobile, Alabama

Foong-Yen Lim, MD
Associate Professor
Department of Surgery
University of Cincinnati
Surgical Director of the Cincinnati Fetal Center
Division of Pediatric, General, and Thoracic and Fetal Surgery
Cincinnati Children's Hospital Medical Center
Cincinnati, Ohio

Nancy C Lintner, MS, ACNS, RNC-OB, CPT
Clinical Program Coordinator for the Diabetes and Pregnancy Program
Division of Maternal-Fetal Medicine
University of Cincinnati College of Medicine
Cincinnati, Ohio

H. Trent Mackay, MD, MPH
Department of Obstetrics and Gynecology
Uniformed Services University of the Health Sciences
Bethesda, Maryland

Kalyani S. Marathe, MD, MPH
Post-Doctoral Clinical Fellow in Dermatology
Pediatric Dermatology
Department of Dermatology
Columbia University Medical Center
New York, New York

Samantha Mast, MD
Instructor
Department of Obstetrics and Gynecology
Maternal-Fetal Medicine Fellow
University of Kentucky
Lexington, Kentucky

Jill G. Mauldin, MD
Associate Professor
Medical Director, Women's Services
Division of Maternal-Fetal Medicine
Department of Obstetrics and Gynecology
Medical University of South Carolina
Charleston, South Carolina

Kathleen McIntyre-Seltman, MD
Professor
Department of Obstetrics
Gynecology and Reproductive Sciences
Division of Gynecologic Specialties
University of Pittsburgh Physicians
Pittsburgh, Pennsylvania

Susan C. Modesitt, MD, FACOG, FACS
Professor and Director
Division of Gynecologic Oncology
Department of Obstetrics and Gynecology
University of Virginia
Charlottesville, Virginia

Michael P. Nageotte, MD
Professor
Department of Obstetrics and Gynecology
Division of Maternal-Fetal Medicine
University of California–Irvine Medical Center
Orange, California

Tondra Newman, MD
Fellow, Maternal-Fetal Medicine
Department of Obstetrics and Gynecology
University of Cincinnati Medical Center
Cincinnati, Ohio

Tifany Nolan, MD
Instructor of Clinical Obstetrics and Gynecology
University of Cincinnati College of Medicine
Cincinnati, Ohio

Errol Norwitz, MD, PhD
Professor and Chairman
Department of Obstetrics and Gynecology
Tufts University School of Medicine
Boston, Massachusetts

David M. Pariser, MD
Professor
Department of Dermatology
Eastern Virginia Medical School
Norfolk, Virginia

Samuel Parry, MD
Associate Professor
Department of Obstetrics and Gynecology
University of Pennsylvania School of
  Medicine
Chief, Maternal-Fetal Medicine Division
Department of Obstetrics and Gynecology
Hospital of the University of
  Pennsylvania
Philadelphia, Pennsylvania

Ruth Anne Queenan, MD, MBA
Assistant Professor
Department of Obstetrics and
  Gynecology
University of Rochester
Chief
Department of Obstetrics and Gynecology
Highland Hospital
Rochester, New York

Raymond W. Redline, MD
Professor
Department of Pathology and Reproductive
  Biology
Case Western Reserve University
Staff Pathologist
Department of Pathology
University Hospitals Case Medical Center
Cleveland, Ohio

Jodi Regan, MD
Fellow, Maternal-Fetal Medicine
Division of Maternal-Fetal Medicine
University of Cincinnati College of Medicine
Cincinnati, Ohio

Julian N. Robinson, MD
Associate Professor of Obstetrics and
  Gynecology and Reproductive Biology
Department of Obstetrics and Gynecology
Brigham and Women's Hospital
Boston, Massachusetts

Reena Shah, MD
Assistant Professor
Department of Neurology
University of Cincinnati Medical Center
Cincinnati, Ohio

Tushar A. Shah, MD, MPH
Assistant Professor
Department of Pediatrics
Eastern Virginia Medical School
Staff Neonatologist
Division of Neonatology
Children's Hospital of The King's
  Daughters
Norfolk, Virginia

Baha M. Sibai, MD
Director, Maternal-Fetal Medicine
  Fellowship Program
Department of Obstetrics, Gynecology and
  Reproductive Sciences
The University of Texas Medical School at
  Houston
Professor
Department of Obstetrics, Gynecology and
  Reproductive Sciences
Memorial Hermann Hospital-Texas
  Medical Center
Houston, Texas

Brett H. Siegfried, MD
Assistant Professor
Department of Pediatrics
Eastern Virginia Medical School
Neonatologist
Division of Neonatology
Children's Hospital of the King's
  Daughters
Norfolk, Virginia

Nicole A. Smith, MD, MPH
Assistant Professor of Obstetrics, Gynecology
  and Reproductive Biology
Department of Obstetrics, Gynecology and
  Reproductive Biology
Brigham and Women's Hospital
Boston, Massachusetts

Julie Sroga, MD
Assistant Professor of Obstetrics and
Gynecology
Division of Reproductive Endocrinology and
Infertility
University of Cincinnati College of Medicine
Cincinnati, Ohio

Amy Thompson, MD, FACOG
Assistant Professor of Obstetrics and
Gynecology
The Clarence R. McLain Chair of Medical
Student Education
University of Cincinnati College of Medicine
Cincinnati, Ohio

Loralei L. Thornburg, MD
Assistant Professor
Department of Obstetrics and Gynecology
University of Rochester
Maternal-Fetal Medicine Division
Obstetrician and Gynecologist
Department of Obstetrics and Gynecology
Strong Memorial Hospital
Rochester, New York

Kenneth F. Tiffany, MD
Assistant Professor
Department of Pediatrics
Eastern Virginia Medical School
Neonatologist
Division of Neonatology
Children's Hospital of the King's Daughters
Norfolk, Virginia

Amy M. Valent, DO
Fellow, Maternal-Fetal Medicine
Department of Obstetrics and Gynecology
University of Cincinnati College of Medicine
Department of Obstetrics and Gynecology
University of Cincinnati Medical Center
Cincinnati, Ohio

Catherine Van Hook, MD
Associate Professor
Department of Obstetrics and Gynecology
University of Cincinnati College of Medicine
Cincinnati, Ohio

James W. Van Hook, MD
Professor and Executive Vice Chair, Director
Division of Maternal-Fetal Medicine
Department of Obstetrics and Gynecology
Director, Maternal-Fetal Medicine
Department of Obstetrics and Gynecology
University of Cincinnati Medical Center
Cincinnati, Ohio

Carri R. Warshak, MD
Assistant Professor of Obstetrics and
Gynecology
Division of Maternal-Fetal Medicine
University of Cincinnati College of
Medicine
Cincinnati, Ohio

Selman I. Welt, BS, MD
Professor
Department of Obstetrics and Gynecology
East Tennessee State University
Obstetrics Director
Department of Obstetrics and Gynecology
Johnson City Medical Center
Johnson City, Tennessee

Jason J. Woo, MD, MPH,
FACOG
Attending Consultant
Department of Obstetrics and Gynecology
MedStar Washington Hospital Center
Washington, District of Columbia

John D. Yeast, MD
Vice Chair
Department of Obstetrics and Gynecology
University of Missouri-Kansas City School
of Medicine
Vice President of Medical Education and
Research
Saint Luke's Hospital of Kansas City
Kansas City, Missouri

Preface

The eighth edition of the *Manual of Obstetrics* is changing to meet the digital expectations and needs of health care providers. We all want to have choices for how we access information. Clinical situations and personal preferences dictate different solutions at different times. We began the process to provide access to both print and electronic book formats with the seventh edition of the *Manual of Obstetrics*. The style and presentation were reformatted to be tighter, more compact, and more accessible. The eighth edition brings this process to completion with convergence of print and digital formats allowing the Manual to be available as a traditional printed book or, for the first time, as an e-book on computers and smart devices. Our goal is to make the Manual available to you in the format that works best for you as you care for your patients.

The entire eighth edition of the Manual has been carefully updated. A new chapter, Fetal Therapy, has been added in response to the emergence of the fetus as a bona fide individual patient. This chapter recognizes that the fetus has its own principles of care and standards of management. This rapidly evolving specialty area is truly at the cutting edge of obstetric care. A basic understanding of the capabilities and limitations of fetal care is an important new addition to our standard of obstetric care. Several other chapters have been thoroughly revised and updated. Both of the chapters on endocrine disorders have significant additions including insulin pump therapy for pregestational diabetes, choices for gestational diabetes screening and diagnostic testing, thyroid disease management, and complications of adrenal disease with pregnancy. The Neurologic Diseases chapter has been extensively revised and expanded as has Disease of the Placenta. The Preeclampsia chapter contains the most up-to-date version of the new ACOG definitions of, criteria for, and management of preeclampsia. Finally, the chapter on spontaneous preterm birth includes updated recommendations for screening and treatment of preterm labor and preterm rupture of membranes. It also provides new insight for the contemporary management of cervical insufficiency and the short cervix.

For the eighth edition, Dr. Emily DeFranco has joined the *Manual of Obstetrics* as the Associate Editor. Dr. DeFranco is Associate Professor of Obstetrics and Gynecology at the University of Cincinnati College of Medicine. She is an academic clinician-scientist and a specialist in Maternal-Fetal Medicine. Her research focus is spontaneous preterm birth and evidence-based medicine. We have worked together for many years, and it is a great pleasure to have her join the editorial staff of the eighth edition of the Manual. I am confident that Dr. DeFranco will be a significant contributor to the success of the *Manual of Obstetrics* for many editions to come.

We are greatly indebted to the distinguished physicians who serve as our chapter authors. The eighth edition of the *Manual of Obstetrics* would not be possible without their efforts and thoughtful contributions. We note the passing since the last edition of three of the Manual's long-standing chapter authors, Dr. Richard Oi, Dr. Gary Karlowicz, and Dr. Thomas Pellegrino. Notably, Dr. Oi was the author of "Disease of the Placenta" since the first edition in 1980. We also recognize, in his well-deserved retirement, Dr. Ken Niswander, the founding author of the Manual and editor of the first three editions.

We thank Lippincott Williams & Wilkins (LWW) and their editorial staff for their continued support in the production process. Two individuals have been particularly integral to the creation of the eighth edition. Ashley Fischer, the LWW Product Development Editor, has expertly guided the entire project. Debbie Stormer, my academic assistant, managed the complex process of coordinating chapter development between the authors and editors. Without their combined efforts, the eighth edition of the Manual would not have come to fruition.

The *Manual of Obstetrics* is intended to be used by all levels of obstetric providers. We hope that you will find the eighth edition to be a useful guide for making clinical decisions and a stimulus for excellence in obstetric and fetal care.

Arthur T. Evans, MD
Emily DeFranco, DO, MS

Contents

PART I

Obstetric Care

Prenatal Care
Elizabeth A. Kelly

KEY POINTS
- Prenatal care is designed to provide preventive care, active intervention for acute medical problems and identification of social determinants with referral to appropriate programs and assistance for two patients.
- Advances in technology have allowed the fetus to become a separate and distinct patient.
- Patient education is an important component of prenatal care.

BACKGROUND
- Prenatal care is unique:
  - It provides care simultaneously to two interdependent patients.
- There are many components of prenatal care:
  - Confirming the diagnosis of pregnancy and establishing the estimated gestational age, which allows the estimated date of confinement to be accurately assigned.
  - Obtaining a full history and conducting a physical examination with laboratory evaluation.
  - Conducting regular periodic examinations with ongoing patient education.
  - Assessing and performing well woman health maintenance and preventative care.
  - Identifying and addressing pregnancy complications as well as acute medical and psychosocial problems.
- All information obtained should be recorded in a concise manner that is accessible to other members of the health care team in the electronic health record.

DIAGNOSIS OF PREGNANCY AND ACCURATE DATING
- Early pregnancy diagnosis and accurate dating are essential for establishing a prenatal care plan, addressing risk factors, identifying medical complications, and determining appropriate timing of the delivery.
- The diagnosis of pregnancy is facilitated by both presumptive and probable signs.
  - *Presumptive signs* lead a woman to believe that she is pregnant.
  - *Probable signs* are highly suggestive of the diagnosis of pregnancy.
  - Note that these signs do not differentiate between an ectopic and an intrauterine pregnancy.

Presumptive Signs

- Amenorrhea is often the first sign of possible conception but may result from other factors, such as anovulation, premature menopause, thyroid disease, or elevated prolactin.
- Subjective signs and symptoms of early pregnancy include breast fullness and tenderness, skin changes, nausea, vomiting, urinary frequency, and fatigue.
- Between 12 and 20 weeks' gestation, a woman will note an enlarging abdomen and perceive fetal movement.

Probable Signs

- Uterine enlargement
- Softening of the uterine isthmus (Hegar sign)
- Vaginal and cervical cyanosis (Chadwick sign)
- Pregnancy tests:
  - Urine pregnancy tests used today are very sensitive and may be positive as early as 5 days after embryo implantation.
  - Radioimmunoassay for serum testing of the beta subunit of human chorionic gonadotropin (hCG) may be accurate up to a few days after implantation (or even before the first missed period). hCG production is at its maximum between 60 and 70 days of gestation and declines thereafter.
  - These tests do not differentiate between normal pregnancy, gestational trophoblastic disease, ectopic pregnancy, and abnormal intrauterine pregnancy.
  - Other bioassay techniques used in the past, such as progesterone withdrawal, are of historic interest only.

Positive Diagnostic Signs

- Fetal heart tones can be detected as early as 7 weeks from the last menstrual period (LMP) by Doppler technology. The nonelectronic fetoscope detects fetal heart tones at 18 to 20 weeks from the LMP.
- Fetal movements ("quickening") are generally first felt by the patient at approximately 16 to 18 weeks. They are a valuable indication of fetal well-being.
- Ultrasound examination will demonstrate an intrauterine gestational sac at 5 to 6 weeks and a fetal pole with movement and cardiac activity at 6 to 8 weeks. Vaginal probe ultrasonography has made these early measurements even more accurate. Fetal age can be estimated by crown–rump length, and the number of fetuses may be identified. After 12 to 14 weeks of gestation, fetal biometric measurements, including biparietal diameter and femur length, can be used to estimate fetal age accurately. In the second trimester, fetal anatomy, placental location, and amniotic fluid volume can be evaluated. There is no evidence that diagnostic ultrasound exposure has adverse effects on the developing human fetus.

Estimated Date of Delivery

- The expected duration of pregnancy, calculated from the LMP to estimated date of delivery (EDD) is 280 days, or 40 weeks.
- Naegele's rule is used to calculate the EDD:
  - To the 1st day of the LMP, add 7 days and then subtract 3 months.
  - Deviations from this calculation may be made for various reasons (e.g., irregular or prolonged menstrual cycles, known single sexual exposure, or known conception date via artificial reproductive technologies, such as in vitro fertilization).
  - If the date of the LMP is unknown or does not correlate with uterine size at the first visit, ultrasonography should be used to establish the EDD.

EVALUATION

A complete history and physical examination are performed after the diagnosis of pregnancy is established. An important goal is to develop a trusting, working relationship between the patient and the health care team.

History

- Menstrual and contraceptive history:
  - Reliable menstrual history is the most accurate predictor of EDD.
- Gynecologic history: Previous sexually transmitted infections, abnormal Papanicolaou (Pap) smear, gynecologic surgeries, and hospitalization for gynecologic conditions should be recorded.
- Obstetric history:
  - The obstetric history is recorded as gravidity and parity. Gravidity is the total number of pregnancies. Parity is expressed as four serial numbers: term deliveries, premature deliveries, abortions and ectopic pregnancy, and living children.
  - Details of previous pregnancies, such as character and length of labor, mode of delivery, pregnancy and delivery complications, newborn health, and birth weight, should be noted. Recurrent first-trimester losses may suggest genetic abnormalities in the conceptus or parents while a history of second-trimester losses may suggest genetic abnormalities or cervical insufficiency.
  - If the patient has had a cesarean delivery, it is important to document the prior uterine scar type to assist with counseling for delivery mode and timing.
- Medical and surgical history and prior hospitalizations:
  - Preexisting medical problems or diagnoses are important for pregnancy risk assessment and management.
  - Previous surgeries and hospitalizations should be elicited and evaluated.
- Environmental exposures, medications taken in early pregnancy, history of reactions to medications, legal and illicit drug use, and allergic history.
- Family history of medical illnesses, heritable conditions, genetic abnormalities, mental retardation, congenital anomalies, and multiple gestation.
- Social history:
  - Home environment, family and social support, and history of physical or mental abuse should be assessed and appropriate referrals made.
  - Assessment of tobacco, alcohol and substance use, abuse, or dependence.
- Review of systems as related to pregnancy: nausea, vomiting, abdominal pain, constipation, headaches, syncopal episodes, vaginal bleeding or discharge, dysuria or urinary frequency, swelling, varicosities, and hemorrhoids.

Physical Examination

- Complete physical examination with attention to specific organ systems as directed by any positive findings in the history:
  - Measurement of height, weight, blood pressure, pulse and documentation of prepregnancy body mass index (BMI); funduscopic examination; examination of thyroid, lymph nodes, lungs, heart, breasts, and abdomen, with fundal height and presence of fetal heart tones, extremities; and a basic neurologic exam
- Pelvic examination:
  - External genitalia—Evidence of previous obstetric injury should be noted.
  - Vagina—Under hormonal influence of pregnancy, cervical secretions are increased, thus raising the vaginal pH, which may cause a change in the bacteriologic flora of the vagina. No treatment is necessary unless diagnosis of a specific infection is made (see "Treatment of Common Lesions and Infections" later in this chapter).
  - Cervix—A Pap test as indicated and testing for *Chlamydia* and gonorrhea are routinely performed.
    - Cervical softening and eversion (ectropion) is normal.
    - Nabothian cysts are of no consequence.
    - Dilatation of the external os is common in multiparous patients and is a nonpathologic finding. Significant cervical effacement or dilation of the internal os is abnormal, except near term, and may indicate premature labor or cervical insufficiency.

- ○ Morphologic cervical changes (ridges, hood, or collar), or vaginal adenosis may indicate DES exposure in utero. These women have a higher incidence of cervical insufficiency and preterm delivery and should be evaluated accordingly.
- Uterus—Estimating gestational age by gauging uterine size is one of the most important elements of the initial obstetric examination.
  - ○ A normal, nongravid uterus is firm, smooth, and approximately 3 × 4 × 7 cm. The uterus will not change noticeably in consistency or size until 5 to 6 weeks after the LMP, or 4 weeks after conception.
  - ○ Gestational age from the LMP is estimated by uterine volume (i.e., 8 weeks, twice normal size; 10 weeks, three times normal; 12 weeks, four times normal). At 12 weeks, the uterus fills the pelvis so that the fundus of the uterus is palpable at the symphysis pubis. By 16 weeks, the uterus is midway between the symphysis pubis and the umbilicus. At 20 weeks, the uterine fundus is at the level of the umbilicus. Thereafter, there is a rough correlation between weeks of gestation and centimeters of fundal curvature when measured from the top of the symphysis pubis to the top of the uterine fundus (MacDonald measurement).
  - ○ After correcting for minor discrepancies resulting from adiposity and variation in body shape, a uterine size that exceeds the anticipated gestational age by 3 weeks or more, as calculated from the last normal menstrual period, suggests multiple gestation, molar pregnancy, leiomyomata, uterine anomalies, adnexal masses, or simply an inaccurate date for the LMP. Ultrasonography is the best diagnostic tool for this situation.
  - ○ Smaller than expected uterine size for gestational age may indicate inaccurate dating or early pregnancy loss.
- Adnexa are difficult to evaluate because the fallopian tubes and the ovaries are lifted out of the pelvis by the enlarging uterus. Any questionable masses should be confirmed by ultrasound evaluation.
- Clinical pelvimetry is performed as part of the initial bimanual exam to assess the general adequacy of the pelvis for vaginal delivery.

Laboratory Evaluation
A history positive for certain illness or abnormalities in other screening tests should be investigated with further tests as indicated.
- A routine initial screen includes a complete blood count, ABO blood typing and Rh factor, red blood cell antibody screening, urinalysis and culture, serologic test for syphilis, rubella titer, Pap test as indicated, cervical testing for gonorrhea and *Chlamydia*, hepatitis B surface antigen, and testing for HIV.
- Group B *Streptococcus* (GBS) (see Chapter 23):
  - Screening is not indicated in early pregnancy, nor is it based on risk factors. Women with a urine culture positive for GBS do not require screening between 35 and 37 weeks as they will require antibiotic prophylaxis in labor.
  - All women except those with GBS bacteriuria in the current pregnancy should be screened for GBS at 35 to 37 weeks' gestation by a culture obtained from a swab of the rectum and the lower third of the vagina. Patients with positive results are treated with appropriate antibiotics during labor.
- Specialized screening tests:
  - Hemoglobin electrophoresis should be used to identify hemoglobinopathies in specific groups of women:
    - ○ Sickle hemoglobinopathies, beta-thalassemia, and alpha-thalassemia in persons of African descent
    - ○ Beta-thalassemia in persons of Mediterranean descent
    - ○ Beta-thalassemia and alpha-thalassemia (if microcytic anemia is present) in persons of Southeast Asian descent

- Screening for Tay-Sachs disease, familial dysautonomia, cystic fibrosis, and Canavan disease should be offered to persons of Ashkenazi Jewish (European Jewish) background.
- Cystic fibrosis carrier screening should be discussed with all patients and offered to all who are at risk, with highest risk prevalence in Caucasian women.
- Herpes cultures for purposes of screening are not recommended. Cultures may be helpful for confirming diagnosis when active lesions are present; however, they have little value in predicting whether the fetus is at risk.
- Urine or blood toxicology screening may be indicated for the evaluation of illicit substance use.
- Fetal ultrasound as a routine screening test without indications is not currently considered a standard of care in uncomplicated pregnancies. However, most physicians consider an obstetric ultrasound examination to be an essential part of prenatal evaluation and care for all pregnant women.
- Aneuploidy screening for trisomy 13, 18, and 21 can be offered in the first trimester at 10 to 14 weeks' gestation by early aneuploidy screening. This is a combination of ultrasound nuchal translucency and two serum analytes values (pregnancy associated plasma protein-A (PAPP-A) and free or total beta-hCG). Combined early aneuploidy screening with nuchal translucency and serum analytes provides better screening accuracy for selected trisomies compared to later individual screening tests, such as the second trimester quad screen or ultrasound screening alone.
- First plus send trimester screening tests
  - Aneuploidy screening for trisomy 13, 18, and 21 can also be accomplished through tests which utilize a combination of first trimester and second trimester screening results. The tests depend on the desire of the patient after counseling and the need for additional screening to assist with follow-up counseling. These screening options are integrated screening, stepwise sequential screening, and contingent screening.
- Mid-trimester screening tests:
  - Risk assessment for trisomy 13, 18, and 21 and open neural tube defects (NTDs) can be accomplished through the quadruple serum screening tests. These tests use a combination of serum analyte levels to provide an aneuploidy and NTD risk estimate rather than a definitive diagnosis. The quad screen is the preferred over the triple screen because the combination of maternal serum (MS)-alpha-fetoprotein, beta-hCG, estriol, and inhibin A provides greater sensitivity for aneuploidy detection. Blood should be drawn between the 15th and 20th weeks of gestation (16 to 18 weeks is preferred). Abnormal results are further evaluated by ultrasonography and consultation with a maternal–fetal medicine specialist.
  - At 24 to 28 weeks, a 1-hour glucola screen (blood glucose measurement 1 hour after a 50-g oral glucose load) is obtained to screen for gestational diabetes.
    - A 1-hour glucola screen value >140 mg/dL is considered abnormal and requires definitive testing with a 3-hour 100-g oral glucose tolerance test.
    - A universal screening approach may be used in which all pregnant women are screened.
    - Alternatively, a screening scheme can be used that excludes women who are at low risk for gestational diabetes by meeting all of the following criteria:
      - Younger than 25 years of age
      - Not a member of a racial or ethnic group with high prevalence of gestational diabetes
      - BMI < 25
      - No history of abnormal glucose tolerance
      - No previous history of adverse pregnancy outcomes associated with gestational diabetes
      - No known diabetes in first-degree relatives
    - Women with a particular risk (e.g., previous gestational diabetes or fetal macrosomia, family history of first degree relative with DM, obesity, glycosemia, polycystic ovarian syndrome [PCOS]) should receive a GCT before 20 weeks gestation.

- Repeat hemoglobin and hematocrit may be obtained at 26 to 30 weeks to determine whether iron supplementation is needed.
- At 28 to 30 weeks, an antibody screen is obtained in Rh-negative women, and an $Rh_o(D)$ immunoglobulin (RhoGAM) is administered.
- Repeat third-trimester screening for gonorrhea, *Chlamydia*, syphilis serology, and HIV is recommended in populations with increased prevalence of sexually transmitted infections.

TREATMENT OF COMMON LESIONS AND INFECTIONS THAT MAY BE ENCOUNTERED ON PELVIC EXAMINATION

Bartholin Gland Abscess
- A painful, erythematous, cystic enlargement on either side of the lateral vaginal introitus may indicate obstruction and infection of the Bartholin gland.
- Treatment includes sitz baths, analgesic, and, when fluctuant, incision and drainage. Cyst formation may result from incomplete resolution of an abscess. Marsupialization after the puerperium may be advisable for recurrent problems.

Condylomata Acuminata
- Venereal warts are hyperkeratotic, flat, or polypoid lesions found in the vulvar or perineal areas, vagina, or cervix and caused by infection with the human papillomavirus (HPV). Certain viral types are associated with the development of dysplasia and epithelial carcinoma.
- Pregnancy may stimulate proliferation of these lesions, which may become friable. Cesarean delivery is indicated if the pelvic outlet is obstructed or if vaginal delivery would result in hemorrhage.
- Transmission of HPV to the infant is very rare but may result in respiratory papillomatosis. The mode of transmission is unknown (transplacental, perinatal, or postnatal). Cesarean should not be performed to prevent HPV transmission to the infant.
- Treatment options in pregnancy are limited.

Herpes Simplex Viral Infections
- Characteristic lesions are small, painful, superficial, erythematous vesicles that ulcerate.
- Treatment is symptomatic. The safety of the antiviral agents acyclovir, famciclovir, and valacyclovir has not been definitively established, but available data do not indicate an increased incidence in congenital anomalies in women treated with acyclovir.
- If lesions are present at the time delivery is indicated, cesarean is recommended.
- Acyclovir, famciclovir, and valacyclovir are all FDA category B medications and are all approved for treatment of genital HSV in pregnancy.
- Women with recurrent genital HSV in pregnancy should be given suppressive therapy with acyclovir from 36 weeks of gestation until delivery to decrease the risk of acute lesions that will necessitate cesarean delivery.

Monilial Vulvovaginitis
- Monilial (also known as *Candida* or yeast) infection with the characteristic curdy, white, itchy discharge is common. Hyphal structures are seen on wet mount.
- This infection can be treated safely during pregnancy with nystatin or miconazole nitrate creams or suppositories or fluconazole in the usual dose regimens.

Trichomonas vaginalis Infection
- Vulvar or vaginal burning or itching with an abnormal discharge is a frequent finding with this infection. Confirmation of the diagnosis is by visualization of the organisms on wet mount.

- Metronidazole (Flagyl) is the treatment of choice. Clotrimazole suppositories (one nightly for 1 week) have been used, with an improvement in symptoms but only a 70% cure rate. The sexual partner should be referred for treatment or treated depending on the law in the state where one practices medicine.

Bacterial Vaginosis
- Bacterial vaginosis (BV) produces an abnormal discharge that may cause puritis. Characteristic clue cells are noted on wet mount, with amine discharge on potassium hydroxide preparation.
- Metronidizole or clindamycin may be used for treatment. Treatment of the sexual partner has not been found to be useful in routine cases.
- Some studies have suggested an association between BV and preterm labor or P PROM risk in women with a prior history of preterm birth. Treatment has not been shown to reduce the risk, and therefore routine screening for BV in pregnancy is not recommended.

Neisseria gonorrhoeae Infection
- Symptoms may include dysuria, burning, or vaginal discharge. Many patients are asymptomatic. Gram stain of endocervical specimens is not sufficient to detect infection and is not recommended.
- Usual treatment regimens may be administered; however, tetracycline is contraindicated in pregnancy. The sexual partner should be treated or referred for treatment.
- It is recommended that women with gonorrheal infection be treated for *Chlamydia* (see below). Routine cotreatment may also decrease the development of antimicrobial resistant *N. gonorrhoeae*.

Chlamydia trachomatis Infection
- Symptoms of the infection from this obligatory intracellular parasite include vaginal discharge. Diagnosis can be made through urine, vaginal, or endocervical specimens.
- The infection can be transmitted to the newborn in the form of conjunctivitis or pneumonia.
- The recommended treatment regimen is azithromycin 1 g orally.
- The sexual partner should be treated or referred for treatment, and a test-of-cure 3 to 4 weeks after therapy should be obtained.

COMPLICATIONS
Risk Assessment
Risk assessment is an important components of prenatal care. It is a continuous evaluation that must take into account aspects of the patient's medical and social complications. Designation of a pregnancy as low risk or high risk creates specific expectations and requirements for prenatal management.
- *Low risk* implies expectation of a term delivery without maternal or infant morbidity or mortality.
- *High risk* implies a need for increased surveillance, special care, and appropriate referrals. Categories of increased risk that should be identified and given appropriate attention include
  - Preexisting medical illness
  - Previous pregnancy complications, such as stillbirth, neonatal or infant mortality, preterm birth, fetal growth restriction, congenital malformations, placental abruption, and maternal hemorrhage
  - Prepregnancy BMI less than 18.5 or greater than 40
  - Onset of complicating events that may transition a low-risk pregnancy to a high-risk pregnancy

Genetics Referral

- Congenital anomalies and genetic abnormalities are major causes of infant morbidity and mortality.
- Indications for genetic referral include
  - Maternal age 35 years or older at the time of the EDD
  - Family history of congenital anomalies or heritable medical disorders
  - Developmental delay or mental retardation of a previous child
  - Ethnic background associated with increased risk of specific heritable diseases
  - Exposure to teratogens
  - Three or more prior spontaneous abortions

SUBSEQUENT PRENATAL CARE

Regular prenatal visits allow ongoing evaluation and assurance that the pregnancy is progressing normally.

- For low-risk pregnancies, the recommended frequency of prenatal visits is monthly up to 32 weeks, every 2 weeks up to 36 weeks, and then weekly until delivery.
- Standard assessment at each prenatal visit includes maternal weight, blood pressure, uterine size, auscultation of fetal heart tones, and evaluation for proteinuria and glucosuria. After 18 to 20 weeks, the patient should be questioned about fetal movements. At 32 weeks and beyond, the presenting fetal part should be documented.
- Ongoing patient education appropriate to the gestational age of the fetus is incorporated into these visits.
- All prenatal care information should be recorded on a standardized form.

GUIDELINES FOR PATIENTS

- Nutrition: A balanced approach is necessary because there are many limitations to our understanding of the nutritional needs of pregnancy.
  - Suggestions include eating foods from each of the major food groups, consuming adequate liquids (especially water), adding fiber, and ensuring adequate calcium intake.
  - For a woman whose weight is normal before pregnancy (BMI 18.5 to 24.9), normal pregnancy weight gain is 25 to 35 lb based on IOM recommendations. This is usually achieved by eating a well-balanced diet containing 60 to 80 g of protein, 2400 or more calories, low sugars and fats, high fiber, and at least three glasses of milk or other dairy equivalents daily. An underweight woman is at an increased risk for poor fetal growth, and more weight gain is often required. Excessive weight gain and preexisting maternal obesity (BMI $\geq$ 30) may be associated with increased risk of fetal macrosomia, cesarean delivery, and gestational diabetes and pre eclampsia.
  - Routine prescription of prenatal vitamins is probably not necessary. Practically all diets that supply adequate caloric intake for appropriate weight gain will also provide enough minerals. There are two exceptions:
    - Folic acid supplementation preconceptually and throughout the first twelve weeks of pregnancy has been shown to decrease the incidence of fetal NTDs.
    - Iron supplementation is recommended after 14 weeks' gestation because increased iron requirements in the latter part of pregnancy may be difficult to meet via a normal diet.
- Working during pregnancy: Most women can safely work until term without complications.
  - Pregnant women may work full time. Activity limitations have not been shown to decrease risk of spontaneous preterm birth in women at high risk and are not routinely recommended for prevention of preterm birth in asymptomatic patients.
- Exercise: Women may exercise if they have no complicating factors.

- Exercise recommendations should be tailored according to the level of physical activity of the patient before she became pregnant and according to her level of physical fitness. A trained athlete can continue rigorous training during pregnancy but should avoid raising her core temperature or becoming dehydrated.
- Smoking should be discontinued during pregnancy.
  - It is important to counsel patients about antenatal smoking risks and cessation recommendations and to record their compliance.
  - The potentially harmful effects of cigarette smoking during pregnancy include
    1. Intrauterine growth restriction
    2. Placenta previa
    3. Abruptio placentae
    4. Low birth weight
    5. Preterm premature rupture of membranes
    6. Ectopic pregnancy
  - An evidence-based team approach to tobacco cessation in pregnancy allows a higher rate of cessation. This approach includes the use of motivational interviewing, the Five A's, support groups, the use of a quit line and individual counseling with a health educator.
  - Tobacco cessation before fifteen weeks gestation yields the greatest benefit for the woman and fetus, however quitting at any gestation can be beneficial.
- Alcohol use should be discontinued in pregnancy, including social and binge drinking.
  - There may be a linear relationship between alcohol consumption and fetal damage, which would explain why even limited fetal exposure to alcohol through social or binge drinking can be damaging.
  - Fetal alcohol syndrome (FAS) is the result of chronic fetal alcohol exposure.
    ○ With alcohol use throughout pregnancy, the risk of FAS is 20% to 40%.
    ○ Variants of FAS may also result from binge drinking or persistent social drinking.
    ○ FAS occurs as a characteristic pattern of physical abnormalities that includes fetal growth restriction and mental retardation. As such, it is an important cause of poor fetal growth and abnormal development.
    ○ FAS includes
      – Cardiac malformations
      – Central nervous system anomalies such as microcephaly and NTDs
      – Micrognathia, cleft lip/cleft palate, and other facial abnormalities
      – Skeletal and truncal abnormalities including diaphragmatic hernia
      – Genitourinary malformations
- Seat belt use is the same as for the nonpregnant automobile passengers: The lap belt is worn low and snugly across the hip bones; the shoulder harness is worn over one shoulder and under the opposite arm, loosely enough to place a clenched fist between the sternum and the belt.
- Sexual intercourse: There are no restrictions for the patient without complications.
- Fetal movement is generally discernible by the mother at 18 to 20 weeks' gestation.
  - Fetal activity is cyclic in nature and will normally vary in frequency and intensity throughout the day.
  - Decreased fetal movement is best evaluated by a nonstress test or biophysical profile.
- Warning signs of preterm labor
  - Studies have suggested that patient education regarding the warning signs for preterm labor leads to improved rates of early diagnosis of preterm labor. Self-identification allows these patients to seek the attention of the health care staff earlier in their preterm delivery course.
  - The following symptoms should prompt the patient to seek medical recommendations for evaluation:
    1. Contractions every 10 minutes for one hour
    2. Vaginal bleeding
    3. Rupture of membranes

- Somatic problems are a result of a normal pregnancy. After investigating to rule out a serious pathologic condition, treatment may be directed to symptomatic relief.
  - Headache and backache. Acetaminophen (Tylenol), 325 to 650 mg every 3 to 4 hours, is usually sufficient.
  - Nausea and vomiting:
    - ○ Nausea and vomitting may be relieved by eating frequent, and small meals.
    - ○ Severe, persistent symptoms may require hospitalization and intravenous fluids. The antiemetics, promethazine (Phenergan), diphenhydramine (Benadryl), and several other antihistamines (2) are considered safe for use in pregnancy and have no known association with birth defects.
    - ○ The first line therapy for nausea and vomitting during pregnancy is pyridoxine.
  - Constipation:
    - ○ A high-fiber diet, increased fluid intake, and regular exercise are recommended. Stool softeners such as docusate sodium (Colace) or psyllium hydrophilic mucilloid (Metamucil) may help.
    - ○ Mild laxatives should be used sparingly and only if the prior measures fail.
  - Varicosities: Support stockings and leg elevation are recommended.
  - Other important information for patients to know:
    - ○ When and where to call if they have questions or problems
    - ○ Availability of childbirth classes
    - ○ Signs of the onset of labor
    - ○ Obstetric analgesic options
    - ○ Indications for cesarean delivery
    - ○ Home safety
    - ○ Infant care and feeding, including breast-feeding
    - ○ Access to consumer education (e.g., infant safety products, furniture, car seats)
    - ○ Birth control counseling

PATIENT EDUCATION

- Effective prenatal care requires patient-centered, targeted patient education.
- One of the primary goals of prenatal care is to address the social determinants of health.
- Each woman's personal socioeconomic situation and support system must be explored and taken into account as part of her prenatal plan of care.
- Empowering women through education allows them to participate in decision making regarding the course of the pregnancy and labor.

REFERENCES

1. American College of Obstetricians and Gynecologists. ACOG committee opinion number 558. Integrating immunizations into practice: tetanus, diphtheria, and pertussis vaccination. *Obstet Gynecol.* 2013;121:897–903.
2. Rasmussen KM, Abrams B, Bodnar LM, et al. Recommendations for weight gain during pregnancy in the context of the obesity epidemic. *Obstet Gynecol.* 2010;116(5): 1191–1195.
3. DeFranco EA, Stamilo DM, Boslaugh SE, et al. A short interpregnancy interval is a risk factor for preterm birth and its recurrance. *Am J Obstet Gynecol* 2007;197: 264.e1–264.e6.
4. Hauck FR, Thompson JMD, Tanabe KO, et al. Breastfeeding and reduced risk of sudden infant death syndrome: a meta-analysis. *Pediatrics.* 2011;128(1):103–110.
5. DeFranco EA, Lian M, Muglia LA, et al. Area-level poverty and preterm birth risk: a population-based multilevel analysis. *BMC Public Health.* 2008;8:316.
6. Mangesi L, Hofmeyr GJ. Fetal movement counting for assessment of wellbeing (Review). *Cochrane Library.* 2008;(3).

7. Task Force on Sudden Infant Death Syndrome. SIDS and other sleep-related deaths: expansion of recommendations for a safe infant sleeping environment. *Pediatrics*. 2011; 128;1030.

8. American Academy of Pediatrics, American College of Obstetricians and Gynecologists. *Guidelines for perinatal care*. Elk Grove Village, IL: American Academy of Pediatrics; 2002.

9. Behrman RE. *Preterm birth: causes, consequences, and prevention*. Washington, DC: National Academies Press, 2007.

10. Cunningham FG, Williams JW. *Williams obstetrics*. New York: McGraw-Hill, 2007.

11. Creasy RK, Gummer BA, Liggins GC. System for predicting spontaneous preterm birth. *Obstet Gynecol*. 1980;55:692–695.

12. Briggs GG, Freeman RK, et al. *Drugs in pregnancy and lactation*. 7th ed. Philadelphia, PA: Lippincott Williams & Wilkins, 2005.

Normal Labor

Jodi Regan and Catherine Van Hook

KEY POINTS

- Labor and delivery are normal physiologic processes.
- Careful evaluation of both the mother and fetus upon presentation to the labor and delivery suite is important due to the possibility of acute changes in status.
- Attention to the principles of normal labor and maternal–fetal physiology is imperative to avoid unnecessary interventions.
- Continuous electronic fetal monitoring has not been shown to be beneficial in any prospective, randomized controlled study. Nonetheless, its utilization is customary in many labor and delivery suites (1).
- Maternal request is sufficient justification for providing pain relief during labor.
- Routine use of episiotomies is not recommended as it has not been shown to improve outcomes. Restricted use is preferable (2,3).

BACKGROUND

Definition

- Labor is the process by which contractions of the gravid uterus expel the fetus.
- A term pregnancy delivers between 37 and 42 weeks from the last menstrual period (LMP).
- Preterm delivery is birth that occurs before 37 completed weeks of gestational age.
- Postterm pregnancy occurs after 42 weeks of gestation and requires careful monitoring secondary to increased perinatal morbidity and mortality (4).
- Termination of pregnancy before 20 weeks of gestation is defined as either spontaneous or elective abortion.

EVALUATION OF THE LABORING PATIENT

- Evaluation of the patient presenting with symptoms of labor includes
  - History
  - Physical examination
  - Selected laboratory tests
  - Fetal assessment
- A clinical impression and management plan are formulated from the information obtained.

History

History of the Present Labor

- Contractions:
  - The onset, frequency, duration, and intensity of uterine contractions should be determined.
  - Contractions that effect progressive cervical effacement and dilation are usually regular and intense (the patient may no longer be able to walk or talk during these contractions). They may be accompanied by a "bloody show," the passage of blood-tinged mucus from the effacing cervix.
  - Braxton-Hicks contractions are commonly experienced by many women during the last weeks of pregnancy. These are usually irregular, mild, not well organized, and do not result in cervical change.
  - Factors that differentiate true labor from false or *prodromal* labor are listed in Table 2-1.

Table 2-1	Differentiating True Labor and False Labor	
Factors	**True labor**	**False labor**
Contractions	Regular intervals	Irregular intervals
Interval between contractions	Gradually shortens	Remains long
Intensity of contractions	Gradually increases	Remains same
Location of pain	In back and abdomen	Mostly in lower abdomen
Effect of analgesia	Not terminated by sedation	Frequently abolished by sedation
Cervical change	Progressive effacement and dilation	No change

- Rupture of membranes:
  - The status of the fetal membranes must be determined if it is not reported as part of the initial presentation.
  - The patient may present with leaking fluid alone or in conjunction with uterine contractions. The time of occurrence is important, because prolonged membrane rupture increases the risk of chorioamnionitis (5). Color of the amniotic fluid may suggest the presence of meconium or blood.
  - The patient may report a large gush of fluid with continued leakage, which would lead to a high suspicion for ruptured membranes.
  - The patient may report merely increased moisture on her underclothes, which leads to uncertainty about whether this moisture represents urine, vaginal secretions, cervical mucus, or amniotic fluid.
  - Confirmation of rupture of membranes (ROM) may include physical examination, laboratory testing (nitrazine or fern test), ultrasonography, and/or other laboratory screening tests such as AmniSure (6).

Vaginal Bleeding
- The extent, if any, of vaginal bleeding should be ascertained.
- Spotting or blood-tinged mucus is common in normal labor.
- Heavy vaginal bleeding merits complete investigation because it may be abnormal and reflect a significant complication (see Chapter 32).

Fetal Movement
- The initial assessment of the patient reporting symptoms of labor should include questions about the level of her fetus's movement. Most patients are aware of their fetus's baseline level of activity.
- If the patient reports a significant or progressive decrease in fetal movement from her normal baseline, fetal well-being must be ascertained.
- Such evaluations can involve fetal monitoring with a nonstress test (NST), a contraction stress test (CST), or biophysical profile (BPP) (see Chapter 32).
- Fetal movement-counting protocols (aka "kick counts") are commonly used in the third trimester as a screen for fetal well-being (7).

History of Current Pregnancy
- The history of the present pregnancy should be obtained by interviewing the patient in labor and by reviewing the prenatal record (8).
- The prenatal record may be from one's own institution or from an outside source. The patient, of course, may have had no prenatal care or have no record of it.
- If a prenatal record is available, important items should be verified with the patient.

Gestational Age
- Gestational age is best determined from data in the prenatal record including ultrasound data.
  - The later the patient presents for initial prenatal care, the more difficult it becomes to accurately determine the estimated gestational age (EGA).
  - Patients presenting for initial prenatal care at ≥24 weeks of gestation are considered to have inherently unreliable dates.
- Important landmarks for determining gestational age include
  - The 1st day of the LMP—the estimated date of confinement (EDC) is calculated as 40 weeks or 280 days from this date, based on regular 28-day cycles
  - The date of last ovulation (as determined by an ovulation prediction kit or basal body temperature chart), or the date of conception (if known precisely), with the EDC calculated as 38 weeks from this date
  - Early ultrasound measurement of crown–rump length at 6 to 12 weeks of gestation (accurate to within 3 days) (9)
  - The average of multiple biometric measurements on fetal ultrasound between 12 and 20 weeks of gestation (accurate to within 10 days)
  - Fetal heart tones, first heard with a Doppler instrument at 10 to 12 weeks of gestation or with a fetoscope at 18 to 20 weeks of gestation
  - Quickening (maternally perceived fetal movement), which first occurs at approximately 18 to 20 weeks of gestation in primigravidas
  - Uterine size on pelvic examination before 16 weeks of EGA, as determined by an experienced clinician
- Accurate dating requires evaluation during the first half of pregnancy.
  - The patient presenting in labor with an uncertain LMP and no prenatal care may be difficult to date with accuracy.
  - Uncertain gestational age presents a significant problem because of different management strategies for term, preterm, and postterm pregnancies. In these situations, the only alternative is to use ultrasonography in the labor and delivery suite, realizing that it may, at best, be accurate to within only ±3 weeks of gestation in the last trimester.
  - Amniocentesis to assess fetal lung maturity can be considered to help guide delivery decisions when gestational age is uncertain.

Medical Problems Arising during Gestation
- The patient should be questioned specifically regarding any medical problems arising during the pregnancy.
- Hospitalizations should be noted, as well as any new medications prescribed.
- A history of genital herpes, bleeding, abnormal placentation, hepatitis B/C, HIV, group B streptococcus (GBS) carrier status, recurrent urinary tract infections and pyelonephritis, or any infectious diseases requiring treatment should be elicited.
- A history of glucose intolerance and treatment with diet or insulin should be noted.
- If any blood pressure elevation has been recorded during the pregnancy, the time of onset, severity, and treatment should be determined.
- Seizure history, noting frequency and medications, is pertinent for obstetric care.
  - Any drug usage with illicit or prescription drugs should also be discussed.

Review of Systems
- An obstetrically oriented review of symptoms should be carried out.
- Severe headaches, scotomata, hand and facial edema, or epigastric pain may suggest preeclampsia.
- Generalized pruritus may be secondary to intrahepatic cholestasis of pregnancy or hepatitis.
- Dysuria, urinary frequency, or flank pain may indicate cystitis or pyelonephritis.

History of Past Pregnancies

Each past pregnancy and its duration and outcome should be reviewed.

- Particular attention should be paid to preterm deliveries, operative deliveries, prolonged or difficult labors, shoulder dystocias (up to 16.7% risk of recurrence) (10,11), malpresentation, hypertensive disorders of pregnancy (4% in the general population with a high recurrence rate) (12), placental abruption (20-fold increased risk of recurrence) (13) or placenta previa (risk increases with age, parity, and prior cesarean deliveries) up to 3% for three or more cesarean deliveries (14), and blood loss requiring transfusion.
- Other medical facilities may need to be contacted for records to verify or clarify certain points.

Medical History

- All active medical problems should be evaluated and the extent of the disease determined (i.e., epilepsy, hypertension, asthma, diabetes, heart disease, etc.).
- The stress of labor can aggravate many medical problems and jeopardize both maternal and fetal well-being and may require appropriate consultations from subspecialists.

Psychosocial and Emotional History

- Labor is a stressful physical and psychological event, and understanding the patient's psychosocial and emotional status and history will help in planning for her care and maintaining her sense of control.
- How the patient wishes to be addressed should be determined.
- Her preparation and plans for labor and birth should be discussed.
- The patient's labor support person(s) and their preparation should be identified.
- Questions about substance and alcohol use or abuse, intimate partner violence, and diagnosis and treatment of psychiatric disorders should be included. This part of the history must be obtained from the patient without any family or support persons present.
  - Plans for breast-feeding after delivery regardless of mode of delivery should be discussed prior to delivery.

Physical Examination

- Although active labor is not the optimal setting for a comprehensive physical examination, a focused examination with emphasis on the abdomen and pelvis can be performed between painful contractions.
- Any signs of intercurrent medical illness or abnormalities of major organ systems should be elicited and carefully noted.
- Special note should be taken of those parts of the physical examination that may generate abnormal findings because of that individual patient's history.

General Examination

Vital Signs

- A complete set of vital signs should be taken immediately on admission including a pulse oximeter for oxygen saturation if possible.
- Blood pressure should be taken between contractions in the upright or left lateral recumbent position with the patient's arm at the level of the heart. The appropriate size cuff should be utilized with the cuff length 1.5 times the upper arm circumference or cuff with a bladder enclosing 80% of the arm (15). Abnormal readings should be rechecked.
- An elevated body temperature, especially if associated with ruptured membranes, may indicate chorioamnionitis.
- An elevated pulse or respiratory rate in the absence of any other abnormality is commonly observed in healthy patients in active labor.

Head and Neck

- Funduscopy may be indicated to rule out vascular abnormalities, hemorrhages, or exudates that may suggest such diseases as diabetes or hypertension.
- Pale conjunctivae (or nail beds) may suggest anemia.

- Facial, most notably periorbital, edema can be found—in preeclampsia.
- The thyroid gland should be palpated to rule out goiter or other masses and to determine if anesthesia should be involved for any concerns related to airway management.
- Distended neck veins suggest congestive heart failure, which, although rare, is a serious complication of labor and should be recognized early so that proper therapy may be initiated.

Chest
- Examination of the chest may reveal the presence of a pneumonic process or significant cardiac murmurs (other than the physiologic systolic ejection murmur common in pregnancy) and provides a baseline in case complications such as pulmonary edema develop.
- Auscultation of the lungs for rales, crackles, and wheezes is especially important in patients with asthma or hypertension or at risk for pulmonary edema.

Abdomen
- An attempt should be made to palpate major abdominal viscera for pain or masses, although this is difficult with a term-sized uterus.
- Epigastric tenderness may suggest preeclampsia or HELLP (*h*emolysis, *e*levated *l*iver enzyme levels, and a *l*ow *p*latelet count) syndrome.

Extremities
- Examination of extremities should include an assessment of peripheral edema.
  - Although mild ankle edema commonly is found near term in normal pregnancies, severe lower extremity or hand edema may suggest preeclampsia. Unilateral edema also may suggest underlying VTE (venous thromboembolism).
  - A brief neurologic examination should be performed because the presence of deep-tendon hyperreflexia and clonus may suggest a lowered threshold for seizure activity.

The Gravid Uterus
- A general examination includes assessment for the size of the uterus, presence of tenderness, globular masses (i.e., fibroids), estimated fetal weight (EFW), and fetal presentation and lie.
- Presence of uterine tenderness may by indicative of chorioamnionitis, uterine rupture, or placenta abruption, all of which require prompt attention.

Uterine Size
- After 20 weeks, the size of the uterus is anticipated to correlate with the number of centimeters from the pubis to the top of the fundus in a singleton pregnancy.
- Correlation of these findings lessens as the pregnancy approaches term due to variation in fetal size and pelvic engagement.
- Significant lack of correlation raises concern for the presence of a fetal growth or amniotic fluid disorder or multiple gestation. Size date discrepancy can also be due to the influence of pelvic engagement.
- Ultrasonography is indicated to resolve concerns of size date discrepancy.

Leopold Maneuvers
- Leopold maneuvers (Fig. 2-1) are a technique used to palpate the gravid uterus to determine fetal presentation and fetal lie. It can also be used to estimate fetal weight (mentally adjusting for maternal habitus, amniotic fluid, and proportion of fetus engaged in the pelvis). Ultrasound can be used for primary assessment of these clinical factors or as confirmation of the Leopold maneuvers.
- The first maneuver determines which fetal pole occupies the uterine fundus (e.g., the breech with a vertex presentation). The breech moves with the fetal body. The vertex is rounder and harder and feels more globular than the breech and can be maneuvered separately from the fetal body.

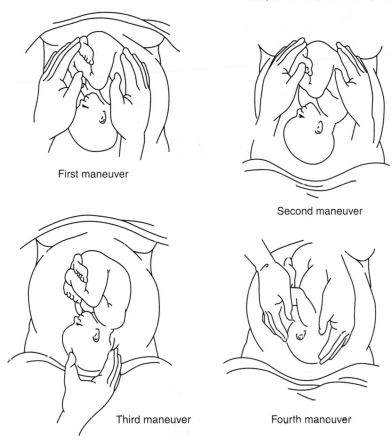

First maneuver

Second maneuver

Third maneuver

Fourth maneuver

Figure 2-1. Leopold maneuvers to diagnose fetal presentation and position of the fetus. (Gibbs RS, Karlan BY, Haney AF, et al. *Danforth's obstetrics and gynecology.* 10th ed. Lippincott Williams & Wilkins, 2008:22–41, Figure 6.)

- With the second maneuver, the lateral aspects of the uterus are palpated to determine on which side the fetal back or fetal extremities, or "small parts," are located. The back is firm and smooth.
- The third maneuver is performed with the examiner facing caudally, and the presenting part is made to move from side to side. If this is not done easily, engagement of the presenting part probably has occurred.
- The fourth maneuver reveals the presentation. With the fetus presenting by vertex, the cephalic prominence may be palpable on the side of the fetal small parts, confirming flexion of the fetal head (occiput presentation). Extension of the head (face presentation) is suspected when the cephalic prominence is on the side of the fetus opposite the small parts.

Fetal Lie
- The *lie* of the fetus is a description of the relationship of the long axis of the fetus to the long axis of the mother. The lie is longitudinal with a vertex or breech presentation or otherwise transverse or oblique, as with a shoulder presentation.

Presentation
- Designates the part of the fetus lowest in the pelvis.
- Cephalic denotes the fetal head presenting to the pelvis.
  - Vertex, presentation of the occipital fontanelle due to flexion of the fetal head to the fetal chest is the most common.
  - Deflexion of the fetal head leads to sinciput (presentation of anterior fontanelle), brow (bregma), or face presentations.
- Breech presentations are classified by presentation of the buttocks with or without the feet.
  - Frank breech presentation: Both hips are flexed with the knees extended.
  - Complete breech: Both hips are flexed with one or both knees flexed.
  - Incomplete breech: One or both hips deflexed with one or both feet or knees below the buttocks.
  - Footling breech is an incomplete breech with one or both feet located below the buttocks.
- Shoulder presentation is found with transverse lie.
- Compound presentation is presentation of an extremity with the presenting part.

Estimated Fetal Weight
- EFW can be assessed with palpation of the gravid uterus and mentally adjusting for maternal habitus, amniotic fluid, and proportion of fetus engaged in the pelvis.
- Discrepancy between the gestational age and anticipated fundal height suggests growth or fluid volume abnormality or multiple gestation. Ultrasound examination will be necessary for resolution.
- EFW calculated by ultrasound has a margin of error of up to 20% (9,16).

Fetal Heart Tones
- Documentation of the fetal heart tones must be performed on admission.
- Continuous electronic fetal heart rate monitoring (CEFM) is performed as an initial evaluation at many institutions. The baseline heart rate, variability, accelerations, and decelerations are carefully assessed, and categorization of the tracing is performed accordingly (1,17,18) (see Chapter 22).
- If a reassuring tracing is obtained, the patient may continue to be managed with CEFM or may be a candidate for intermittent fetal heart rate monitoring by auscultation.

Pelvic Examination
- Inspection and palpation of the perineum and the pelvis are critically important in evaluating the laboring patient.
- Information needed includes
  - Presence or absence of perineal, vaginal, and cervical abnormalities (including herpes or human papillomavirus infections)
  - Adequacy of the bony pelvis
  - Integrity of the fetal membranes
  - Degree of cervical dilation and effacement
  - Station of the presenting part
- The presence of third-trimester vaginal bleeding or preterm premature rupture of the membranes will preclude digital examination of the cervix until further evaluation is performed, which may include bedside ultrasound.

Inspection
- The perineum should be inspected for herpetic or syphilitic lesions, large vulvar varicosities, large condylomas, or other altered vulvar anatomy, that is, female genital mutilation.
- If there is any question of active genital herpes, a speculum examination of the vagina or cervix is necessary.

- Diagnosis of ruptured membranes may sometimes be visually confirmed by inspection, but it is often necessary to perform a sterile speculum examination to determine the status of the fetal membranes.
  - Using sterile technique, a sterile speculum is inserted into the vagina, and a light source is positioned so the cervix and posterior vagina can be visualized.
  - Gross pooling of amniotic fluid in the posterior fornix is consistent with the diagnosis of ROM. It is important to note the color and consistency of the fluid, the presence of purulence, blood, or meconium.
  - Direct transcervical visualization of fetal scalp, feet, umbilical cord, or other fetal parts confirms ruptured membranes definitively.
  - If uncertain about ROM, any fluid pooled in the posterior vaginal fornix is sampled with a sterile cotton swab, smeared on a glass slide, and viewed with the aid of a microscope. Other laboratory methods for the evaluation of ROM are available, that is, AmniSure (6).
    - Ferning of the air-dried fluid under the microscope suggests amniotic fluid (Fig. 2-2).
    - Ultrasound may be used to evaluate amniotic fluid volume if the status of the membranes is still uncertain after physical and laboratory testing.
  - If bloody amniotic fluid is noted (port-wine fluid), further investigation to rule out abruptio placentae should be undertaken.
  - The absence or presence of meconium (fetal stool) in the amniotic fluid should be noted.
    - The incidence of meconium-stained amniotic fluid increases with advancing gestational age.
- Cultures are obtained when preterm labor or chorioamnionitis is suspected.
- With preterm ROM at 32 to 34 weeks, a sample of amniotic fluid from the vaginal pool can be obtained to evaluate fetal lung maturity to assist with management decisions regarding expectant management (19).

Palpation of the Cervix
- Palpation of the cervix should be done when the patient is between contractions to ensure accuracy and to minimize the patient's discomfort.
- Dilation of the cervix describes the degree of opening of the internal cervical os. The cervix can be described as undilated or closed (0 cm), fully dilated (10 cm), or any point between these two extremes (0 to 10 cm).
- Effacement of the cervix describes the process of thinning that the cervix undergoes before or during labor (Fig. 2-3).
  - The thick prelabor cervix is approximately 3 cm long and is said to be uneffaced or to have 0% effacement. With complete or 100% effacement, the cervix is paper thin.
- As a general rule, primiparous women begin to efface the cervix before dilation begins, whereas multiparous women begin to dilate before significant effacement has been reached.

Palpation of the Fetal Presenting Part
- Identification of fetal presentation should be confirmed by digitally palpating the fetal presenting part. The novice often assumes it to be a vertex, but identification must be positively made on every occasion.
  - Vertex presentation can be confirmed by palpating the suture lines of the fetal skull. If the suture lines cannot be identified with certainty, other presentations must be considered.
  - Palpation of the fetal buttocks, feet, face, or arms is confirmatory.

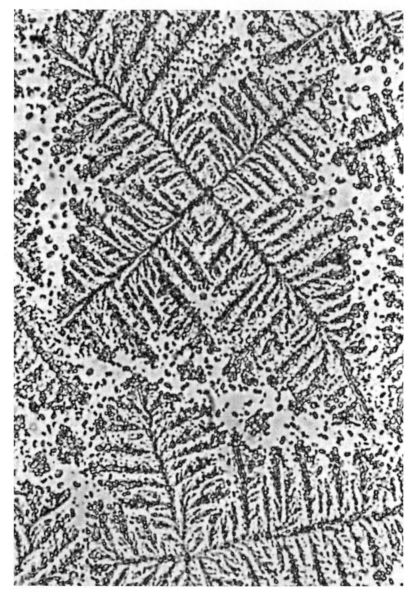

Figure 2-2. "Ferning" in smear from the vagina suggests that amniotic fluid is present in the vagina.

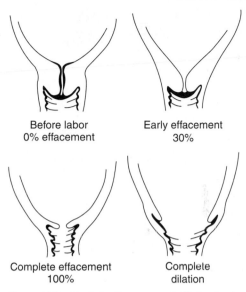

Figure 2-3. Cervical effacement and dilation in the primigravida. (LifeART image copyright (c) 2013 Lippincott Williams & Wilkins. All rights reserved.)

- Inability to positively identify the presenting part is an indication for expeditious ultrasound examination.
- *Station* refers to the relationship between the fetal presenting part and pelvic landmarks.
  - When the presenting part is at zero station, it is at the level of the ischial spines, which are the landmarks for the midpelvis. This is important in the vertex presentation because it implies that the largest dimension of the fetal head, the biparietal diameter, has passed through the smallest dimension of the pelvis, the pelvic inlet.
  - In 1988, the American College of Obstetricians and Gynecologists introduced a classification dividing the pelvis into 5-cm segments above and below the ischial spines:
    - If the presenting part is 1 cm above the spines, it is described as −1 station.
    - If it is 2 cm below the spines, the station is +2.
    - At −5 station, the presenting part is described as floating.
    - At +5 station, the presenting part is on the perineum, and it may distend the vulva with a contraction and be visible to an observer.
    - In practice, this system has not been widely adopted, and many physicians still describe station on the basis of dividing the maternal pelvis below the spines into thirds. An approximation would be, for example, +4 cm = +2/3.
  - Position of the presenting part is described as the relationship between a certain landmark on the fetal presenting part and the maternal pelvis (Fig. 2-4), as follows:
    - Anterior, closest to the symphysis pubis
    - Posterior, closest to the coccyx
    - Transverse, closest to the left or right vaginal sidewall

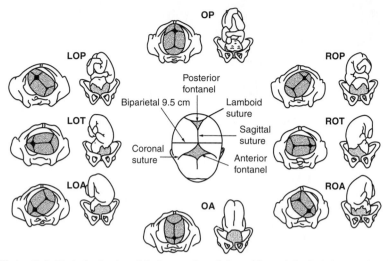

Figure 2-4. Vaginal palpation of the large and small fontanelles and the frontal, sagittal, and lambdoidal sutures determines the position of the vertex. Various vertex presentations. LOP, left occiput posterior; LOT, left occiput transverse; LOA, left occiput anterior; ROP, right occiput posterior; ROT, right occiput transverse; ROA, right occiput anterior. (Beckmann CRB, Frank W, et al. *Obstetrics and gynecology.* 5th ed. Philadelphia: Lippincott Williams & Wilkins, 2006.)

- º The index landmark in a vertex presentation is the occiput, which is identified by palpating the lambdoid sutures forming a Y with the sagittal suture; it is the sacrum in a breech presentation and the mentum (or chin) in a face presentation.
- º The designations of anterior, posterior, left, and right refer to the maternal pelvis. Therefore, right occiput transverse implies that the occiput is directed toward the right side of the maternal pelvis.
- Breech and face presentations are described in a similar fashion (e.g., right sacrum transverse, right mentum transverse).

Evaluation of Pelvic Adequacy
- The shape of the maternal pelvis may be visualized as a cylinder with a gentle anterior curve toward the outlet. The curve forms because the posterior border of the pelvis (the sacrum and the coccyx) is longer than the anterior border (the symphysis pubis). The lateral borders (the innominate bones) are more or less parallel in the normal female pelvis.
- Dystocia may be encountered when abnormalities of the pelvis are present. Pelvic adequacy can be judged clinically by measuring pelvic diameters at certain levels.
- Even when conducted by the most experienced clinicians, clinical pelvic measurements are merely estimations.
  - Unless the maternal pelvis is grossly contracted, adequacy is proven only by a trial of labor.
  - Despite this, the pelvis must be evaluated at admission for an estimate of adequacy or documentation of abnormalities.
- The maternal pelvis is one of three factors that determine the success of labor. These factors have been referred to as the three P's: Pelvis, Power, and the Passenger. A macrosomic fetus or inadequate uterine contractions, even with an adequate pelvis, may preclude vaginal delivery.

Inlet
- The inlet of the true pelvis is limited by the symphysis pubis anteriorly, the sacral promontory posteriorly, and the iliopectineal line laterally.
- The anteroposterior (AP) diameter of the inlet may be estimated by determining the diagonal conjugate measurement. The diameter (the distance from the sacral promontory to the inner inferior surface of the symphysis pubis) is measured clinically by attempting to touch the sacral promontory with the vaginal examining finger while simultaneously noting where the inferior border of the symphysis touches the examining finger. A measurement greater than 12 cm suggests adequacy.

Midpelvis
- The midpelvis is bordered anteriorly by the symphysis pubis, posteriorly by the sacrum, and laterally by the ischial spines. A gently curved concave sacrum increases the adequacy of the midpelvis.
- The interspinous diameter is estimated by palpating the ischial spines. An estimated distance less than 9 cm suggests midpelvis contraction. Experience is required to estimate this diameter with accuracy.

Outlet
- The outlet is limited anteriorly by the arch of the symphysis pubis, posteriorly by the tip of the coccyx, and laterally by the ischial tuberosities.
- This transverse diameter of the outlet can be estimated by placing a clenched fist between the two ischial tuberosities. A measurement of 8 cm or more suggests an adequate diameter.
- The AP measurement is estimated by judging the prominence of the tip of the sacrum and by noting the angle made by the pubic rami. A narrow pelvic arch decreases the effective AP diameter.
- Dystocia as a result of an abnormal outlet alone is unusual, although with midpelvic inadequacy, the outlet is also usually inadequate.

Laboratory Tests

All prenatal laboratory tests should be reviewed when the patient is admitted for labor. If the patient has not had any prenatal care, or if the care has been incomplete, prenatal laboratory tests should be drawn at the time of hospital admission.

Results of the patient's routine prenatal labs should be available at the time of presentation of labor (for list of these, see Chapter 1 Prenatal Care). If the set of routine prenatal lab results is not available, these tests should be redrawn at the time of evaluation.

- Additional laboratory evaluations, such as testing for sexually transmitted infections (STIs), may be indicated in high-risk populations. Gonorrhea, chlamydia, hepatitis B surface antigen, syphilis, and HIV are among the most routinely assessed STIs in pregnancy.
- If the patient is diabetic or of unknown status, fingerstick blood glucose testing is appropriate upon evaluation in labor.
- Patients with a history of glucose intolerance or diabetes should have serial blood glucose determinations. Often, this can be done with a glucometer in the labor and delivery suite.
- If preeclampsia is a possibility, a complete blood cell count including platelets and an expanded hepatic function panel should be ordered.
- Fibrinogen and clotting parameters should be measured if the diagnosis of abruptio placentae is being considered.
- If a patient has a history of postpartum hemorrhage, preexisting anemia, grand multiparity, or high likelihood for cesarean, a type and screen can be obtained to facilitate rapid crossmatching of blood.
- Cervical cultures and perianal cultures for GBS should be obtained for patients who may be preterm or who have symptoms of chorioamnionitis (20,21).
- Other specific laboratory tests should be ordered as required for specific physical findings, diseases, or complications.

Formulation of Impression and Plan

- With the pertinent information from the history, examination, and laboratory testing, a clinical impression is formulated.
- The process of deciding which patients require invasive procedures, such as placement of internal fetal monitors or intensive care–level monitoring of maternal vital functions begins with the initial clinical impression. The practitioner must be cognizant of and show respect for the patient's desires regarding her birthing process, while not compromising the level of care given to the mother and fetus.
- The high-risk patient presenting in labor needs detailed counseling regarding the nature of her problems, the rationale for tests and procedures, and any options that are available for her medical management. Any needed specialists should then be involved in the care according to the plan for the medical management. Anesthesia should be appropriately notified of the admission as indicated.

MANAGEMENT OF NORMAL LABOR

- Pregnancy is not a disease, and labor is the normal physiologic consequence of the completion of pregnancy. Nonetheless, complications can occur, such as nonreassuring fetal status, intrapartum fetal death, dysfunctional labor, uterine rupture, chorioamnionitis, maternal and fetal hemorrhage, and even maternal death.
- Management of labor should achieve delivery in a reasonable period of time while providing maternal and fetal support and avoiding any significant compromise to the mother or fetus.

Distinguishing Normal from Abnormal Progress in Labor

Stages of Labor

- The first stage of labor encompasses the interval of time from the onset of labor until the cervix has become fully dilated (10 cm). This stage is further subdivided into a latent and an active phase.
  - The latent phase is characterized by slow dilation of the cervix to a point at which the rate of change in cervical dilation begins to increase (active phase of labor). Historically, the latent phase has ended with achievement of 4 cm dilation. Newer evidence supports 6 cm as the onset of the active phase of labor (22,23).
  - The active phase is characterized by more rapid dilation until 10 cm is achieved.
- The second stage of labor begins with complete dilation of the cervix and ends with delivery of the infant.
- The third stage of labor denotes the interval from delivery of the infant to delivery of the placenta (afterbirth).

Assessment of Progress in Labor

- Assessment requires periodic digital examination of the cervix to assess changes in effacement, cervical dilation, and descent of the presenting part. Vaginal examinations should be timed often enough to determine the progress of labor, while still being limited for the sake of patient comfort and to minimize the risk of infection.
- Assessment of the strength of the uterine contractions can be done manually, with tocometry or with an internal uterine pressure catheter (IUPC).
  - Manual assessment relies on experienced labor and delivery staffing.
  - Tocometry or external monitoring is limited to onset and completion of the contractions and is suboptimal for measurement of strength of contractions in the presence of labor that is not progressing.
- IUPC provides direct assessment of onset, completion as well as strength of the contractions. Montevideo units (MVUs) are an objective assessment of uterine contraction strength. During a 10-minute window, the MVU difference between the baseline uterine

tone and the peak of each contraction is added together. Greater than 200 MVUs is considered an adequate contraction pattern (24).

- The modern spontaneous labor curve differs from the classic Friedman curve (22), which has been used for decades previously. For nulliparous and multiparous patients, acceleration of cervical dilation occurs with active labor at 6 cm dilation (as opposed to 4 cm previously described in the Friedman curve). Once active labor is entered, the multiparous acceleration is more rapid than that of the nulliparous patient.
- Defining the duration of the latent phase of labor is difficult due to its onset prior to arrival to the labor unit.
- The number of hours from admission to 6 cm varies by the cervical dilation upon presentation (22).
- For a nulliparous patient admitted at 2 cm dilation, the median number of hours to reach 6 cm is 6 hours (with 95% percentile at 15.7 hours). Admission at 3 cm corresponded to reaching 6 cm of dilation by a median of 4.2 hours (95% at 12.5 hours) (22).
- Diagnosis of an arrest disorder in the first stage of labor (24):
- The patient is 6 cm or more dilated with ROM without cervical change, and
  - Has had an adequate contraction pattern (greater than 200 montevideo units) for 4 or more hours or
  - Has had an inadequate contraction pattern for 6 or more hours
- The patient may persist in latent labor, making a diagnosis of an arrest of labor prior to 6 cm of dilation difficult and could require extended time, if maternal and fetal status permit (24).
- The average second stage of labor is influenced by parity and presence of regional anesthesia.
  - Absent specific maternal or fetal indications, second stage arrest is defined as ≥3 hours in a nulliparous woman without an epidural and for ≥4 hours with an epidural. In a multiparous woman, the intervals to define a second-stage arrest disorder are ≥2 hours and ≥3 hours, respectively (22).
  - Some authorities believe that the second stage should be divided into two phases and that expulsive efforts should not be encouraged until the head has descended well into the pelvis and the patient feels the urge to push (if the feeling is not obliterated by epidural anesthesia). This is often described as allowing the patient to "labor down." In practice, this theory has shown few clinical differences, especially in high-quality studies (25) (see Chapter 10 regarding management of abnormal labor).

Amniotomy

Amniotomy, or artificial rupture of the membranes (AROM), is usually accomplished by puncturing the amniotic membranes with a sterile plastic instrument that is guided between two gloved fingers.

- Indications for amniotomy may include
  - Visualizing the amniotic fluid for quantity and evidence of meconium or blood
  - Gaining direct access to the fetus for placement of internal fetal monitors
  - Attempting to induce labor or restore (augment) progress in labor
  - Impending second stage of labor where the provider wants to minimize the risk of exposure to body fluids during the birth
- Special considerations for avoidance of amniotomy include
  - Infection with HIV, hepatitis B or C (8)
  - Polyhydramnios—initial confirmation of engagement of the fetal head is essential
  - Preterm gestation without medical indication for delivery
  - Concern for placenta previa or vasa previa
  - Noncephalic presentations (i.e., breech, compound). Unstable fetal lie or unengaged fetal vertex

- Amniotomy is the only definitive way to visualize the amniotic fluid and to gain direct access to the fetal scalp.
- The effect of amniotomy on the duration of labor is controversial:
  - Most studies suggest that amniotomy performed in the active phase of labor significantly shortens labor (4,26,27,28–29). At the National Maternity Hospital in Dublin, amniotomy is performed by protocol once the diagnosis of active labor has been confirmed.
  - Amniotomy performed during the latent phase of labor in nulliparous women undergoing labor induction has been shown to shorten the duration of time to delivery without increase in adverse maternal or neonatal complications (30).
- Risks of amniotomy include possible complications:
  - Rupture of a fetal vessel traversing the fetal membranes (vasa previa) at the site of amniotomy is rare but can cause fetal exsanguination and death.
  - Prolapse of the umbilical cord between the presenting part and the cervix or below the presenting part can occur at time of amniotomy and cause severe fetal compromise unless operative delivery is performed rapidly.
  - The risk of cord prolapse can be minimized by avoiding amniotomy until the fetal head is engaged in the pelvis and is exerting significant pressure against the cervix. Cord prolapse can also occur with spontaneous ROM.
- Several studies have suggested that one of the side effects from amniotomy is an increased incidence of variable fetal heart rate decelerations in the active phase of labor (29). However, there were no differences in nonreassuring fetal heart rate patterns nor operative deliveries (29,31,32).
- In summary, the various applications for amniotomy have rendered it integral to the practice of modern obstetrics, and it is used frequently at most institutions.
  - There is little disagreement that amniotomy is indicated as part of induction of labor and as an intervention for protraction and arrest of labor disorders.
  - The procedure has risks, and these must be weighed against the expected benefits each time artificial ROM is contemplated.
  - It should be understood that, when amniotomy is performed to hasten labor, no randomized controlled study has proven that an accelerated labor provides better fetal or maternal outcomes than a natural labor without interventions.

Mechanisms of Labor in the Vertex Presentation

- The process of labor and delivery is marked by characteristic changes in fetal position or cardinal movements in relation to the maternal pelvis. These spontaneous adjustments are made to effect efficient passage through the pelvis as the fetus descends (Fig. 2-5).
- *Engagement* is the descent of the largest transverse diameter, the biparietal diameter, to a level below the pelvic inlet. An occiput below the ischial spines is engaged.
- Descent of the head is a discontinuous process occurring throughout labor. Because the transverse diameter of the pelvic inlet is wider than the AP diameter and because the greatest diameter of the unflexed fetal head is the AP diameter, in most instances, the fetus enters the pelvis in an occiput transverse alignment.
- Flexion decreases the AP diameter of the fetal head. It occurs as the head encounters the levator muscle sling, thereby decreasing the diameter by approximately 1.5 to 2.5 cm (occipitomental, 12.0 cm, to occipitofrontal, 10.5 cm). Later, further flexion occurs, reducing the diameter to 9.5 cm (suboccipitobregmatic).
- Internal rotation occurs in the midpelvis. The architecture of the midpelvic passageway changes so that the AP diameter of the maternal pelvis at this level is greater than the transverse diameter. The fetus accommodates to this change by rotation of the head from a transverse orientation (occiput transverse) to an AP alignment (usually occiput anterior), thus accomplishing internal rotation. Further descent to the level of the perineum occurs with the head aligned in the AP plane.

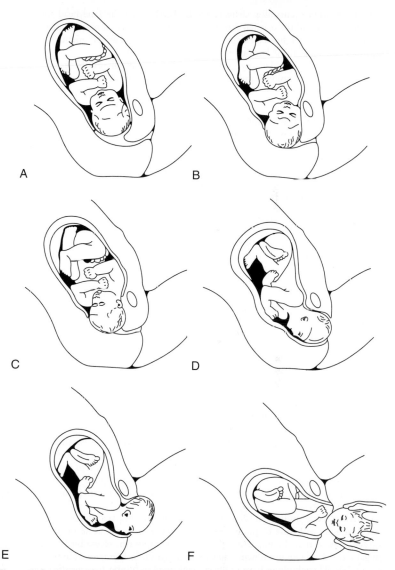

Figure 2-5. Cardinal movements of labor. (Wolters Kulwer©2013.)

- Extension of the head allows delivery of the head from the usual occiput anterior position through the introitus. Little actual descent occurs with extrusion of the head because the head is delivered by a reversal of the flexion that occurred as it entered the pelvis. The face appears over the perineal body, while the symphysis pubis acts as a fulcrum where it impinges on the occiput.

- External rotation occurs after delivery of the head, when the fetal head rotates back or restitutes, toward the original transverse orientation (external rotation or restitution) when the bisacromial diameter (fetal shoulders) is aligned in an AP orientation with the greatest diameter of the pelvic outlet.
- The remainder of the delivery proceeds with presentation of the anterior shoulder beneath the symphysis pubis and the posterior shoulder across the posterior fourchette.

Intrapartum Fetal Assessment

- Some form of evaluation of fetal well-being during labor is recommended to minimize the risk of intrapartum fetal death and intrapartum fetal asphyxia.
- The two choices are intermittent auscultation and CEFM.
- The clinical decision concerning the use of intermittent auscultation of the fetal heart rate versus continuous electronic fetal monitoring (external or internal) is usually based on risk status of the patient at admission and patient desires.

Intermittent Auscultation of the Fetal Heart Rate

- If no risk factors are present at the time of admission, a standard approach to fetal monitoring is to determine and record the fetal heart rate (8).
  - At least every 30 minutes or just after each contraction in the active phase of the first stage of labor, and
  - At least every 15 minutes in the second stage of labor
- If risk factors are present at admission, or if they become apparent during the course of labor, continuous electronic fetal monitoring should be considered.
- At most institutions, some degree of continuous fetal heart rate monitoring is conducted. Because intermittent auscultation is not commonly used, many labor and delivery nurses do not have experience with this method of fetal assessment.
- Intermittent auscultation requires a higher registered nurse-to-patient ratio than electronic fetal monitoring, which limits its use in many institutions.

Continuous Electronic Fetal Monitoring

- The application and interpretation of CEFM are discussed in Chapter 32.
- CEFM was developed to decrease the risk of cerebral palsy, which is now known to be infrequently associated with intrapartum events.
- No prospective, randomized controlled studies have clearly demonstrated the value of CEFM. The use of CEFM compared to intermittent auscultation did not reduce the risk of CP in these study populations. However, CEFM was found to increase the incidence of operative delivery (cesarean section and assisted vaginal delivery), decrease the risk of neonatal seizures, and had no effect on reduction of perinatal mortality (1,17,18,32–34).
- Two retrospective studies published in the early 1980s compared the outcome of monitored patients with that of premonitoring-era patients in the same institution. These studies showed that the incidence of intrapartum stillbirth, severe birth asphyxia, low Apgar scores, and long-term neurologic damage significantly improved in the monitored group (32). These findings have not been confirmed in prospective investigations.
- All patients should be considered for CEFM.
- Internal fetal electrodes and intrauterine pressure monitors are used when it is necessary to precisely assess the fetal heart rate pattern and the amplitude, duration, and frequency of uterine contractions. Internal fetal monitors may be used for
  - Patients who are obese or who are difficult to monitor externally
  - Patients whose labor has been augmented with oxytocin for arrest disorders
  - Patients whose external tracing is not reassuring
  - Patients undergoing trial of labor after a prior cesarean delivery

Risks and Complications
- Intermittent auscultation imparts no direct risk to the fetus, except that evolving fetal compromise may be not be detected at an early stage. Potentially significant deceleratory fetal heart rate patterns could escape notice when using auscultation, allowing a decompensating fetus to be subjected to continued labor (32,34).
- CEFM likewise has no direct ill effect on the mother or fetus. It does tend to restrict patient activity and often results in strict bed rest. The main risk is difficult and/or inaccurate fetal heart rate pattern interpretation, thereby allowing either a compromised fetus to go unrecognized or, conversely and more commonly, precipitating unnecessary intervention in the case of a healthy fetus.
- Internal fetal monitoring complications include
  - Fetal scalp cellulitis but with an incidence of less than 1% in most studies (35).
  - Even more rare, serious complications include cranial osteomyelitis, generalized gonococcal sepsis, and cerebrospinal fluid leakage with associated meningitis, ocular injury, or disseminated HSV infection (36–39).
    o Avoidance of fetal scalp electrode is warranted in those with maternal HIV, hepatitis B or C, or other perinatal infection with concern for vertical transmission.
- The benefits must be carefully weighed against the risks.

Maternal Preparation, Position, Anesthesia, and Analgesia
Physical Preparation
- General considerations for delivery:
  - Patients with poor personal hygiene and for whom delivery is not imminent are encouraged to shower.
  - A constipated patient or one who has hard stool palpable in the rectum can be offered an enema.
  - Shaving of the perineum is not routinely performed. It has no effect on infection rate in episiotomy and laceration repairs and may increase the patient's risk of morbidity.
  - Patients in active uncomplicated labor may be candidates for some clear liquid intake (40)—Intravenous (IV) infusion should be considered in some laboring patients.
  - An IV catheter facilitates rapid administration of medications, anesthetic agents, and blood if clinically indicated.
  - IV fluids administered in labor are usually Ringer lactate or 0.45% normal saline with or without 5% dextrose.
  - Gastric emptying is reduced during pregnancy but especially during labor, and keeping the stomach empty for the possibility of emergency general endotracheal anesthesia should be considered.

Maternal Position
- Maternal position in labor has consequences for both maternal comfort and fetal well-being. The dorsal supine position with the gravid uterus resting on the aorta and inferior vena cava can cause decreased cardiac output and relative placental hypoperfusion.
- Patients in the latent phase of labor frequently are most comfortable if they are allowed to ambulate. No significant risk of fetal compromise exists, as long as an initial monitoring strip is reassuring and the membranes are intact or the presenting part is well applied to the cervix.
  - A randomized controlled trial (RCT) comparing patients who were ambulatory during the active phase of labor versus those who were confined to bed found no differences in the duration of labor, need for oxytocin, use of analgesia, operative vaginal delivery, or cesarean. Neonatal outcomes were also similar (41).
- Patients who have freedom of movement in labor will find positions that are most comfortable to them and thereby improve their tolerability of labor. The patient's labor support person, doula, or registered nurse is critical in helping the patient become

comfortably positioned during labor. If it becomes necessary, bed rest on the patient's side rather than on her back is recommended and allows intermittent or continuous fetal monitoring to be performed.

- One study (42) showed that continuous fetal monitoring may be carried out in the ambulatory patient by telemetry with no difference in fetal outcome but significantly less subjective pain compared to control subjects.

Analgesia and Anesthesia

- Management of discomfort and pain during labor and delivery is a necessary part of good obstetric practice. For a detailed discussion of this topic, see Chapter 3.
- The *Guidelines for Perinatal Care*, published by the American College of Obstetricians and Gynecologists, states that maternal request is sufficient justification for providing pain relief during labor (8). The goal of pain relief in labor is to provide the patient sufficient comfort to experience her birth process fully while avoiding fetal compromise.
- The modalities that meet these needs include psychoprophylaxis and alternative pain management strategies, narcotic and analgesic drugs, and regional anesthesia.
- The first step in pain management should be antepartum counseling and childbirth education classes regarding the different modalities. These should set realistic expectations for labor pains, review nonpharmacologic techniques, and discuss the controversy regarding the association of epidurals with increased risk for cesarean delivery.

Alternative Pain Management Strategies

- Alternative pain management strategies include the use of a trained lay support person, such as a doula, and relaxation techniques such as massage and acupressure, therapeutic touch, hydrotherapy, music, aromatherapy, self-hypnosis, and alternative positioning techniques, including use of a birthing ball, and breathing techniques (i.e., Lamaze).
- In a number of studies, the use of a doula has been shown to reduce the length of the active phase of labor, reduce requests for narcotic analgesia and regional anesthesia, and reduce the rate of operative interventions including cesarean delivery, while maintaining optimal maternal and fetal outcome (43).
- Other studies have shown lower intervention rates for women using certified nurse–midwives, particularly when they are able to function in a one-on-one situation with the laboring patient (44).

Analgesic Medications and Regional Anesthesia (See Chapter 3)

Trial of Labor after Cesarean Delivery

Patients with one or two prior low transverse cesarean deliveries may be offered a trial of labor and vaginal delivery (45–47). Current evidence supports the premise that a properly selected and managed patient undergoing trial of labor after cesarean delivery (TOLAC) is associated with decreased maternal morbidity and a decreased risk of complications with future pregnancy.

Candidates for a TOLAC include (45)

- Patients who have undergone one or two previous cesarean deliveries with low transverse uterine incision
- Patients with pelvis that is clinically adequate for the EFW
- Patients with no other uterine scars (i.e., myomectomy or classical hysterotomy) or history of uterine rupture
- Patients delivering at a facility capable of performing emergency cesarean delivery which includes availability of support staff (delivering physician, anesthesia, nursing, and pediatrics) as well as blood products

Success Rates for TOLAC
- Reports over the past several years suggest that 60% to 80% of women undergoing trial of labor after previous cesarean delivery achieve a successful vaginal birth (14,45–48).
- If the prior cesarean delivery was performed for an arrest disorder, then the probability for success is less than when the first cesarean delivery was for a nonrecurring indication (e.g., breech presentation) (15,45–58).
  - Factors associated with increased likelihood of success of vaginal birth after caesarean (VBAC) are a prior vaginal birth and spontaneous labor.

TOLAC Risks
- The potential of uterine rupture or dehiscence is the complication of greatest concern and the outcome associated with TOLAC that most significantly increases the chance of additional maternal and neonatal morbidity (45–48).
  - Location of prior incision on the uterus influences the potential chance of uterine rupture. One prior low transverse incision has reported clinically determined uterine rupture rates of approximately 0.5% to 1.0% after TOLAC. In women with two prior cesareans, the risk of uterine rupture increased from 0.9% to 1.7% (46,47). Two large studies that reported the risks for women with two previous cesarean deliveries undergoing TOLAC reported some increased risk in morbidity, but the chances of achieving VBAC appear to be similar compared to women with one prior cesarean delivery (48–50).
- The TOLAC candidate should be counseled that the risk of uterine rupture is 0.5% to 1% (46). Additionally, in the event of uterine rupture, there is a 6.2% risk of hypoxic ischemic encephalopathy (HIE) and a neonatal death rate of 1.8% (45–49). If uterine rupture does occur, there is an approximately 4% risk of hysterectomy (48).
  - Epidural may be utilized as part of TOLAC, and no causal relationship has been shown to decrease the rate of successful VBAC (14,48).
  - Twins who attempt TOLAC have similar rates of success in VBAC compared to their singleton counterparts (14,45). Therefore, any patient with one prior low transverse cesarean may be counseled regarding the option of TOLAC.
  - Induction of labor remains an option for those women undergoing a TOLAC, but the usage of cervical ripening agents such as Cervidil or misoprostol should be discouraged secondary to increased risk of uterine rupture (14,45).
  - In any patient undergoing an induction, the patient should be counseled on the potential increased rate of uterine rupture and the decreased success rate of achieving a successful VBAC (14,45).

Procedure
- It is essential that an operating room and surgical staff, anesthesiologist, and blood bank services are immediately available on a 24-hour basis and that obstetricians are on site to respond appropriately to the potential uterine rupture in the patient attempting VBAC.
- Patients attempting VBAC are admitted to the labor floor, an IV catheter is placed, and a blood type and screen is obtained to facilitate the possibility of blood component transfusion. Internal monitoring with either an electronic fetal scalp electrode or an intrauterine pressure catheter has not been shown to assist in the prediction of uterine rupture (14,45).
- Acute signs and symptoms of uterine rupture may be variable and accurate predictors do not exist. However, any fetal heart rate changes (particularly late or severe variable decelerations), increased uterine contractions, vaginal bleeding, loss of fetal station, or new onset of intense pain require careful evaluation. The most common sign associated with uterine rupture is fetal heart rate changes, which occur in up to 70% of uterine ruptures (14,45).
- Manual exploration of the uterus after the third stage of labor has not been shown to improve outcomes (45).

NORMAL DELIVERY
Management of Spontaneous Delivery of the Infant
Preparation
- As the multiparous patient approaches complete dilation or the nulliparous patient begins to crown the fetal scalp with a push, preparations are made for delivery. If delivery is to take place in a combined labor and delivery room, equipment is opened and materials are readied to receive the newborn.

Maternal Position
- The mother's position on a traditional delivery room table is usually restricted to the dorsal lithotomy position with left lateral tilt (to displace the uterus from the great vessels). This position has been encouraged to allow the clinician adequate access to the perineum.
- In a labor and delivery room setting, patients may naturally tend to push and deliver on their sides, sitting, squatting, on all fours, or in the knee–chest position.
- Relatively few controlled comparisons have been published reporting the benefits of various delivery positions with or without an epidural.
  - One study (50) advocated the "half-sitting" position that can be used in a delivery room setting with stirrups. Benefits were that patients found this position more comfortable, it led to fewer operative deliveries, and it had equivalent fetal outcomes to controls.
  - There are insufficient data to support specific patient positioning recommendations in those patients with epidural anesthesia (51).

Procedure
- The perineum need not be prepared in a manner similar to that for a surgical procedure. In fact, povidone iodine (Betadine) has never been shown to be indicated for mucous membranes. Warm water or saline irrigation is sufficient to minimize maternal fecal contamination of the perineum.
- If not already addressed, delivery anesthesia is chosen at this time. Many deliveries may be performed without anesthesia if it is the patient's and clinician's preference. (A pudendal block or local infiltration may be utilized for the delivery if necessary.)
- Restricting the use of episiotomy to specific fetal and maternal indications reduces the risk of posterior perineal trauma. Midline episiotomy may increase the risk of third- and fourth-degree lacerations when compared to mediolateral episiotomy (2,3,52).

Maneuvers of Delivery from an Occiput Anterior Position
Delivery of the Head
- The fetal head is delivered by extension. As the flexed head passes through the vaginal introitus, the smallest diameter (occipitobregmatic) is presented if the vertex is maintained in a state of flexion. Maintaining flexion and pushing the perineum back over the face and under the chin before the head is allowed to extend appeared to be the least traumatic method in one study (53). Extending the fetal head by lifting the fetal chin with a towel-covered hand on the perineum (Ritgen maneuver) can accelerate the delivery process but may be more traumatic to the perineum. A multicenter RCT showed that there was no difference in risk of perineal trauma between the "hands on" and "hands poised" techniques of delivery. Once the fetal head has been delivered, external rotation and restitution to the occiput transverse position occurs.
  - Updated NRP 2010 guidelines suggest not using the bulb syringe to suction the nares and oropharynx of the fetus, even in the face of meconium-stained fluid. Allowing the fetus to cry and clear secretions on its own is recommended if the infant is vigorous. However, in the special circumstance of meconium, if the infant is not vigorous, there is insufficient evidence to recommend a change in the current practice that tracheal suctioning should be performed immediately after delivery (54).

- A finger should be insinuated into the vagina along the fetal neck to evaluate for a nuchal cord. If one is present, it can usually be reduced over the vertex or over the body. If this cannot be accomplished easily, the cord should be doubly clamped and divided between the clamps on the perineum and the remainder of the delivery carried out promptly. If multiple loops of cord are encountered, the adjacent clamps should be placed on just a single loop.

Delivery of the Shoulders

- Delivery of the anterior shoulder is accomplished by gentle downward traction on the fetal head toward the floor in association with maternal expulsive efforts. Flexion of the maternal thighs against the abdomen (McRoberts maneuver) (55) will often facilitate delivery of the anterior shoulder. With the anterior shoulder delivered, the posterior shoulder is delivered with vertical traction directed upward on the vertex. In general, gentle traction should be exerted coincident with the long axis of the fetus to avoid undue stretching of the brachial plexus. The perineal body should be supported to avoid extensions of the episiotomy or to avoid lacerations. When both shoulders have passed through the introitus, the remainder of the delivery requires little assistance in most cases.

Final Steps

- Grasping the infant around the back of the neck and head with one hand and gliding the other hand toward the vagina to the baby's buttocks, the operator delivers the infant. Care should be taken not to compress the blood vessels of the baby's neck and to keep the baby's head downward to facilitate drainage of nasopharyngeal secretions. The infant can usually be cradled in one arm and tucked against the operator's abdomen, leaving the other hand free to perform the steps that follow. The umbilical cord is then doubly clamped and divided, leaving 2 to 3 cm of cord with the infant.
- If the infant appears stable and healthy, an alternative to holding the infant, clamping, and cutting the cord is to place the infant directly into the mother's arms and onto her abdomen. Delaying the cord clamping and cutting until the cord stops pulsating allows for a placental transfusion to newborn. Neither method, early or delayed cord clamping, has been shown to be superior (54,56). Delay of up to 60 seconds can be considered as it may increase total body iron stores and blood volume; these potential benefits must be weighed against the increased risk of neonatal jaundice (56). The 2010 American Heart Association Neonatal Resuscitation Guidelines suggest cord clamp delay (54).
- Examination of the proximal end of the cord will prevent clamping part of an omphalocele or umbilical hernia.
- If the infant has not been given to the mother, the infant is transferred to the mother's abdomen for initial bonding. All efforts should be made to keep the mother and the newborn together for a prolonged period after birth. Breast-feeding can be initiated at this time and should be encouraged in most cases. Most routine newborn care can be given by the nursing staff while the infant is on the mother's abdomen. If resuscitative efforts are necessary, then the infant should be placed in the appropriate location needed to render such care.

Episiotomy

- Episiotomy has traditionally been one of the most frequently performed obstetric procedures and has been one of the more controversial (2,3,55). This incision of the perineum enlarges the vaginal orifice at the time of delivery. The incision may be made with scissors or a knife and may be made in the midline (medial episiotomy) or begun in the midline and extended laterally (mediolateral episiotomy).
- Routine use of episiotomies has not been shown to improve outcomes for patients and can actually be harmful. Routine or liberal use of episiotomies increases the risk that the

patient will have a surgical incision that is larger than if she experiences a spontaneous laceration at birth (2,3,52).

- It is recommended that episiotomies should be used selectively and only when clinically indicated.

Complications of Episiotomy
- As with any other surgical procedure, the risks of episiotomy must be compared with the benefits.
- Refraining from routine performance of episiotomy in some cases has resulted in an increased incidence of first- and second-degree periurethral and vaginal lacerations.
- Although an episiotomy may be simpler to repair than a spontaneous laceration, it is associated with a higher incidence of third- and fourth-degree lacerations. Even when recognized and repaired appropriately, these have lifelong implications, most significantly in regard to continence of flatus and stool (2,3,52,57,58).
- Pain and edema are the most frequent postepisiotomy complaints. These usually resolve within a few days, particularly if a regimen of sitz baths several times a day is encouraged in the immediate postpartum period.
- Dyspareunia may be noted by some women. Evaluation for abnormal healing, lactation-associated atrophy, or other causes is necessary.
- Infection can be one of the most serious complications of episiotomy, leading to significant morbidity and, rarely, maternal mortality (2,3,52,57,58).

Method
- Episiotomy timing is important. It should be performed when a 3- to 4-cm diameter of fetal scalp is visible during a contraction. Excessive blood loss can occur if it is performed earlier, whereas if performed too late, excessive stretching of the perineum and vagina may already have occurred.
- With adequate local, pudendal, or regional anesthetic in place, the perineum is separated from the fetal head usually by insertion of the provider's fingers between the perineum and fetal head. Medial episiotomy is performed by incising the triangularly shaped perineum toward the anus and into the vagina. An adequate incision should be made for the episiotomy to be of value. Care must be taken to avoid cutting into the anal sphincter or the rectum, unless this degree of exposure is deemed necessary. If a short perineum is encountered or third- or fourth-degree extension likely, a mediolateral episiotomy should be considered (2,3,52).
- Delivery is performed with care taken by the clinician to prevent extension of the episiotomy by applying pressure at the perineal apex with a towel-covered hand.
- The critical part of the procedure is the decision to perform the episiotomy. Most deliveries can be performed without episiotomy, and the proposed benefits of episiotomy have never been proven (2,3,52).

Delivery of the Placenta
Delivery of the placenta can be accomplished by either expectant or active management of the third stage of labor.

Expectant Management
- Normally, the placenta separates spontaneously from the uterine wall within approximately 5 minutes of delivery but may take as long as 20 to 30 minutes. No attempt should be made to extract the placenta before its separation.
- Separation is indicated by
  - The fundus changing to a globular shape and firm consistency
  - The appearance of a gush of blood
  - Lengthening of the umbilical cord

- When separation has occurred, gentle fundal massage and firm but gentle traction on the cord sometimes will effect rapid delivery of the placenta.
- In the Brandt-Andrews maneuver, cephalad stabilizing pressure is exerted with the abdominal hand on the lower segment of the uterus while traction on the cord is simultaneously exerted. The abdominal hand should prevent uterine inversion.
- An advantage of expectant management of the third stage is that it does not interfere with the normal delivery processes and requires no special medications or supplies. Disadvantages of this method are that the third stage of labor is longer, and there is possible increased risk of postpartum hemorrhage compared with active management of this stage (59).

Active Management
- After delivery of the anterior shoulder, or immediately after birth of the infant, the patient is administered an uterotonic drug to stimulate uterine contraction.
- Clamp and cut the cord.
- Wait for a strong uterine contraction and then apply controlled cord traction while applying countertraction above the pubic bone.
- If the placenta is not delivered, wait until the next contraction.
- Advantages of active management of the third stage include decreased length of third stage, decreased maternal blood loss of less than 1000 mL (59), possible lower risk for postpartum hemorrhage and anemia, and decreased need for transfusion.
- Disadvantages of this method are increased incidence of maternal diastolic blood pressure, nausea, vomiting, increased pain, and increased use of analgesia from time of birth until hospital discharge (59).

Manual Extraction
- If the placenta has not delivered after 30 minutes, or if separation has occurred without delivery of the placenta, manual removal may be performed to reduce excessive blood loss. Intrauterine bacterial contamination is a theoretical risk of manual extraction but is not a common complication.
- Procedure: Adequate anesthesia should be assured. One hand should grasp the fundus and hold it downward firmly. Physicians should avoid contamination by using an extended-cuff glove and arm cover. With the other hand, reach into the uterine cavity and gently insinuate the fingers between the placenta and the maternal surface in a circumferential fashion until separation is complete. The placenta can now be removed. Vigorous fundal massage and the use of a uterotonic agent, preferably oxytocin, will minimize subsequent bleeding.
- Several studies document an increased risk of postpartum endometritis after manual removal of the placenta during a cesarean section. Although it is a common practice to administer prophylactic antibiotics to patients who deliver vaginally and have manual placental extraction, there is no evidence to support this practice (60).

Examination of the Placenta
- The placenta should be examined for missing cotyledons or other evidence of undelivered remnants.
- The membranes should be inspected for vessels that run blindly to an edge, suggesting a succenturiate lobe that may not have been removed.
- The cut end of the cord should be examined for the presence of two arteries and a vein. The absence of one umbilical artery may suggest a congenital anomaly in the newborn.
- When abnormalities of the placenta are suspected, pathologic evaluation is warranted.

Active Prophylaxis against Postpartum Atony
- Although the fundus usually contracts well after delivery, this is not always the case. A poorly contracted uterus can lead to rapid and severe blood loss. Therefore, it is wise to take measures to avoid excessive blood loss caused by postpartum uterine atony.

- Gentle but firm external fundal message should always be part of postpartum management.
- It is usually is wise to give an oxytocic agent either intramuscularly with the delivery of the anterior shoulder (10 U oxytocin) or in an IV drip after the delivery of the placenta (10 to 20 U in 1000 mL of isotonic IV fluid). The latter route is preferable because it allows for a more controlled third stage. Oxytocin can cause marked hypotension if administered as an IV bolus. Occasionally, oxytocin is insufficient, and other drugs must be considered.
- Misoprostol, 600 to 1000 μg placed in the rectum, is a very effective treatment for excessive bleeding due to uterine atony. However, shivering, pyrexia, and vomiting are more common with misoprostol, this is usually self-limited (61).
- Methylergonovine maleate (Methergine), 0.2 mg intramuscularly, often produces sufficient uterine contractility to correct atony. Methylergonovine is contraindicated in patients who are hypertensive (hypertension may be aggravated), who are HIV-positive patients on any of the protease or reverse transcriptase inhibitors (e.g., delavirdine, indinavir, nelfinavir), coronary artery disease, and should be avoided as well in patients who are hypotensive (further peripheral vasoconstriction in a patient in hypovolemic shock may result in digit loss secondary to vascular insufficiency) or have recently received ephedrine for hypotension.

Repair of Lacerations and Episiotomy
Lacerations of the Birth Canal
- After delivery of the placenta, the clinician should inspect the birth canal for lacerations.
  - The vaginal sidewalls and fornices should be palpated and inspected.
  - Lacerations involving the periurethral tissues can be missed unless the labia minora are separated.
  - Lacerations usually are linear and cephalad and may be repaired in an interrupted or continuous fashion.
- By placing the palm of one hand into the vagina as a retractor, the cervix can be exposed. The anterior lip of the cervix should be examined and elevated to allow visualization of the entire cervix. If a cervical laceration is present, visualization can often be improved by having an assistant exert caudad pressure on the uterine fundus. Use of retractors by an assistant may also be necessary. Exposure of vaginal vault lacerations can sometimes be improved by using the initially placed suture for traction to assure visualization and control of the cephalad apex.
- Absorbable synthetic suture has been found to reduce short-term pain and dyspareunia (62).

Episiotomy
- The episiotomy is repaired with 2-0 or 3-0 absorbable suture material. Interrupted sutures may be required to approximate the deep tissues of the perineal body. Running interlocking sutures are used to repair the vaginal mucosa, with care being taken to include its apex. The perineum is reapproximated with subcutaneous and subcuticular running sutures with attention to landmarks such as the hymeneal ring.
- A laceration extending through the anal sphincter (third degree) should be repaired with interrupted sutures, incorporating the fascia of the muscle for strength. The overlapping technique has not been shown to be more effective than the end-to-end technique.
- When the rectal mucosa is involved (fourth degree), it should be reapproximated in two layers with interrupted absorbable suture no more than 0.5 cm apart reinforced with the overlying fascia using a continuous synthetic absorbable suture. Care should be taken to avoid including suture material in the luminal surface of the intact mucosa. The remainder of the repair is routine. Performing fourth-degree repairs in the operating room with assistants and lighting for adequate exposure should be considered. Liberal irrigation with isotonic saline during the repair may also facilitate healing.
  - Although not extensively studied, the use of a single dose of second-generation cephalosporin or clindamycin, if penicillin allergic, was protective of perineal wound complications (62).

Assisted Delivery

- When it is not possible to achieve spontaneous vaginal delivery, operative delivery may be necessary.
- This may be either by cesarean delivery or an instrumented vaginal delivery. The latter entails the use of either forceps or a vacuum extractor.
- Operative delivery options and considerations are discussed in detail in Chapter 10.

PATIENT EDUCATION

- Patient education for labor and delivery begins during prenatal care and should include the mother's key support person(s).
- Patients should be strongly encouraged to enroll in childbirth preparation classes.
- Throughout the pregnancy, health care providers should reinforce the concept that labor, birth, and breast-feeding are normal physiologic processes.
- Patient education may be given to the patient by the clinicians and/or the registered nurses responsible for her care.
- Information that patients need includes
  - Signs and symptoms of labor
  - How and when to contact the labor and delivery suite
  - Routines in the labor and delivery suite
  - Analgesia and anesthesia options
  - Breast-feeding support immediately after birth
- Throughout the labor process, the patient and support person(s) must be kept aware of her progress and status.
- Informed consent needs to be obtained from the patient before any interventions, procedures, analgesia, or anesthetics are administered.

REFERENCES

1. American College of Obstetricians and Gynecologists. AGOG Practice Bulletin No. 106: intrapartum fetal heart rate monitoring: nomenclature, interpretation, and general management principles. *Obstet Gynecol.* 2009;114(1):192–202.
2. American College of Obstetricians and Gynecologists. ACOG Practice Bulletin No. 71: Episiotomy. Clinical Management Guidelines for Obstetrician-Gynecologists. *Obstet Gynecol.* 2006;107(4):957–962.
3. Carroli G, Mignini L. Episiotomy for vaginal birth [Review]. *Cochrane Database Syst Rev.* 2009;(1):CD00081.
4. Greene MF, Creasy RK, Resnik R, Lockwood CL, Moore T. *Creasy and Resnik's maternal-fetal medicine: principles and practice.* Cambridge University Press, New York, 2008.
5. ACOG Practice Bulletin No. 8: premature rupture of membranes. Clinical management guideline for obstetrician-gynecologists. *Obstet Gynecol.* 2007;109(4):107–119.
6. Abdelazim IA, Makhlouf HH. Placental alpha microglobulin-1(Amnisure® test) for the detection of premature rupture of fetal membranes. *Arch Gynecol Obstet.* 2012;285(4):985–989.
7. ACOG practice bulletin No 9: Antepartum fetal surveillance. *Int J Gynaecol Obstet.* 2000;68(2):175–185.
8. *Guidelines for perinatal care.* 7th ed. Washington: American Academy of Pediatrics and the American College of Obstetricians and Gynecologists, 2012.
9. American College of Obstetricians and Gynecologists. ACOG practice bulletin No. 101: Ultrasonography in pregnancy. *Obstet Gynecol.* 2009;113(2 Pt 1):451–461.
10. Lewis DF, Raymond RC, Perkins MB, Brooks GG, et al. Recurrence rate of shoulder dystocia. *Am J Obstet Gynecol.* 1995;172:1369–1371.
11. ACOG practice bulletin No 40: Shoulder dystocia. *Int J Gynaecol Obstet.* 2003;80(1):87–92.
12. Hjartardottir S, Leifsson BG, Geirsson RT, et al. Recurrence of hypertensive disorder in second pregnancy. *Am J Obstet Gynecol.* 2006;194:916–920.

13. Ananth CV, Savitz DA, Williams MA. Placental abruption and its association with hypertension and prolonged rupture of membranes: a methodologic review and meta-analysis. *Obstet Gynecol.* 1996;88:309–318.
14. Cunningham FG, Bangdiwala SI, Brown SS, et al. National Institutes of Health Consensus Development Conference Statement vaginal birth after cesarean: new insights March 8–10, 2010. *Semin Perinatol.* 2010;34(5):351–365.
15. ACOG Committee on Practice Bulletins–Obstetrics. ACOG practice bulletin No 33: diagnosis and management of preeclampsia and eclampsia. *Obstet gynecol.* 2002;99(1):159–167.
16. Hadlock FP, Deter RL, Harrist RB, et al. Estimating fetal age: computer assisted analysis of multiple fetal growth parameters. *Radiology.* 1984;152:497–501.
17. Macones GA, Hankins GD, Spong CY, et al. The 2008 National Institute of Child Health and Human Development workshop report on electronic fetal monitoring: update on definitions, interpretation, and research guidelines. *Obstet Gynecol.* 2008;112(3):661–666.
18. AGOG Practice bulletin No. 116: management of intrapartum fetal heart rate tracings. *Obstet Gynecol.* 2010;116(5):1232–1240.
19. Mercer BM, Crocker LG, Boe NM, et al. Induction versus expectant management in premature rupture of the membranes with mature amniotic fluid at 32 to 36 weeks: a randomized trial. *Am J Obstet Gynecol.* 1993;169:775–782.
20. Verani JR, McGee L, Schrag SJ; Division of Bacterial Diseases, National Center for Immunization and Respiratory Diseases, Centers for Disease Control and Prevention. Prevention of perinatal group B streptococcal disease-revised guidelines from CDC, 2010. *MMWR Recomm Rep.* 2010;59(RR-10):1–36.
21. American College of Obstetricians and Gynecologists Committee on Obstetric Practice. ACOG Committee Opinion No. 485: prevention of early-onset group B streptococcal disease in newborns. *Obstet Gynecol.* 2011;117(4):1019–1027.
22. Zhang J, Landy HJ, Branch DW, et al.; Consortium on Safe Labor. Contemporary patterns of spontaneous labor with normal neonatal outcomes. *Obstet Gynecol.* 2010;116:1281–1287.
23. Zhang J, Troendle J, Reddy UM, et al.; the Consortium on Safe Labor. Contemporary cesarean delivery practice in the United States. *Am J Obstet Gynecol.* 2010;203:e1–e10.
24. Spong CY, Berghella V, Wenstrom KD, et al. Preventing the first cesarean delivery: Summary of a joint Eunice Kennedy Shriver National Institute of Child Health and Human Development, Society for Maternal-Fetal Medicine, and American College of Obstetricians and Gynecologists Workshop. *Obstet Gynecol.* 2012;120:1181–1193.
25. Tuuli MG, Frey HA, Odibo AO, et al. Immediate compared with delayed pushing in the second stage of labor: a systematic review and meta-analysis. *Obstet Gynecol.* 2012;120(3):660–668.
26. Fraser WD, Turcot L, Krauss I, et al. Amniotomy for shortening spontaneous labor. *Cochrane Database Syst Rev.* 2006;(3): CD00015.
27. Rouse DJ, McCullough C, Wren AL, et al. Active-phase labor arrest: a randomized trial of chorioamnion management. *Obstet Gynecol.* 1994;83:937–940.
28. American College of Obstetrics and Gynecology Committee on Practice Bulletins-Obstetrics. ACOG Practice Bulletin No. 49: Dystocia and augmentation of labor. *Obstet Gynecol.* 2003;102(6):1445–1454.
29. Garite TJ, Porto M, Carlson NJ, et al. The influence of elective amniotomy on fetal heart rate patterns and the course of labor in term patients: a randomized study. *Am J Obstet Gyneol.* 1993;168:1827–1831.
30. Macones GA, Cahill A, Stamilio DM, Odibo AO. The efficacy of early amniotomy in nulliparous labor induction: a randomized controlled trial. *Am J Obstet Gynecol.* 2012;207(5):403.e1–e5.
31. Ingemarsson E, Ingemarsson I, Svenningson HW. Impact of routine fetal monitoring during labor and fetal outcome with long-term follow-up. *Am J Obstet Gynecol.* 1981;141:29–38.
32. Mueller-Heubach E, MacDonald HM, Joret D, et al. Effects of electronic fetal heart rate monitoring on perinatal outcome and obstetric practices. *Am J Obstet Gynecol.* 1980;137:758–763.
33. Hon EH, Petrie RH. Clinical value of FHR monitoring. *Clin Obstet Gynecol.* 1975;18:(4):1–23.

34. Girvell RM, Alfirevic Z, Gyte GM, et al. Antenatal cardiotocography for fetal assessment. *Cochrane Database Syst Rev.* 2012;12:DC007863.
35. Wagener MM, Rycheck RR, Yee RB, et al. Septic dermatitis of the neonatal scalp and maternal endomyometritis with internal fetal monitoring. *Pediatrics.* 1984;74:81–85.
36. Nieburg P, Gross SJ. Cerebrospinal fluid leak in a neonate associated with fetal scalp electrode monitoring. *Am J Obstet Gynecol.* 1983;147:839.
37. Overturf GD, Balfour G. Osteomyelitis and sepsis: severe complications of fetal monitoring. *Pediatrics.* 1984;74:81–85.
38. Miyashiro MJ, Mintz-Hittner HA. Penetrating ocular injury with a fetal scalp monitoring spiral electrode. *Am J Ophthalmol.* 1999;128(4):526–528.
39. Amann ST, Fagnant RJ, Shartrand SA, et al. Herpes simplex infection associated with short-term use of a fetal scalp electrode. A case report. *J Reprod Med.* 1992;37(4):372–374.
40. Committee on Obstetric Practice, American College of Obstetricians and Gynecologists. ACOG committee opinion No. 441: oral intake during labor. *Obstet Gynecol.* 2009;114(3):714.
41. Bloom SL, McIntire DD, Kelly MA, et al. Lack of effect of walking on labor and delivery. *N Engl J Med.* 1998;339:76–79.
42. Haukkamaa M, Purhonen M, Teramo K. The monitoring of labor by telemetry. *J Perinat Med.* 1982;10:17–22.
43. Kennell J, Klaus M, McGrath S, et al. Continuous emotional support during labor in a US hospital. *JAMA.* 1991;265:2197–2201.
44. Butler C, Abrams K, Parker J. Supportive nurse midwife care associated with reduced incidence of cesarean section. *Am J Obstet Gynecol.* 1993;168:404–413.
45. American College of Obstetricians and Gynecologists. ACOG Practice bulletin no. 115: vaginal birth after previous cesarean delivery. *Obstet Gynecol.* 2010;116(2 Pt 1):450–463.
46. Landon MB. Vaginal birth after cesarean delivery. *Clin Perinatol.* 2008;25(3):491–504.
47. Landon MB, Spong CY, Thom E, et al. Risk of uterine rupture during a trial of labor in women with multiple and single prior cesarean delivery. National Institute of Child Health and Human Development Maternal-Fetal Medicine Units Network. *Obstet Gyncol.* 2006;108:12–20.
48. Tahseen S, Griffiths M. Vaginal birth after two caesarean sections (VBAC-2)- a systematic review with meta-analysis of success rate and adverse outcomes of VBAC-2 versus VBAC-1 and repeat (third) caesarean sections. *BJOG.* 2010;117:5–19.
49. Landon MB, Hauth JC, Leveno KJ, et al. Maternal and perinatal outcomes associated with a trial of labor after prior cesarean delivery. National Institute of Child Health and Human Development Maternal-Fetal Medicine Units Network. *N Engl J Med.* 2004;351:2581–2589.
50. Marttila M, Kajanoja P, Ylikorkala O. Maternal half-sitting position in the second stage of labor. *J Perinat Med.* 1983;11:286–289.
51. Kemp E, Kingswood CJ, Kibuka M, Thorton JG. Position in the second stage for labour for women with epidural anaesthsia. *Cochrane Database Syst Rev.* 2013;(1):CD008070.
52. Coats PM, Chan KK, Wilkins M, Beard RJ. A comparison between midline and mediolateral episiotomies. *Br J Obstet Gynaecol.* 1980;87(5):408–412.
53. Goodlin RC. On protection of the maternal perineum during birth. *Obstet Gynecol.* 1983;62:393.
54. Kattwinkel J, Perlman JM, Aziz K, et al. Neonatal resuscitation: 2010 American Heart Association Guidelines for Cardiopulmonary resuscitation and Emergency Cardiovascular Care. *Pediatrics.* 2010;126(5):e1400–e1413.
55. Gonik B, Stringer CA, Held B. An alternate maneuver for management of shoulder dystocia. *Am J Obstet Gynecol.* 1983;145:882–884.
56. Committee on Obstetric Practice, American College of Obstetricians and Gynecologists. Committee Opinion No. 543: timing of umbilical cord clamping after birth. *Obstet Gynecol.* 2012;120(6):1522–1526.
57. Poen AC, Felt-Bersma RJ, Strijers RL, et al. Third-degree obstetric perineal tear: long-term clinical and functional results after primary repair. *Br J Surg.* 1998;85:1433–143.

58. Anthony S, Buitendijk SE, Zondervan KT, et al. Episiotomies and the occurrence of severe perineal lacerations. *Br J Obstet Gynaecol.* 1994;101:1064–1067.

59. Begley CM, Gyte GM, Devane D, McGuire W, Weeks A. Active versus expectant management for women in the third stage of labour. *Cochrane Database Syst Rev.* 2011;(11):CD007412.

60. American College of Obstetricians and Gynecologists. ACOG Practice Bulletin No. 120: use of prophylactic antibiotics in labor and delivery. *Obstet Gynecol.* 2011;117(6):1472–1483.

61. Badejoko OO, Ljarotimi AO, Awowole IO, Loto OM, Bedejoko BO, et al. Adjunctive rectal misoprostol versus oxytocin infusion for prevention of postpartum hemorrhage in women at risk: a randomized controlled trial. *J Obstet Gynaecol Res.* 2012;38(11):1294–1301.

62. Hale RW, Ling FW. *Episiotomy: Procedure and Repair Techniques. Amer College of Obstetricians and Gynecologists.* 2007.

3 Obstetric Anesthesia
Regina Fragneto

KEY POINTS
- The physiologic changes of pregnancy are a significant factor in the anesthetic care of women during childbirth and sometimes increase the risks of anesthesia.
- Neuraxial anesthesia procedures, including epidural and combined spinal–epidural (CSE) analgesia, provide excellent pain relief during labor and are used in the majority of childbirths in the United States.
- Both neuraxial and general anesthesia techniques provide effective anesthesia for cesarean delivery. Historically, anesthesia-related maternal mortality has been greater when general anesthesia is used, but the difference in mortality rate between general and regional anesthesia has narrowed in the United States.
- Ensuring maternal safety and maintaining adequate uteroplacental perfusion and fetal oxygenation are the most important goals when anesthesia is administered for nonobstetric surgery during pregnancy.

BACKGROUND
Obstetric anesthesia is an important component in the care of most women during childbirth. Many women choose to receive neuraxial analgesia while in labor, and all women who undergo cesarean delivery require some type of anesthesia. Anesthesia care is also provided to the many women who require other surgical procedures while pregnant.

Pathophysiology
- The physiologic changes of pregnancy have a significant impact on the administration of both regional and general anesthesia to women during childbirth.
- Sensitivity of nerves to local anesthetics is enhanced during pregnancy (1).
  - As a result, the local anesthetic dose requirements for both spinal anesthesia during surgery and epidural labor analgesia are decreased in pregnant women (2,3).
- The sedative effects of increased progesterone levels and the activation of the endorphin system during pregnancy also decrease general anesthesia requirements.
  - The minimum alveolar concentration of halogenated volatile anesthetic agents, which is defined as the drug concentration at which 50% of patients do not move when exposed to a noxious stimulus, is decreased by approximately 30% in women during pregnancy (4).
  - The dose of intravenous propofol needed to induce general anesthesia is also decreased in pregnant women (5).
- The physiologic changes of pregnancy may affect the safety of administering anesthesia to pregnant women.
  - Aortocaval compression from the gravid uterus decreases venous return and can result in significant hypotension when a pregnant woman assumes the supine position, especially during late pregnancy.
  - The sympathetic block produced by spinal and epidural anesthesia causes vasodilatation that results in a further decrease in venous return.
  - The sympathectomy induced by neuraxial anesthesia impairs a pregnant woman's ability to compensate via vasoconstriction for the decreased venous return caused by aortocaval compression. As a result, the degree of hypotension that occurs during neuraxial anesthesia is significantly greater in pregnant compared to nonpregnant women.

- Anesthesia-related maternal mortality is more common during general anesthesia than regional anesthesia although the difference in mortality rate between the anesthetic techniques has declined since 1990.
  - A study of anesthesia-related maternal mortality in the United States between 1991 and 2002 found that the overall rate was 1.2 per million live births, which was a 59% decrease from 1979 to 1990; and 86% of those deaths occurred during cesarean delivery.
  - The anesthesia-related case fatality rate for cesarean delivery under general anesthesia was 16.8 per million anesthetics from 1991 to 1996 with a decrease to 6.5 per million anesthetics for 1997–2002.
  - The anesthesia-related case fatality rate for cesarean delivery under regional anesthesia was 2.5 per million regional anesthetics for 1991–1996 and 3.8 per million anesthetics for 1997–2002.
  - Therefore, the risk of anesthesia-related mortality was 6.7 times greater for pregnant women receiving general anesthesia compared to regional anesthesia for 1991–1996, but the risk ratio had decreased to 1.7 for the period 1997–2002 (6).
  - The majority of deaths during general anesthesia resulted from airway management problems, such as failed intubation and aspiration, while high neuraxial block was the most common cause of regional anesthesia-related deaths (6).
- The physiologic changes of pregnancy play a significant role in the increased risk of general anesthesia for pregnant women.
  - Airway edema caused by pregnancy-induced capillary engorgement of the mucosa can distort airway anatomy and contributes to the increased incidence of difficult intubation in pregnant women.
  - One study found that the incidence of difficult or failed intubation was approximately eight times greater in obstetric patients compared to nonpregnant patients (7).
  - Respiratory changes of pregnancy, including decreased functional residual capacity and increased oxygen consumption, result in a more rapid development of hypoxemia when apnea occurs (8). Therefore, when difficult intubation is encountered during the induction of general anesthesia, an obstetric patient will become hypoxemic more quickly than a nonobstetric patient.
- A variety of physiologic factors contribute to the risk of aspiration in parturients.
  - Gastric emptying is prolonged during labor (9,10). In addition, anatomic changes resulting from displacement of the stomach by the gravid uterus and decreased lower esophageal sphincter tone, caused by increased progesterone levels, produce an increased incidence of gastroesophageal reflux in pregnant women.
  - Both delayed gastric emptying and gastroesophageal reflux are risk factors for gastric aspiration during the induction of general anesthesia.
  - Aspiration is more likely to occur when difficult airway management is encountered and securing of the airway with tracheal intubation is delayed.

Epidemiology

- The majority of pregnant women in the United States will receive obstetric anesthesia.
  - All patients undergoing cesarean delivery require anesthesia, and the cesarean delivery rate in the United States continues to rise; it had reached 32.8% of all deliveries in 2010 and 2011 (11).
  - Approximately 75% of women who deliver at a hospital in the United States with greater than 1500 deliveries per year receive neuraxial analgesia during labor (12).
  - Finally, based on estimates of the rate of surgery during pregnancy (0.3% to 2.2%), as many as 87,000 pregnant women in the United States undergo anesthesia for non–pregnancy-related surgical procedures each year (13).

EVALUATION

History

- Before providing obstetric anesthesia care, the anesthesiologist must perform a focused history and physical examination.
- Important components of the patient's medical history include the presence of serious underlying medical conditions—especially cardiovascular, pulmonary, and neurological disorders. The anesthesiologist must also be aware of any current pregnancy complications because the presence of these complications will affect decisions concerning anesthetic management.
  - Crucial medical history information for the anesthesia care provider includes any available information concerning previous general or regional anesthetics. The anesthesiologist will seek any evidence of technical difficulties with regional or general anesthesia procedures, including a history of failed or difficult intubation.
  - Adverse reactions to anesthetic drugs and a history of anesthesia-related inheritable disorders in the patient or her relatives, such as malignant hyperthermia and atypical pseudocholinesterase, should be noted.

Physical Examination

- The anesthesiologist's focused physical examination of the obstetric patient will include auscultation of the heart and lungs and careful assessment of the airway.
- When a neuraxial anesthesia technique is planned, examination of the back is also essential.
- Most anesthesiologists would agree that the most important component of the physical examination in healthy pregnant women is airway assessment. Evaluation of the airway includes mouth opening, neck movement, thyromental distance, Mallampati classification, and the upper-lip bite test.
  - The Mallampati airway classification system evaluates the size of the tongue relative to the size of the oropharyngeal cavity. Patients are assigned an airway class based on the pharyngeal structures that can be visualized when the patient opens her mouth wide and sticks out her tongue (Fig. 3-1). A correlation exists between Mallampati airway class and ease of intubation (14).

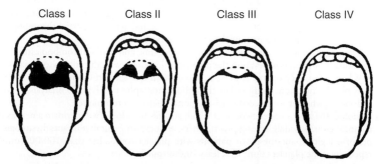

Class I   Class II   Class III   Class IV

Figure 3-1. Mallampati classification of the airway based on pharyngeal structures that are visible with mouth open. *Class I:* the soft palate, uvula, and tonsillar pillars are visualized. *Class II:* the uvula is only partially visualized, and the tonsillar pillars are not visualized. *Class III:* soft palate only is visualized. *Class IV:* not even the soft palate is visualized. (Reprinted from Chestnut DH. *Obstetric anesthesia: principles and practice.* 3rd ed. Philadelphia: Mosby, 2004, with permission.)

Table 3-1	Risk Factors for Difficult Intubation

Morbid obesity
Short neck
Increased neck circumference
Small mouth opening
Mallampati Class III or greater
Upper-lip bite test Class III
Congenital craniofacial abnormalities
Receding chin
Protruding maxillary incisors
Thyromental distance <3 fingerbreadths
Limited cervical spine mobility

- Airway classification using the upper-lip bite test, which assesses a patient's ability to cover the upper lip with the lower incisors, has also been shown to correlate with ease of intubation (15).
- Patient factors that increase the risk of difficult intubation are listed in Table 3-1.
- The anesthesiologist's preanesthetic evaluation also involves an assessment of fetal status because fetal condition is an important factor when deciding upon an anesthetic plan of care.

Laboratory Tests
- Healthy women who have received comprehensive prenatal care that included routine laboratory testing with normal results do not usually require additional laboratory tests before proceeding with regional or general anesthesia.
- If obstetric or other factors place the patient at increased risk for hemorrhage during delivery, a complete blood count and a blood type and screen or type and cross are indicated.
- Because the incidence of thrombocytopenia is increased in patients with preeclampsia, platelet count should be measured in these patients before performing regional anesthesia or surgery.
  - If the platelet count is greater than 100,000/mm^3, no other coagulation testing is required (16).
  - If the patient does have a platelet count less than 100,000/mm^3 or abnormal liver function tests, some anesthesiologists do request other coagulation studies, including prothrombin time, international normalized ratio, and activated partial thromboplastin time before initiating neuraxial anesthesia procedures.
    - There are data suggesting routine prothrombin time and partial thromboplastin time testing is not necessary, even in the preeclamptic patient with thrombocytopenia (17).
    - When thrombocytopenia is present, some anesthesia care providers perform testing of platelet function, using either thromboelastography or PFA-100 analysis, before deciding whether to proceed with a regional anesthesia technique.
  - Although the lowest platelet count at which an anesthesiologist will perform a neuraxial technique varies widely among practitioners, an increasing number of anesthesiologists perform regional anesthesia for patients with platelet counts less than 100,000/mm^3, especailly if the platelet count is at least 70,000/mm^3.

LABOR ANALGESIA
Background
- Labor pain and approaches to its relief have been controversial for thousands of years. In the 15th century, midwives were burned at the stake for offering pain relief. Some advocates of psychoprophylaxis have suggested that labor pain is minor.

- In reality, the experience of labor pain varies widely among women.
  - Although nearly a quarter of the women in one study reported their labor pain as minimal or mild, another 23% rated the pain as severe or intolerable (18).
  - Using a questionnaire developed by one of the pioneers of modern pain research, labor pain was rated as more painful than cancer pain. Using this same questionnaire, nulliparous women who had not received prepared childbirth training rated their labor pain as nearly as painful as traumatic amputation of a digit (19).
- Since approximately 75% of women in labor in the United States receive neuraxial labor analgesia, one can safely assume that the majority of pregnant women do consider labor pain significant.

Pathophysiology
- To provide adequate labor analgesia, an understanding of the physiology and mechanisms of labor pain is necessary.
- First stage: The pain women experience during the first stage of labor is primarily visceral pain caused by cervical dilation. These visceral afferents travel via the T10-L1 nerve roots. Therefore, analgesia during the first stage of labor can be provided via blockade of these peripheral afferents using either epidural block of the T10-L1 dermatomes or paracervical block. Pain during the first stage of labor can also be relieved via blockade of pain transmission within the spinal cord using the subarachnoid injection of opioids and/or local anesthetics.
- Second stage: During the second stage of labor, patients continue to experience the visceral pain described above. In addition, they experience somatic pain that results from stretching of the vagina and perineum as the fetal head traverses through the birth canal. These somatic pain impulses travel via the pudendal nerve, which is composed of nerve fibers from the S2-S4 nerve roots. Blockade of these pain impulses can be achieved by extending epidural or subarachnoid block to include the S2-S4 dermatomes or by performing a pudendal nerve block.

TREATMENT
Medications
Opioids
- Although several studies have shown that neuraxial analgesia techniques provide superior pain relief and cause less neonatal depression than do systemic opioids, the use of parenteral medications to provide labor analgesia remains relatively common for several reasons.
  - Some hospitals, especially those with few obstetric patients, do not have sufficient anesthesia care providers available to provide daily, 24-hour neuraxial labor analgesia services.
  - Some patients have medical contraindications to regional anesthesia, and some patients refuse neuraxial procedures.
- Several different opioids can be used to provide labor analgesia. The obstetrician should be aware of the advantages and disadvantages, as well as the duration of action for each drug when deciding which systemic opioid to administer to a woman in labor.
  - Table 3-2 describes the recommended dosing, onset time, and duration of action for commonly used systemic opioid medications.

Table 3-2	Commonly Used Systemic Opioids for Labor Analgesia		
Drug	Recommended dose (mg IV)	Onset time (min)	Duration of action (h)
Morphine	2–5	5	3–4
Butorphanol	1–2	5–10	3–4
Nalbuphine	10–20	2–3	3–6

- All systemic opioids rapidly cross the placenta and gain access to the fetus.
- Some adverse effects of systemic opioids are common to all of the medications, although to a greater or lesser extent depending on which drug was administered. These include decreased fetal heart rate variability and both maternal and neonatal respiratory depression.
- Meperidine has previously been one of the most widely used systemic opioids for labor analgesia in the United States and remains a commonly used systemic analgesic. There are significant disadvantages to this drug, however.
  - Metabolism of meperidine and its active metabolite, normeperidine, is prolonged in newborns due to their immature livers. Compared to a maternal half-life of 2.5 to 3 hours, the half-life of meperidine in the newborn is 18 to 23 hours (20). The half-life of normeperidine in newborns is approximately 60 hours (21).
  - These prolonged half-lives are responsible for the subtle neurobehavioral changes that have been reported in infants for as long as 5 days after maternal administration of meperidine (22).
  - If meperidine is used for labor analgesia, attention should be paid to the anticipated time interval between drug administration and delivery. Maximal fetal uptake of the drug occurs 2 to 3 hours after administration, and increased risk of respiratory depression has been noted in infants who were born 2 to 3 hours after meperidine administration (23).
- Butorphanol and nalbuphine have become the systemic analgesics of choice in many labor and delivery suites.
  - Butorphanol and nalbuphine are mixed agonist/antagonist opioids and provide analgesia similar to that provided by meperidine.
  - One advantage of these drugs is that a ceiling effect on respiratory depression is reached as the dose of the drug is increased.
  - Many women who receive these drugs during labor experience significant sedation.
  - Agonist/antagonist opioids should not be administered to patients who are opioid dependent because they could precipitate withdrawal symptoms.

Patient-Controlled Analgesia
- Although parenteral medications provide less effective labor analgesia than do neuraxial analgesia techniques, improved pain relief has been achieved with the administration of intravenous patient-controlled analgesia (IV PCA) using potent, short-acting opioids such as fentanyl and remifentanil.
- In one study that used fentanyl IV PCA, 65% of women were satisfied with their labor analgesia and reported that they would use the technique again. Among these women, no maternal respiratory depression or significant sedation occurred. Although the authors reported no adverse neonatal outcomes, 16% of the newborns did receive naloxone (24).
- Remifentanil is an ultra-short-acting drug that would be expected to produce less neonatal depression than do other opioids. Its use for labor analgesia has increased significantly over the past few years. Because it is such a potent opioid requiring increased patient monitoring, most anesthesiologists prefer to offer this technique only to patients in whom neuraxial anesthesia is contraindicated. Some labor and delivery units have been successful in offering it as an analgesic option to all laboring women (25).
- In a recent study that compared IV PCA with remifentanil, fentanyl, or meperidine, women who received remifentanil reported lower pain scores and higher satisfaction with their labor analgesia (26).
- In the most recent study of remifentanil PCA in laboring parturients, 91% of women were satisfied with their pain management. Moderate maternal sedation occurred, and 27% of women did require supplemental oxygen for oxygen saturation less than 92%. No adverse neonatal effects were reported (27).

Table 3-3	Recommended Dosing for Intravenous Patient-Controlled Labor Analgesia		
Drug	**PCA dose (µg)**	**Lockout interval (min)**	**Basal infusion**
Fentanyl	50	10	None
Remifentanil	20 (may increase by 5 µg every 15 min, not to exceed 1500 µg /h)	3	None

PCA, patient-controlled analgesia.

- Recommended dosing strategies for both fentanyl and remifentanil IV PCA are listed in Table 3-3.
  - Because both of these drugs are significantly more potent than are other opioids commonly used for labor analgesia, caution is necessary when administering these medications in order to avoid serious respiratory depression.
  - Administration of fentanyl and remifentanil should be supervised by health care providers experienced in the use of these drugs.
  - Continuous pulse oximetry monitoring and close nursing surveillance are also needed.

Procedures
- Table 3-4 describes the techniques that are effective in providing pain relief during the first and second stages of labor.
- Epidural analgesia is the most common technique anesthesiologists use to provide labor analgesia. Every study that has compared epidural analgesia to systemic opioids for labor analgesia has found that epidural analgesia provides superior pain relief.
- CSE analgesia is another procedure commonly performed by anesthesia care providers to deliver excellent pain relief during labor.
- Continuous spinal analgesia is another acceptable procedure for providing labor analgesia in certain situations.
- Nerve blocks performed by the obstetrician can also be useful for achieving labor pain relief.

Epidural Analgesia
- Epidural analgesia is the anesthetic procedure most commonly used in the United States to provide labor analgesia. In a recent national survey, hospitals that had more than 1500 births per year reported that 61% of their laboring patients received epidural analgesia (12).
- The advantages of epidural analgesia that make it so popular among anesthesiologists, patients, and obstetricians include an excellent quality of pain relief and versatility.
  - With appropriate dosing, a segmental block from T10-L1 can be achieved early in labor with the block being extended over time to include the sacral nerve roots once the second stage of labor has been reached.

Table 3-4	Procedures for Providing Effective Labor Analgesia	
Procedure	**First stage of labor**	**Second stage of labor**
Epidural analgesia	Effective	Effective
CSE analgesia	Effective	Effective
Continuous spinal analgesia	Effective	Effective
Paracervical block	Effective	Ineffective
Pudendal block	Ineffective	Effective

- By increasing the dose and concentration of drugs administered, epidural labor analgesia can be converted to a more dense, extensive block that provides anesthesia when a cesarean or operative vaginal delivery is necessary.
- A variety of dosing techniques have been used to provide effective pain relief during labor. The goal of the anesthesiologist when administering epidural labor analgesia is to provide effective analgesia while minimizing motor block, so the woman's expulsive efforts during the second stage of labor are not adversely affected.
  - One study found that the administration of higher concentrations of local anesthetic (bupivacaine 0.25%) for labor analgesia resulted in an increased incidence of operative vaginal deliveries (28). As a result, there has been a trend over the past 20 years to use lower concentrations of local anesthetics.
  - Lipid-soluble opioids are commonly added to the local anesthetic solutions because they decrease local anesthetic requirements while achieving an equivalent quality of labor analgesia (29).
  - Local anesthetics that produce relatively less motor block at equianalgesic doses, such as bupivacaine and ropivacaine, are also preferred for providing labor analgesia.
  - A continuous infusion technique is commonly used (sometimes in conjunction with patient-controlled epidural analgesia [PCEA]) to provide labor analgesia. Recent data, however, suggest that programmed intermittent epidural boluses provide equivalent pain relief and higher patient satisfaction compared with a continuous infusion while using less local anesthetic (30). Epidural pumps that can be programmed to deliver automated boluses have recently become commercially available.
- Suggested dosing regimens for providing epidural labor analgesia with a continuous infusion technique are listed in Table 3-5. The degree of pain experienced by women in labor varies widely, and the dosing regimen used for individual patients should be titrated to meet their pain-relief requirements.
- The use of PCEA is an ideal technique for providing pain relief that can be individualized to meet each woman's needs throughout labor. Many anesthesiologists prefer using PCEA rather than a continuous infusion.
  - Several studies have compared PCEA with continuous infusion epidural analgesia during labor. A meta-analysis of randomized controlled trials showed that women who received PCEA used less local anesthetic, developed less motor block, and required less interventions by anesthesia personnel. Despite using less local anesthetic, women who received PCEA achieved pain relief equivalent to that of women who received continuous infusions. Although some anesthesiologists have suggested that the patient's ability to actively participate in her pain management will lead to increased satisfaction, a meta-analysis showed no difference in maternal satisfaction between women receiving PCEA or continuous infusion epidural analgesia. In addition, no differences in obstetric outcomes have been found between these two techniques of epidural analgesia, despite the use of less local anesthetic in women receiving PCEA (31).

Table 3-5	Recommended Dosing for Continuous Infusion Epidural Labor Analgesia	
Drug solution		**Infusion rate (mL/h)**
Bupivacaine, 0.0625%–0.125% + fentanyl 2 µg/mL		8–15
Bupivacaine, 0.065%–0.125% + sufentanil 0.33–0.5 µg/mL		8–15
Ropivacaine, 0.1%–0.2% + fentanyl 2 µg/mL		8–15
Ropivacaine, 0.1%–0.2% + sufentanil 0.33–0.5 µg/mL		8–15

Table 3-6	Suggested Dosing Strategies for PCEA	
Basal infusion (mL/h)	**PCA dose (mL)**	**Lockout interval (min)**
None	5	10
4–5	5	10–15
8–10	5	15

PCA, patient-controlled analgesia.

- A variety of dosing strategies have been suggested for the PCEA technique, and currently, no consensus exists on whether use of a basal infusion is worthwhile.
  - Several recommended options for PCEA dosing during labor are listed in Table 3-6. The same drug solutions used for continuous infusion epidural analgesia are usually also used for PCEA.
  - One study reported no benefit from using a basal infusion (32), but another study found that less physician-administered boluses were required when a basal infusion of 6 mL/h was included in the PCEA dosing regimen (33).
  - The need for a basal infusion during PCEA is largely determined by the motivation level of patients to be actively involved in their pain management.
- The newest dosing strategy for epidural labor analgesia is PCEA + automated intermittent mandatory boluses. Compared to PCEA with basal infusion, this technique has been shown to increase patient satisfaction and decrease total local anesthetic dose (34). Larger boluses administered over longer time intervals (10 mL bolus every 60 minutes) provide equivalent pain relief with less local anesthetic consumption compared to smaller boluses administered over shorter intervals (2.5 mL every 15 minutes or 5 mL every 30 minutes) (35). Because commercially available pumps that can be programmed for this dosing technique have just recently been approved for use in the United States, it is not yet clear how frequently used this labor analgesia technique will become.

Combined Spinal–Epidural Analgesia
- CSE analgesia is another commonly used technique for labor analgesia.
- This procedure requires the anesthesiologist to first insert an epidural needle into the lumbar epidural space. A long spinal needle is then introduced through the epidural needle into the subarachnoid space. An opioid or opioid/local anesthetic combination is injected into the subarachnoid space. The spinal needle is then removed, and an epidural catheter is advanced through the epidural needle into the epidural space. The epidural catheter is later used to administer epidural analgesia when the analgesia produced by the spinal drugs has resolved.
- This technique has increased in popularity over the last 10 years because it provides the versatility of epidural analgesia while delivering a more rapid onset of analgesia (1 to 3 minutes compared to 10 to 15 minutes for epidural analgesia alone) and minimal or no motor block, which may allow women to ambulate during labor.
  - The CSE technique is especially well suited for low-risk, multiparous patients in advanced labor who are expected to deliver within the next 1 to 2 hours. When these patients receive CSE analgesia, they are nearly guaranteed of receiving pain relief before delivery has occurred and often do not require the administration of any drugs through the epidural catheter.
  - Another subset of patients who may benefit from CSE analgesia is women in early labor (less than 4 cm dilation) who request pain relief. A large study found that the first stage of labor was 90 minutes shorter in women who received intrathecal fentanyl via a CSE technique in early labor than in women who received systemic opioids in early labor followed later by the initiation of epidural analgesia (36).

- The anesthesiologist must consider certain factors when choosing which drugs to administer into the subarachnoid space, including cervical dilation and whether the patient wishes to ambulate during labor.
  - Opioid alone may be the optimal choice for women who are in early labor or plan to ambulate.
  - When CSE analgesia is initiated during advanced labor, the administration of both opioid and a small dose of local anesthetic provides excellent analgesia. The addition of a local anesthetic prolongs the duration of spinal analgesia while producing little motor block.
  - Anesthesiologists generally use the same epidural infusion solution used for traditional epidural analgesia when the epidural component of the CSE technique is initiated after resolution of the spinal analgesia.
- Because CSE provides a rapid onset of analgesia with minimal or no motor block, some consider it the ideal analgesic technique for women in labor.
  - Some anesthesiologists use CSE as their technique of choice for all low-risk laboring women.
  - CSE labor analgesia is not recommended for patients at high risk for either cesarean delivery or general anesthesia. This would include women with severe preeclampsia, multiple gestation, nonreassuring fetal heart rate tracing, morbid obesity, women undergoing trial of labor after cesarean, or anticipated difficult airway.
  - The recommendation against using CSE in high-risk obstetric patients is due to the following considerations:
    - Because CSE analgesia is initially achieved with the administration of subarachnoid drugs, proper functioning of the epidural catheter remains unproven during the duration of intrathecal analgesia. If emergent cesarean delivery is required during this time period, dosing of the epidural catheter may provide ineffective anesthesia for surgery. General anesthesia would then be required. While many anesthesiologists still consider this a reason to avoid CSE in high-risk parturients, study data have reported that failure of the epidural catheter is more likely to occur with an epidural-only technique (37). Failure of the catheter will be recognized immediately after placement with the epidural-only procedure, though, allowing prompt replacement with a functioning epidural catheter.
    - CSE analgesia is associated with higher rates of uterine hypertonus and fetal heart rate abnormalities compared to epidural analgesia (38).
- Table 3-7 lists suggested CSE dosing regimens.

Continuous Spinal Analgesia
- Continuous spinal analgesia is another procedure that is occasionally used to provide labor analgesia.

Table 3-7	Dosing Strategies for CSE Analgesia during Labor	
Opioid	**Local anesthetic**	**Recommended patient types**
Fentanyl 15–25 µg	None	Early labor or ambulation planned
Sufentanil 2.5–5 µg	None	Early labor or ambulation planned
Fentanyl 15–25 µg	Isobaric bupivacaine 1.25–2.5 mg	Advanced labor
Sufentanil 2.5–5 µg	Isobaric bupivacaine 1.25–2.5 mg	Advanced labor

- With this technique, the anesthesiologist inserts an epidural needle into the subarachnoid space and then places a catheter into the subarachnoid space instead of the epidural space. Most commonly, this procedure is performed when the dura is unintentionally punctured during a planned epidural technique ("wet tap").
- The dosing strategy is similar to the intrathecal dosing component of the CSE technique.
- With a spinal catheter in place, the injection of intrathecal opioids and local anesthetics can be repeated throughout labor (unlike a CSE technique where only one spinal dose can be administered) or a continuous infusion of opioid + low-dose local anesthetic can be used to provide effective analgesia without producing significant motor block.
  - Sympathetic blockade and the associated vasodilation that can lead to maternal hypotension are avoided when labor analgesia is provided with spinal opioids alone instead of epidural local anesthetics.
  - Correct placement of the intrathecal catheter is definitively established by the aspiration of cerebrospinal fluid. In morbidly obese women, the ability to objectively confirm correct catheter placement is a significant advantage of this technique over epidural analgesia, where a somewhat subjective "loss of resistance" is used to confirm correct catheter placement. One study found that the failure rate for the initial placement of an epidural catheter in morbidly obese women in labor was 42% (39).
- Continuous spinal analgesia with opioids may also be preferred in seriously compromised cardiac patients. Because sympathetic blockade and its associated hemodynamic changes, including decreased systemic vascular resistance, are avoided, hemodynamic stability can more easily be maintained in these fragile patients.
- The major disadvantage of continuous spinal analgesia is the unacceptably high incidence of spinal headache.
  - Because the technique requires that the dura be punctured with a large-gauge epidural needle, the incidence of spinal headache is 50% or greater.
  - For this reason, the technique is generally limited to use in morbidly obese parturients with an anticipated difficult airway, women with serious cardiac disease, and patients who have received an unintended wet tap during attempted epidural catheter placement.

NEURAXIAL ANALGESIA COMPLICATIONS
Hypotension
- Hypotension induced by sympathetic blockade is the most common adverse effect associated with epidural labor analgesia.
- Hypotension may also occur after the administration of intrathecal opioids during CSE and continuous spinal analgesia. However, intrathecal opioids do not cause a sympathetic block, and the decrease in blood pressure appears to be related to the pain relief itself.
- Regardless of the etiology of hypotension, uteroplacental perfusion may be compromised and could lead to fetal hypoxia and acidosis.
- In the majority of women who receive epidural analgesia, hypotension can be prevented by intravenous volume expansion and left uterine displacement to avoid aortocaval compression.
- When hypotension does occur, it is rapidly treated with the administration of additional intravenous fluids and vasopressors.
  - Previously, ephedrine was considered the vasopressor of choice in obstetric patients.
  - Recent data show that phenylephrine can also be used to treat hypotension in laboring women without adversely affecting the fetus. In fact, the mean umbilical artery pH has been shown to be higher in newborns whose mothers received phenylephrine to treat hypotension than in newborns whose mothers received ephedrine (40).

Pruritus

Pruritus is the most common side effect of neuraxial opioids.

- The incidence of pruritus is much higher with intrathecal opioid administration than with epidural administration. Although it is not a serious adverse effect, the itching can be very bothersome to women in labor. Although most parturients can tolerate this annoying side effect without treatment, the careful titration of small doses of intravenous naloxone or nalbuphine can produce prompt relief of symptoms without significantly affecting the patient's pain relief.

Dural Puncture

- Unintended dural puncture, or "wet tap," during a planned epidural technique is an uncommon but significant complication of epidural analgesia.
- The wet tap rate is dependent on the experience of the anesthesiologist and is approximately only 1% among anesthesiologists who have performed more than 100 epidural procedures (41). Because epidural needles are large-gauge needles that produce a large dural hole, approximately 50% to 70% of patients who experience an unintended dural puncture during epidural placement will develop a postdural puncture headache.
- Spinal headache is also a complication of intended dural puncture with a small-gauge spinal needle during a CSE technique. The incidence of spinal headache after dural puncture with the 27-gauge, specialized noncutting spinal needles currently used to perform CSE is less than 1% (42).
- A Cochrane Database Systematic Review of epidural versus CSE labor analgesia reported no difference in the incidence of postdural puncture headache between the two techniques (43).

Spinal Headache

- A spinal headache can be very painful and often interferes with a mother's ability to care for her newborn infant. Therefore, prompt diagnosis and treatment of this complication is essential.
- A postdural puncture headache is usually localized to the frontal and occipital regions. The headache worsens when the patient is in the upright position and improves when she assumes the supine position.
- For mild headache, conservative therapy, including hydration, analgesic medication, and caffeine, often provides successful relief of symptoms.
- For severe headache, definitive treatment with an epidural blood patch should be offered to the patient.

Neurologic Injury

- Neurologic injury following neuraxial labor analgesia is a rare complication but commonly feared by women in labor.
- Epidural hematoma and abscess are potentially catastrophic complications that could lead to serious and permanent neurologic deficits.
  - Fortunately, these are rare complications in the obstetric population.
  - An analysis of large studies (greater than 10,000 patients) performed after 1990 demonstrated an estimated rate of epidural hematoma in obstetric patients of 1 in 183,000 women and an estimated rate for epidural abscess of 1 in 145,000 women (44).
  - Symptoms of an epidural hematoma or abscess include lower extremity weakness, sensory deficits of the lower extremities, severe back pain, and bladder dysfunction. If a postpartum patient experiences these symptoms, the anesthesiologist should be notified, and emergent magnetic resonance imaging should be obtained.
  - If surgical decompression of an abscess or hematoma does not occur within 6 to 8 hours of the onset of symptoms, permanent neurologic injury is likely.

- Obstetric nerve palsies involving nerve injuries of the lower extremities are relatively common.
  - A prospective survey reported an approximate 1% incidence of lower extremity nerve injuries after labor and delivery.
  - Patients and health care providers often assume neuraxial analgesia is the cause of these nerve injuries, but obstetric factors are more likely etiologies.
  - Risk factors identified in a recent survey included nulliparity and a prolonged second stage of labor, but neuraxial analgesia was not found to be an independent risk factor (45).

Labor Progression

- One of the most controversial issues in the past related to epidural labor analgesia was its effect on the progress and outcome of labor.
- Several retrospective and prospective studies as well as meta-analyses have investigated the effects of epidural analgesia on the duration of labor and mode of delivery.
  - A meta-analysis determined that the first stage of labor was not prolonged and the second stage of labor was prolonged by approximately 15 minutes in women who received epidural analgesia compared with women who received intravenous opioids (46).
  - An individual patient meta-analysis reported that nulliparous women receiving epidural analgesia had a first stage of labor that was approximately 30 minutes longer than that of women receiving intravenous opioids. Similar to the previously mentioned meta-analysis, the second stage of labor was approximately 15 minutes longer in women who received epidural analgesia (47).
- Several retrospective studies have reported that epidural analgesia is associated with an increased incidence of cesarean delivery for dystocia (48–50). However, women who choose to receive epidural analgesia during labor often have other risk factors for cesarean delivery, such as increased pain, less favorable cervical dilation on admission, and larger babies, which may also contribute to their decisions to undergo epidural analgesia.
  - These retrospective studies were then followed by a small clinical trial in which women who were randomized to receive epidural analgesia had a 10-fold increase in cesarean delivery rate compared with women randomized to receive intravenous meperidine (51).
  - Many subsequent prospective, randomized studies and meta-analyses performed since the completion of that initial study have found no significant association between epidural analgesia and an increased rate of cesarean delivery (46,47,52–54).
  - It is currently generally accepted that epidural analgesia does not substantially prolong the duration of labor, nor does it increase the risk of cesarean delivery.
- Controversy has previously existed concerning the timing of epidural analgesia and its effects on labor outcome.
  - Many obstetricians in the past required women to reach 4 to 5 cm cervical dilation before they would allow the administration of epidural analgesia.
  - A meta-analysis of eight studies found that early initiation of epidural analgesia did not increase the rate of cesarean delivery compared to late initiation of epidural analgesia (55).
  - A randomized controlled trial of nearly 13,000 patients investigated early versus late initiation of epidural labor analgesia. Women in the early group (at least 1 cm dilation) had a median cervical dilation of 1.6 cm when epidural analgesia was begun. Women assigned to the late group had to reach at least 4 cm cervical dilation before epidural analgesia was begun; the median cervical dilation was 5.1 cm in this group. The duration of labor and rate of cesarean delivery did not differ between the early and late epidural groups (56).
  - Although the American College of Obstetricians and Gynecologists had previously recommended that nulliparous women not receive epidural analgesia before 4 cm cervical dilation, this more recent evidence prompted them to revise their Committee Opinion on Analgesia and Cesarean Delivery Rates by removing the recommendation that a specific cervical dilation be reached before initiating epidural labor analgesia (57).

Likewise, the American Society of Anesthesiologists Practice Guidelines for Obstetric Anesthesia state that women should not have to reach an arbitrary cervical dilation before they can receive neuraxial analgesia (58).

PATIENT EDUCATION
- Education and discussion about pain relief options for labor and delivery should occur in the antepartum period when a woman is not distracted by the discomforts of labor.
- Many childbirth classes include detailed discussions of pain-relief options. Publications from the American Society of Anesthesiologists and the American College of Obstetricians and Gynecologists are also available to help educate women about their options.
- The decision about whether or not to use labor analgesia and what type to use is a personal one; health care providers should be available to advise and support women as they make these decisions before and during labor.

ANESTHESIA FOR CESAREAN DELIVERY
Background
- As the incidence of cesarean delivery increases, anesthesia for cesarean delivery is accounting for an increasing proportion of the patient care provided by anesthesiologists to pregnant women. Certain aspects of this anesthesia care apply to all patients regardless of the type of anesthesia used.
- Aspiration prophylaxis is recommended for all women undergoing cesarean delivery. This prophylaxis should at least include administration of a nonparticulate antacid, such as citric acid (Bicitra). Many anesthesia care providers also administer metoclopramide and a histamine$_2$-receptor antagonist. In addition to providing aspiration prophylaxis, metoclopramide decreases the risk of intraoperative nausea and vomiting during cesarean delivery performed under regional anesthesia (59).
- Maintenance of uterine displacement is necessary during cesarean delivery to avoid aortocaval compression, especially since both regional and general anesthesia will produce vasodilatation and thus impair the patient's vasoconstrictive compensatory mechanisms.
- Finally, intraoperative monitoring must include the routine monitors required by the American Society of Anesthesiologists *Standards for Basic Anesthetic Monitoring* (60), as well as any special monitoring that is dictated by an individual patient's medical condition.

Treatment
Selection of Anesthetic Technique
- A key component of the anesthesiologist's anesthetic plan for cesarean delivery is deciding whether regional or general anesthesia should be administered.
- The urgency of surgery, the patient's medical status, and patient preference are all important factors to be considered when making this decision.
- Because anesthesia-related maternal mortality is relatively higher with general anesthesia, most anesthesiologists believe regional anesthesia should be used whenever feasible.

Procedures
- Once the anesthesiologist decides to perform regional anesthesia for cesarean delivery, the specific technique must then be chosen. Spinal, CSE, and epidural anesthesia all provide effective surgical anesthesia.
- Regardless of the technique used, a sensory level of at least T6 must be achieved to ensure adequate anesthesia; a sensory level of T4 may provide improved anesthesia compared to a lower sensory level.
- Patient and surgical characteristics as well as the preference of the anesthesiologist will determine which procedure is used for a particular parturient.

Spinal Anesthesia

- Spinal anesthesia is by far the most common regional anesthesia technique used in the United States for both elective and emergent cesarean deliveries (12). Several advantages are associated with the use of spinal anesthesia:
  - It provides a rapid onset (generally within 5 minutes) of dense surgical anesthesia.
  - Adequate anesthesia is achieved more quickly, and total operating room time is shortened when spinal anesthesia is administered for cesarean delivery compared with epidural anesthesia (61,62).
  - Spinal anesthesia is also considered by most anesthesiologists to be a technically easier procedure that provides a better quality of anesthesia than an epidural technique.
  - Because dense anesthesia is obtained with a very small dose of local anesthetic, the risk of maternal systemic local anesthetic toxicity is essentially nonexistent, and transfer of drug to the fetus is minimal.
- The rapid onset of neural blockade, including sympathetic blockade, that occurs with spinal anesthesia has raised concerns that detrimental maternal hypotension could occur, especially in women with preeclampsia or cardiac disease.
  - Spinal anesthesia should be avoided in patients with serious cardiac disorders in which a rapid decrease in systemic vascular resistance or venous return could be catastrophic due to the pathophysiology of the disease.
  - Current data do not support the long-held belief by many anesthesiologists and obstetricians that spinal anesthesia should be avoided in preeclamptic patients. Spinal anesthesia–induced hypotension is actually less likely to occur in preeclamptic patients than in healthy patients (63,64).
  - Several local anesthetics can be administered to provide spinal anesthesia during cesarean delivery, but bupivacaine is the most commonly used drug. Typical doses utilized for cesarean delivery range from 8 to 12 mg. Opioids, including fentanyl 10 to 25 μg and morphine 0.1 to 0.2 mg, are frequently added to the spinal local anesthetic to improve the quality of intraoperative anesthesia and provide postoperative analgesia. A duration of anesthesia between 1 and 2 hours is achieved with spinal bupivacaine.

Epidural Anesthesia

- Epidural anesthesia provides effective anesthesia for cesarean delivery and is usually the technique of choice for women who are already receiving epidural analgesia for relief of labor pain. The flexibility gained by having an epidural catheter in place during surgery makes it the preferred procedure for other subsets of patients as well.
- When the duration of surgery is expected to be prolonged, an epidural technique is preferred over spinal anesthesia because anesthesia can be maintained for an indefinite period of time by administering additional local anesthetic through the epidural catheter. If a spinal block dissipates before the completion of surgery, the anesthesiologist would need to induce general anesthesia and expose the patient to the risks of two anesthetics.
- The presence of an epidural catheter also allows the local anesthetic to be administered in incremental doses, with the total dose titrated to the desired sensory level. The slower onset of blockade that occurs with this incremental dosing may decrease the risk of hypotension, especially in women with serious cardiovascular disease.
- In patients considered to be at increased risk for general anesthesia, such as a patient with an anticipated difficult airway, epidural anesthesia is the anesthetic technique of choice. Unlike spinal anesthesia, the anesthesiologist can maintain adequate anesthesia with additional dosing through the epidural catheter if unforeseen circumstances lead to prolonged surgery.
- In emergent situations, there are disadvantages of epidural anesthesia compared to spinal anesthesia:

- Performance of an epidural procedure is more involved and usually takes longer than performance of a spinal procedure.
- The slower onset of sensory blockade may also be disadvantageous, although adequate anesthesia can often be achieved within 5 minutes when 3% 2-chloroprocaine is administered through an epidural catheter that had previously been placed for labor analgesia.
- Anesthesiologists use a variety of local anesthetic drugs to provide epidural anesthesia for cesarean delivery, including lidocaine, 2-chloroprocaine, bupivacaine, and ropivacaine. The urgency of surgery, expected duration of surgery, and maternal and fetal condition are all considered when choosing which drug to administer.
  - For elective cesarean deliveries, 2% lidocaine with epinephrine 1:200,000 is probably the most commonly administered local anesthetic in the United States. It has an intermediate onset of action with duration of approximately 60 to 90 minutes.
  - For an emergent cesarean delivery with nonreassuring fetal status, 3% 2-chloroprocaine is the drug of choice. It has the most rapid onset of action, less risk of systemic toxicity with rapid injection, and avoids ion trapping of the drug in an acidotic fetus. Because maternal and fetal metabolism of 2-chloroprocaine is so rapid, placental transfer of this drug is not increased by fetal acidosis (65).
  - Bupivacaine and ropivacaine have slower onset of action compared to lidocaine or chloroprocaine, so they should be used whenever maternal condition requires a slow onset of sympathetic blockade.
  - Opioids are frequently administered with epidural local anesthetics to improve the quality of anesthesia.

Combined Spinal–Epidural Anesthesia
- CSE anesthesia has gained popularity as an anesthetic technique for cesarean delivery. It combines the advantages of spinal anesthesia, including rapid onset and better quality of anesthesia, with the versatility of epidural anesthesia.
- It is an ideal procedure when both a rapid onset of neural blockade and the ability to extend the duration of anesthesia are desired.
- However, because the anesthesiologist cannot determine that the epidural catheter is functional until the spinal block has begun to resolve, the CSE technique is not recommended for pregnant women who are considered at increased risk for general anesthesia, such as morbidly obese patients and patients with an anticipated difficult airway.
- When performing a CSE technique for cesarean delivery, most anesthesiologists administer the same dose of local anesthetic described above for spinal anesthesia. If a prolonged duration of surgery requires the initiation of epidural anesthesia as the spinal block is resolving, small incremental doses of local anesthetic should be administered to avoid the development of a block that is too high.

General Anesthesia
- Although anesthesiologists prefer to avoid general anesthesia in pregnant women because of the increased risks associated with this technique, there are situations where general anesthesia for cesarean delivery is indicated. These include
  - Severe maternal hemorrhage
  - Coagulopathy
  - Inadequate regional anesthesia
  - Patient refusal of regional anesthesia
  - Some nonreassuring fetal heart rate patterns
- Neuraxial techniques can also often provide rapid-onset surgical anesthesia, however. Therefore, an urgent delivery indication, such as nonreassuring fetal heart rate pattern, does not always necessitate exposing a woman to the increased morbidity and mortality associated with general anesthesia.

- When a woman has preexisting epidural labor analgesia, rapid extension of the epidural block is acceptable, even in the setting of fetal bradycardia.
- Spinal anesthesia can also be obtained rapidly and is acceptable when cesarean delivery is required for nonreassuring fetal status. However, when the fetal status is ominous, delivery should not be delayed to initiate regional anesthesia, and general anesthesia should be performed.
- Even in emergent situations, the anesthesiologist needs to obtain a brief anesthetic history and assess the patient's airway, as well as administer a nonparticulate antacid to decrease the risk of aspiration pneumonitis.
  - Maternal well-being should not be jeopardized in an effort to expedite delivery.
  - If the anesthesiologist anticipates a difficult intubation based on history or physical examination, the anesthesiologist should secure the patient's airway while she is still awake and breathing spontaneously or have equipment immediately available for alternative airway techniques, such as video laryngoscopy, before proceeding with induction of general anesthesia.
- Adequate preoxygenation is essential before induction of general anesthesia because pregnant women develop hypoxemia more rapidly than do nonobstetric patients during periods of apnea.
- To minimize placental transfer of anesthetic agents to the fetus, anesthesia should not be induced until the abdomen has been prepared and draped and the obstetrician is ready to begin surgery.
- To decrease the risk of gastric aspiration, a rapid sequence induction of general anesthesia is required in pregnant women. Such an induction involves no positive pressure ventilation before insertion of the endotracheal tube, and the application of cricoid pressure to occlude the esophagus until correct placement of the tube has been confirmed.
- Several drugs are available for the induction of general anesthesia (Table 3-8), and the anesthesiologist should choose a drug based on maternal status. To avoid neonatal depression, the lowest possible dose needed to induce anesthesia is administered.
  - Thiopental has a long record of safety in obstetric patients. At the dose usually administered to parturients, data suggest that fetal drug concentrations are not high enough to produce significant depression (66). While the drug is a preferred induction agent for obstetrics and still widely used in some areas of the world, it is no longer available in the United States.
  - Propofol is now the most commonly used induction agent for parturients undergoing general anesthesia in the United States. Studies that have investigated the use of propofol for cesarean delivery have not found significant hypotension associated with its use for induction of anesthesia (67,68).
  - When significant maternal hemorrhage or hypovolemia is present, induction agents that maintain hemodynamic stability, such as ketamine and etomidate, are typically administered.
  - Unless contraindicated, succinylcholine (1 to 1.5 mg/kg) is the muscle relaxant of choice for rapid sequence induction because it provides optimal conditions for intubation more quickly than does any other neuromuscular blocking drug.

Table 3-8	General Anesthesia Induction Drugs
Induction drug	**Dose (mg/kg)**
Thiopental	4
Propofol	2
Ketamine	1
Etomidate	0.3

- Until delivery of the infant is accomplished, most anesthesiologists maintain general anesthesia with a combination of 50% nitrous oxide/50% oxygen and 0.5 to 1.0 minimum alveolar concentration of a halogenated volatile anesthetic, such as desflurane, sevoflurane, or isoflurane. After the infant has been delivered, the concentration of nitrous oxide is often increased, and intravenous opioids are administered. Many anesthesiologists also decrease the concentration of the volatile anesthetic agent after delivery because high concentrations of these drugs could contribute to decreased uterine tone.
- At the completion of surgery, extubation of the patient's trachea can be performed when she is able to respond appropriately to verbal commands and shows evidence that she has regained her airway protective reflexes. Ensuring these criteria are met prior to extubation is crucial as recent data have suggested that airway-related anesthetic deaths in parturients now occur more frequently during anesthesia emergence and recovery than during induction (69).

Complications Associated with Anesthesia for Caesarean Delivery

- Many of the complications of neuraxial labor analgesia discussed above, including hypotension, pruritus, and spinal headache, can also occur when regional anesthesia is used for cesarean delivery. Because anesthesia for cesarean delivery requires a higher and denser block than is required for effective labor analgesia, the incidence and severity of hypotension may be greater.
- Women who receive spinal or CSE anesthesia for cesarean delivery occasionally experience a high or total spinal block. Management of a total spinal block requires ventilatory and cardiovascular support until resolution of the block occurs.
- Some risk of maternal systemic local anesthetic toxicity exists when epidural anesthesia is administered for cesarean delivery because large doses of local anesthetics are required to achieve adequate surgical anesthesia.
  - Initial signs and symptoms of systemic toxicity include tinnitus, perioral numbness, and dizziness.
  - As higher plasma concentrations of local anesthetic are reached, seizures and cardiovascular collapse can occur.
  - The best treatment for local anesthetic toxicity is prevention, which can be achieved by administering small incremental doses of local anesthetic through the epidural catheter. This allows inadvertent intravascular injection to be identified before life-threatening effects of local anesthetic toxicity can develop.
  - If serious cardiovascular and neurologic toxicity does occur, in addition to cardiovascular resuscitation, intravenous lipid emulsion should be administered as several case reports have reported patient rescue (70).
- As discussed previously, anesthesiologists prefer to avoid general anesthesia for cesarean delivery whenever possible because the risk of maternal mortality and morbidity is relatively greater compared to regional anesthesia.
- The majority of serious complications during general anesthesia result from airway management problems, including gastric aspiration and difficult or failed intubation, which lead to hypoxemia.
- Although the most recent U.S. data show that the risk of death from complications of general anesthesia is 1.7 times higher than that for regional anesthesia, it is important to understand that the incidence of mortality related to general anesthesia is still rare, with an incidence of only 6.5 deaths per million general anesthetics (6).
- Anesthesiologists and obstetricians should be aware that cesarean delivery is one of the surgical procedures considered high risk for awareness during general anesthesia (71).
- If a woman reports to the obstetrician any perioperative experiences that suggest recall during surgery, the anesthesiologist should be informed. If awareness during general

anesthesia is likely to have occurred, the patient should be offered appropriate assistance and counseling.

ANESTHESIA FOR NONOBSTETRIC SURGERY DURING PREGNANCY
Evaluation
- Preanesthetic evaluation of the pregnant woman undergoing nonobstetric surgery is similar to the evaluation of women receiving anesthesia for labor and delivery.
- In addition to the components of history and physical examination that are emphasized for the patient presenting for delivery, the anesthesiologist must focus on the medical condition that is necessitating surgery and its impact on anesthetic management.
- The anesthesiologist should consult with the patient's obstetrician before surgery to identify any pregnancy-related complications and to document the presence of fetal heart activity before surgery and anesthesia.

Diagnosis
- To develop an appropriate anesthetic plan for the pregnant woman undergoing nonobstetric surgery, the anesthesiologist must have a clear understanding of the patient's medical and surgical diagnoses and the effects of pregnancy on her disease state. The physiologic changes of pregnancy, however, can produce symptoms and changes in the physical examination that might make correct diagnosis difficult, especially when abdominal pathology is suspected.

Treatment
- Several issues must be addressed when the anesthesiologist develops an anesthetic plan for nonobstetric surgery during pregnancy.
- Although patients and surgeons often worry about the effects of anesthetic drugs on the fetus, the most important aspects of anesthetic management include maintaining uteroplacental perfusion and fetal oxygenation and ensuring maternal safety. The obstetrician and anesthesiologist must decide whether intraoperative fetal monitoring will be performed. Left uterine displacement, adequate fluid resuscitation, and avoidance of a deep level of general anesthesia or a high epidural or spinal block will help maintain uteroplacental perfusion by preventing maternal hypotension.
  - Normal maternal oxygenation and ventilation are necessary to ensure adequate fetal oxygenation and normal acid–base status. Maternal hyperventilation that results in respiratory alkalosis can compromise fetal Pao_2 by shifting the maternal oxyhemoglobin dissociation curve to the left and causing uterine artery vasoconstriction. Maternal hypercarbia can produce fetal acidosis and myocardial depression.
- When intraoperative fetal monitoring is used, the physicians should decide before surgery how they will proceed if persistent fetal heart rate abnormalities are noted during the perioperative period.
  - The obstetrician should understand that even if delivery of the infant is not planned in the event of nonreassuring fetal status, continuous fetal monitoring can be a valuable tool to help the anesthesiologist optimize fetal status throughout surgery.
  - When fetal heart rate changes are noted, the anesthesiologist can assess maternal status and make modifications to her anesthetic care that will lead to improved uteroplacental perfusion and fetal oxygenation.
  - Many anesthetic drugs will produce a decrease in fetal heart rate variability and small changes in baseline fetal heart rate. Fetal bradycardia or decelerations, however, are not expected effects of anesthetic agents. When these fetal heart rate changes occur, they require action by the anesthesiologist to optimize maternal and fetal status.
- Women undergoing nonobstetric surgery during pregnancy often express concern that the administration of anesthetic drugs could lead to fetal loss or congenital malformations. Currently, no anesthetic drugs, including local anesthetics, general anesthesia

induction agents, and halogenated volatile anesthetics, are proven human teratogens, although no prospective studies have been performed. Some controversy does exist about the fetal effects of certain drugs:

- All benzodiazepines are classified as category D drugs by the Food and Drug Administration's use-in-pregnancy rating. Category D drugs are defined as having positive evidence of human fetal risk, but the potential benefits of the drugs may warrant their use. Benzodiazepines received this rating based on retrospective studies that found an association between maternal diazepam use and cleft lip and/or palate (72). A subsequent prospective study did not find an increased risk of congenital malformations in newborns whose mothers received benzodiazepine therapy (73). There are no data suggesting that a single dose of midazolam administered during anesthesia causes congenital malformations.
- Poorly designed surveys performed several years ago suggested an association between volatile anesthetics and increased risk for spontaneous abortion and congenital anomalies (74,75). More recently, better designed studies have found no association between halogenated anesthetic agents and an increased rate of congenital malformations (76,77).
- Studies that have investigated the risks associated with nitrous oxide exposure have also found no increase in the incidence of congenital anomalies (78,79).
- Women who require surgery and anesthesia during pregnancy do have a slight increased incidence of spontaneous abortion compared to other pregnant women, but data do not support a direct causal relationship between miscarriage and anesthetic drugs.
- The anesthesiologist must consider several factors when deciding whether to perform regional or general anesthesia for nonobstetric surgery. These include maternal condition, type and duration of surgery, patient position, and patient preference.
- When feasible, regional anesthesia is often preferred to avoid the pregnancy-related increased risks of general anesthesia.
- Many patients and anesthesiologists also prefer regional anesthesia because it minimizes exposure of the fetus to anesthetic drugs.
- No association between a specific anesthetic technique or drug and improved fetal outcome has ever been proven. In addition, the nature of many surgeries performed during pregnancy require general anesthesia.

REFERENCES

1. Flanagan HL, Datta S, Lambert DH, et al. Effect of pregnancy on bupivacaine-induced conduction blockade in the isolated rabbit vagus nerve. *Anesth Analg.* 1987;66:123–126.
2. Camorcia M, Capogna G, Columb MO. Effect of sex and pregnancy on the potency of intrathecal bupivacaine: determination of ED50 for motor block with the up-down sequential allocation method. *Eur J Anaesthesiol.* 2011;28:240–244.
3. Fagraeus L, Urban BJ, Bromage PR. Spread of epidural analgesia in early pregnancy. *Anesthesiology.* 1983;58:184–187.
4. Gin T, Chan MT. Decreased minimum alveolar concentration of isoflurane in pregnant humans. *Anesthesiology.* 1994;81:829–832.
5. Mongardon N, Servin F, Perrin M, et al. Predicted propofol effect-site concentration for induction and emergence of anesthesia during early pregnancy. *Anesth Analg.* 2009;109:90–95.
6. Hawkins JL, Chang J, Palmer SK, et al. Anesthesia-related maternal mortality in the United States: 1979–2002. *Obstet Gynecol.* 2011;117:69–74.
7. Samsoon GLT, Young JRB. Difficult tracheal intubation: a retrospective study. *Anaesthesia.* 1987;42:487–490.
8. Archer GW, Marx GF. Arterial oxygen tension during apnoea in parturient women. *Br J Anaesth.* 1974;46:358–360.
9. Carp H, Jayaram A, Stoll M. Ultrasound examination of the stomach contents of parturients. *Anesth Analg.* 1992;74:683–687.

10. Whitehead EM, Smith M, Dean Y, et al. An evaluation of gastric emptying times in pregnancy and the puerperium. *Anaesthesia.* 1993;48:53–57.
11. Hamilton Be, Hoyert DL, Martin JA, et al. Annual summary of vital statistics: 2010–2011. *Pediatrics.* 2013;131:548–58.
12. Bucklin BA, Hawkins JL, Anderson JR, et al. Obstetric anesthesia workforce survey: twenty-year update. *Anesthesiology.* 2005;103:645–53.
13. Van de Velde M. Nonobstetric surgery during pregnancy. In: Chestnut DH, ed. *Obstetric anesthesia: principles and practice.* 4th ed. Philadelphia: Mosby, 2009:337–358.
14. Mallampali SR, Gatt SP, Gugino LD, et al. A clinical sign to predict difficult intubation: a prospective study. *Can J Anaesth.* 1985;32:429–434.
15. Khan ZH, Kashfi A, Ebrahimkhani E. A comparison of the upper lip bite test (a simple new technique) with modified Mallampati classification in predicting difficulty in endotracheal intubation: a prospective blinded study. *Anesth Analg.* 2003;96:595–599.
16. Ledue L, Wheeler JM, Kirshen B, et al. Coagulation profile in severe preeclampsia. *Obstet Gynecol.* 1992;79:14–18.
17. Prieto JA, Mastrobattrsta JM, Blanco JD. Coagulation studies in patients with marked thrombocytopenia due to severe preeclampsia. *Am J Perinatol.* 1995;12:220–222.
18. Melzack R, Taenzec P, Feldman P, et al. Labour is still painful after prepared childbirth training. *Can Med Assoc J.* 1981:125:357–363.
19. Melzack R. The myth of painless childbirth. *Pain.* 1984;19:321–337.
20. Kuhnert BR, Kuhnert PM, Tu AL, et al. Meperidine and normepcridine levels following meperidine administration during labor. *Am J Obstet Gynecol.* 1979;133:904–913.
21. Caldwell J, Wakile LA, Notarianni LJ, et al. Maternal and neonatal disposition of pethidine in childbirth: a study using quantitative gas chromatography-mass spectrometry. *Life Sci.* 1978;22:589–596.
22. Kuhnert BR, Linn PL, Kennard MJ, et al. Effects of low doses of meperidine on neonatal behavior. *Anesth Analg.* 1985;63:301–308.
23. Shnider SM, Moya F. Effect of meperidine on the newborn infant. *Am J Obstet Gynecol.* 1964;89:1008–1115.
24. Campbell DC. Parenteral opioids for labor analgesia. *Clin Obstet Gynecol.* 2003;46:616–622.
25. Hughes D, Hodgkinson P. Remifentanil PCA for labour analgesia. *Anaesthesia.* 2013;68:298.
26. Douma MR, Verwey RA, Kam-Endtz CE, et al. Obstetric analgesia: a comparison of patient-controlled meperidine, remifentanil, and fentanyl in labour. *Br J Anaesth.* 2010;104:209–215.
27. Tveit TO, Halvorsen A, Seiler S, et al. Efficacy and side effects of intravenous remifentanil patient-controlled analgesia used in a stepwise approach for labour: an observational study. *Int J Obstet Anesth.* 2013;22:19–25.
28. Comparative Obstetric Mobile Epidural Trial (COMET) Study Group UK. Effect of low-dose mobile versus traditional epidural techniques on mode of delivery: a randomized controlled trial. *Lancet.* 2001;358:19–23.
29. Lyons G, Columb M, Hawthorne L, et al. Extradural pain relief in labour: bupivacaine sparing by extradural fentanyl is dose dependent. *Br J Anaesth.* 1997;78:493–496.
30. George RB, Allen TK, Habib AS. Intermittent epidural bolus compared with continuous epidural infusions for labor analgesia: a systematic review and meta-analysis. *Anesth Analg.* 2013;116:133–144.
31. Vandervyver M, Halpern S, Joseph G. Patient-controlled epidural analgesia versus continuous infusion for labour analgesia: a meta-analysis. *Br J Anaesth.* 2002;89:459–465.
32. Paech MJ. Patient-controlled epidural analgesia in labour—is a continuous infusion of benefit? *Anaesth Intensive Care.* 1992;20:15–20.
33. Ferrante FM, Rosinia FA, Gordon C, et al. The role of continuous background infusions in patient-controlled epidural analgesia for labor and delivery. *Anesth Analg.* 1994;79:80–84.
34. Leo S, Ocampo CE, Lim Y, et al. A randomized comparison of automated intermittent mandatory boluses with a basal infusion in combination with patient-controlled epidural analgesia for labor and delivery. *Int J Obstet Anesth.* 2010;19:357–364.

35. Wong CA, McCarthy RJ, Hewlett B. The effect of manipulation of the programmed intermittent bolus time interval and injection volume on total drug use for labor epidural analgesia: a randomized controlled trial. *Anesth Analg.* 2011;112:904–911.

36. Wong CA, Scavone BM, Peaceman AM, et al. The risk of cesarean delivery with neuraxial analgesia given early versus late in labor. *N Engl J Med.* 2005;352:655–665.

37. Norris MC. Are combined spinal-epidural catheters reliable? *Int J Obstet Anesth.* 2000;9:3–6.

38. Abrao KC, Francisco RP, Miyadahira S, et al. Elevation of uterine basal tone and fetal heart rate abnormalities after labor analgesia; a randomized controlled trial. *Obstet Gynecol.* 2009;113:41–47.

39. Hood DD, Dewan DM. Anesthesia and obstetric outcome in morbidly obese parturients. *Anesthesiology.* 1993;79:1210–1218.

40. Veeser M, Hofmann T, Roth R, et al. Vasopressors for the management of hypotension after spinal anesthesia for elective caesarean section. Systematic review and cumulative meta-analysis. *Acta Anaesthesiol Scand.* 2012;56:810–816.

41. Gaiser RR. Postdural puncture headache: a headache for the patient and a headache for the anesthesiologist. *Curr Opin Anaesthesiol.* 2013;26:296–303.

42. Landau R, Ciliberto CF, Goodman SR, et al. Complications with 25-gauge and 27-gauge Whitacre needles during combined spinal-epidural analgesia in labor. *Int J Obstet Anesth.* 2001;10:168–171.

43. Simmons SW, Taghizadeh N, Dennis AT, et al. Combined spinal-epidural versus epidural analgesia in labour. *Cochrane Database Syst Rev.* 2012;10:CD003401.

44. Ruppen W, Derry S, McQuay H, et al. Incidence of epidural hematoma, infection, and neurologic injury in obstetric patients with epidural analgesia/anesthesia. *Anesthesiology.* 2006;105:394–399.

45. Wong CA, Scavone BM, Dugan S, et al. Incidence of postpartum lumbosacral spine and lower extremity nerve injuries. *Obstet Gynecol.* 2003;101:279–288.

46. Leighton BL, Halpern SH. The effects of epidural analgesia on labor, maternal, and neonatal outcomes; a systematic review. *Am J Obstet Gynecol.* 2002;186:S69–S77.

47. Sharma SK, McIntire DD, Wiley J, et al. Labor analgesia and cesarean delivery: an individual patient meta-analysis of nulliparous women. *Anesthesiology.* 2004;100:142–148.

48. Thorp JA, Paris VM, Boylan PC, et al. The effect of continuous epidural analgesia on cesarean section for dystocia in nulliparous women. *Am J Obstet Gynecol.* 1989;161:670–675.

49. Thorp JA, Eckert LO, Ang MS, et al. Epidural analgesia and cesarean section for dystocia: risk factors in nulliparas. *Am J Perinatol.* 1991;8:402–410.

50. Lieberman E, Lang JM, Cohen A, et al. Association of epidural analgesia with cesarean delivery in nulliparas. *Obstet Gynecol.* 1996;88:993–1000.

51. Thorp JA, Hu PH, Albin RM, et al. The effect of intrapartum epidural analgesia on nulliparous labor: a randomized, controlled, prospective trial. *Am J Obstet Gynecol.* 1993;169:851–858.

52. Sharma SK, Srdawi JE, Ramin SM, et al. Cesarean delivery: a randomized trial of epidural versus patient-controlled meperidine analgesia during labor. *Anesthesiology.* 1997; 87:487–494.

53. Loughnan BA, Carli F, Romney M, et al. Randomized controlled comparison of epidural bupivacaine versus pethidine for analgesia in labour. *Br J Anaesth.* 2000;84:715–719.

54. Halpern SH, Muir H, Breen TW, et al. A multicenter randomized controlled trial comparing patient-controlled epidural with intravenous analgesia for pain relief in labor. *Anesth Analg.* 2004;99:1532–1538.

55. Marucci M, Cinnella G, Perchiazzi G, et al. Patient-requested neuraxial analgesia for labor: impact on rates of cesarean and instrumental vaginal delivery. *Anesthesiology.* 2007;106:1035–1045.

56. Wang F, Shen X, Guo X, et al. Epidural analgesia in the latent phase of labor and the risk of cesarean delivery: a five-year randomized controlled trial. *Anesthesiology.* 2009;111:871–880.

57. American College of Obstetricians and Gynecologists Committee on Obstetric Practice. ACOG committee opinion no. 339: analgesia and cesarean delivery rates. *Obstet Gynecol.* 2006;107:1487–1488.

58. American Society of Anesthesiologists Task Force on Obstetric Anesthesia. Practice guidelines for obstetric anesthesia: an update report by the American Society of Anesthesiologists Task Force on Obstetric Anesthesia. *Anesthesiology.* 2007;106:843–863.
59. Mishriky BM, Habib AS. Metoclopramide for nausea and vomiting prophylaxis during and after Caesarean delivery: a systematic review and meta-analysis. *Br J Anaesth.* 2012;108:374–383.
60. American Society of Anesthesiologists. *Standards for basic anesthetic monitoring.* Amended October 2010. Available at: www.asahg.org. Accessed 05/27/13.
61. Riley ET, Cohen SE, Macario A, et al. Spinal versus epidural anesthesia for cesarean section: a comparison of time efficiency, costs, charges and complications. *Anesth Analg.* 1995;80:709–712.
62. Ng K, Parson J, Cyna AM, et al. Spinal versus epidural anaesthesia for caesarean section. *Cochrane Database Syst Rev.* 2004;(2):CD003765.
63. Aya AG, Vialles T, Tanoubi I, et al. Spinal anesthesia-induced hypotension: a risk comparison between patients with severe preeclampsia and healthy women undergoing preterm cesarean delivery. *Anesth Analg.* 2005;101:869–875.
64. Visalyaputra S, Rodanant O, Somboonviboon W, et al. Spinal versus epidural anesthesia for cesarean delivery in severe preeclampsia: a prospective randomized, multicenter study. *Anesth Analg.* 2005;101:862–868.
65. Philipson EH, Kuhnert BR, Syracuse CD. Fetal acidosis, 2-chloroprocaine, and epidural anesthesia for cesarean section. *Am J Obstet Gynecol.* 1985;151:322–324.
66. Finster M, Morishima HO, Mark LC, et al. Tissue thiopental concentrations in the fetus and newborn. *Anesthesiology.* 1972;36:155–158.
67. Abboud TK, Zhu J, Richardson M, et al. Intravenous propofol vs. thiamylal-isoflurane for caesarean section: comparative maternal and neonatal effects. *Acta Anaesthesiol Scand.* 1995;39:205–209.
68. Moore J, Bill KM, Flynn RJ, et al. A comparison between propofol and thiopentone as induction agents in obstetric anaesthesia. *Anaesthesia.* 1989;44:753–757.
69. Mhyre JM, Riesner MN, Polley LS, et al. A series of anesthesia-related maternal deaths in Michigan, 1985–2003. *Anesthesiology.* 2007;106:1096–1104.
70. Ozcan MS, Weinberg G. Update on the use of lipid emulsions in local anesthetic systemic toxicity: a focus on differential efficacy and lipid emulsion as part of advanced cardiac life support. *Int Anesthesiol Clin.* 2011;49:91–103.
71. American Society of Anesthesiologists Task Force on Intraoperative Awareness. Practice advisory for intraoperative awareness and brain function monitoring. *Anesthesiology.* 2006;104:847–864.
72. Safra MJ, Oakley OP. Association between cleft lip with or without cleft palate and prenatal exposure to diazepam. *Lancet.* 1975;2:478–480.
73. Shiono PH, Mills JL. Oral clefts and diazepam use during pregnancy. *N Engl J Med.* 1984;311:919–920.
74. Cohen EN, Belville JW, Brown BW. Anesthesia, pregnancy, and miscarriage: a study of operating room nurses and anesthetists. *Anesthesiology.* 1971;35:343–347.
75. Knill-Jones RP, Moir DD, Rodrigues LU, et al. Anaesthetic practice and pregnancy: Controlled survey of women anesthetists in the United Kingdom. *Lancet.* 1972;2:1326–1328.
76. Ericson HA, Kallen B. Hospitalization for miscarriage and delivery outcome among Swedish nurses working in operating rooms 1973–1978. *Anesth Analg.* 1985;64: 981–988.
77. Spence AA. Environmental pollution by inhalation anaesthetics. *Br J Anaesth.* 1987; 59:96–103.
78. Crawford JS, Lewis M. Nitrous oxide in early human pregnancy. *Anaesthesia.* 1986; 41:900–905.
79. Aldridge IM, Tunstall ME. Nitrous oxide and the fetus: a review and the results of a retrospective study of 175 cases of anaesthesia for insertion of a Shirodkar suture. *Br J Anaesth.* 1986;58:1348–1356.

4

Postpartum Care
Tifany Nolan and Amy M. Thompson

KEY POINTS
- Life-threatening emergencies and serious complications may occur during the postpartum period. These must be recognized and managed efficiently.
- Health care providers caring for postpartum women should be sensitive to the initiation of family bonding, a special process that should not be disturbed unless maternal or neonatal complications arise.

BACKGROUND
Definition
The postpartum period is traditionally defined as the 6 weeks following parturition.

Pathophysiology
Reproductive Organs
- Contraction of the uterine myometrium occurs immediately after delivery of the placenta and serves to compress dilated vessels supplying the placental site. By 2 weeks postpartum, the uterus involutes sufficiently to again be a pelvic organ, and by 4 weeks postpartum, the uterus returns to nonpregnant dimensions. Within days of delivery, the superficial decidua necroses and sloughs in the form of lochia. New endometrium is regenerated from the basal layer within 7 to 10 days, with the exception of the placental site. The placental site is slowly exfoliated by the undermining growth from the surrounding regenerating endometrium.
- The cervix regains tone within 2 to 3 days after delivery and remains dilated 2 to 3 cm. By 1 week postpartum, the cervix regains a nonpregnant appearance.
- The vagina remains edematous and enlarged for approximately 3 weeks. Involution is usually complete by 6 weeks postpartum.
- Ovulation occurs on the average at 10 weeks in the nonlactating woman (1). The first menstrual cycle is frequently anovulatory. In nonlactating women, the mean time to first menses is 7 to 9 weeks, and 70% will menstruate by 12 weeks postpartum (2). In lactating women, time to ovulation and menstruation is highly variable and depends on the duration and frequency of breast-feeding.
- The breasts are prepared for lactation during pregnancy by estrogen, progesterone, cortisol, prolactin, placental lactogen, and insulin, while actual lactation is suppressed by high levels of placental steroids. The rapid fall in progesterone postpartum allows expression of α-lactalbumin, which stimulates milk lactose production and initiates lactation. Initial milk production consists mostly of colostrum, which is richer in proteins and immunoglobulins than is mature milk. Prolactin appears to be the single most important maintenance hormone necessary for continued milk production (3).

Systemic Changes
- Circulating blood volume returns to nonpregnant levels by the 10th day postpartum. Dilated blood vessels supplying the uterus during pregnancy undergo involution, and extrauterine vessels decrease their diameter to nonpregnant dimensions. In contrast, cardiac output increases immediately after delivery but then slowly declines, reaching late pregnancy levels 2 days postpartum and decreasing by only 16% 14 days after delivery (4).

This occurs as a consequence of increased stroke volume from increased venous return, despite a quick fall in the pulse rate by about 10 beats/min.

- The bladder demonstrates increased capacity and decreased volume sensitivity. This may result in transient urinary retention. This is also aggravated by increased urine production as a consequence of infused fluid during labor and withdrawal of the antidiuretic effect of oxytocin administered in large doses after delivery. Renal function decreases to non-pregnant levels by 6 weeks postpartum. A postpartum diuresis occurs within 1 to 2 weeks after delivery and compensates for water retention during pregnancy. Anatomic changes of pregnancy such as ureteral and calyceal dilatation may persist for several months.

- The enlarged thyroid gland returns to prepregnancy dimensions over a 12-week period (5). Previously increased thyroid-binding globulin, total thyroxine, and total triiodothy-ronine return to normal levels by 4 to 6 weeks postpartum.

- In late pregnancy, the pancreas exhibits an enhanced insulin response to glucose chal-lenge, accompanied by higher postprandial glucose levels. The insulin response curve returns to the nonpregnant state 2 days after delivery. The glucose curve normalizes by 8 to 10 weeks postpartum.

- Hemoglobin concentration rises on the first postpartum day and then decreases, reaching a nadir on the 4th or 5th day. A gradual increase in hemoglobin then ensues, approaching day 1 values on the 9th day. Mean leukocyte count steadily increases during pregnancy, reaching about 10,000 in the third trimester. There is a further increase during and immediately after delivery. The leukocyte count returns to nonpregnant values by the 6th day postpartum. Platelet count, in contrast, decreases steadily during pregnancy. For 2 days after delivery, platelets decrease further and then rise rapidly thereafter secondary to release of fresh platelets with increased adhesiveness. A hypercoagulable postpartum state results and lasts about 7 weeks. Several clotting factors including fibrinogen rise during first postpartum days. The fibrinolytic enzyme system, on the other hand, is depressed during pregnancy but returns rapidly to the nonpregnant state after delivery.

NORMAL POSTPARTUM CARE

History and Physical

- Vital signs should be assessed every 4 hours for the first 24 hours, including measurement of urine output.
- Uterus and lochia
  - The quantity of bleeding in the first several days postpartum should be similar to the menses. The uterus should be slightly below the umbilicus and firm. If it is not, the patient may be experiencing significant bleeding, either concealed in the uterus or in the vagina. The uterus should be evaluated for any unusual degree of tenderness that might suggest endometritis.
  - Lochia should be assessed for unusual odor. Lochia rubra, seen for the first several days, consists mainly of blood and necrotic decidual tissue. Lochia serosa follows and is lighter, as there is less blood. After several weeks, the patient notices only a leukorrhea known as lochia alba.
  - Immediately postpartum, nursing staff and patients should be instructed to perform uterine massage to decrease uterine bleeding.
- The abdomen should be examined for distension and the presence of bowel sounds, especially in patients who had cesarean deliveries.
  - Postcesarean patients usually experience a return of coordinated bowel function by the 2nd or 3rd day. Failure to do so strongly suggests an ileus.
  - Following cesarean section, oral intake may resume immediately as tolerated. Early feeding has been shown to shorten hospital stay without increasing vomiting or ileus in women after major abdominal gynecologic surgery (6).
- The perineum should be inspected for hematoma formation, signs of infection, or break-down. Hemorrhoids may also be noted on examination.

- Perineal care consists of gentle cleansing and warm sitz baths initiated on the first postpartum day.
- Local anesthetics such as witch hazel pads or benzocaine spray may be used. Hydrocortisone and local anesthetic preparations may be applied to hemorrhoids.
- Stool softeners such as docusate sodium and osmotic laxatives are usually prescribed, especially in cases of third or fourth degree lacerations. Shorter-interval follow-up is recommended for these patients.
- Bladder function should be assessed by noting urine output and any symptoms of urinary retention.
  - Patients at risk for urinary retention include those receiving regional anesthesia and/or experiencing perineal pain from genital tract injury at delivery. Catheterization may be required if the patient is unable to void within 6 hours. Failure to urinate for greater durations of time increases the risks of bladder dysfunction.
  - Postcesarean section patients generally have their Foley catheter removed approximately 18 to 24 hours after surgery. It may be removed once the effects of regional anesthesia have disappeared and there are no signs of internal hemorrhage.
- Anatomical barriers to successful breast-feeding should be identified. Observation of a nursing session can distinguish patients likely to benefit from lactational support. The breasts should be examined for engorgement or signs of infection.
- The lungs should be evaluated in all postpartum patients because they are an important source of postoperative fever.
  - Patients should receive instruction and encouragement in the use of incentive spirometry during the postoperative period. Use of splinting during coughing can minimize pain associated with this important aspect of pulmonary function.
- The extremities should be evaluated for signs of increasing edema and calf pain.
  - Unilateral edema and calf pain warrant investigation for thrombus.

Lactational Support
Background
- Human milk is the preferred infant nutrition except in very rare infant metabolic disorders (7).
  - There are numerous infant and maternal benefits to human milk and breast-feeding. These include decreased infant infection and infant mortality, decreased chronic childhood diseases, and decreased childhood obesity. Maternal benefits include a decrease in postpartum hemorrhage, a lower average weight compared to non–breast-feeding women, and possibly decrease in breast and ovarian cancer (7,8).
  - Maternal milk obtained by either direct breast-feeding or expression is encouraged except in cases of maternal HIV or certain maternal medication/drugs. These drugs include chemotherapeutic, anticonvulsant, and psychiatric medications or illicit drugs and should be carefully evaluated on an individual basis.
- Infant feeding should be initiated within 1 hour of birth.
  - On-demand feeding, or unrestricted nursing, ensures an adequate supply of milk is available for the infant.
  - Infants innately possess the reflexes that confer the ability to breast-feed—rooting, suckling, and swallowing.
- A good infant latch is imperative to successful breast-feeding.
  - Much of the areola of the mother's nipple should be included in the infant's mouth during suckle, which places the nipple at the infant's hard palate.
- Patients who elect not to breast-feed should have their breasts tightly bound to inhibit lactation.
  - Bromocriptine is no longer used to suppress lactation due to reported cases of hypotension, hypertension, seizures, and strokes (9).

• Every effort should be made to provide a postpartum atmosphere that supports breast-feeding, including lactational consultants if available.
  • Ongoing support will need to be provided throughout the duration of breast-feeding especially if a mother will be physically absent for long periods of time such as returning to work.
• Evaluation of infant latch should be observed early when feeding concerns occur.
  • Large breasts, previous breast surgery, or inverted nipples can make latch difficult and may require supportive care or education on positioning.
  • Infant anatomical abnormalities such as cleft lip/palate, restrictive frenulum, and muscular weakness can cause difficult nursing and should be evaluated for treatment.
  • Appropriate breast care during lactation can ensure the nipples remain pain free.
  • Breast support should not include underwire, and lanolin cream can ease soreness.
  • Cracked nipples should be evaluated promptly for infection.
  • If there is a concern for low supply of breast milk, galactogogues such as metoclopramide or domperidone can be used to stimulate lactation.
• Should breast-feeding prove very difficult, the patient should be educated on expression of breast milk either manually or via electric pump to be fed to the infant.
• Breast engorgement can occur resulting in maternal discomfort or poor infant latch.
  • This may need to be relieved by either manual expression or use of a breast pump.
• Development of a clogged lactational duct can cause maternal pain and should be treated with continued nursing or milk expression.
  • Warm compresses and gentle massage of the area are important if a palpable lump is present.
  • It is imperative to differentiate this from mastitis, which is discussed more extensively in the section on postpartum infection.

Laboratory Tests and Immunizations
• Complete blood count on the first postpartum day.
• Blood type and screen (to administer RhoGAM to nonsensitized Rh-negative patients).
• Rubella titer if not previously known, to assess need for immunization postpartum.
• Influenza and TDap vaccination are universally recommended in the postpartum period if not administered antepartum (10–12).

COMPLICATIONS IN POSTPARTUM CARE
Postpartum Hemorrhage
Background
• Hemorrhage is the most common cause of maternal mortality worldwide.
  • Postpartum hemorrhage has been defined as either a 10-point decrease in hematocrit between admission and postpartum or a need for erythrocyte transfusion. The classical definition of postpartum hemorrhage of total blood loss greater than 500 mL at vaginal delivery and greater than 1000 mL at cesarean delivery suffers from the limitations of clinical estimation of blood loss during delivery. Average blood loss following vaginal delivery, cesarean section, and cesarean hysterectomy was estimated by Pritchard et al. (13) to be approximately 500, 1000, and 1500 mL, respectively. It has been demonstrated that assessment of blood loss during delivery is oftentimes underestimated (14).

Differential Diagnosis
Early
• Atony (in about 90% of patients)
• Genital tract trauma (in about 7%)
• Coagulopathy (in about 2% to 3%)
• Retained placental fragments, placenta accreta, increta, and percreta
• Uterine inversion (rare)
• Uterine rupture

Late
• Retained placental fragments
• Subinvolution of the placental bed
• Endomyometritis
• Coagulopathy

Treatment
Prevention
• Avoid genital tract trauma.
• Prophylactically use oxytocic agents at the onset of the third stage of labor.
• Actively manage the third stage of labor (with controlled cord traction after signs of placental separation have occurred) (15) (Fig. 4-1).

Uterine Atony
Background
• Uterine atony is responsible for approximately 90% of postpartum hemorrhages.

Diagnosis
• The diagnosis is usually made in the presence of a soft uterus on abdominal examination and vaginal bleeding.
• Risk factors include polyhydramnios, multiple gestation, fetal macrosomia (probably secondary to uterine over distention), rapid or prolonged labor, oxytocin use, high parity, chorioamnionitis, and myometrial relaxing agents (magnesium sulfate, terbutaline, halogenated anesthetic agents, and nitroglycerine) (16,17).

Treatment
Massage
• Bimanual uterine massage is performed by applying compression between a hand on the abdomen and a hand in the vagina.

Medications
• If massage is unsuccessful, the next measure is medical therapy. Many labor and delivery units have an emergency medicine kit that is readily accessible in these situations. The following are commonly used uterotonic agents that can be administered once drug-specific contraindications are identified (14).
  • Oxytocin intravenously (10 to 40 U/L up to 500 mL in 10 minutes), intramuscularly, or intramyometrially (10 U). There are no contraindications to the use of oxytocin. Side effects such as nausea, vomiting, and water intoxication secondary to its antidiuretic effect are rare.
  • Methylergonovine intramuscularly, intravenously, or intramyometrially (0.2 mg every 2 to 4 hours). Methylergonovine is contraindicated in patients with hypertension. Side effects of hypertension, hypotension, nausea, and vomiting have been reported.
  • 15-Methylprostaglandin $F_{2\alpha}$ intramuscularly or intramyometrially (0.25 mg every 15 to 90 minutes up to 8 doses). This medication has been used to correct uterine atony unresponsive to other agents (18,19). Prostaglandins of the F series should be used with great caution in patients with bronchospasm, renal or hypertensive disorders, and pulmonary hypertension. Common side effects including fever, vomiting, diarrhea, hot flushes, and chills. Prostaglandins can also cause bronchoconstriction, pulmonary vasoconstriction, hypotension, hypertension, and arterial oxygen desaturation.
  • Prostaglandin E_2 (dinoprost) is administered as a vaginal or rectal suppository (20 mg every 2 hours). It may be particularly helpful in cases of refractory, persistent postpartum atony (20). It does not cause severe pulmonary vasocongestion or bronchoconstriction, thus providing a potentially safer alternative for patients with heart and lung

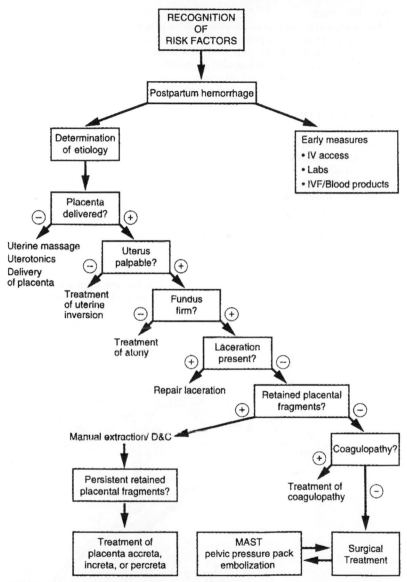

Figure 4-1. Management of postpartum hemorrhage.

disease. It shares other side effects with prostaglandin $F_{2\alpha}$ and has been reported to cause vasodilation and hypotension.

• Prostaglandin E1 (misoprostol) 800 to 1000 mcg rectally once. It is most likely to cause GI distress, nausea, vomiting, diarrhea, or fever. Shares side effects such as hypotension common to the prostaglandins.

Uterine Tamponade

- When uterotonics do not provide adequate uterine contraction to inhibit bleeding, uterine tamponade can provide direct pressure especially to temporize and reduce blood loss (14).
  - Uterine packing with 4-inch gauze with or without thrombin can reduce blood loss especially if tightly packed. If thrombin is available, the gauze can be soaked in a solution of 5000 U of thrombin in 5 mL saline.
  - Commercial balloon tamponade devices such as the Bakri (Fig. 4-2) or Ebb balloons can be inserted up to the uterine fundus and filled with saline to provide direct intrauterine pressure (21).

Surgery

- Surgical intervention via laparotomy is indicated when uterine bleeding does not respond to massage or medication. Each of these interventions may also be performed at the time of cesarean delivery.
  - The B-Lynch stitch was first described by Christopher B-Lynch (22–24) and is a useful tool in the armamentarium for uterine atony because it is simple to apply, preserves fertility, and does not obliterate the uterine or cervical lumen. The utility of the technique is first verified by an assistant who observes resolution of vaginal bleeding under the operative drape as the surgeon applies manual compression to the atonic uterus on the surgical field. The hysterotomy incision is then reopened, and a 36-inch suture of chromic catgut is obtained. Due to the tension placed on the suture, the suture must be at least of 2-0 size. The suture is placed anterior across the hysterotomy incision and is brought up over the uterine fundus (Fig. 4-3A). The next surgical bite is placed horizontally in the posterior aspect of the uterus, at the level of the uterine incision (Fig. 4-3B). The suture is then returned over the contralateral side of the uterine fundus to the anterior lower uterine segment. The third surgical bite is then made perpendicular across the hysterotomy incision and the suture tied below the incision, achieving manual uterine compression (see Fig. 4-3C).

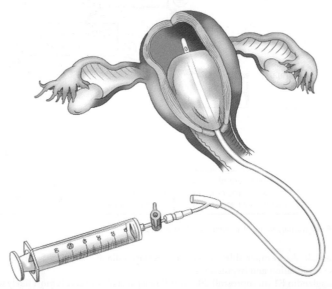

Figure 4-2. Bakri tamponade balloon. (Lippincott's Nursing Advisor 2013. Available at: http://thepoint.lww.com. Lippincott Williams & Wilkins, 2013.)

- Uterine artery ligation was first described by O'Leary and O'Leary (25) and has proven to be safe, easily performed, often effective, and preservative of fertility. The technique, designed to control postcesarean hemorrhage, uses single mass ligation of the uterine artery and vein with a no. 1 chromic suture on a large atraumatic needle placed at the level of the vesicouterine peritoneal reflection. The vessels are not divided, and recanalization with subsequent normal pregnancy can be expected (26). When combined with ligation of utero-ovarian vessels, the procedure has been reported to be successful in 95% of cases. Both procedures work by reducing uterine perfusion. Bilateral ovarian artery ligation may adversely affect future fertility and does not enhance the effectiveness of the preceding measures because more than 90% of the uterine blood flow in pregnancy passes through the uterine arteries.
- Bilateral hypogastric artery ligation is indicated in hemodynamically stable patients with placenta accreta, uterine atony, or laceration associated with uterine incision when

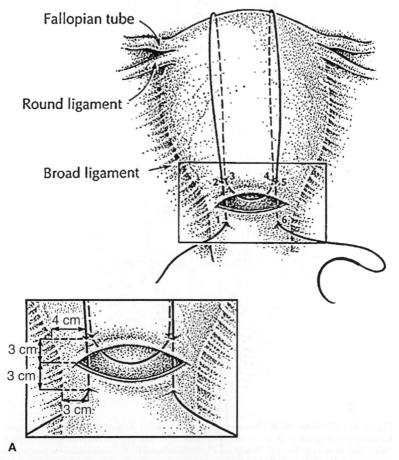

Figure 4-3. A: Anterior uterine wall with B-Lynch suture in place and an enlarged drawing (inset) of lower uterine segment with B-Lynch suture in place.

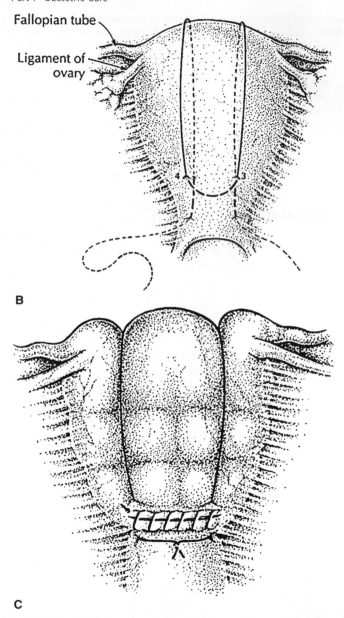

Fallopian tube

Ligament of ovary

B

C

Figure 4-3 *(Continued).* **B:** Posterior uterine wall with B-Lynch suture in place before tying. **C:** Compressed uterus with the hysterotomy incision closed and the B-Lynch suture in place. (Reprinted from Ferguson JM, Bourgeois FJ, Underwood PB. B-Lynch suture for postpartum hemorrhage. *Obstet Gynecol.* 2000;95:1020–1022, with permission.)

future fertility is of great concern. It reduces pulse pressure to pelvic organs. Its success rate is reported to be less than 50%. It is performed after division of the round ligament and exposure of the pelvic side wall (27). Clinically it requires advanced surgical skills and is a rarely utilized technique as its success rate is less than 50%.

- Hysterectomy is used to treat postpartum hemorrhage when other surgical techniques have failed. It is thus the procedure of choice in unstable patients or to stop very severe bleeding. In many situations, a supracervical hysterectomy is sufficient and preferred. Clark et al. (28) reported an average blood loss of approximately 3500 mL, mean operating time of more than 3 hours, and mean hospital stay of 7 to 8 days. These figures may have been magnified by unsuccessful attempts of conservative surgical management.

Other Maneuvers
- Other maneuvers are applied when medical and surgical treatments are unsuccessful in controlling postpartum hemorrhage.
  - Selective arterial embolization is indicated in stable patients when preservation of fertility is a goal. Prior ligation of the hypogastric artery will reduce access for embolization. Fever, contrast media toxicity, and buttock claudication have all been reported to complicate this procedure (29).
  - Pelvic pressure pack has been proposed for treatment of persistent posthysterectomy bleeding with associated coagulopathy.
  - Military antishock trousers have been used in patients with persistent postpartum hemorrhage or when reexploration must be avoided.

Supportive Measures
- Essential supportive measures include adequate fluid resuscitation via two large-bore IVs, replacement of blood products as needed, and anesthesia consultation in the event emergent laparotomy is necessary.

GENITAL TRACT TRAUMA
Background
- Genital tract trauma constitutes approximately 7% of postpartum hemorrhages.

Diagnosis
Clinical Manifestations
- The diagnosis of genital tract trauma should be considered when hemorrhage is present despite firm uterine tone. Bleeding accompanying laceration is usually bright red. Examination of the genital tract will reveal presence of lacerations or hematoma. In the rare situation in which a hematoma forms above the pelvic diaphragm, it cannot be palpated and presents as pelvic pain, inability to void, urge to defecate, unexplained tachycardia and hypotension, anemia, and finally shock.

Risk Factors
- Risk factors for genital trauma include abnormal presentation, operative delivery, use of episiotomy, precipitous delivery, obstructed labor, fetal macrosomia, multiple gestation, and history of female genital mutilation.

Treatment
- Treatment first involves a systematic examination of the genital tract, starting superiorly for optimal visualization. Use of vaginal retractors and single forceps blades aid in this process. The uterine cavity is palpated to assure its integrity. Ensuring adequate patient anesthesia is essential to accomplishing a thorough and effective examination. On occasion, delivery room lighting is not adequate for this examination and the patient should be transferred to the operating room.

- Full-thickness mucosal repair should begin above the apex because bleeding vessels tend to retract. Continuous interlocking absorbable suture is generally used. Consideration must be given to the size and type of needle and the appropriate suture chosen based on location and severity of laceration. When suturing in the proximity of the urethra, insertion of a catheter is advisable to avoid injury of this structure.
- Management of an expanding hematoma consists of incision, removal of clots, ligation of bleeding vessels, and obliteration of the defect with interlocking absorbable sutures. Antibiotics and a vaginal pack may be beneficial for 24 hours after evacuation of large vaginal hematomas, keeping in mind that the pack may provide a false sense of security to care providers. Tight vaginal packing can cause voiding difficulty for the patient, and a Foley catheter should be placed. This will also facilitate monitoring urine output. Serial laboratory studies are necessary. Packing should be removed in a controlled environment where the patient can be observed for any residual bleeding.
- Subperitoneal hematomas are rare but may cause shock. When conservative measures fail to achieve improvement, laparotomy is indicated. Attempts to ligate bleeding vessels or perform bilateral hypogastric artery ligation may be difficult because of the distorted anatomy caused by the expanding hematoma. An alternative is selective arterial embolization (29).

RETAINED PLACENTAL TISSUE

Diagnosis

Clinical Manifestations
- The diagnosis of retained placental tissue should be suspected when bleeding persists in the absence of apparent lacerations or atony. The expelled placenta should be carefully inspected for completeness following each delivery.

Risk Factors
- Risk factors for retained placental fragments include deliveries with aggressive early cord traction (before signs of placental separation); placenta accreta, increta, and percreta; and succenturiate lobe.
    - Placenta accreta has recently reported to be as common as 1 in 533 deliveries, a significant increase from the pre-1972 estimate of 1 in 7000 deliveries (30). This marked increase is due to the increasing rate of cesarean delivery. Placenta accrete consists of a relatively superficial attachment of the placenta to the myometrium. More invasive attachment (placenta increta or percreta) is less common.
    - Predisposing factors are cesarean delivery, previous postpartum curettage, hysterotomy from myomectomy, placenta previa, advanced maternal age, previous endometrial ablation, or uterine artery embolization. Ideally, this condition is identified before delivery so that delivery may take place in a center with anesthesia support and transfusion capabilities (31).

Treatment
- Should the diagnosis not be made antepartum, treatment after delivery may first involve manual intrauterine exploration or curettage with a Banjo or Hunter curette under adequate anesthesia. Some providers use ultrasound guidance for this procedure if it is available. Care must be taken to avoid uterine perforation, and when perforation is suspected, the patient must be observed closely and laparotomy performed if bleeding is excessive or hemodynamic indices deteriorate. In this situation, placenta accreta, increta, or percreta should be suspected. Treatment usually requires hysterectomy for these abnormal placentations. In rare instances, curettage or conservative surgical management (with manual removal and packing) can be attempted. Maternal morbidity and mortality are high if surgical therapy is necessary. On occasion, the placenta can be left in situ and the patient treated with methotrexate and placental removal performed at a later date. However, this should only be reserved for rare cases when fertility is strongly desired or when immediate hysterectomy would have greater maternal risk (32).

COAGULOPATHY

Diagnosis

Clinical Manifestations

- The diagnosis of coagulopathy should be suspected when a patient presents with persistent vaginal bleeding without signs of uterine atony, genital tract trauma, or retained placental tissue.

Laboratory Tests

- Laboratory evaluation should include fibrinogen, prothrombin time, partial thromboplastin time, platelet count, fibrin split products, and clot retraction test.
- Initially, the fibrinogen level will fall rapidly while the platelet count and tests of functional coagulation remain normal. Fibrinogen levels less than 100 mg/dL in this clinical setting assist with confirmation of the diagnosis. The platelet count and other coagulation tests will only become abnormal late in the course of the abruption.

Risk Factors

- Risk factors for coagulopathy include abruptio placentae, large acute blood loss, amniotic fluid embolism, intrauterine fetal demise, preeclamptic syndromes, inherited coagulopathy, sepsis, and anticoagulant therapy.

Treatment

- Treatment involves the administration of blood products to correct developing clotting abnormalities (33,34).
  - Fresh frozen plasma or cryoprecipitate is used when fibrinogen concentration is less than 100 mg/dL.
  - Platelet concentrate is used for platelet count less than 50,000/mm³ and bleeding time greater than 8 minutes.
  - Recombinant Factor VIIa may have a role in avoiding hysterectomy or achieving hemostasis after hysterectomy. The dose is 90 mcg/kg as a single IV bolus over 3 to 5 minutes. A second dose can be administered 20 minutes later if bleeding continues and fibrinogen and platelets have been replaced above the levels previously mentioned (35).

UTERINE INVERSION

Diagnosis

Clinical Manifestations

- Uterine inversion is a rarely encountered complication following vaginal delivery. Patients typically manifest vaginal bleeding, hypotension, diaphoresis, and anxiety. The incidence has been estimated to be 1 in 20,000 vaginal births (36). The diagnosis of uterine inversion is confirmed when abdominal examination reveals the uterine fundus to be inverted or missing. Vaginal inspection confirms the diagnosis when the prolapsing endometrium is visualized. The fundus may be inverted to varying degrees and in severe cases can be found entirely outside the vulva.

Risk Factors

- Risk factors for uterine inversion include fetal macrosomia, fundal placentation, use of oxytocin, uterine anomalies, and placenta accreta. Fifty percent of reported cases occur spontaneously in primiparous patients.

Treatment

- Successful treatment depends on early recognition, manual replacement, and intravascular volume replacement (37). If the placenta has not been removed, the physician should attempt to replace the uterus by applying pressure to the inverted fundus without removing the placenta and increasing natural oxytocin. If manual replacement succeeds, the placenta can be manually removed, the uterus explored, and uterine contraction assured by massage and oxytocin infusion. If manual replacement fails, this can be repeated with the aid of uterine relaxing agents (terbutaline, magnesium sulfate) or general anesthesia (38). When all the above measures fail, laparotomy is indicated to correct the inversion using Allis clamps along round ligaments (Huntington procedure) or by incision of the posterior wall over the constriction ring (37).

UTERINE RUPTURE
Diagnosis
Clinical Manifestations
- The diagnosis of uterine rupture is suspected in the presence of tachycardia, shock, fetal distress, disappearance of presenting part from the pelvis, and a variable amount of pain and vaginal bleeding. Complete rupture involves rupture of visceral peritoneum and results in intraperitoneal bleeding. Incomplete rupture occurs when the visceral peritoneum remains intact over ruptured myometrium.
- Uterine rupture during trial of labor after cesarean section results in significant maternal and neonatal morbidity and mortality (39). Large blood loss is expected during rupture as well as possible injury to the maternal genitourinary tract. Risk of neonatal death is 1.8%, and risk of hypoxic ischemic encephalopathy is 6.2% (40).

Risk Factors
- Risk factors include obstructed labor, multiple gestation, abnormal fetal lie, and high parity. However, uterine rupture is most commonly associated with prior uterine surgery (deep myomectomy, prior cesarean delivery, especially with classical uterine incision). Other risk factors include use of oxytocin, prostaglandins, spontaneous uterine hyperstimulation, internal podalic version, and breech extraction.

Treatment
- Treatment consists of intravascular volume and blood replacement and immediate laparotomy.
- Repair of uterine rupture may be possible. However, emergency hysterectomy is more often necessary (28).

LATE POSTPARTUM HEMORRHAGE
Background
- Late postpartum hemorrhage is defined as any sudden loss of any amount of fresh blood occurring after the first 24 hours of delivery and within 6 weeks postpartum.

Differential Diagnosis
- Retained placental tissue
- Subinvolution of the placental bed
- Endometritis
- Vulvar hematoma (rare)
- Uterine scar dehiscence (rare)
- Gestational trophoblastic disease (rare)

Treatment
- Treatment options include uterotonics, curettage, and antibiotics. If the bleeding is not severe, antibiotics make a good first choice, and if bleeding persists, curettage should be implemented. In the case of severe bleeding, uterine evacuation should be arranged.

PUERPERAL INFECTIONS
Background
- Puerperal febrile morbidity was defined by the U.S. Joint Committee on Maternal Welfare as "a temperature of 100.4°F (38°C), the temperature to occur in any two of the first 10 days postpartum, exclusive of the first 24 hours, and to be taken by mouth by a standard technique at least four times daily" (41).

- The overall rate of postpartum infection is difficult to ascertain, but it is estimated to be 1% to 8%.
- Transient, low-grade fever is common in the postpartum period and will resolve spontaneously in the majority of patients who delivered vaginally. In patients who undergo cesarean delivery, only 30% of fevers will resolve spontaneously, reflecting the greater risk for development of infection after surgery (41).

Differential Diagnosis (42,43)
- Endometritis
- Wound infection
- Urinary tract infection
- Mastitis
- Septic pelvic thrombophlebitis
- Pelvic abscess
- Other (pneumonia, viral infection, HIV, connective tissue disorder, bacterial endocarditis)

Evaluation
History and Physical
- Thorough review of patient's antepartum, intrapartum, and postpartum history
- Physical examination focusing on lungs, breast, uterine fundus, abdomen for incision infections, perineum, costovertebral angles, lower extremities

Laboratory Tests
- Complete blood count with differential.
- Urinalysis with culture.
- Blood cultures may be considered.
- Sputum for Gram stain and culture if respiratory infection is suspected.

ENDOMETRITIS
Background
- Endometritis is infection of the endometrium, whereas endomyometritis also involves the myometrium. Endoparametritis includes infection of the parametrium, although clinically these conditions are difficult to distinguish.

DIAGNOSIS
Clinical Manifestations
- The criteria for diagnosis usually includes fever, uterine tenderness, foul or purulent lochia, elevated white cell count, and lack of other localizing symptoms. Symptoms generally appear within 5 days of delivery. Early onset is defined as within 48 hours of delivery, and late onset is defined as infection occurring up to 6 weeks postpartum (44).
- Endometrial cultures may be obtained in refractory cases but are generally not necessary for initial evaluation and diagnosis because the infection is generally polymicrobial, and therapy is empirical with broad-spectrum antibiotics.

Risk Factors
- Risk factors include cesarean delivery, prolonged duration of ruptured membranes, prolonged labor, and low socioeconomic status and chorioamnionitis. Prolonged internal fetal monitoring and multiple vaginal examinations are also associated with endometritis (45,46). The risk of developing postcesarean endometritis in laboring and nonlaboring patients can be reduced by administering prophylactic antibiotics (47).

Organisms
- Implicated organisms are typically polymicrobial with mixed aerobic and anaerobic types. Commonly isolated pathogens include aerobic gram-negative bacilli (*Escherichia coli*, *Klebsiella* sp., *Proteus* sp.), aerobic gram-positive streptococci (group B *Streptococcus*,

enterococcus), anaerobic gram-negative bacilli (*Bacteroides bivius, Bacteroides mela-ninogenicus, Bacteroides fragilis, Fusobacterium*), and anaerobic gram-positive cocci (*Peptostreptococcus, Peptococcus*) (48).

Treatment
- Historically, treatment after vaginal delivery consisted of a combination of penicillin and aminoglycoside resulting in a 95% response rate. Addition of antibiotics effective against anaerobic bacteria such as clindamycin or metronidazole in primary treatment failures will increase the cure rate to 98%. Treatment of postcesarean endometritis consists of clindamycin and an aminoglycoside (48,49). Single-agent and multiagent regimens have been proposed.
- Treatment must consider the probability of streptococci, Enterobacteriaceae, and obligate anaerobes (50). A recent Cochrane database review concluded that an aminoglycoside and clindamycin is an appropriate first choice. There were not enough studies to determine if antibiotic choice should differ based on method of delivery (51). Aminoglycoside levels and renal function should be monitored.
- All patients are treated with intravenous antibiotics until they are afebrile for more than 48 hours. A course of oral antibiotics is not needed.
- Treatment failures with this regimen usually result from inadequate aminoglycoside dosage (Table 4-1) (50) or from a resistant organism such as enterococcus. Care should be taken to administer appropriate weight-based doses. In treatment failures with therapeutic aminoglycoside levels, ampicillin is generally added empirically to the regimen.

Complication
- Complications of refractory cases include septic pelvic thrombophlebitis, pelvic abscess, and septic shock. Cases associated with pelvic abscess may decrease future fertility; however, most uncomplicated cases of endometritis are not associated with infertility (52).

WOUND INFECTIONS
- Wound infections most commonly involve an abdominal incision after cesarean delivery. They occur less commonly following episiotomy incision or perineal laceration from vaginal delivery.

Diagnosis
Clinical Manifestations
- Patients report pain, incision site erythema, and drainage. The diagnosis of a postcesarean wound infection is usually made clinically by 3 to 8 days postoperatively. Temperature elevation is variable. The overlying skin is frequently erythematous, and there may be tenderness and palpable fluctuance. Drainage of purulent material allows for culture and definitive diagnosis. Postepisiotomy wound infection manifests as local edema and erythema with purulent exudate.

Table 4-1	Antibiotic Dosage in the Postpartum Patient	
Antibiotic	**Dose**	**Interval (h)**
Ampicillin	2 g	4–6
Cefazolin	1–2 g	8
Gentamicin	Loading, 2 mg/kg; maintenance, 1.5–1.75 mg/kg (23)	8
Clindamycin	900 mg	8

Risk Factors
- Risk factors for postcesarean wound infection include chorioamnionitis, obesity, prolonged surgery, emergency surgery, diabetes, corticosteroid therapy, and malnutrition.

Organisms
- The organisms isolated from a typical postcesarean wound infection are those found in the healthy lower genital tract or skin flora. Wound infection presenting with extensive cellulitis within the first 48 hours after surgery suggests necrotizing fasciitis and may be caused by group A streptococci or *Clostridium perfringens*. In the latter case, a bronze discoloration of the skin with a watery discharge may be noted.

Treatment
- Treatment for the usual postcesarean wound infection is local. The wound is opened and cleansed, and nonviable tissue is debrided. Generally, the wound is left open to heal by secondary intention. Antibiotic therapy is not necessary unless extensive overlying cellulitis is present. For larger wound separation, negative pressure wound therapy can decrease healing time.
- Early-onset infection, as described, should be treated with penicillin and extensive debridement.
- Suspected episiotomy infection is treated with sitz baths. If this treatment is unsuccessful, the wound is opened and debrided and allowed to heal secondarily. Infections affecting third- and fourth-degree lacerations require debridement and anatomical repair of the anal sphincter to prevent long-term sequelae.

Complications
- Complications include superficial fascial necrosis, necrotizing fasciitis, and myonecrosis. Treatment for the above complications is high-dose antibiotic therapy including penicillin and early extensive debridement.

URINARY TRACT INFECTION

Diagnosis

Clinical Manifestations
- The diagnosis of cystitis is suspected in patients with dysuria, urgency, and frequency. As these are common complaints in the postpartum patient, the diagnosis should be confirmed with a positive urinalysis or urine culture.
- Pyelonephritis is diagnosed in the patient with fever, flank pain, and a positive urine culture. Infection develops in the right kidney in the majority of pregnant patients with pyelonephritis.

Risk Factors
- Risk factors for the development of pyelonephritis in the postpartum patient include the physiologic hydroureter of pregnancy, catheterization during labor or for cesarean delivery, and preexisting asymptomatic bacteriuria (occurs in 2% to 12% of pregnant women).

Organisms
- The most commonly isolated etiologic organisms are the gram-negative bacilli *E. coli, Klebsiella enterobacter, Proteus* sp., and *Enterobacter* sp.; less commonly implicated are the gram-positive cocci, enterococcus, and group B *Streptococcus*.

Treatment
- Treatment for simple cystitis includes oral antibiotics. Treatment for more severe infections should consist of a first-generation cephalosporin such as cefazolin, given intravenously, as many gram-negative bacilli are resistant to ampicillin. If the patient appears

septic, an aminoglycoside should be added to the initial regimen. Renal imaging should be considered. Further therapy is guided by results to culture sensitivities. Intravenous therapy should be continued until the patient remains afebrile for 48 hours.
• Following completion of parenteral antibiotics, an oral antibiotic agent should be given to complete a 10- to 14-day course of therapy.

Complications
• Complications include septic shock and pulmonary capillary leak syndrome.

MASTITIS
Background
• Mastitis is an infection of the parenchyma of the mammary gland, usually occurring 2 to 3 weeks postpartum. Breast engorgement can cause low-grade fever in the early postpartum period, but other diagnoses must be carefully excluded before ascribing fever to this noninfectious cause.

Diagnosis
Clinical Manifestations
• Patients typically report breast pain, erythema, malaise, myalgias, and chills. The diagnosis of mastitis is based on the physical finding of a localized area of cellulitis, frequently V shaped, which delineates the infected lobule. The fever is usually higher than 102°F.

Risk Factors
• Risk factors include breast-feeding, recent weaning, fissures of the areola, and blocked duct.

Organisms
• The most common etiologic organism is *Staphylococcus aureus.* Other organisms include group A and B streptococci, *Haemophilus influenzae,* and *Haemophilus parainfluenzae.*

Treatment
• Treatment includes continued breast-feeding or pumping from the affected side, ice packs, and support. The antibiotic chosen should be active against penicillinase-producing *S. aureus,* such as dicloxacillin (250 to 500 mg, orally every 6 hours) or a cephalosporin such as cephalexin (250 to 500 mg, orally every 6 hours). Antibiotic therapy should be prescribed for 7 to 10 days.

Complications
• Complications such as a breast abscess may develop. This may be diagnosed on exam or via ultrasound imaging in refractory cases. This requires incision and drainage. Breast-feeding on the affected side should be stopped as long as purulent drainage continues.

SEPTIC PELVIC THROMBOPHLEBITIS
• Septic pelvic thrombophlebitis is the development of ovarian vein thrombosis in a patient with a preceding pelvic soft tissue infection. Incidence following vaginal delivery has been reported to be 1:9000; incidence following cesarean section is 1:800 (53).

Diagnosis
Clinical Manifestations
• The diagnosis of septic pelvic thrombophlebitis is suspected in a patient with persistent postpartum fever in spite of appropriate antibiotic therapy for endometritis. In actuality, the patient will not have other clinical signs of sepsis. Abdominal tenderness may be appreciated, and rarely, a palpable mass may extend from the uterine cornua laterally and cephalad, usually on the right side.

- Computed tomography (CT) or magnetic resonance imaging (MRI) may be utilized to support the diagnosis, with MRI offering better imaging of the soft tissue. Pelvic ultrasound can be used to follow the progress of the disease (53). But imaging may be inconclusive. The diagnosis is made clinically and is not dependent on imaging for verification.

Risk Factors
- Risk factors include endometritis, cesarean section, traumatic delivery, major vulvovaginal hematomas, and low socioeconomic status.

Organisms
- The most commonly implicated organisms are aerobic and anaerobic streptococci, staphylococci, *Proteus* sp., and *Bacteroides* sp.

Treatment
- Treatment includes broad-spectrum antibiotic coverage and therapeutic anticoagulation with heparin (see Chapter 22) for 7 to 10 days. Brown et al. (54) compared antibiotic therapy alone to antibiotic therapy with heparin and found no significant difference in the length of the febrile morbidity. Surgical therapy is reserved for medical failures.

Complications
- Complications include pelvic abscess and septic pulmonary thromboembolism.

PELVIC ABSCESS
- Pelvic abscess may result from an infected hematoma, septic thrombophlebitis, or prior pelvic soft tissue infection such as endomyometritis or tuboovarian infection.

Diagnosis
- The diagnosis of pelvic abscess is suspected when a patient has high spiking fevers that are unresponsive to broad-spectrum antibiotic therapy. A mass may be felt on pelvic examination. The diagnosis may be confirmed by ultrasound, CT scan, or MRI.
- Risk factors are the same as those for endometritis.
- Implicated organisms are the same as for endometritis.

Treatment
- Treatment consists of broad-spectrum antibiotic therapy. Surgery is reserved for those patients who fail to respond to conservative measures. If the mass is pointing into the cul-de-sac, it may be drained vaginally by colpotomy incision.

Complications
- Complications include abscess rupture with peritonitis and septic shock.

OTHER POSTPARTUM COMPLICATIONS
- Amniotic fluid embolism may occur immediately postdelivery (see Chapter 14).
- Thromboembolic events may occur as pregnancy is a hypercoagulable state. This risk is even further increased in the puerperium, with an incidence of 0.1% to 1.0% (see Chapter 22).
- Eclampsia complicates approximately 0.5% of pregnancies, and one-third of seizures occur postpartum. Treatment in the postpartum period is simplified by the absence of a fetus, allowing more aggressive antihypertensive and antiseizure therapy (see Chapter 11).
- Known medical conditions that preceded the pregnancy (i.e., chronic hypertension, thyroid disease) should undergo appropriate monitoring and necessary adjustments made to drug dosages.

POSTPARTUM PSYCHIATRIC PROBLEMS

Postnatal Blues

• *Postnatal blues* is estimated to occur in up to 75% of postpartum women.

Diagnosis or Clinical Manifestations

• The diagnosis of postnatal blues is suspected when crying, emotional lability, sleep disturbance, poor concentration, restlessness, headaches, and feelings of vulnerability and rejection are reported during the first 7 to 10 days after delivery. The condition is defined as a mood disorder that is probably related to hormonal changes occurring after delivery.

Risk Factors

• There are no known obstetric or social risk factors for mild blues. More severe blues can be anticipated in patients with a previous history of depression or relationship issues (55).

Treatment

• Treatment relies on reassurance of the patient, and antenatal preparation is of benefit in severe cases; follow-up is essential to evaluate for postpartum depression.

Postpartum Depression

Diagnosis

• This occurs in up to 20% of patients in the year following delivery. Typical onset is 1 to 3 months following delivery.

• Universal screening is necessary, and validated instruments such as the Edinburgh Postnatal Depression Scale are available and should be administered to all patients at their postpartum visit (56). Screening is mandated in some states.

• Diagnostic and Statistical Manual of Mental Disorders V states that the symptoms begin in the first 4 weeks following delivery (57); most clinicians agree that a major depressive episode occurring up to a year after delivery should be considered to be postpartum depression. Five or more of the following symptoms must be present for at least 2 weeks: insomnia or hypersomnia, psychomotor agitation or retardation, fatigue, changes in appetite, feelings of worthlessness, decreased concentration, and suicidal ideation. The patient must also have either depressed mood or loss of interest/pleasure.

• Risk factors include adverse life events before or during pregnancy, marital conflict or domestic violence, ambivalent attitude toward pregnancy, and history of depression. Its occurrence is not related to obstetric factors other than unplanned pregnancy.

Treatment

• Treatment depends on patient preference and severity of illness and may include supportive psychotherapy, counseling, and antidepressant medications.

Postpartum Psychosis

Background

• Postpartum psychosis has an incidence of 1 in 500 to 800 deliveries. It generally begins 2 to 7 days after delivery and peaks in severity at 2 weeks (58).

Diagnosis

• The diagnosis of postpartum psychosis is based on psychotic symptoms (delusions, hallucinations, cognitive impairment, etc.) that fluctuate and frequently are preceded by insomnia.

• Risk factors include a history of psychosis, bipolar disorder, marital discord, and possibly primiparity (58).

Treatment

• Treatment requires hospitalization of the mother, as the risk of suicide increases by 70-fold in the first postpartum year. Homicidal thoughts are also more common in women affected by postpartum psychosis compared to women affected by other postpartum mood disorders.

- Recurrence is less likely if the psychotic symptoms start within the 1st month after delivery or in the background of bipolar disease. Patients who present early often times have more severe hallucinations and delusions but respond better to treatment. For patients with baseline schizophrenia, the recurrence of psychotic symptoms is as high as 30% to 50% (58).

NEUROLOGIC ABNORMALITIES

- Common peroneal nerve compression with foot drop from improper positioning in stirrups.
- Sacral plexus neuralgia from pressure of the fetal head.
- Sensory loss of skin surrounding Pfannenstiel incision, with usual resolution by 6 months.
- Separation of symphysis pubis or iliosacral synchondroses presenting as pain and inability to walk.

PATIENT EDUCATION

- Postpartum information should be provided to patients as part of their education during pregnancy.
- After delivery and before discharge, women should be given specific instructions regarding complications that might occur and how to contact their care provider.
- Women who develop a postpartum wound infection or mastitis should be instructed on the proper home care of their complication.
- After delivery, all women should receive information about postpartum depression and how to recognize it.
- Contraceptive counseling is an important part of the postdelivery hospitalization period and should include information about resumption of menses and return of fertility.

REFERENCES

1. Lyon RA, Stamm MJ. The onset of ovulation during the puerperium. *Calif Med.* 1946;65: 99–103.
2. Sharman A. Menstruation after childbirth. *Br J Obstet Gynaecol.* 1951;58:440–445.
3. Howie PW. The physiology of the puerperium and lactation. In: Chamberlain G, ed. *Turnbull's obstetrics.* 2nd ed. Edinburgh: Churchill Livingstone, 1995.
4. Robson SC, Dunlop W, Hunter S. Haemodynamic changes during the early puerperium. *BMJ.* 1987;294:1065.
5. Rasmusen NG, Hornnes PJ, Hegedus L. Ultrasonographically determined thyroid size in pregnancy and postpartum: the goitrogenic effect of pregnancy. *Am J Obstet Gynecol.* 1989;160:1216–1220.
6. Charoenkwan K, Phillipson G, Vutyavanich T. Early versus delayed oral fluids and food for reducing complications after major abdominal gynaecologic surgery. *Cochrane Database Syst Rev.* 2007;4:1–27.
7. World Health Organization. Infant and young child feeding: model chapter for textbooks for medical students and allied health professionals. Available at: http://www.who.int/maternal_child_adolescent/documents/9789241597494/en/. Accessed April 30, 2013.
8. Johnston M, Landers S, Noble L, et al. American Academy of Pediatrics Policy Statement: breastfeeding and the use of human milk. *Pediatrics.* 2012;129(3):e827–e841.
9. Postpartum hypertension, seizures, strokes reported with bromocriptine. *FDA Drug Bull.* 1984;14:3–4.
10. Centers for Disease Control and Prevention. Postpartum Tdap vaccination as an option. Available at: http://www.cdc.gov/vaccines/vpd-vac/pertussis/tdap-pregnancy-hcp.htm#postpartum. Accessed April 30, 2013.
11. Centers for Disease Control and Prevention. Seasonal influenza (flu): additional information about vaccination of specific populations. Available at: http://www.cdc.gov/flu/professionals/acip/specificpopulations.htm. Accessed April 30, 2013.

12. Centers for Disease Control and Prevention. Immunization and pregnancy: vaccines keep a pregnant woman and her growing family healthy. Available at: http://www.cdc.gov/vaccines/pubs/downloads/f_preg_chart.pdf. Accessed April 30, 2013.

13. Pritchard JA, Baldwin RM, Dickey JC, et al. Blood volume changes in pregnancy and the puerperium. II. Red blood cell loss and changes in apparent blood volume during and following vaginal delivery, cesarean section, and cesarean section plus total hysterectomy. *Am J Obstet Gynecol.* 1962;84:1271–1282.

14. American College of Obstetricians and Gynecologists. Practice Bulletin #76: Postpartum hemorrhage (reaffirmed 2011). *Obstet Gynecol.* 2006;108(4):1039–1048.

15. Begley CM, Gyte GM, Devane D, et al. Active versus expectant management of the third stage of labor. *Cochrane Database Syst Rev.* 2011;11:CD007412.

16. Combs CA, Murphy EL, Laros RK, Jr. Factors associated with postpartum hemorrhage with vaginal birth. *Obstet Gynecol.* 1991;77:69–76.

17. Combs CA, Murphy EL, Laros RK, Jr. Factors associated with hemorrhage in cesarean deliveries. *Obstet Gynecol.* 1991;77:77–82.

18. Herbert WN, Cefalo RC. Management of postpartum hemorrhage. *Clin Obstet Gynecol.* 1984;27:139–147.

19. Hayashi RN, Castillo MS, Noah ML. Management of severe postpartum hemorrhage with a prostaglandin $F_{2\alpha}$ analogue. *Obstet Gynecol.* 1984;63:806–808.

20. Hertz RH, Sokol RJ, Dierker LJ. Treatment of postpartum uterine atony with prostaglandin E2 vaginal suppositories. *Obstet Gynecol.* 1980;56(1):129–130.

21. Bakri YN, Amri A, Abdul Jabbar F. Tamponade-balloon for obstetrical bleeding. *Int J Gynecol Obstet.* 2001;74:139–142.

22. Lynch C, Coker A, Lawal AH, et al. The B-Lynch surgical technique for the control of massive postpartum haemorrhage: an alternative to hysterectomy? Five cases reported. *Br J Obstet Gynecol.* 1997;104:372–375.

23. Ferguson JM, Bourgeois FJ, Underwood PB. B-Lynch suture for postpartum hemorrhage. *Obstet Gynecol.* 2000;95:1020–1022.

24. Sarojo CSM, Nankani A, El-Hamamy E. Uterine compression sutures, an update: a review of efficacy, safety and complications of B-Lynch suture and other uterine compression techniques for postpartum hemorrhage. *Arch Gynecol Obstet.* 2010;281:581–588.

25. O'Leary JL, O'Leary JA. Uterine artery ligation for control of postcesarean section hemorrhage. *Obstet Gynecol.* 1974;43:849–853.

26. O'Leary JA. Pregnancy following uterine artery ligation. *Obstet Gynecol.* 1980;55:112–113.

27. Burton R, Belfast MA. Etiology and management of hemorrhage. In: Dildy GA, ed. *Critical care obstetrics.* Massachusetts: Blackwell Science, 2004:298–311.

28. Clark SL, Yeh SY, Phelan JP, et al. Emergency hysterectomy for obstetric hemorrhage. *Obstet Gynecol.* 1984;64:376–380.

29. Glickman MG. Pelvic artery embolization. In: Berkowitz RL, ed. *Critical care of the obstetric patient.* New York: Churchill-Livingstone, 1983:165–187.

30. Wu S, Kocherginsky M, Hibbard JU, et al. Abnormal placentation: twenty-year analysis. *Am J Obstet Gynecol.* 2005;192:1458–1461.

31. Miller DA, Chollet JA, Goodwin TM, et al. Clinical risk factors for placenta precia-placenta accreta. *Am J Obstet Gynecol.* 1997;177:210–214.

32. Wortman AC, Alexander JM. Obstetric emergencies: placenta accreta, increta, percreta. *Obstet Gynecol Clin North Am.* 2013;40(1):137–154.

33. Romero R. The management of acquired hemostatic failure during pregnancy. In: Berkowitz RL, ed. *Critical care of the obstetric patient.* New York: Churchill-Livingstone, 1983:219–284.

34. James AH, McLintock C, Lockart E. Postpartum hemorrhage: when uterotonics and sutures fail. *Am J Hematol.* 2012;87:S16–S22.

35. Welsh A, McLintock C, Gatt S, et al. Guidelines for the use for recombinant Factor VII in massive obstetric hemorrhage. *Aust N Z J Obstet Gynaecol.* 2008;48:12–16.

36. Wittereen T, vanStralen G, Zwart J, et al. Puerperal uterine inversion in the Netherlands: a nationwide cohort study. *Acta Obstet Gynecol Scand.* 2013;92(3):334–337.

37. Harris BA. Acute puerperal inversion of the uterus. *Clin Obstet Gynecol.* 1984;27:134–138.
38. Kovacs BW, DeVore GR. Management of acute and subacute puerperal uterine inversion with terbutaline sulfate. *Am J Obstet Gynecol.* 1984;150:784–786.
39. American College of Obstetricians and Gynecologists. Practice Bulletin: 115 Vaginal birth after previous cesarean delivery (reaffirmed 2013). *Obstet Gynecol.* 2010;116(2 Pt 1): 450–463.
40. Landon MD, Hauth JC, Leveno KJ, et al. Maternal and perinatal outcomes associated with a trial of labor after cesarean delivery. *N Engl J Med.* 2004;351(25):2581–2589.
41. Filker R, Monif GRG. The significance of temperature during the first 24 hours postpartum. *Obstet Gynecol.* 1979;53:358–361.
42. Maharaj D, Teach DT. Puerperal pyrexia: a review. Part I. *Obstet Gynecol Surv.* 2007;62(6):393–399.
43. Maharaj D, Teach DT. Puerperal pyrexia: a review. Part II. *Obstet Gynecol Surv.* 2007;62(6):400–406.
44. Faro S. Postpartum endometritis. *Clin Perinatol.* 2005;32:803–814.
45. Gibbs RS. Postpartum infections. In: Sweet RL, Gibbs RS, eds. *Infectious diseases of the female genital tract.* Baltimore: Williams & Wilkins, 1985:277–292.
46. Newton ER, Prihoda TJ, Gibbs RS. A clinical and microbiologic analysis for puerperal endometritis. *Obstet Gynecol.* 1990;75(3 Pt 1):402–406.
47. Smaill F, Gyte GM. Antibiotic prophylaxis for cesarean section. *Cochrane Database Syst Rev.* 2010;(1):CD007482.
48. Duff P. Pathophysiology and management of postcesarean endomyometritis. *Obstet Gynecol.* 1986;67:269–276.
49. Gibbs RS, Rodgers PJ, Castaneda YS, et al. Endometritis following vaginal delivery. *Obstet Gynecol.* 1980;56(5):555–558.
50. Chaim W, Burstein E. Postpartum infection treatments: a review. *Expert Opin Pharmacother.* 2003;4(8):1297–1313.
51. French L, Smaill FM. Antibiotic regimens for endometritis after delivery. *Cochrane Database Syst Rev.* 2012;8:1–91.
52. Hurry DJ, Larsen B, Charles D. Effects of post cesarean section febrile mobility on subsequent fertility. *Obstet Gynecol.* 1984;64(2):256–260.
53. Garcia J, Aboujaoude R, Apuzzio J, et al. Septic pelvic thrombophlebitis: diagnosis and management. *Infect Dis Obstet Gynecol.* 2006;2006:1–4.
54. Brown CE, Stettler RW, Twickler O, et al. Puerperal septic thrombophlebitis: incidence and response to heparin therapy. *Am J Obstet Gynecol.* 1999;181(1):143–148.
55. Beck CT. Postpartum depression—it isn't just the blues. *Am J Nurs.* 2006;106(5):40–50.
56. Cox JC, Holden JM, Sagovsky R. Detection of postnatal depression: developing a 10-item Edinburgh Postnatal Depression Scale. *Br J Psychiatry.* 1987;150:782–786.
57. American Psychiatric Association. *Diagnostic and Statistical Manual of Mental Disorders.* 5th ed. Arlington: American Psychiatric Association. 2013.
58. Sit D, Rothchild AJ, Wisner KL. A review of postpartum psychosis. *J Womens Health (Larchmt).* 2006;15(4):352–368.

5

Contraception, Sterilization, and Abortion

Jason J. Woo and H. Trent Mackay

KEY POINTS

- Fertility control and family planning should be considered an integral part of health care.
- Contraception should be readily available to any individual or couple that desires it.
- There are a wide variety of effective contraceptive methods available, and most individuals and couples will be able to find a method that fits their needs.
- Long-acting reversible contraception (LARC), including intrauterine devices (IUDs) and contraceptive implants, have seen an encouraging increase in use and hold great promise to reduce the unintended pregnancy rate in the United States and globally.

CONTRACEPTION

Contraceptive Effectiveness

Background

- Table 5-1 presents data on contraceptive effectiveness collected from a variety of sources by Trussell (1).
  - The *perfect use* rates represent the author's "best guess" of the failure rate during the first 12 months of use among couples who use the method perfectly.
  - The *typical use* rate is the rate of failure in the 1st year of use among average users who may use the method incorrectly or inconsistently.
- In counseling patients about contraceptive choice, it is important to recognize one's own biases about the methods. It is fairly common for counselors to quote *perfect use* failure rates for methods that they favor while quoting *typical use* rates for those they disfavor.
- In the United States, over a third of all women who have used at least one method of contraception have discontinued due to dissatisfaction, but there is a wide variation in discontinuation among specific methods. Good follow-up is essential to ensure users are comfortable with their choice of contraceptive method.

Evaluation

- Although no perfect contraceptive exists, a wide range of methods are available, and almost every user and couple should be able to find a method that suits their needs.
- To choose a contraceptive method that will be effective for them, couples and individuals need information and advice from their medical care provider. This should include method-specific information on:
  - Efficacy
  - Side effects
  - Risks
  - Potential benefits
  - Convenience
  - Expense
- Providers need to evaluate prospective users for contraindications (2).

Table 5-1	Contraceptive Failure Rates	
	Percentage of women experiencing an unintended pregnancy in the 1st year of use	
Method	**Perfect use**	**Typical use**
No method	85	85
Withdrawal	4	22
Spermicides	18	28
Fertility awareness methods		24
Standard days	5	—
Two day	4	—
Ovulation method	3	—
Symptothermal	0.4	—
Withdrawal	4	22
Sponge		
Parous women	20	24
Nulliparous women	9	12
Diaphragm	6	12
Condom		
Female	5	21
Male	2	18
Intrauterine device		
Mirena	0.12	0.12
TCu 380A or ParaGard (copper T)	0.6	0.8
Combined pill and mini-pill	0.3	9
Evra patch	0.3	9
NuvaRing	0.3	9
Depo-Provera	0.32	6
Implanon	0.05	0.05
Female sterilization	0.50	0.50
Male sterilization	0.10	0.15

Adapted from Trussell J. Contraceptive efficacy. In: Hatcher RA, Trussell J, Stewart F, et al., eds. *Contraceptive technology*. 20th ed. New York: Ardent Media, 2011.

Hormonal Contraception
Combined Oral Contraceptives (COC)
Background
- Oral contraceptives prevent pregnancy primarily by inhibiting ovulation, although thickening of cervical mucus, endometrial changes, and reduction of tubal motility may also contribute.
- Combination hormone preparations:
  - With combination therapy, a tablet containing both an estrogen and a progestin is taken for 21 days, beginning between the 1st and 5th days of the menstrual cycle or on the first Sunday after the menses begin.
  - The primary antifertility effect is mediated by the progestin, which prevents ovulation and effects changes in the endometrium and the cervical mucus.
  - The estrogen is added principally to decrease the number of days of vaginal bleeding experienced by the patient.

- Triphasic pills contain different doses of progestin, and in some cases estrogen, in each 7-day segment of the cycle and allow a reduction in hormone dose from the levels in the monophasic pills.
- A formulation, Seasonale, is approved in the United States to reduce a women's menstrual cycle to four times a year instead of the usual 13 times. Previously, women were instructed to continue taking the active birth control pills without placebo to delay their periods.
- Combined oral contraceptives (COCs) do not protect against STI/HIV. If there is a risk of STI/HIV, consistent and correct condom use is recommended, either alone or with another contraceptive method.

Effect on Various Organ Systems

- In addition to their effect on fertility, oral contraceptives exert effects on many other organ systems. Some of these effects may be beneficial (11), while others may be unwanted. For example, certain organ function tests are altered substantially by oral contraceptives, thus complicating the diagnosis of disease in these organs during oral contraceptive use.
- Contraindications to the use of contraceptive pills frequently are based on the drug's effects on a particular organ system. The side effects of the pills may result from an undesirable action of the drug on certain organs.

Effect on Reproductive Organs

- COCs prevent ovulation, thus decreasing the incidence of functional ovarian cysts, although there is less suppression of ovarian cysts with the low-dose monophasic and multiphasic pills. COCs are an effective treatment for patients with polycystic ovarian syndrome (PCOS) (3).
- Breast effects:
  - Oral contraceptives decrease the incidence of benign breast disease.
  - There is no evidence of an overall increase in the risk of breast cancer with pill use (4). Among users with a family history of breast cancer, there is no increased risk of breast cancer compared with non-COC users with a family history of breast cancer.
  - Breast tenderness is a well-recognized side effect of oral contraceptives, caused primarily by the estrogen component.
- If given during the postpartum period, combination (but not progestin-only) pills may decrease milk production, as well as the milk's protein and fat content.

Effect on Other Endocrine Organs

- Estrogen increases the amount of circulating binding globulins, thus increasing the total amount of bound circulating hydrocortisone and thyroxine. Because these increases are in the bound (inactive) fraction of the hormone, no recognized change occurs in either adrenal or thyroid function.
- Although low-dose oral contraceptives may cause a slight decrease in glucose tolerance, there is no evidence of an increased risk of developing overt diabetes.
  - Women with a history of gestational diabetes may safely use oral contraceptives.
  - Women under age 35 with overt diabetes of less than 20 years' duration, without vascular disease, may safely use oral contraceptives with appropriate monitoring (2).

Effect on Other Organ Systems

- Minimal changes in certain blood-clotting factors have been reported with low-dose oral contraceptives. There is a small increase in the risk of venous thromboembolism (VTE), primarily in the 1st year of use.
- The hypertension that occurs in a small number of patients taking oral contraceptives may be mediated through changes in the renin–angiotensin system. The blood pressure usually returns to normal when the pills are discontinued.
- Liver effects:
  - Some liver function tests may show elevated levels, but this change is of no known clinical significance.

- COCs are metabolized by the liver, and their use may adversely affect women whose liver is already compromised. COC use has not been shown to inhibit the action of other drugs, but some medications can clinically interfere with the action of COCs, including barbiturates, sulfonamides, cyclophosphamide, and rifampin. While evidence of a clear negative impact on the contraceptive effectiveness of COCs is lacking, it is prudent to suggest use of an alternative or additional contraceptive method when using these other medications.
- Cholestasis may occur with use of oral contraceptives, just as it may occur during pregnancy.
- Hyperpigmentation of the face in a butterfly distribution (melasma) occurs in a few patients taking oral contraceptives. This may not disappear completely after discontinuation of pill use.

Side Effects

- Because oral contraceptives are potent agents capable of exerting effects on virtually all organ systems, it is not surprising that side effects are common. Most are merely annoying, but a few are life threatening.
- Counseling patients who choose oral contraception must include a description of the possible serious complications and an estimation of the risk for the patient.

Major Considerations
Vascular Complications

- Studies have shown a two- to sevenfold increased risk of VTE in users of combined hormonal contraceptives (CHCs) compared with women who do not use CHCs (5).
- COCs containing third-generation progestogens (desogestrel, norgestimate, and gestodene) or the progestin drospirenone have a greater risk of VTE (1.5- to 3-fold increase over levonorgestrel).
- The most important risk factor for thromboembolism appears to be inherited thrombophilia. Routine screening is NOT appropriate because of the rarity of the conditions and the high cost of screening (6).
- Recent meta-analysis studies have shown an increased risk of stroke and myocardial infarction (MI) even with current low-dose OC formulations containing second- and third-generation progestogens. Age, apart from cardiovascular risk factors, appears to be the predominant factor in this increased risk, so use of low-dose OCs in healthy women should not increase the incidence of these adverse outcomes (7).
- Women with underlying vascular disease have an increased risk of arterial thrombosis with COC use and should not use COCs. Because of the association of vascular-type headaches and stroke, women who develop migraine headaches associated with aura also should not use COCs (2).
- The risk of developing a blood clot from a CHC is higher than when not using CHC but still remains lower than the risk of developing blood clots in pregnancy and in the postpartum period (8).

Liver Tumors

- Oral contraceptive use has been associated with the development of a rare liver tumor, benign hepatocellular adenoma. These tumors appeared to be related to the estrogenic component and are related to both historically higher-dose formulations and extended duration of use of oral contraceptives. More recent data show an emerging role of obesity as a contributing factor rather than current COC formulations (9).
- Although some of the tumors have been resected successfully, they will usually regress spontaneously if oral contraceptives are discontinued.

Breast Cancer

- Although the majority of studies to date, including the large Cancer and Steroid Hormone study (10), show no overall increase in breast cancer risk, several studies have suggested a small increased risk of premenopausal breast cancer among current oral contraceptive users.

- A study that analyzed various formulations of oral contraceptives found no evidence that breast cancer risk varies significantly by OC formulation, and no specific OC formulation was associated with a significantly increased risk of breast cancer (4).

Endometrial and Ovarian Cancer

- Oral contraceptive use has been shown to decrease the incidence of both endometrial and ovarian cancers (8). Almost all of the studies on both these cancers and oral contraceptive use have shown a protective effect.
  - For women who have used oral contraceptives for at least 1 year, the relative risk of endometrial cancer is 0.5.
  - The relative risk of ovarian cancer is 0.6, and a protective effect is seen with as little as 3 to 6 months of use.
- For both cancers, the protective effect continues for at least 15 to 20 years after the last use of oral contraceptives.

Cervical Cancer

- The association of oral contraceptive use and cervical cancer remains controversial. A large systematic review of the literature showed a significantly increased risk with more than 5 years of use by women who are positive for human papillomavirus (12).
- Most studies of oral contraceptive use and the risk of cervical dysplasia, carcinoma in situ, and invasive cancer have found a small increase in risk. Unfortunately, many of the studies failed to control for at least a few of the known risk factors related to the risk of cervical cancer, such as number of sexual partners, age at first intercourse, and smoking history.

Hypertension

- Oral contraceptives appear to be associated with a small increase in the incidence of hypertension.
  - In most women who experience hypertension with oral contraceptives, the rise in blood pressure is small.
  - A few women may experience a more severe elevation in blood pressure, presumably as a result of a derangement in the renin–angiotensin system.
- Among women with preexisting hypertension, smoking, along with oral contraceptive use, is associated with an increased risk of cardiovascular disease, particularly in women over the age of 35. Women over the age of 35 who smoke should not use COCs. Nonsmoking women with well-controlled hypertension can usually use oral contraceptives safely (2).
- A history of pregnancy-induced hypertension is not a contraindication to oral contraceptive use.
- Blood pressure monitoring is important for all oral contraceptive users, particularly in the first few months of use.

Minor Side Effects

- Certain minor but troublesome side effects are associated with oral contraceptive use. These symptoms include breakthrough bleeding, nausea, vomiting, and weight gain (13).

Intermenstrual Bleeding

- Intermenstrual bleeding is common during the first 3 months of oral contraceptive use and will usually abate by the 4th month of use.
- After the first 3 months of use, bleeding that occurs early in the cycle may be related to the low estrogen content of the pill, and bleeding that occurs late in the cycle may be the result of a deficient progestin content.
- Although the bleeding may disappear spontaneously, switching to a different pill with an appropriate balance of hormones will usually solve the problem.

Nausea and Vomiting
- Nausea and vomiting are related to the estrogen content of the pill. They occur most commonly during the first few months of pill use.
- The symptoms may be eliminated by switching to a pill with a lower estrogen content or by simply having the patient take the pill consistently with the evening meal or at bedtime.

Weight Gain
- Weight gain is reported frequently with oral contraceptives, although scientific evidence does not support a causal association between COCs or a combination skin patch and weight change (13).
- Most comparisons of different combination contraceptives show no substantial difference in weight changes.

Continuous Use and Postpill Amenorrhea
- Use of OCPs in a continuous manner, where patients remain on active hormonal contraceptive pills without a week of placebo pills, is a treatment for primary dysmenorrhea or endometriosis and may induce amenorrhea throughout the treatment period (14).
- The occurrence of post-OC amenorrhea has been estimated to range from 0.2% to 3.1% depending on the definition of the duration of amenorrhea; however, there does not seem to be any significant difference between the occurrence of spontaneous and post-OC amenorrhea.
- A diagnostic investigation is indicated if amenorrhea continues for 6 months or more or is associated with galactorrhea.

Contraindications
Absolute Contraindications
- Use of the combination oral contraceptives is not recommended if any of the following is present (2):
  - Known thrombophilia, history of or current thrombophlebitis, pulmonary embolus, cerebral hemorrhage, coronary artery disease, or valvular heart disease with complications
  - Current markedly impaired liver function
  - History of or current hepatic adenoma or carcinoma
  - Known or suspected carcinoma of the breast or other estrogen-dependent tumor
  - Pregnancy
  - Diabetes with vascular disease or diabetes of greater than 20 years' duration
  - Lactation less than 6 weeks postpartum
  - Migraine headaches with aura
  - Age over 35 and smoking greater than 15 cigarettes per day
  - Uncontrolled hypertension
  - Surgery or orthopedic injury requiring prolonged immobilization

Caution
- Caution should be exercised in prescribing oral contraceptives for patients who have the following conditions:
  - Hypertension
  - Gallbladder disease
  - Diabetes
  - Migraine without aura
  - Cholestasis during pregnancy
  - Cardiac or renal disease
  - Planned elective major surgery
  - Family history of hyperlipidemia or MI in a parent or sibling younger than 50 years
  - Undiagnosed genital bleeding
  - Sickle cell disease or sickle C disease
  - Active gallbladder disease

Choice of Medication

Initial Prescription

- When a patient has decided to take oral contraceptives, a pill with as low a dose of estrogen as the patient will tolerate should be prescribed because most of the serious complications are related to the estrogen component.
- When prescribing the pill, be certain that the patient does not have an absolute contraindication. If a relative contraindication exists, inform the patient and encourage her to consider other contraceptive methods (2).
- The patient who is just beginning to use oral contraception should be given sufficient medication for a 3-month period, and she should be encouraged to read the package insert. Any symptom of thrombophlebitis, pulmonary embolism, coronary occlusion, cerebrovascular accident, or an eye problem should be reported immediately.
- The patient may start using the pill the day she receives the medication (Quick Start) or wait until the start of her next period. Evidence suggests that neither the risk of inadvertently starting COCs in a woman who is pregnant nor the risk of pregnancy after COC initiation are affected by the cycle day on which COCs are started. While starting CHCs via Quick Start may initially increase continuation compared with more conventional starting strategies, evidence suggests that this difference disappears over time (15).
- If the patient reports no problems, she should be seen at 3 months, at which time
  - A history should be obtained regarding headaches, blurred vision, and leg, chest, or abdominal pain.
  - Blood pressure should be checked.
  - The patient should be encouraged to raise any concerns that may affect her willingness to continue with her current choice.
- The patient should then be seen at 12-month intervals, at which time a history of possible complications and blood pressure are taken, and, if indicated, a brief physical examination, including breast, abdominal, and pelvic examination as well as health screening tests as indicated.

Nonoral Combined Hormonal Contraceptives

Transdermal Patch

Background

- The Ortho Evra patch contains ethinyl estradiol and the progestin norelgestromin. The patch is used weekly for 3 weeks on with 1 week off.
- The patch has the potential for improved compliance as a woman does not have to remember to take a pill daily. Studies have demonstrated an improvement of 5% to 15% perfect compliance rate with the patch over oral contraceptives (16).

Effects

- Efficacy, contraindications, side effects, and complications are similar to those with COCs. Skin irritation from the patch also occurs in up to 20% of users.

Complications

- Concern has arisen about the patch's potential for a higher risk of cardiovascular complications because of a higher steady state concentration and area under the curve (AUC), and a lower peak concentration of ethinyl estradiol in comparison with 35 µg oral contraceptives.
- There appears to be a slightly higher increased risk of thrombotic events from use of the patch than with COCs, but, as with COCs, this risk is the risk attributed to age and other cardiovascular risk factors (7).

Vaginal Ring

Background

- The NuvaRing is a 54-mm flexible vaginal ring that contains ethinyl estradiol and etonogestrel. The ring is placed in the vagina for 3 weeks and then removed for 1 week.

- Progering is a progesterone vaginal ring currently available in Latin America for use by breast-feeding women. One ring may be used for up to 3 months.
- Although not recommended, the ring may be removed during sexual intercourse for a period of up to 2 hours.

Effects
- The efficacy, contraindications, side effects, and complications of the vaginal ring are similar to those with COCs.
- Cycle control, compliance, and continuation rates are equal or higher than with COCs (17).

Complications
- Expulsion of the ring is reported by 4% to 20% of women.
- Approximately 6% of women using the ring complain of vaginal discharge.

Progestin-Only Hormonal Contraception
Progestin-Only Pill
Background
- The progestin-only pill (or mini-pill) may be appropriate for patients who have a contraindication to an estrogen-containing pill. In the United States, norethindrone (Camila) is the only currently available progestin-only pill, while in Europe, both norethindrone (Micronor) and desogestrel (Cerazette) are available as progestin-only pills.
- The progestin-only pill is recommended over regular birth control pills for women who are breast feeding because the mini-pill does not affect milk production.

Effects
- The mini-pill has not been popular in the United States because of a relatively high frequency of intermenstrual bleeding and irregular menses, in addition to slightly reduced effectiveness compared with COCs. However, it is still a highly effective form of contraception and may be appropriate for selected patients.

Complications
- The major advantage of these pills is that they lack side effects caused by estrogen, so there are fewer serious complications than with COCs.
- The incidence of breakthrough bleeding is substantially higher than with CHCs.

Subdermal Capsules (Implanon/Jadelle/Norplant)
Background
- Norplant, a six-rod system, was the original implantable hormonal contraceptive system approved in the United States but was discontinued in 2002. Norplant II, or Jadelle, is the successor to the original Norplant and consists of two silicone rods each containing 75 mg of levonorgestrel but, though approved by the U.S. Food and Drug Administration (FDA) for up to 5-year use, is not currently marketed in the United States.
- Implanon, a single-rod implant containing etonogestrel, is approved and available in the United States for contraceptive protection for up to 3 years. In 2011, the FDA also approved Nexplanon (Implanon NXT) that is essentially identical to Implanon but with the rod containing barium so that it is detectable by x-ray. Nexplanon also includes a specialized insertion kit to reduce incorrect placements.

Effects
- When Implanon is placed correctly, it is very effective with a failure rate of 0.05%.
- Implanon works primarily by stopping ovulation but also induces changes in the cervical mucus and the uterine lining to keep sperm from reaching the egg.
- Women who are seeking long-term contraception but do not desire sterilization are ideal candidates for Implanon.

Complications

- The most common problems leading to the removal of Implanon include irregular bleeding, headache, and weight gain. Thorough counseling about side effects will reduce the likelihood of early removal.
- Complications with Implanon are fewer than associated with the earlier subdermal capsules, largely because these are related to insertion and removal, including hematoma, slight bleeding, and difficulty with removal due to incorrect insertion.

Medroxyprogesterone Acetate
Background

- Depot medroxyprogesterone acetate (DMPA) is an extremely effective injectable progestin contraceptive.
- DMPA is available as a 150-mg intramuscular dose (Depo-Provera) or 104-mg subcutaneous dose (Depo-subQ Provera 104).

Effects

- The failure rate of DMPA is approximately 0.3 per 100 woman-years at the standard contraceptive dose of 150 mg intramuscularly every 3 months (1).
- Most women using DMPA experience amenorrhea. However, the most common reason for discontinuation is irregular bleeding.
- Women using DMPA generally experience bone loss, but the loss is regained within a few years after discontinuation.
- Other side effects include weight gain, headache, and mood changes. As with Implanon, counseling about potential side effects is important.
- Pregnancy should be ruled out before use, and women with unexplained abnormal vaginal bleeding should not be started on DMPA. There does not appear to be any reason to restrict the use of DMPA in either adolescents or perimenopausal women (18).

Intrauterine Devices
Background

- The history of the IUD dates back to the early 1900s. The modern IUD shaped as a capital "T" did not arrive until the 1960s and has greatly decreased rates of expulsion and dissatisfaction due to cramping or pain. The inventions of the copper IUD and hormonal IUD have further improved the effectiveness of the IUD in preventing pregnancy.
- The IUD is currently the most widely used form of reversible contraception worldwide.

Choice of Device

- Two types of IUDs are currently available in the United States:
  - ParaGard or TCu 380A, a copper-containing device
  - Mirena, a levonorgestrel-releasing IUD

ParaGard

- The ParaGard or TCu 380A is a T-shaped device with copper wire wound around the vertical arm and copper sleeves on the horizontal arms.
- It is approved by the U.S. FDA for 10 years' use.
- The typical failure rate is 0.8 pregnancies per 100 woman-years.

Mirena Intrauterine System

- The Mirena Intrauterine System releases levonorgestrel at the rate of 20 µg/d, and it is approved by the FDA for 5 years' use.
- The typical failure rate is 0.1 per 100 women-years.
- While irregular bleeding is common during the first 6 to 12 months, most women subsequently experience reduced menstrual blood loss or amenorrhea.
- Mirena is also approved by the FDA for treatment of menorrhagia.

Effectiveness
- The typical failure rate with the IUD is approximately 1 to 2 pregnancies per 100 woman-years, and the lowest reported rate is 0.6 to 1.5 pregnancies. Because the method does not depend on the user to any significant degree after placement of the device, the method failures are largely those of unrecognized expulsions or incorrect insertion.
- The exact mechanism of action of the IUD is uncertain. Neither ovulation nor steroidogenesis is affected. Before studies of the IUD were completed, it was believed that the device functioned primarily as an abortifacient—that it prevented implantation of the fertilized egg. However, there is considerable evidence that the IUD acts before fertilization, possibly by affecting ovum transport or by immobilizing sperm.

Complications
- The only relatively serious complications of IUDs are uterine perforation, pregnancy, and pelvic inflammatory disease (PID). Minor complications, such as cramps and bleeding, are serious only if they require removal of the device, with subsequent loss of pregnancy protection.
- Spontaneous expulsion occurs in 1% to 10% of users during the 1st year of use and is particularly likely during the first 3 months.
  - Expulsion may occur without symptoms, and so the patient must be instructed to palpate the string protruding from the cervix regularly, especially during the first 3 months of use and routinely after menses.

Uterine Perforation
- Uterine perforation is rare when the IUD is placed by an experienced clinician.
- Perforation is usually asymptomatic.
  - Perforation is suspected first when the tail of the device cannot be palpated or seen or when pregnancy occurs. If perforation is suspected, the IUD can be located by one of several methods: an ultrasound of the pelvis or an x-ray film of the pelvis with or without another IUD in the uterus.
  - Although the risk of bowel obstruction is small, IUDs should be surgically removed from the peritoneal cavity. The device may be removed either through laparoscopy, through an incision in the posterior cul-de-sac if the device is behind the uterus, or by laparotomy, if necessary.

Pregnancy with Intrauterine Device in Place
- Ectopic pregnancy should be ruled out, as the pregnancy is more likely to be ectopic than in a patient not using an IUD.
- There is an increased risk of first- or second-trimester spontaneous abortion (including life-threatening septic abortion), as well preterm delivery if the device is left in place.
- If the strings are visible or retrievable, the IUD should be removed. If the IUD cannot be removed, the patient should be informed of the risks associated with continuing the pregnancy and be offered the possibility of a therapeutic termination.
- If she continues the pregnancy, she should be warned to seek care immediately if she experiences bleeding, cramping, lower abdominal pain, abnormal vaginal discharge, or fever (19).

Pelvic Inflammatory Disease
- Women currently using an IUD are more likely to experience PID than those using barrier methods, oral contraceptives, or no method of contraception. However, there has been much confusion about the relation of IUD use to PID.
- In one study (20), reanalyzing information from the Women's Health Study, there was no increased risk of PID in women using an IUD who had only one recent sexual partner and who were either married or cohabiting. Among previously married women, the relative risk was slightly elevated at 1.8, and among never-married women, the relative risk was significantly elevated at 2.6. Single women are probably more likely to have multiple sexual partners and to be exposed to the risk of sexually transmitted pelvic infections.

- The risk of PID with the IUD is also related to the length of time since insertion. Several studies have shown a transient but statistically significant increase in the risk of PID in the 1st month of use, which then falls gradually over the next few months (21).
- Although infections that occur at the time of insertion or in the first few months of use may be related to bacterial contamination at the time of IUD insertion, infections occurring after this time are probably caused by sexually transmitted organisms.
  - A recent study of nearly 2000 women receiving IUDs showed a very low rate of pelvic infection in women at low risk of sexually transmitted infections.
  - Although some studies have suggested that prophylactic antibiotics may reduce early infection with IUDs, the risk appears to be negligible in women at low risk of sexually transmitted diseases (22).
- Any IUD user who complains of fever, pelvic pain, abdominal tenderness, cramping, or unusual vaginal bleeding should be suspected of harboring a pelvic infection. The patient should be instructed to report to her physician when any of these symptoms appears.
  - If pelvic examination reveals suspected PID, appropriate diagnostic tests should be performed.
  - The IUD does not have to be removed (19).
  - If the infection appears to be mild, the patient need not be hospitalized.

Intrauterine Device Insertion
- Insertion is an outpatient procedure that should be performed only by trained health care professionals.
- IUDs are considered appropriate for the majority of women, including nulliparous women and adolescents.
- There is fair evidence indicating that timing of IUD insertion has little effect on contraceptive continuation, effectiveness, or safety (23). Both immediate postpartum insertion (within 10 minutes of placental delivery) and delayed postpartum insertion (within 4 weeks of placental delivery) are acceptable. Similarly, postabortion (spontaneous or elective) insertion is acceptable.

Contraindications
Absolute Contraindications
- Active or recent pelvic infection.
- Suspected pregnancy. To avoid inadvertent insertion into a pregnant uterus, it is best to perform insertion during menses or in the first 2 weeks of the cycle. However, if it is certain that the patient is not pregnant, insertion may be performed at any time in the cycle.
- Severely distorted uterine cavity due to conditions such as leiomyomata, endometrial polyps, or a bicornuate uterus.
- Undiagnosed abnormal vaginal bleeding, suspicion of genital malignancy, or an unresolved abnormal Papanicolaou test.

Relative Contraindications
- Active liver disease (Mirena only)
- Risk factors for PID, such as exposure to sexually transmitted diseases, including a recent postabortal infection or puerperal endometritis, multiple sexual partners, or an impaired response to infection such as occurs with human immunodeficiency virus (HIV) or steroid treatment

Barrier Methods
Diaphragm and Spermicide
Background
- The diaphragm is a dome-shaped device that is inserted over the cervix before coitus. The dome is molded of a thin layer of latex and is surrounded by a firm ring formed by a circular, rubber-covered spring. The device is squeezed to allow insertion through the

introitus into the vagina, where it assumes its original shape because it fits the contours of the vagina. The diaphragm is available in diameters ranging from 50 to 95 mm and must be properly fitted by a health care provider to the individual patient.

- The device prevents pregnancy by the dual mechanism of a partial physical barrier between the sperm and the cervix and the spermicidal action of the vaginal cream or jelly used with the diaphragm. Use of the diaphragm without the spermicidal agent is associated with a high failure rate.

Effects

- The device has a *perfect use failure rate* of six pregnancies per 100 woman-years, with a *typical failure rate* of 16.
- No serious side effects are definitely associated with diaphragm use, although there have been reports of nonfatal toxic shock syndrome associated with the device.

Complications

- There appears to be an approximately twofold increase in the risk of urinary tract infections among diaphragm users, probably related to changes in vaginal flora and the pressure of the diaphragm on the urethra (24).
- Concerns about the teratogenicity of nonoxynol-9 spermicidal preparations have largely been put to rest by several reports (25).

Method of Use

- The clinician estimates the distance from the posterior fornix of the vagina to the posterior surface of the symphysis pubis by careful pelvic examination. The diaphragm prescribed should be the largest one that will fit comfortably between these two points.
- Diaphragms come in several different styles, including flat spring, coil spring, and arcing spring, and it is important to fit the patient with the specific style that she will use.
- Before insertion, an appropriate amount of spermicidal jelly or cream is placed on the surface of the dome that is fitted against the cervix.
- The diaphragm may be inserted from a few minutes to an hour or more before intercourse and should be removed no sooner than 6 to 8 hours after intercourse. If a second coital episode occurs during the 6-hour interval, additional spermicide should be inserted without removing the diaphragm.

Contraindications

- Severe vaginal prolapse, cystocele, and urethrocele may interfere with a good fitting of the device, and pelvic relaxation constitutes a relative contraindication.
- Women who have previously had toxic shock syndrome, who have latex allergy, or who have recurrent urinary tract infections are not good candidates for diaphragms.

Cervical Cap
Background

- The cervical cap is a cup-shaped device that is inserted directly onto the cervix before coitus. Proper fitting is critical to effective use, as is use with a spermicide cream or jelly.
- FemCap is the only cervical cap currently marketed in the United States.

Effects

- The effectiveness of the cervical cap is higher in nulliparous women than in parous women, with approximately a 14% and 29% failure rate, respectively.

Complications

- Most women can use the cervical cap with no problems. Minor side effects such as vaginal irritation or discomfort may occur.

Method of Use

- The FemCap must be carefully fitted to the cervix because it maintains its position by suction, and a loose-fitting cap will not stay in place. The cap should be one-third filled with spermicidal jelly or cream.

- The cap may be inserted many hours in advance of coitus and remain effective for 48 hours after insertion.
- The cap should be checked for dislodgement after intercourse and left in place for at least 6 hours but no longer than 24 hours after intercourse.
- The cap should be removed by breaking the seal on the cervix with pressure on one side of the rim.
- The cap should not be used with any kind of vaginal bleeding, including during menses.

Contraindications
- Contraindications to cap use include the inability to fit a cap or the inability of the woman to insert the cap properly.
- Significant structural abnormalities of the cervix, allergy to latex or spermicide, and a history of toxic shock syndrome are also contraindications.

Contraceptive Sponge
Background
- After a number of years off the market, the Today sponge has been reapproved by the FDA and is now available as an over-the-counter contraceptive. Pharmatex and Protectaid are other contraceptive sponges available outside of the United States.
- The sponge is composed of polyurethane foam impregnated with nonoxynol-9.

Effects
- The *perfect use effectiveness rate* is approximately 90%, and there is no difference in the effectiveness between nulliparous and parous women.

Complications
- Improper use, such as leaving the sponge in too long, can result in toxic shock syndrome.
- Some women may be allergic to the spermicide used in the sponge.

Method of Use
- The sponge should be moistened with tap water and inserted with the concave side toward the cervix. It can be removed by grasping the string loop on the opposite side.
- It may be placed in the vagina up to 24 hours before intercourse and should be left in place for 6 hours after intercourse. It should not remain in the vagina for more than 30 hours.
- The sponge should not be used with any kind of vaginal bleeding, including during menses.

Male Condom
Background
- In addition to its contraceptive effect, the condom is an effective barrier to the transmission of some sexually transmitted diseases, including HIV, gonorrhea, chlamydia, and Trichomonas, and it may reduce transmission of other sexually transmitted diseases (26).

Effects
- Condoms have a *perfect use failure rate* of 2 pregnancies per 100 woman-years. The *typical failure rate* is 15 pregnancies per 100 woman-years.

Complications
- No known serious complications are associated with the use of the condom.
- A few patients experience an allergy to latex. Some patients will complain that use of a condom results in a decrease in sensation during intercourse; these couples should be encouraged to use another method of contraception.

Method of Use
- Because the condom depends on physical factors for its effectiveness, it is important to discuss the technique of use in some detail with patients who plan to use this form of contraception.
- The patient should be given the following instructions:

- Place the condom on the erect penis before any penile penetration of the vagina is permitted.
- Immediately after ejaculation and before the erection is lost, withdraw the penis, taking care to hold the rim of the condom so it cannot slip off the penis.
- A contraceptive jelly, cream, or foam may be used to increase the contraceptive effectiveness of the condom. Do not use petroleum jelly as a lubricant.

Female Condom
Background
- The first female condom, FC1, was made from polyurethane. The current female condom, FC2, was approved by the FDA in 2009 and is made from synthetic nitrile.
- The majority of female condoms have been purchased by donor agencies and distributed in 100 countries across the world.

Effects
- Effectiveness is similar to that of other female barrier methods, with a *typical use failure rate* of 21% and *perfect use failure rate* of 5% (1).
- The female condom also reduces the risk of acquisition of many sexually transmitted infections, including HIV.

Complications
- Minor side effects include irritation of the vagina, vulva, penis, or anus.
- The condom may slip into the vagina during intercourse.

Method of Use
- To insert the female condom:
  - Spermicide or lubricant is first placed on the outside of the closed end.
  - The sides of the inner ring (at the close end) are squeezed and inserted into the vagina like a tampon, then pushing the inner ring up to the cervix with the index finger. The outer ring remains on the outside of the vagina.
- The penis should be guided into the female condom in order to ensure that it does not slip into the vagina outside the condom.
- The female condom should not be used at the same time as a male condom because the friction between them may cause the condoms to break.

Spermicides
Background
- A number of different spermicidal preparations are available, including foams, creams, gels, suppositories, and film. Each of the preparations contains nonoxynol-9 in varying quantities and concentrations.

Effects
- Pregnancy rates associated with *perfect use* are about 18%, and rates associated with *typical use* are 29% or higher.

Complications
- Spermicides are free of serious side effects, although irritation is common, and the unpleasant taste of the preparations may interfere with pleasurable orogenital contact.
- Spermicides have been demonstrated to interfere with the normal vaginal flora and promote overgrowth of pathogenic organisms associated with urinary tract infections.
- Spermicides containing nonoxynol-9 appear to have a small protective effect against bacterial sexually transmitted diseases, but current evidence shows no effect against HIV. There is concern that epithelial disruption associated with frequent spermicide use could increase the risk of HIV transmission, and a study of prostitutes, using spermicide up to 20 times per day, actually demonstrated an increased risk of HIV transmission compared to a placebo compound (27).

Method of Use

• Most spermicidal preparations may be used alone or with a condom, and some are meant to be used only with a diaphragm. Most preparations are effective for up to 1 hour after insertion. The film and suppository require 15 minutes to melt and disperse before intercourse, and the foams, creams, and gels are effective immediately after insertion.

• The foams, creams, and gels are inserted high into the vagina with an applicator, and the film and suppositories are placed high in the vagina, next to the cervix, with the index or middle finger.

• If intercourse is repeated, a new application of spermicide is necessary, and the preparation must remain in the vagina for at least 6 hours before rinsing or douching.

Natural Family Planning

Background

• Several methods of natural family planning are based on the detection of ovulation with periodic abstinence during the fertile period.

• Because these methods require abstinence for varying periods during the cycle, they require a high degree of motivation as well as careful training of the users.

• These methods have the approval of the Roman Catholic Church, a factor that may be of importance to some couples.

Calendar Method

• In the calendar method, a woman records the length of her menstrual cycle for 6 to 12 months.

• Because ovulation occurs 12 to 16 days before the 1st day of the next menstrual period, and the life span of the ovum is 24 hours and that of sperm is 48 hours, the fertile period can be calculated in the following way:

  • The beginning of the fertile period can be estimated by subtracting 18 days (16 days plus 2 days sperm survival) from the shortest cycle.

  • The end of the fertile period can be estimated by subtracting 11 days (12 days minus 1 day ovum survival) from the length of the longest cycle.

• For instance, if a woman has cycles varying from 24 to 34 days in length, she should abstain from day 6 of her cycle (24 − 18 = 6) to day 23 (34 − 11 = 23), a total of 17 days of abstinence in each cycle. These dates theoretically should encompass all possible pregnancy exposure dates.

• The more irregular the cycles, the longer the period of abstinence should be.

• There are widely varying reports of efficacy with this method, but well-designed studies show a typical use failure rate of approximately 13 per 100 woman-years.

Basal Body Temperature Method

• If a woman takes her temperature under the same conditions and at the same time every morning, that is, under basal conditions, a biphasic curve will be recognized if she is menstruating normally.

• Shortly after ovulation, the basal temperature rises 0.6°F to 0.88°F, and when the temperature rise has been sustained for 3 days, this is good evidence that ovulation has occurred, and the remainder of the month is a "safe" period.

• Although this technique may be used alone as a method of contraception, it is frequently used in conjunction with the mucous method.

Mucous Method

• The mucous method is based on the recognition of changes in vaginal secretions, from the thick, tenacious cervical secretions of the preovulatory and postovulatory periods to the thin, watery secretions of the ovulatory period. It is safe to have intercourse when the ovulatory mucus is no longer present.

• Confusion can result from the presence of vaginal discharge resulting from infection or from the use of intravaginal medications.

Symptothermal Method
- The symptothermal method combines several of the previously natural family planning methods and adds some additional techniques.
- In general, both the basal body temperature and cervical mucus are monitored. With this method, the 1st day of mucus change would indicate the need for abstinence until 3 days after the rise in basal body temperature or 4 days after the peak mucus.
- In addition, women may watch for symptoms that precede or accompany ovulation such as mittelschmerz, spotting, vulvar swelling, or breast tenderness. Softening and dilation of the cervix and movement of the cervix to a position higher or deeper in the vagina may also be detected.

Standard Days Method
- The standard days method uses a set of beads to remind couples to avoid intercourse on days 8 through 19. The beads are color-coded to differentiate between days when pregnancy may be a risk and "safe" days. A movable ring is repositioned to a new bead each day.
- The method has a *perfect use failure rate* of 5% and a *typical use failure rate* of 12% in women with 29- to 32-day cycles (28).

Two-Day Method
- The two-day method may be used by women with any cycle length. Each day, the woman determines whether she is having cervical secretions that day and if she had them the previous day. If she is without cervical secretions for two consecutive days, she can consider herself "safe."
- This method has a *perfect use failure rate* of 4% and a *typical use rate* of 14% (29).

Miscellaneous Methods
Withdrawal
- Withdrawal as a method of contraception is very old but unreliable. The method has a *perfect use rate* of 4% and a *typical failure rate* of 27%.
- The risks of the method are that (a) preejaculatory secretions of the male frequently contain sperm, (b) precise male control is difficult to achieve, and (c) the method may exert an adverse emotional impact on one or both partners.
- The advantage of the method is that it is available under all circumstances and at no cost.

Lactation Amenorrhea Method (LAM)
- Lactation may provide effective contraception in the postpartum period. Breast-feeding women may not ovulate for as long as 24 months after delivery, although lactational amenorrhea depends on the pattern of breast-feeding.
- During the first 6 months postpartum, women who are breast-feeding with little or no supplementation and whose menses have not returned, have a pregnancy rate of less than 2% (30).

Postcoital/Morning-After/Emergency Contraception
- Postcoital, also referred to as "morning-after" or "emergency" contraception, is a safe and relatively effective way to prevent pregnancy after unprotected intercourse.
- Several choices are available to the physician under these circumstances, but no method is completely satisfactory or always effective.

Hormonal Postcoital Contraception
- Hormonal postcoital contraception has been used with a high degree of effectiveness.
- The Yuzpe regimen, developed by Dr. Albert Yuzpe in 1974, used a combination of 100 µg of ethinyl estradiol and 50 mg of levonorgestrel taken in two doses 12 hours apart within 72 hours of unprotected intercourse. This method prevents approximately 75% of the pregnancies (2% pregnancy rate) that might be expected in the absence of treatment. Modifications of this regimen using various brands of oral contraceptives with different progesterone components have also been utilized with similar results.

- Subsequent studies have shown levonorgestrel alone to be more successful than the combination with ethinyl estradiol, and this has become the standard method in most countries. The current product available in the United States is Plan B, or Plan B One-Step, that contains levonorgestrel 0.75 mg in two doses to be taken 12 hours apart. Taking both doses of levonrogestrel at one time (1.5 mg) is at least as effective as the two-dose regimen. While approved for use within 72 hours (3 days) of unprotected intercourse, it is acceptable to take this regimen for up to 120 hours (5 days) after unprotected intercourse, although there is some diminution of efficacy with time from intercourse (31). Plan B is available over the counter for women age 17 or older.
- Another product, Ella (ellaOne in Europe) was approved in 2010 and contains the selective progesterone receptor modulator (SPRM) ulipristal acetate. It is approved for use within 120 hours (5 days) after unprotected intercourse and has shown to prevent about 60% of expected pregnancies (2.1% pregnancy rate). It is available by prescription only in the United States and Europe.

Copper Intrauterine Device
- Copper-bearing IUDs have been shown to be 99.9% effective as a postcoital contraceptive if inserted within 5 days of unprotected intercourse.
- While more expensive and invasive upfront, the IUD may be left in as an extremely effective birth control for years if effective for emergency contraception (EC).
- Because of the risk of pelvic infection, the IUD should not be used as a postcoital contraceptive for rape victims unless accompanied by prophylactic antibiotic therapy.

STERILIZATION
Epidemiology
- Surgical sterilization has become the most common method of contraception for married couples in the United States. Approximately 1 million sterilization procedures are performed annually in the United States. About 60% of the procedures are performed on women.
- The perceived risks of other highly effective methods of contraception, such as oral contraceptives or the IUD, often lead couples or individuals to choose sterilization when childbearing has been completed.

Legal Requirements
- Legal requirements for sterilization have been introduced by many states, and stringent requirements were introduced by the federal government in 1979 for patients whose medical care is funded by the government. Physicians performing sterilization procedures should be aware of the applicable legal requirements.
- The federal requirements are rigid and include the following restrictions:
  - The patient must be at least 21 years old at the time consent is obtained.
  - The patient must be mentally competent.
  - A 30-day waiting period must expire between the time of consent and the surgical procedure. A reduction in this waiting period to 72 hours is allowed in the case of an individual who consents to be sterilized preceding premature delivery or an emergency abdominal operation. In no case can the 72-hour delay be reduced.
  - The consent cannot be obtained during labor or when a patient is seeking to obtain an abortion.

Procedures
Female Sterilization
- Nearly all operations intended to sterilize women interrupt the continuity of the fallopian tubes. An exception occurs when there is a significant pathologic condition of the uterus. In this case, hysterectomy may be viable option.

- Sterilization may be done in the immediate postpartum period or as an interval procedure.
  - During the postpartum period, a subumbilical minilaparotomy with some variation of the Pomery technique, removing a segment of the fallopian tube, is the most widely used procedure.
  - Laparoscopic tubal ligation using rings, clips, or electrocoagulation is currently the most common interval sterilization approach used in the United States.
  - Minilaparotomy under local or general anesthesia can also be used.
- Complications are rare after sterilization procedures, and mortality is approximately 1 or 2 per 100,000 procedures. If sterilization fails, approximately 30% of the pregnancies will be ectopic.
- For established procedures, failure rates vary with the specific procedure used, but overall at 12 months are approximately 5 per 1000 procedures. A large U.S. prospective study of more than 10,000 women showed an overall sterilization failure rate of 18 per 1000 procedures at 10 years. Some of the procedures with higher failure rates included in this study are no longer in use, so the long-term failure rates with current procedures may be lower.
- A transcervical sterilization procedure (Essure) approved by the FDA in 2003 can be performed in the office with minimal anesthesia.
  - Under hysteroscopic guidance, a tiny coiled wire is placed in each fallopian tube.
  - Over 3 months, the body works with the wire to form a natural barrier within the fallopian tubes. A hysterosalpingogram is performed after 3 months to confirm complete obstruction of the fallopian tubes.
  - When confirmed, Essure has a 5-year 99.8% effectiveness rate.
- Regret about sterilization is relatively common:
  - The incidence is up to 20% in some studies.
  - A much smaller number of women actually seek reversal procedures.
  - Successful reversal has been reported in 51% to 73% of cases, but only 20% to 30% of women are candidates for reversal.

Male Sterilization

- Approximately 40% of the sterilization procedures in the United States are performed on men. The procedure is usually done in the physician's office under local anesthesia.
- Through small scrotal incisions, each vas deferens is identified and ligated at two points with transection between the points of ligature. The cut ends usually are cauterized.
- The mortality associated with the operation is virtually zero, although a few complications such as hematoma formation can occur.
- The *failure rate* is less than 1%. Although operative reversibility frequently is successful, the patient should regard the procedure as permanent.

LEGAL ABORTION
Background
- Legal abortion is the intentional termination of pregnancy before the fetus is viable in a manner consistent with current law or custom.
- At present, in the United States, the law established by the U.S. Supreme Court in 1973 allows abortion to be performed through the second trimester of pregnancy. Many states have legislated restrictions on access to abortion, and the Supreme Court is continuing to review cases that could result in further restrictions.
- In 2009, approximately 784,000 abortions in the United States were reported to the Centers for Disease Control and Prevention. This represented the largest single year decrease during 2000–2009, and the lowest total number, rate, and ratio of abortions since 1984 (31).
- In 2009, approximately 64% of abortions occurred at 8 weeks' gestation or earlier, and 92% of abortions occur at 13 weeks or earlier. About 1.3% of abortions were performed at greater than 21 weeks' gestation.

- Since 1995, the abortion rate has steadily declined over the previous 10 years but has remained essentially unchanged since 2000.
- In 2008, the most recent year for which data are available, 12 women were reported to have died as a result of complications from known legal abortion. There were no reported deaths associated with known illegal abortion.

Selection of Abortion Technique

- The choice of abortion technique will depend primarily on the length of gestation and the presence of a diagnosis that contraindicates a particular technique. The earlier an abortion is performed, the safer the procedure. The later the abortion is performed, the greater is the risk of excessive blood loss or uterine perforation.
- The currently available techniques include
  - Vacuum aspiration
  - Dilation and evacuation
  - Medical abortion with mifepristone or methotrexate, usually combined with a prostaglandin
  - Intravaginal or intra-amniotic use of various agents
- Hysterotomy may be indicated under certain rare circumstances but is almost never performed because of a markedly increased risk of morbidity and mortality.
- Medical abortion, with oral mifepristone, 200 to 600 mg, followed by misoprostol, 400 to 800 mg, orally or vaginally, can be performed up to 9 weeks. Success rates at 63 days range from 82% to 96%, depending upon the dose and route of administration of misoprostol.
  - Methotrexate with misoprostol or misoprostol alone can be used if methotrexate is not available.
  - Because medical abortion does not have a 100% success rate, access to surgical abortion must be available as a backup.
- Abortion with either a handheld syringe and flexible cannula or mechanical suction can be used through 14 to 15 weeks' gestation.
- Dilation and evacuation, requiring instrumental removal of the fetus and placenta, is the most common method after 15 weeks.
- Some physicians continue to prefer other methods for late abortion, notably vaginal prostaglandins.
- Whenever an abortion is performed on an Rh-negative patient whose blood is not sensitized to the Rh factor, $Rh_0(D)$ immunoglobulin should be given.
  - If the pregnancy is 12 gestational weeks or less, a dose of 50 mg within 72 hours of the procedure is sufficient.
  - With later abortion, 300 mg is used.

PATIENT EDUCATION

- The choice of a contraceptive method should be made by the individual after suitable counseling about method technique, safety, and effectiveness.
- Contraceptive counseling should be based on the individual's lifestyle.
- Women need to understand that contraceptive effectiveness depends heavily on personal motivation, perhaps even more than on the effectiveness of the device itself.
- Appropriateness of contraceptive options change for each woman throughout her reproductive lifetime. The health care provider should review these options at each annual visit.
- Sterilization by tubal ligation requires specific counseling and informed consent.

REFERENCES

1. Trussell J. Contraceptive efficacy. In: Hatcher RA, Trussell J, Stewart F, et al., eds. *Contraceptive technology*. 20th ed. New York: Ardent Media, 2011.
2. Centers for Disease Control and Prevention. U.S. medical eligibility criteria for contraceptive use, 2010. *MMWR Recomm Rep.* 2010;59(No. RR-4):1–85.

3. Artini PG, Di Beradino OM, et al. Best methods for identification and treatment of PCOS. *Minerva Medica.* 2010;62(1):33–48.
4. Marchbanks PA, et al. Oral contraceptive formulation and risk of breast cancer. *Contraception.* 2012;85(4):342–350. [PMID: 22067757]
5. Rott H. Thrombotic risks of oral contraceptives. *Curr Opin Obstet Gynecol.* 2012;24(4):235–240.
6. Grimes DA, Stuart GS, Levi EE. Screening women for oral contraception: can family history identify inherited thrombophilias? *Obstet Gynecol.* 2012;120(4):889–895.
7. Lidegaard O, et al. Thrombotic stroke and myocardial infarction with hormonal contraception. *New Engl J Med.* 2012;366(24):2257–2266.
8. FDA Drug Safety Communication: updated information about the risk of blood clots in women taking birth control pills containing drospirenone. 2012 April 10.
9. Chang CY, et al. Changing epidemiology of hepatocellular adenoma in the United States: review of the literature. *Int J Hepatol.* 2013;2013:604860. doi: 10.1155/2013/604860. Epub 2013 Feb 24. [PMID: 23509632]
10. Collaborative Group on Hormonal Factors in Breast Cancer. Breast cancer and hormonal contraceptives: collaborative reanalysis of individual data on 53,297 women with breast cancer and 100,239 women without breast cancer from 54 epidemiological studies. *Lancet.* 1996;347:1713–1727.
11. Huber JC, Bentz EK, Ott J, et al. Non-contraceptive benefits of oral contraceptives. *Expert Opin Pharmacother.* 2008;9(13):2317–2325.
12. International Collaboration of Epidemiological Studies of Cervical Cancer. Cervical cancer and hormonal contraceptives: collaborative reanalysis of individual data for 16,573 women with cervical cancer and 35,509 women without cervical cancer from 24 epidemiological studies. *Lancet.* 2007;370(9599);1609–1621. [PMID: 17993361]
13. Gallo MF, et al. Combination contraceptives: effects on weight. *Cochrane Database Syst Rev.* 2011;(9);CD003987.
14. Dmitrovic R, Kunselman AR, Legro RS. Continuous compared with cyclic oral contraceptives for the treatment of primary dysmenorrhea: a randomized controlled trial. *Obstet Gynecol.* 2012;119(6):1143–1150.
15. Brahmi D, Curtis KM. When can a woman start combined hormonal contraceptives (CHCs)?: a systemic review. *Contraception.* 2012. Pii:S0010-7824(12)00820-7.
16. O'Connell K, Burkman RT. The transdermal contraceptive patch: an updated review. *Clin Obstet Gynecol.* 2007;50(4):918–926.
17. Roumen FJ, Mishell DR. The contraceptive vaginal ring, Nuvaring, a decade after its introduction. *Eur J Contracept Reprod Health Care.* 2012;17(6):415–427.
18. Committee on Adolescent Health Care Long-Acting Reversible Contraception Working Group; the American College of Obstetricians and Gynecologists. Committee Opinion No. 539: Adolescents and long-acting reversible contraception: implants and intrauterine devices. *Obstet Gynecol.* 2012;120(4):983–988. [PMID: 22996129]
19. American College of Obstetricians and Gynecologists. ACOG Practice Bulletin No. 121: Long-acting reversible contraception: implants and intrauterine devices. *Obstet Gynecol.* 2011;118(1):184–196. [PMID: 21691183]
20. Lee NC, Rubin GL, Borucki R. Type of intrauterine device and the risk of pelvic inflammatory disease revisited: new results from the Women's Health Study. *Obstet Gynecol.* 1988;72:1–6.
21. Farley TM, Rosenberg MJ, Rowe PJ, et al. Intrauterine devices and pelvic inflammatory disease: an international perspective. *Lancet.* 1992;339:785–788.
22. Grimes DA, Schulz KF. Prophylactic antibiotics for intrauterine device insertion: a meta-analysis of randomized controlled trials. *Contraception.* 1999;60:57–63.
23. Whiteman MK, et al. When can a woman have an intrauterine device inserted? A systemic review. *Contraception.* 2012. Pii:S0010-7824(12)00744-5.
24. Hooten TM, Hillier S, Johnson C, et al. *Escherichia coli* bacteriuria and contraceptive method. *JAMA.* 1991;265:64–69.
25. Einarson TR, Koren G, Mattice D, et al. Maternal spermicide use and adverse reproductive outcome: a meta-analysis. *Am J Obstet Gynecol.* 1990;162:655–660.

26. Holmes KK, Levine R, Weaver M. Effectiveness of condoms in preventing sexually transmitted infections. *Bull World Health Organ.* 2004;82:454–461.

27. Van Damme L, Ramjee G, Alary M, et al. Effectiveness of COL-1492, a nonoxynol-9 vaginal gel, on HIV-1 transmission in female sex workers: a randomized controlled trial. *Lancet.* 2002;28:971–977.

28. Arevalo M, Jennings V, Sinai I. Efficacy of a new method of family planning: the standard days method. *Contraception.* 2002;65:333–338.

29. Arevalo M, Jennings V, Nikula M, et al. Efficacy of a new TwoDay method of family planning. *Fertil Steril.* 2004;82:885–892.

30. Labbock MH, Hight-Laukaran V, Peterson AE, et al. Multicenter study of the Lactational Amenorrhea Method (LAM): I. Efficacy, duration, and implications for clinical application. *Contraception.* 1997;55:327–336.

31. Gemzell-Danielsson K, Rabe T, Cheng L. Emergency contraception. *Gynecol Endocrinol.* 2013;29(suppl 1):1–14. [PMID: 23437846]

32. Pazol K, et al.; Centers for Disease Control and Prevention. Abortion surveillance—United States, 2009. *MMWR Surveill Summ.* 2012;61(8):1–44. [PMID: 23169413]

PART II

Obstetric Complications

Pregnancy Loss and Spontaneous Abortion

Charles C. Coddington and Albert Asante

KEY POINTS

- Spontaneous abortion is the most common complication of early pregnancy.
- Chromosome abnormalities account for a large percentage of all spontaneous abortions.
- Habitual abortion becomes an issue only after three documented (by pathology or ultrasound with heart beat) consecutive spontaneous abortions.
- Septic abortion remains a relatively rare but potentially lethal complication that requires careful management.

BACKGROUND

Definition

- Abortion is the termination of pregnancy by any means, resulting in the expulsion of an immature, nonviable fetus.
- A fetus of 500 g or less that correlates with 20 to 22 weeks' gestational age (from the 1st day of the last menstrual period), is considered an abortus (1). Note that although "fetus" is the term used in this text for the sake of simplicity, the actual terminology should be "embryo" for any gestation that is 10 weeks or less.
- The term "miscarriage," although imprecise, has been used for all types of pregnancy losses up to a gestational age of 20 to 22 weeks. Often, its use is preferred in discussions with patients, as the word abortion has undesirable connotations for many people.
- Miscarriage is often classified as either a clinical or a biochemical pregnancy loss. Clinical pregnancies are those that can be identified by ultrasound or histological evidence, while biochemical pregnancies occur earlier and can only be identified by a raised quantitative beta-hCG. In practice, the majority of biochemical pregnancy losses go unnoticed.

Etiology

- Although spontaneous abortion has multiple etiologies, chromosome abnormalities are present in up to 60% of abortuses in some studies (2).
- Abortuses after 12 weeks are less likely to be karyotypically abnormal.

Factors that are known to increase the risk for spontaneous abortion include advanced maternal age, alcohol, cigarette smoking, previous spontaneous abortion, and uterine anomalies.

Epidemiology

- The incidence of spontaneous abortion is believed to be 15% to 20% of all pregnancies. Some have estimated the true incidence to be as high as 50% to 78% (3).
- Fetal loss is higher in women in their late 30s and older irrespective of reproductive history. The risk of a spontaneous abortion by age group: age 20 to 30 years: 9% to 17%; age 30 to 35 years: 20%; age 35 to 40 years: 40%; age 40 to 45 years: 80% (4).

THREATENED ABORTION

Laboratory Tests

- Blood count if bleeding has been heavy.
- Serum β-human chorionic gonadotropin (hCG) level if pregnancy is undocumented or unknown location. Positive tests may occur in nonviable gestations because β-hCG may persist in the serum for several weeks after fetal death (5). Serum levels of β-hCG also help discriminate intrauterine from extrauterine pregnancy.
- In the discriminatory hCG zone concept, the level of hCG is defined above which an intrauterine gestational sac should be identifiable by ultrasound for an intrauterine pregnancy. Failure to identify a gestational sac in the uterus defines the pregnancy as being extrauterine. Ultrasound performed at hCG levels below the zone cutoff will not be expected to demonstrate a gestational sac and therefore, will not be able to distinguish between intra- and extrauterine pregnancies.
  - Levels of β-hCG greater than 2500 IU/mL should reflect a greater than 90% chance of intrauterine pregnancy that can be identified by transvaginal ultrasound. Levels greater than 6500 IU/mL should reflect the same capability for transabdominal scans.
- The discriminatory zone is based on a singleton pregnancy. Multiple gestations have proportionately higher hCG levels at any given gestational age. Therefore, the best "discriminatory zone" is a gestation age and not hCG alone (6).
- In pregnancies of 5.5 weeks of gestation or greater (when conception occurs under close observation), transvaginal ultrasonography should identify a viable intrauterine pregnancy with almost 100% accuracy (7,8).
  - In a normal pregnancy, the serum β-hCG level should double every 48 to 72 hours. However, in normal pregnancies, the increase may be as low as 50% over the same 48 to 72 hours (9).
  - Fetal cardiac activity is normally identifiable by ultrasonography at 6 to 7 weeks of gestation by crown–rump length measurement.
  - Absence of fetal heart motion in gestations of 9 weeks or longer predicted nonviable fetuses virtually 100% of the time. Irregular menses and poor or uncertain dates may confuse this evaluation. In such cases, ultrasound should be used to date the pregnancy by crown–rump length (CRL) and use this dating to correlate with the expected rise in β-hCG (serum).
  - Other hormone measurements have not generally been helpful in establishing pregnancy viability or location.
  - Early pregnancy demise has occurred if there is no cardiac activity with CRL ≥7 mm or a gestational sac of ≥25 mm and no embryo or fetal pole identifiable (10).

Diagnosis

Differential Diagnosis

- Benign and malignant lesions of the genital tract:
  - The pregnant cervix often develops an ectropion that is highly vascular, friable, and bleeds easily. Pressure should be applied for several minutes with a large swab to stop any bleeding. If this fails, cautery with silver nitrate sticks is usually successful.
  - Atypical or suspicious cervical lesions should be evaluated with colposcopy or biopsy.
- Anovulatory bleeding:
  - Patients with irregular menses or amenorrhea may have irregular bleeding that can be confused with threatened abortion. The patient should be questioned about a history of similar episodes of irregular bleeding and cycles greater than 35 days.

- Early symptoms of pregnancy are absent, and the pregnancy test is negative.
- On pelvic exam, the uterus is of normal size and firm; the cervix is firm and not cyanotic.
- Disorders of pregnancy:
  - Hydatidiform mole
    - Patients with a hydatidiform mole usually present with unusually high β-hCG levels and a uterus that is inappropriately large for dates and accentuated by early signs/symptoms of pregnancy.
    - The passage of grapelike vesicles from the cervix/vagina arouse suspicion.
    - The diagnosis is made by ultrasound that shows absence of a fetus (although rarely a fetus and molar pregnancy may occur together) and a white "snow storm" pattern of the hydroptic vesicles.
    - No heart tones are heard or seen, and severe hyperemesis, early-onset preeclampsia, or hyperthyroidism may be present.
    - Large ovarian theca lutein cysts may be palpable.
  - Ectopic pregnancy
    - Consider ectopic pregnancy in every patient who has vaginal bleeding and pain in the first trimester. The possibility of ectopic pregnancy is increased if an intrauterine device is in place (11,12).
    - Ectopic pregnancy is associated with a classical triad of symptoms, usually in both ruptured and unruptured cases: delayed menses, vaginal bleeding, and lower abdominal pain.
    - Abdominal tenderness or pain is a common sign. It may be unilateral or generalized, with or without rebound, and of such intensity as to preclude an adequate examination.
    - Light-headedness or syncope (due to hemorrhage and hypovolemia), rectal or urinary pressure, or shoulder pain (due to diaphragmatic irritation) may occur.
    - Pelvic examination usually reveals cervical motion tenderness and/or a bulging cul-de-sac from the hemoperitoneum. An adnexal mass is palpable 50% of the time.
    - Ultrasound will usually show an adnexal mass, often containing a gestational sac, an embryo, and even a fetal heart beat. The presence of free fluid in the abdomen may be indicative of a tubal rupture. This would suggest a more urgent clinical situation.
    - The serum quantitative test will be positive and is most reliable, as the urine pregnancy test may be falsely negative.

Clinical Manifestations

Vaginal bleeding, with or without menstrual-like cramps, in the first 20 weeks of pregnancy is the most common manifestation of threatened abortion. There is frequently no history of passage of tissue or rupture of membranes.
- Symptoms of pregnancy are often decreased in intensity.
- Physical exam is normal, except that the speculum exam may reveal a small amount of bleeding with a closed cervix and no more than mild discomfort.

Treatment
- Traditional treatment is bed rest and abstinence from intercourse; however, controlled studies supporting the efficacy of bed rest are lacking (13).
- Symptoms are best managed on an outpatient basis with hospital admission reserved for heavy bleeding and/or pain relief.

Medications
- There is no evidence that any hormones or medications alter or improve the outcome of threatened abortion in the first and early second trimester.
- Medications given during the period of organogenesis (days 18 to 55 after conception) may have teratogenic effects on the fetus. This may need to be balanced with the health of the mother.

- A regimen of bed rest and abstinence from sexual intercourse seems more rational for late threatened abortions (after 12 weeks of gestation), although the efficacy of such has not been confirmed.

Patient Education

- Patients can be reassured that bleeding during early pregnancy is very common and that the prognosis for a normal child in those who do not abort is excellent. However, some studies have reported that bleeding early in pregnancy is associated with an increase in abruptio placentae, placenta previa, prematurity and its complications, and a slight increase in anomalies, although perinatal mortality is not affected.
- If there is no cramping, the chances are 50% to 75% that the pregnancy will continue successfully. If the pregnancy is 7 to 11 weeks' gestational age and ultrasound has noted no fetal heart beat, there is a 90% to 96% chance the pregnancy will not continue (14).
- The patient should be told to report increased bleeding (greater than a normal menses), cramping, passage of tissue, or fever.
- Tissue passed should be saved for examination.

INEVITABLE ABORTION

Diagnosis

Clinical Manifestations
- The symptoms of threatened abortion are present, and the internal cervical os is dilated as seen on ultrasound exam.
- The patient usually complains of menstrual-like cramps or pelvic pressure.

Differential Diagnosis
- Threatened abortion:
  - The internal cervical os is closed on ultrasound exam.
  - The cervix should not be examined with instruments, as bleeding may also occur with a normal pregnancy.
- Incomplete abortion:
  - The cervix is dilated and either
    ○ Some tissue has already has passed (by history) or
    ○ Tissue is present in the vagina or the endocervical canal
- Complete abortion:
  - Positive pregnancy test with a history of
    ○ Abortion symptoms
    ○ Passage of tissue via vagina
  - No evidence of tissue or gestational sac in the uterus on ultrasound
- Ectopic pregnancy is a possibility if no tissue is present.
- Incompetent cervix:
  - Cervical dilation without pain or contractions that occur only in the second trimester after 15 weeks of gestation.
  - Transvaginal ultrasound of the cervix may show "funneling" of the internal os or shortening (less than 2.5 cm) of the cervical length.

Treatment

Medications
- $Rh_o(D)$ immunoglobulin (RHoGAM) is administered if the patient is Rh negative.

PROCEDURES

- Surgical evacuation of the uterus is advised in nearly all cases because
  - Progression to complete abortion will occur in a few hours to days
  - Placental tissue is likely to be retained in gestations of 10 to 14 weeks.

INCOMPLETE ABORTION

Laboratory Tests
- Complete blood count.
- Rh typing.
- Consider blood type and cross-match if bleeding is heavy or if vital sign postural changes are present.
- Consider karyotyping products of conception (POC) if there is a history of recurrent losses.

Diagnosis
Differential Diagnosis
Differential diagnosis is the same as that for inevitable abortion.

Clinical Manifestations
- Along with cramping and bleeding, the patient may report the passage of tissue. Caution should be taken not to mistake organized clots for tissue.
- Speculum examination reveals a dilated internal os with tissue present in the vagina or endocervical canal.

Treatment
Medications
- RHoGAM is administered to Rh-negative, unsensitized patients.

PROCEDURES
- Stabilization
  - If the patient has signs and symptoms of heavy bleeding, at least one large-bore intravenous catheter suitable for blood transfusion (16 gauge or larger) is started immediately, if she has unstable vital signs.
  - Ringer lactate or normal saline with 30 U oxytocin per 1000 mL is started at 200 mL/h and increased if necessary to obtain uterine tone (the uterus is less sensitive to oxytocin in early pregnancy). Such doses may depress urine output because of the antidiuretic hormone–like activity of oxytocin and should be discontinued as soon as appropriate.
  - POC should be removed from the endocervical canal and uterus with ring forceps or suction. This maneuver often dramatically decreases the bleeding.
- Curettage
  - The patient is placed in a dorsal lithotomy position in stirrups and suitably prepared, draped (as for vaginal delivery), and sedated.
  - Conscious sedation may be used.
  - Bimanual examination confirms the position and size of the uterus and the direction of the endocervical canal.
  - The cervix is exposed, and the vagina and cervix are cleaned with povidone–iodine solution or Hibiclens if the patient has an allergy to iodine.
  - Paracervical block may be performed with chloroprocaine hydrochloride 1% (Nesacaine) or another agent, 12 mL total, divided into equal doses and injected submucosally into the lateral vaginal fornices, with a 20-gauge spinal needle at 2, 4, 8, and 10 o'clock (3 mL each site).
  - Beware of inadvertent intravenous injection. It this occurs, the patient may note tinnitus or a metallic taste in her mouth. Stop and allow symptoms to resolve.
  - Amount of dilation (in millimeters) of cervix required for a given gestation is equal to the gestational age in weeks (e.g., dilate to no. 9 Hegar for a 9-week pregnancy).
  - Curettage is performed carefully but systematically with a suction instrument. A single-tooth tenaculum or a ring forceps placed on the anterior cervical lip is used for countertraction. Vacuum curettage may be faster and result in less blood loss with advanced

gestations. Use of a vacuum curette that is 1 mm smaller than the measured cervical dilation is recommended. To decrease perforation risk, advance the tip of the curette no farther than the middle of the uterine cavity. Ultrasound guidance may be helpful. Sharp curettage and then exploration with polyp or ring forceps should follow vacuum aspiration to ensure completeness.

- Perforation
  - Great care must be used, especially in gestations exceeding 12 to 14 weeks, to avoid perforation of the uterus.
  - Treatment of perforation depends on
    - ○ The location (midline perforations are less likely to damage large blood vessels)
    - ○ The presence or absence of signs of intraperitoneal bleeding
    - ○ Whether the perforation occurred with the suction curette (which increases the chance of bowel or bladder injury)
    - ○ Whether the abortion has been completed
  - Laparoscopy is indicated for perforations. Completion of abortion may be laparoscopically directed (15).
  - Ultrasound guidance may be used (16).
  - During curettage, the uterine cavity should be explored for myoma, septa, and other anomalies that may be related to abortion (17–19).
- Postcurettage
  - The patient is observed for several hours.
  - Repeat blood count is ordered if bleeding has been excessive or if there is temperature greater than 38°C. One might also observe in the hospital setting.
  - Avoid coitus, douching, or the use of tampons for 2 weeks.
  - Oral ferrous sulfate is prescribed if blood loss has been moderate.
  - Analgesics other than ibuprofen are rarely required.
  - Rh-negative, unsensitized patients are given intramuscular RhoGAM.
  - Methylergonovine (0.2 mg orally every 4 hours for 6 doses) may be prescribed in normotensive patients.
  - Follow-up is scheduled in 2 weeks.

REFERRALS/COUNSELING

- The patient should be allowed to express her feelings (20,21).
- A sympathetic, understanding approach is helpful, as feelings of guilt and depression are common (20). Counseling may be a reasonable step for a short duration.
- When grieving and depression are severe, the patient should be encouraged to attend a support group (e.g., SHARE, Empty Arms) (20).
- Discussions about future pregnancy should be delayed until after the follow-up visit (22).

COMPLETE ABORTION

Diagnosis

Differential Diagnosis

- The differential diagnosis is the same as for incomplete abortion.

Clinical Manifestations

- The passage of POC appears to be complete.
- Bleeding is minimal.
- The cervix may be closed or minimally dilated.
- The uterus, on bimanual examination, is well contracted and small.

Treatment

Medications

- Give RhoGAM (300 mg) if the patient is Rh negative.

PROCEDURES

- Observation without surgical intervention is appropriate if
  - The patient's vital signs are stable and no fever is present
  - The passage of tissue appears to be complete
  - Bleeding is minimal
  - Ectopic pregnancy is not suspected
- If these conditions are not present, then uterine curettage is appropriate as previously described.
- Check β-hCG weekly until levels indicate resolution of the pregnancy.

MISSED ABORTION

Definition

- Missed abortion is defined as the retention of POC after death of the fetus.
- There is no definition of the length of time of retention of the POC.
- Missed abortion may occur without the presence of an identifiable fetus or fetal pole.

Laboratory Tests

- Ultrasonography is essential in confirming the diagnosis of missed abortion.

Clinical Manifestations

- The pregnant uterus fails to enlarge as expected.
- Amenorrhea may persist, or intermittent vaginal bleeding, spotting, or brown discharge may occur.
- Rarely disseminated intravascular coagulopathy (DIC) may rarely develop with a missed abortion that extends for more than 4 or 5 weeks.

Treatment

Medications

- RHoGAM is administered to Rh-negative, unsensitized patients.

PROCEDURES

- Dilation and curettage
  - Dilation and curettage (D&C) is frequently chosen by patients because it is a scheduled surgical procedure that definitively empties the uterus.
  - D&C is available for missed abortions that are less than 12 to 14 weeks' gestation by fetal size on ultrasound. This is based on the degree of fetal bone ossification and the risk of uterine perforation.
  - The procedure is similar to that described for surgical management of incomplete and inevitable abortion.
  - If the cervix is not dilated, then preoperative dilation is accomplished with laminaria or prostaglandin cervical-dilating agents.
- Dilation and evacuation
  - Dilation and evacuation (D&E) is frequently chosen by patients because it is a scheduled surgical procedure that definitively empties the uterus.
  - D&E is available for missed abortions greater than 14 weeks' gestation by fetal size on ultrasound. The D&E procedure is used rather than D&C when there are fetal bones and associated risk for uterine perforation.
  - The largest bore suction curette possible is used. Beir or Sopher forceps may be needed to remove large pieces and amounts of tissue.
  - General anesthesia is helpful.
- Oxytocin induction
  - Oxytocin is administered as per hospital protocol.

- Water intoxication may result because of the antidiuretic hormone–like effect of oxytocin. Therefore, fluid intake and output must be monitored carefully, and the administration of large amounts of hypotonic fluids should be avoided.
- This method may fail to induce passage of the tissue.
- Intra-amniotic prostaglandin $F_{2\alpha}$
  - The technique for administering prostaglandin $F_{2\alpha}$ is similar to that recommended for second-trimester amniocentesis.
  - Under ultrasound guidance, the needle is inserted into the amniotic cavity, a test dose of 1 mL (~6 mg) of the prostaglandin is injected, and the patient is observed for adverse reactions.
  - The remainder of the 40-mg vial is slowly infused, with occasional aspiration to ensure intra-amniotic location of the needle tip.
  - Possible adverse effects are nausea and vomiting, diarrhea, hyperpyrexia, bronchospasm, bradycardia, and cervical rupture.
  - Asthma and hypertension are relative contraindications for the use of prostaglandin.
  - Intra-amniotic injections may be technically difficult in missed abortions because the amniotic fluid volume may be quite low. This may make it impossible for the clinician to inject the prostaglandin.
- Prostaglandin E_2 vaginal suppositories
  - Prostaglandin E_2 suppositories are placed intravaginally every 3 hours until adequate contractions are obtained.
  - The adverse effects of prostaglandins listed above are more common with this route of administration because of substantial systemic absorption of prostaglandin when given intravaginally.
  - Regardless of how prostaglandins are administered, the patient's cervix should be inspected carefully postabortion for lacerations and fistulas.
- Vaginal misoprostol
  - Misoprostol may be used for outpatient treatment of missed or incomplete abortion patients with
    - Stable vital signs
    - No evidence of infection
    - Good reliability
    - Fetus measuring less than 13 weeks' gestation
    - POC with no fetal pole on transvaginal ultrasound
  - Treatment
    - An 800-mg misoprostol dose is 80% to 90% successful up to 13 weeks of gestation.
    - Misoprostol is administered intravaginally as four 200-µg tablets (23–25).
    - Buccal administration is as effective as vaginal administration but is associated with more gastrointestinal side effects.
    - This dose is repeated once after 24 hours if there are no results.
    - Oral analgesics are given for pain.
    - Patients should come to the emergency department if extremely heavy bleeding occurs.
    - Up to 30% of patients may require surgical evacuation (2).
    - Ensure adequate analgesia.
    - Expelled tissue should be evaluated by pathology.

HABITUAL ABORTION

Background

Definition

- Habitual abortion, also known as recurrent pregnancy loss (RPL), is defined as three or more consecutive spontaneous abortions of clinical, previable pregnancies (documented by ultrasound or histopathology). In clinical practice, many couples and physicians will proceed with the clinical evaluation for habitual abortion after two consecutive previable losses (2,19,26,27).

Etiology

Up to 75% of cases of RPL will not have a clearly defined etiology (28). General etiological categories of RPL include anatomic, immunological, genetic, endocrine, and infectious factors.

- Uterine anatomic defects that are implicated causes (17) (note that if one of these anatomic causes is found, it should be treated before proceeding with other treatments):
  - Double uterus
  - Septate uterus
  - Asherman syndrome
  - Endometrial polyps
  - Leiomyomas that impinge on the endometrial cavity
- Cervical anatomic defects:
  - Incompetent cervix (15 weeks and beyond)
- Antiphospholipid syndrome (APS) is the only immunological condition in which pregnancy loss is a diagnostic criterion for the disease. Up to 15% of patients with RPL may have APS (29).
- Genetic abnormalities: Approximately 4% of couples with RPL have a major chromosomal rearrangement (vs. 0.7% of the general population); usually a balanced translocation (30). One or both partners may harbor lethal genes in a heterozygous or balanced combination that does not affect them but causes pregnancy loss when inherited by the embryo in a homozygous or unbalanced state.
- Other possible causes that are less well documented:
  - Endocrine factors such as thyroid dysfunction, luteal phase defect, hyperprolactinemia, and
  - Some infections, such as *Listeria monocytogenes, Toxoplasma gondii,* and cytomegalovirus, are known to cause sporadic pregnancy loss, but no infectious agent has been proven to cause RPL (26).
  - Maternal–fetal human leukocyte antigen (major histocompatibility complex).

Epidemiology

- Habitual abortion accounts for approximately 5% of all spontaneous abortions (32).
- Cytogenetic studies of abortion specimens have demonstrated chromosomal anomalies in 20% to 60% of abortuses (2).
- Approximately 95% of chromosomally abnormal fetuses are less than 8 weeks of developmental age, although they often are retained in utero for much longer periods of time (2).
- Chromosomal anomalies are uncommon among abortuses past 12 weeks of development (2).
- Incidence of chromosomal anomalies in couples with habitual abortion (including losses of fetuses of all developmental ages) is estimated at 6.2% (32).

Evaluation

History and Physical

- Signs, symptoms, and physical findings are the same as detailed for other types of abortion (19).
- Patients may complain of lower abdominal pressure symptoms or urinary frequency and urgency (33).

Laboratory Tests

- Submit tissue for pathologic examination.
- Chromosomal studies using banding techniques are recommended for both the father and mother (2,19).
- The minimum immunology work-up for women with RPL is measurement of anticardiolipin antibody (IgG and IgM) and lupus anticoagulant. Lupus anticoagulant and

anticardiolipin antibodies are uncommon but, when present, are associated with high fetal loss rates secondary to placental thrombosis and infarction (26,34).

Genetics
• The parents should receive genetic counseling for familial assessment and as follow-up if abnormalities are found.

Clinical Manifestations
• Uterine anomalies may present with unique nonobstetrical manifestations.
• Incompetent cervix may present with a history of repeated mid-trimester losses with painless cervical dilation. The diagnosis is difficult and relies on previous obstetrical history and/or history of cervical surgery or trauma (19,27).

Treatment
• Patients with repeated abortions beyond 12 weeks of gestation should be investigated for known maternal causes of abortion.
• Sonohysterogram, hysterosalpingography, or hysteroscopy should be performed to evaluate uterine anatomy.
• There is no generalized treatment for habitual abortion. Specific treatment is directed to any identified causes (19,27).
• Whether low-dose aspirin (60 to 80 mg/d), low-dose heparin, or prednisone (20 to 60 mg/d) improves outcomes is controversial and depends on the specific etiology of each patient's series of habitual abortion. When indicated for specific thrombophilias, subcutaneous low-dose heparin and aspirin have been shown to have equally successful outcomes, with fewer complications compared with prednisone (35).

SEPTIC ABORTION
Background
• Septic abortions with renal failure, disseminated intravascular coagulation, and acute lung injury/acute respiratory distress syndrome (ALI/ARDS) were a source of considerable maternal morbidity and mortality during the 1950s and early 1960s. Perhaps because of improved contraceptive methods and the availability of legal induced abortion, these complications are seen less commonly today.
• When septic abortion occurs, progression to multiple organ failure and death is a serious risk even today.
• Complication rates with septic abortion are high:
  • Acute renal failure in 73% of patients
  • DIC in 31%
  • Septic shock in 32%
  • Septic shock mortality in 19%
• Sepsis should be considered even in the absence of shock (36).

Evaluation
• Patients experiencing septic abortion should be managed in an intensive care setting and evaluated rapidly but thoroughly in collaboration with an intensive care physician familiar with septic shock if available.
• The following findings are associated with a poor prognosis and the need for aggressive treatment:
  • High-spiking fever
  • Hypotension
  • Hypothermia
  • Oliguria
  • Advanced gestational age of pregnancy
  • Signs of infection beyond the uterus (12,37)

History and Physical
- History of nonsterile uterine instrumentation may be difficult to elicit but should always be considered.
- Physical examination is used to define the extent of infection (12,37):
  - Stage 1—endometrial–myometrial involvement
  - Stage 2—adnexal spread
  - Stage 3—generalized peritonitis
- Evaluation of the patient's clinical status should include
  - Vital signs and urine output
  - Pulmonary function
  - Assessment of peripheral circulation
  - Central hemodynamics
  - Central nervous system function

Laboratory Tests
- If clinically indicated, obtain
  - Complete blood count
  - Urinalysis
  - Serum electrolytes
  - Blood urea nitrogen
  - Creatinine
  - Lactate
  - Blood type and Rh factor
  - Crossmatch
  - Platelet count
  - Prothrombin time
  - Partial thromboplastin time
  - Fibrinogen
  - Fibrin split products
  - D-dimer assay
  - Arterial blood gases
  - Lipase
- Perform hemolytic studies (e.g., plasma-free hemoglobin) if *Clostridium perfringens* infection is suspected.
  - A gross test of hemolysis is provided by centrifugation of a blood sample and observation of the serum for a pink tinge.
- Obtain aerobic and anaerobic cultures of blood, urine, endometrium, and POC.
- Gram stain of POC:
  - Obtain sample by endometrial swab.
  - Gram-positive rods with swollen ends suggest *C. perfringens* infection.
- Culture the peritoneal aspirate and perform a Gram stain.
- X-rays for
  - Pulmonary artery and lateral of the chest for possible septic emboli
    - Air under the diaphragm implies uterine perforation.
  - Anteroposterior, supine, and upright films of the abdomen
    - Foreign bodies related to an abortion may be identified.
- Intramyometrial gas ("onionskin" pattern) implies *C. perfringens* infection.
- CAT scan may be helpful to locate any collection of pus for drainage.

Diagnosis
The diagnosis of septic abortion is made when a temperature of at least 100.4°F (38°C) exists in the presence of signs and symptoms of abortion in any stage, assuming other sources of fever have been excluded.

- Septic abortion generally is seen with
  - Prolonged, neglected ruptured membranes
  - Intrauterine pregnancy with an intrauterine device in place
  - History of attempts of the patient to terminate the pregnancy herself (usually by mechanical means, such as intrauterine catheters, or by transcervical injection of soaps or phenolics)

Treatment

- Management should take place in an intensive care unit setting with appropriate consultation by experienced specialists (38).
- Consideration should be given to use of central hemodynamic monitoring with placement of a Swan-Ganz catheter.
- Bolus fluid resuscitation with crystalloids (2 to 4 L in the first hour) may be required. Subsequent fluid resuscitation is given at a rate such that urinary output of at least 30 mL/h is maintained (often 150 to 250 mL/h) (38).
- Watch for pulmonary edema secondary to fluid overload.
- Whole-blood transfusions may be given to maintain the hematocrit between 30% and 35% (38).
- Operative intervention may be necessary.
  - Infected tissue may be removed by D&C or D&E.
  - The operative timing is critical as an increased postoperative incidence of sepsis and hypotension has been reported when curettage is performed on febrile patients (37).
  - Alternatively, laparotomy and total abdominal hysterectomy with bilateral salpingo-oophorectomy may be necessary (39).
- Care can be individualized for low-risk patients:
  - Low-risk patients are those with a temperature less than 103°F, a small uterus, localized infection only, and no indications of shock (38).
  - These patients are best managed with intensive antibiotics.
  - Curettage should be done only if needed, but incomplete abortions should be evacuated as soon as effective antibiotic levels have been achieved.
  - Profuse or continued hemorrhage requires rapid intervention and awareness of possible DIC.

Medications

- Give tetanus toxoid, 0.5 mL subcutaneously, to immunized patients with a history of self-induced abortion.
- Antibiotics for seriously ill patients include
  - Penicillin G sodium, 4 to 8 million U intravenously every 4 hours
  - Ampicillin, 1 to 2 g intravenously every 4 hours
  - Gentamicin sulfate, 1.5 mg/kg given by slow intravenous infusion every 8 hours, with careful monitoring of renal and eighth cranial nerve function. Peak (30 minutes after dose is given) and trough (just before dose is given) serum gentamicin levels should be ordered and dosage adjusted as necessary. If possible, the use of nephrotoxic drugs in oliguric patients should be avoided (40).
  - Clindamycin, 600 mg intravenously every 6 hours
- For less seriously ill patients:
  - Cefoxitin, 2 g intravenously every 6 hours.
  - If *Chlamydia* is suspected, add doxycycline, 100 mg intravenously every 12 hours.

PROCEDURES

Closely monitor vital signs including blood pressure, heart rate, SpO_2, respiratory rate, temperature, and urine output with an indwelling Foley catheter.

- If bulging of the cul-de-sac is detected, consider culdocentesis.
- Administer intravenous fluids (normal saline) through at least one large-bore catheter.

- If lactate is greater than 4 mmol/L (36 mg/L) consider inserting an internal jugular or subcutaneous central venous catheter for fluid administration and measurement of central mixed venous O_2 saturation (ScVO$_2$; expect greater than 70% in sepsis).

SEPTIC SHOCK

Diagnosis

An extensive discussion of the diagnosis and management of septic shock is beyond the scope of this text.
- In the setting of septic abortion or other serious systemic infections, septic shock is suggested by the following, usually preceded by chills and fever (12,27):
  - Oliguria
  - Hypotension
  - Tachypnea and tachycardia
  - Mental confusion
  - Warmth and dryness of the extremities (low peripheral resistance) or cold and cyanotic extremities (increased resistance)

Treatment

- The cornerstones of therapy of septic shock are
  - Early goal-directed resuscitation therapy with crystalloid fluid whole blood, vasoactives, and inotropes
  - Respiratory support, from airway maintenance and administration of oxygen by nasal cannula as a minimal treatment, to endotracheal intubation with assisted ventilation, as necessary
  - A decrease in the endotoxin load with antibiotics directed against the infecting organisms
  - Surgical removal of necrotic tissue where indicated
- Important additional therapies include
  - Recombinant activated protein C replacement (Xigris, 24 µg/kg/h for 96 hours, held for 1 hour before and 12 hours after major surgery)
  - Stress ulcer prophylaxis with histamine H2 receptor antagonists or proton pump inhibitors
  - Venous thromboembolism prophylaxis with subcutaneous heparins and sequential compression devices

PROCEDURES

- Continue aggressive volume resuscitation using urine output, hemodynamics, and ScVO$_2$ as a guide.
- Correct acidosis: volume, ventilatory support (noninvasive or invasive mechanical ventilation) versus sodium bicarbonate (intravenous).
- Support organ perfusion: consider titrated norepinephrine infusion and possibly addition of fixed-dose vasopressin infusion (0.04 U/min).
- Superimposed cardiogenic shock is suggested by low ScVO$_2$, persistent lactate elevation and paradoxical worsening with higher doses of norepinephrine. Consider addition of dobutamine infusion and monitor for tachycardia.
- Evaluate for relative adrenal insufficiency before administering replacement-dose corticosteroids (cosyntropin stimulation test).
  - Consider addition of corticosteroids at moderate, not high doses (hydrocortisone, 50 to 100 mg four times a day).
  - Higher doses of methylprednisolone and possibly L-thyroxin may be required if there is concern about peripartum adrenal hemorrhage or Sheehan syndrome (pituitary infarction).

- Prepare for renal replacement therapy (usually continuous venovenous hemofiltration) if needed. A dialysis catheter will be required. Adjust doses of medicines accordingly in renal failure.
- The presence of ALI/ARDS is suggested by
  - Four-quadrant airspace infiltrates
  - Respiratory failure requiring mechanical ventilation
  - PaO_2: FiO_2 ratio less than 300 in the absence of clinically apparent heart failure, or
  - Pulmonary occlusion pressure greater than 18 mm Hg
- Ensure that low tidal volume (6 mL/kg predicated body weight) with positive end-expiratory pressure at 10 to 15 cm is used during mechanical ventilation.
- Monitor and manage coagulopathy of sepsis that may progress to DIC with appropriate clotting factor and blood product support.
- Early uterine curettage to remove the source of thromboplastins is mandatory.
- Hematology/pathology consultation is helpful.

PATIENT EDUCATION

- Spontaneous abortion is a risk in all pregnancies.
- The majority of spontaneous abortions are due to chromosome abnormalities.
- Chance of a successful subsequent pregnancy if no cause is found (idiopathic):
  - After one abortion, the risk is essentially unchanged at 15% to 20%.
  - After two consecutive abortions, the risk of having a third loss rises somewhat to 11% (20 years) to 40% (45 years), depending on age (41).
  - After three losses, the chance of a fourth is approximately 12% (20 to 25 years) to 52% (45 years) (41). After three consecutive losses, if the appropriate evaluation fails to reveal a cause for RPL, the chances for a successful subsequent pregnancy are approximately 80% on average (22,42). There is variation of results because of age and number of prior miscarriages.

ACKNOWLEDGMENTS

We thank Dr. Douglas Ivor, MICU Intensivist, Denver Health Medical Center, Denver, Colorado.

REFERENCES

1. Goddijn M, Leschot NJ. Genetic aspects of miscarriage. *Baillieres Best Pract Res Clin Obstet Gynaecol.* 2000;14(5):855–865.
2. Fabricant JD, Boullie J, Boullie A. Genetic studies on spontaneous abortion. *Contemp Obstet Gynecol.* 1978;11:73.
3. Roberts CJ, Lowe CR. Where have all the conceptions gone? *Lancet.* 1975;1:636–637.
4. Nybo Andersen AM, Wohlfahrt J, Christens P, et al. Maternal age and fetal loss: population based register linkage study. *BMJ.* 2000;320(7251):1708–1712.
5. Steier JD, Bergsjo P, Myking DL. Human chorionic gonadotropin in maternal plasma after induced abortion, spontaneous abortion, and removed ectopic pregnancy. *Obstet Gynecol.* 1984;64:391–394.
6. Barnhart KT. Early pregnancy failure: beware of the pitfalls of modern management. *Fertil Steril.* 2012;98(5):1061–1065.
7. Condous G, Lu C, Van Huffel SV, et al. Human chorionic gonadotrophin and progesterone levels in pregnancies of unknown location. *Int J Gynaecol Obstet.* 2004;86(3):351–357.
8. Shalev E, Yarom I, Bustan M, et al. Transvaginal sonography as the ultimate diagnostic tool for the management of ectopic pregnancy: experience with 840 cases. *Fertil Steril.* 1998;69(1):62–65.
9. Barnhart KT, Sammel MD, Rinaudo PF, et al. Symptomatic patients with an early viable intrauterine pregnancy: HCG curves redefined. *Obstet Gynecol.* 2004;104(1):50–55.

10. Jeve Y, Rana R, Bhide A, et al. Accuracy of first-trimester ultrasound in the diagnosis of early embryonic demise: a systematic review. *Ultrasound Obstet Gynecol.* 2011;38(5): 489–496.

11. Foreman H, Stadel BV, Schlesselman S. Intrauterine device usage and fetal loss. *Obstet Gynecol.* 1981;58(6):669–677.

12. American Congress of Obstetricians and Gynecologists. Septic shock. *ACOG Tech Bull.* 1995:204.

13. Eriksen PS, Philipsen T. Prognosis in threatened abortion evaluated by hormone assays and ultrasound scanning. *Obstet Gynecol.* 1980;55(4):435–438.

14. Deaton JL, Honore GM, Huffman CS, et al. Early transvaginal ultrasound following an accurately dated pregnancy: the importance of finding a yolk sac or fetal heart motion. *Hum Reprod.* 1997;12(12):2820–2823.

15. Freiman SM, Wulff GJ Jr. Management of uterine perforation following elective abortion. *Obstet Gynecol.* 1977;50(6):647–650.

16. Kaali SG, Szigetvari IA, Bartfai GS. The frequency and management of uterine perforations during first-trimester abortions. *Am J Obstet Gynecol.* 1989;161(2):406–408.

17. Exacoustos C, Rosati P. Ultrasound diagnosis of uterine myomas and complications in pregnancy. *Obstet Gynecol.* 1993;82(1):97–101.

18. Pridjian G, Moawad AH. Missed abortion: still appropriate terminology? *Am J Obstet Gynecol.* 1989;161(2):261–262.

19. Stray-Pederson B, Stray-Pederson S. Etiologic factors and subsequent reproductive performance in 195 couples with a prior history of habitual abortion. *Am J Obstet Gynecol.* 1984;148:140.

20. American Congress of Obstetricians and Gynecologists. Grief related to perinatal death. *ACOG Tech Bull.* 1985:86.

21. American Congress of Obstetricians and Gynecologists. *Pregnancy loss: miscarriage and molar pregnancy.* ACOG, 2002.

22. Poland BJ, Miller JR, Jones DC, et al. Reproductive counseling in patients who have had a spontaneous abortion. *Am J Obstet Gynecol.* 1977;127(7):685–691.

23. Chung TK, Lee DT, Cheung LP, et al. Spontaneous abortion: a randomized, controlled trial comparing surgical evacuation with conservative management using misoprostol. *Fertil Steril.* 1999;71(6):1054–1059.

24. Schreiber CA, Creinin MD, Harwood B, et al. A pilot study of mifepristone and misoprostol administered at the same time for abortion in women with gestation from 50 to 63 days. *Contraception.* 2005;71(6):447–450.

25. Wood SL, Brain PH. Medical management of missed abortion: a randomized clinical trial. *Obstet Gynecol.* 2002;99(4):563–566.

26. ASRM. Definition of experimental procedures: a committee opinion. *Fertil Steril.* 2013;99(5):1197–1198.

27. American Congress of Obstetricians and Gynecologists. Hemorrhagic shock. *ACOG Tech Bull.* 1984:82.

28. ASRM. Evaluation and treatment of recurrent pregnancy loss: a committee opinion. *Fertil Steril.* 2012;98(5):1103–1111.

29. Reindollar RH. Contemporary issues for spontaneous abortion. Does recurrent abortion exist? *Obstet Gynecol Clin North Am.* 2000;27(3):541–554.

30. Franssen MT, Korevaar JC, van der Veen F, et al. Reproductive outcome after chromosome analysis in couples with two or more miscarriages: index [corrected]-control study. *BMJ.* 2006;332(7544):759–763.

31. Quenby SM, Farquharson RG. Predicting recurring miscarriage: what is important? *Obstet Gynecol.* 1993;82(1):132–138.

32. Khuda G. Cryogenics of habitual abortion. *Obstet Gynecol Surv.* 1974;29:229.

33. Toaff R, Toaff ME. Diagnosis of impending late abortion. *Obstet Gynecol.* 1974;43(5):756–759.

34. Lubbe WF, Liggins GC. Lupus anticoagulant and pregnancy. *Am J Obstet Gynecol.* 1988;153:322–327.

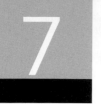

7 Ectopic Pregnancy
Julie M. Sroga and Kathleen McIntrey-Seltman

KEY POINTS
- Ectopic pregnancy is common and can be life threatening.
- Clinical signs and symptoms are nonspecific and are frequently present in healthy pregnancy as well as ectopic pregnancy.
- Serum β-human chorionic gonadotropin levels and ultrasound are used to make early diagnosis.
- Medical or surgical treatment may be used, with similar long-term outcomes in terms of tubal function and future fertility.

BACKGROUND
Definition
An ectopic pregnancy is one in which the fertilized ovum implants at any site other than the endometrial cavity. The fallopian tube is the most common site, accounting for more than 95% of ectopic pregnancies, but other implantation sites include the cervix, abdominal cavity, and ovary (1).

Incidence
The incidence of ectopic pregnancy in the United States has nearly tripled over the past 30 years; whether this is due to increasing recognition because of sensitive diagnostic tools or a true increase is unclear. Currently, ectopic locations are diagnosed in approximately 2% of clinically recognized pregnancies (2). The prevalence of ectopic among women presenting with first-trimester bleeding and/or abdominal pain can be up to 18% (1). Ectopic pregnancy is the most common cause of nonpuerperal maternal mortality and is the leading cause of first-trimester maternal death (2).

Etiology
A number of risk factors for ectopic pregnancy have been identified (Table 7-1), including the following conditions (3):
- Salpingitis. Approximately 50% of ectopic pregnancies can be attributed to a history of salpingitis. Salpingitis has been shown to increase a woman's risk for ectopic pregnancy sevenfold. Chlamydial salpingitis may pose a greater risk than gonorrheal infection.
- Prior ectopic pregnancy. In subsequent pregnancies, there is a 15% to 20% risk of recurrence, in either the same or opposite tube.
- Peritubal adhesions following postabortal or puerperal infections, appendicitis, or endometriosis.
- Tubal surgery, including tubal ligation, tubal reanastomosis, prior surgery for ectopic pregnancy, and tubal reconstruction for fertility.
- Intrauterine device. Intrauterine devices (IUDs) are highly effective at preventing intrauterine pregnancy. Thus, any pregnancy in an IUD user is more likely to be tubal.
- Progestin-only contraceptives. Users of progestin-only oral contraceptives as well as injectable progestins are at increased risk of ectopic pregnancy if pregnancy occurs, possibly because of altered tubal motility.
- History of infertility. Infertile couples have an increased proportion of ectopic pregnancies compared to the total number of pregnancies, regardless of the etiology of the infertility.

Table 7-1	Risk Factors and Relative Risk for Ectopic Pregnancy
Risk factor	**Relative risk**
Prior ectopic pregnancy	3–5
Tubal surgery (repair, ligation)	3–4
History of pelvic infection	3
Current use of progestin contraceptives[a]	1.5
IUD use[a]	1.5
Smoking	2–3
In utero DES exposure	4
Conception via assisted reproductive techniques	1.5

[a]Total number pregnancies decreased, but percentage of ectopic pregnancies increased.
IUD, intrauterine device; DES, diethylstilbestrol.

- Assisted reproductive techniques (ART):
  - Women who have conceived via ART are at increased risk of ectopic pregnancy, regardless of the etiology of their infertility. Approximately 2% of pregnancies occurring as a result of in vitro fertilization, gamete intrafallopian tube transfer (GIFT), gonadotropin-stimulated superovulation, and other methods of assisted reproduction result in ectopic pregnancies (4).
  - Heterotopic pregnancy (simultaneous ectopic and intrauterine pregnancies) occurs at a much higher rate in women treated with assisted reproductive technologies. Up to 2% of ectopic pregnancies in this population are heterotopic.
  - Diagnosis of ectopic pregnancy is more challenging in women receiving reproductive assistance. Women treated with assisted reproductive technologies are more likely to have abdominal pain and spotting early in pregnancy. Even when confronted by a probable ectopic pregnancy, both patients and clinicians are reluctant to interfere with technologically conceived pregnancies, which may result in delay in treatment.
- Developmental abnormalities of the tube, such as diverticula, accessory ostia, and hypoplasia. Women who have been exposed to diethylstilbestrol (DES) have a four to five times greater risk of ectopic pregnancy.
- Increased maternal age.

Pathogenesis
- In tubal pregnancies, the fertilized ovum implants in the epithelium of the tube. The trophoblast invades the tubal muscularis and the maternal blood supply, resulting in bleeding and weakening of the tubal wall. Eventually, the pregnancy either extrudes out the fimbriated end of the tube (tubal abortion) or ruptures the wall of the tube. Either of these situations can cause intra-abdominal bleeding.
- Approximately 80% of tubal pregnancies implant in the ampullary portion of the tube, and 5% implant more distally on the fimbriae.
- Isthmic pregnancies, accounting for approximately 13% of ectopic pregnancies, rupture earlier than do ampullary pregnancies and may result in secondary broad ligament implantation.
- Interstitial pregnancies, although only 2% of ectopics, result in the greatest morbidity because they can grow large and can mimic an intrauterine pregnancy. When these pregnancies rupture, severe hemorrhage may ensue.

DIAGNOSIS
- Ectopic pregnancy should be suspected any time a woman presents with bleeding and/or pain in early pregnancy. While abnormal intrauterine pregnancy is more common than is ectopic pregnancy, ectopic pregnancy is more likely to be life threatening; therefore, it is critical to consider the diagnosis.

- The diagnosis of ectopic pregnancy is not always obvious; initial diagnoses are often incorrect. Women may present with catastrophic intra-abdominal hemorrhage and shock; however, more frequently, they will have ill-defined abdominal pain and minimal vaginal bleeding.
- It is important to carefully evaluate all women of reproductive age with abdominal pain. Early diagnosis before rupture decreases morbidity and allows wider treatment options. More than half of women presenting with life-threatening intra-abdominal bleeding have had at least one visit to a health care provider before rupture.

Clinical Manifestations
- Signs and symptoms with a less catastrophic presentation:
  - Abdominal pain is present in more than 95% of women with ectopic pregnancy. The pain often begins as intermittent, colicky discomfort in one lower quadrant, progressing to more constant, severe pain that generalizes throughout the lower abdomen. The degree of pain may be less than expected, even with a significant hemoperitoneum. Shoulder pain is present in 15% of women with a ruptured ectopic pregnancy as a result of blood irritating the diaphragm.
  - Delayed menses is reported by 90% of women with ectopic pregnancy, varying from a few days to several weeks.
  - Vaginal bleeding, often as spotting, is present in 80% to 90% of women in whom ectopic pregnancy is ultimately diagnosed. However, bleeding is present in about half of all pregnancies, even those with normal outcome. The abnormal bleeding results from low hormonal levels with resulting slough of the endometrium. Bleeding ranges from scant spotting to menstrual-like flow. Some women report passage of tissue, representing decidualized endometrium.
  - Physical examination reveals abdominal tenderness, adnexal tenderness, especially unilateral, and cervical motion tenderness. Up to 10% of women present with intra-abdominal hemorrhage, in which case diffuse abdominal tenderness and rigidity, rebound tenderness, and hypovolemic shock may be present.
    ○ Abdominal tenderness is found in 80% to 90% of women with ectopic pregnancies varying from mild to severe tenderness, guarding, and rebound tenderness.
    ○ Adnexal tenderness on pelvic exam is present in nearly all women with ectopic pregnancies, and it may be associated with cervical motion tenderness.
    ○ Adnexal mass or cul-de-sac mass may be palpable in 50% of women with ectopic pregnancy; however, it is contralateral to the pregnancy nearly half the time and is often a corpus luteum cyst rather than the gestation itself.
    ○ Uterine enlargement, often less than expected relative to the last menstrual period, is present in 25% and does not rule out ectopic pregnancy.
- Women with catastrophic presentation. Women with hemoperitoneum as a result of ruptured ectopic pregnancy will present with an acute abdomen and shock. Often there is a history of vague abdominal pain followed by sudden and worsening acute pain beginning in the lower quadrants and extending to the entire abdomen. Pelvic exam may reveal a doughy mass in the cul-de-sac caused by clotted blood. Assessment of the uterus and adnexa is usually impossible because of abdominal distention and rigidity.

Differential Diagnosis
- *Other pregnancy-related conditions.* Threatened, incomplete, or complete spontaneous abortion, septic abortion, and hydatidiform mole may be confused with ectopic gestations. A normal early intrauterine pregnancy with a bleeding corpus luteum cyst must also be considered. The combination of clinical findings, quantitative human chorionic gonadotropin (β-hCG), and ultrasound can usually help distinguish these conditions.
- *Non–pregnancy-related conditions.* Salpingitis, appendicitis, adnexal torsion, ruptured corpus luteum in the absence of pregnancy, and urinary tract disorders such as infection and stones must be considered. Generally, negative results of a sensitive urine or serum pregnancy test can eliminate ectopic pregnancy when these diagnoses are being considered.

- Intra-abdominal hemorrhage secondary to ruptured spleen or liver may present a diagnostic challenge in the pregnant patient; however, because patients presenting in this manner need urgent surgery, such difficulties in diagnosis may not be problematic.

EVALUATION
Laboratory Tests
- Pregnancy testing. Testing for β-hCG levels is of great value in evaluating a woman with suspected ectopic pregnancy, as virtually all ectopic pregnancies will be associated with detectable levels of β-hCG in blood or urine. These tests should be available in all facilities providing health care to women of reproductive age.
  - Current urine pregnancy tests are sensitive to 20 to 25 IU β-hCG, which is the level excreted in the urine at or before the 1st day of expected menses. β-hCG is detectable in maternal serum within 8 days of ovulation. The β-hCG level rises rapidly, initially doubling in 1 to 1.5 days. By approximately 5 weeks' gestation menstrual age (3 weeks postconception), β-hCG will normally double about every 48 hours. However, a 53% increase in β-hCG value in 48 hours is considered the lower limit of normal and defines a potentially viable intrauterine pregnancy (5).
  - Ectopic pregnancies produce less β-hCG than do normal intrauterine pregnancies at the same gestational age because of a smaller volume of functional trophoblasts. Consequently, the rate of β-hCG rise is slower than in normal intrauterine pregnancies. The failure of serial β-hCG levels to rise at the proper rate can be used to distinguish ectopic pregnancy from normal pregnancy, but a normally rising β-hCG concentration does not exclude ectopic pregnancy (5).
  - If the exact date of conception is known, a single β-hCG level can predict normal versus abnormal placentation; however, an error of even 48 hours in the date of conception can obviously lead to confusing results. Therefore, single β-hCG levels alone are of limited clinical usefulness.
  - In early-pregnancy patients when there is suspicion of ectopic pregnancy, serial β-hCG levels are drawn 48 hours apart to determine if levels are rising appropriately until an intrauterine pregnancy can be determined by pelvic ultrasound.
- Serum progesterone. The use of serum progesterone levels is not generally helpful for distinguishing ectopic pregnancy from abnormal intrauterine pregnancy but can help to distinguish both of these from normal pregnancy.
  - Progesterone initially is made by the corpus luteum of the ovary, with a gradual transition to production by the trophoblast.
  - In a woman with bleeding and/or pain, a serum progesterone level can be helpful in determining normal from abnormal early pregnancy (either miscarriage or ectopic pregnancy).
    - A level greater than 25 ng/mL is associated with normal intrauterine pregnancy.
    - A level less than 5 ng/mL is strongly associated with abnormal pregnancy outcome.
    - However, there is no difference between the level of progesterone associated with abnormal intrauterine pregnancy and ectopic pregnancy.
    - Intermediate levels are nondiagnostic. The majority of results in symptomatic women are in the nondiagnostic range, and an abnormal result does not distinguish the location of the abnormal pregnancy (6).
  - For these reasons, serum progesterone measurement is not widely used in the diagnosis of ectopic pregnancy.
- Other trophoblast markers. A variety of trophoblast markers have been evaluated as possible diagnostic tests for ectopic pregnancy; however, none is clinically available at this time.
- Other laboratory tests. The white blood cell count may be elevated in the range of 10,000 to 15,000. Hemoglobin and hematocrit should be tested; however, these values may be normal even with significant hemoperitoneum.

Ultrasound

Pelvic ultrasound is invaluable in the evaluation of suspected ectopic pregnancy. Verification of an intrauterine pregnancy by ultrasound makes ectopic pregnancy extremely unlikely. Heterotopic pregnancies (multiple gestations with embryos in both the tube and the uterus) are extremely rare, occurring in 1 to 2 per 10,000 spontaneous pregnancies, and in up to 2% of pregnancies conceived with ART.

- Using transvaginal sonography, landmarks consistent with intrauterine pregnancy can be detected as early as 4.5 to 5 weeks menstrual age (Table 7-2). Transabdominal sonography is less sensitive because detection of intrauterine pregnancy is not reliable until 6 weeks' gestation or later.
- Absence of intrauterine pregnancy on ultrasound examination is diagnostic for ectopic pregnancy if the gestational age is known for certain or if the β-hCG level is greater than 2000 IU/mL (7).
- Other ultrasonographic findings associated with ectopic pregnancy include a mass in the tube, which may be echodense or echolucent; free fluid or blood clot in the cul-de-sac; and a "pseudosac" or fluid collection within the uterine cavity. A false or pseudosac may be seen in 10% of women with ectopic pregnancy (8).
- Other sonographic findings suggestive but not diagnostic of ectopic gestation include
  - Mass in the adnexa. This is not specific for ectopic pregnancy because it may be a corpus luteum cyst.
  - Gestational sac in the adnexa. This is seen in 25% of ectopics with vaginal sonography, but false positives can occur. A gestational sac in the adnexa may be easier to detect with color Doppler ultrasound, with the trophoblast appearing as a "ring of fire" surrounding the sac.
  - Fluid in cul-de-sac. This is seen on abdominal scan in 50% and on vaginal ultrasound in 75% of ectopics. It may be associated with unruptured ectopic pregnancy.

Combining Human Chorionic Gonadotropin Levels and Ultrasound: The Discriminatory Zone

- By combining the β-hCG level with information from ultrasound scanning, a diagnosis can frequently be made (Table 7-3).
- An intrauterine pregnancy is reliably visible on ultrasound when it has reached a size associated with a β-hCG level of 6500 IU/mL (abdominal scan) or 1500 to 2000 IU/mL (vaginal ultrasound). This level is known as the discriminatory zone (7).
- Depending on the sensitivity of ultrasound equipment and the experience of the ultrasonographer, the β-hCG representing the discriminatory zone may be lower. It is important for clinicians to be familiar with ultrasound performance in their own institutions.

Culdocentesis

Culdocentesis refers to the insertion of a needle through the vaginal wall posterior to the cervix into the peritoneal cavity and aspiration of contents of the cul-de-sac.

Table 7-2	Intrauterine Pregnancy Landmarks Obtained from Transvaginal Ultrasonography and Corresponding β-hCG Hormone Levels	
	Gestational age (weeks)	**β-hCG (IU/mL)**
Gestational sac	5.0	1500–2000
Yolk sac	5 wk 4 d	3000–4000
Embryo	6.0 (3 mm)	6000–6500
Embryonic cardiac activity	6 wk 3 d	>10,000

β-hCG, β-human chorionic gonadotropin.

Table 7-3	Diagnosis of Ectopic Pregnancy by Ultrasonography and Human Chorionic Gonadotropin Levels	
Variable	**β-hCG level (IU/mL)/ conclusion**	**β-hCG level (IU/mL)/ conclusion**
Abdominal ultrasonogram	6000	>6500
Vaginal ultrasonogram	1500–2000	>2000
Sac in uterus	Probable abortion	Normal intrauterine pregnancy
No sac in uterus	Nondiagnostic	Probable ectopic pregnancy

β-hCG, human chorionic gonadotropin.

- A positive result of culdocentesis is one in which nonclotting blood is obtained and is highly suggestive of an ectopic pregnancy in the presence of symptoms and a positive pregnancy test.
- A negative result is one in which clear serous fluid is obtained, making an ectopic pregnancy unlikely.
- A nondiagnostic test is one in which either no fluid ("dry tap") or a few milliliters of clotting blood are obtained. A nondiagnostic culdocentesis neither confirms nor rules out an ectopic pregnancy.
- Culdocentesis is a readily available, rapid, and low-morbidity procedure; it is also painful, and it has a high frequency of nondiagnostic results. Now that sensitive serum β-hCG screening and vaginal ultrasound are available, culdocentesis is rarely indicated in the diagnosis of ectopic pregnancy.

Diagnostic Dilation and Curettage
- When an abnormal pregnancy is diagnosed by hormone levels and ultrasound, but the location of the pregnancy is unknown, diagnostic dilation and curettage (D&C) is a cost-effective way to distinguish intrauterine pregnancy failure from ectopic pregnancy.
- If chorionic villi are identified on gross or histologic examination, ectopic pregnancy is virtually ruled out. If no products of conception are present, the patient has either an ectopic pregnancy or a completed spontaneous abortion.
- Diagnostic D&C in conjunction with a postprocedure β-hCG concentration can be useful. A decline of β-hCG greater than 30% is suggestive of abnormal intrauterine pregnancy where a rise of β-hCG is suggestive of ectopic (9).
- Some authorities suggest that diagnostic D&C should always precede medical management, but this is controversial.

TREATMENT
Catastrophic Presentation
Ectopic pregnancies can present as life-threatening emergencies. The patient presenting in shock with an acute abdomen should be stabilized and taken to surgery immediately.
- Fluid resuscitation must be carried out immediately. Two large-bore peripheral intravenous lines should be started, and balanced saline solution should be infused rapidly. A Foley catheter should be placed to monitor urine output. In the absence of complicating medical conditions, central venous monitoring is generally not needed.
- Laboratory tests needed are minimal. Blood should be drawn for hematocrit and cross-matched for four units of red cells. A β-hCG level should be obtained, but it is not necessary to wait for the results.
- Surgical approach.
  - The patient should be taken to surgery as quickly as possible. In some women with massive hemorrhage and severe shock, it may be necessary to proceed to surgery while the patient is being stabilized.

- Either a low midline vertical incision or a Pfannenstiel incision can be used.
- After the abdomen has been entered, rapid palpation of the uterus and both adnexa will usually localize the pregnancy. Upward traction on the uterus coupled with digital pressure on the involved tube will stop the bleeding so that fluid resuscitation, including transfusion if needed, can be completed. Only then should the hemoperitoneum be cleared and the involved adnexum stabilized in the operative field. The tube should be clamped across the mesosalpinx, the tube excised, and the mesosalpinx suture ligated. There is no need to remove the ipsilateral ovary.
- Hysterectomy is not indicated unless the ectopic pregnancy is interstitial or cornual, and the uterine rupture is so severe that it cannot be repaired.

Less Acute Presentation
In the hemodynamically stable patient with an ectopic pregnancy, there are three possible strategies for management: expectant, surgical, and medical.
- Expectant management:
  - Many ectopic pregnancies will end in tubal abortion, with cessation of trophoblast growth, separation of the products of conception from the tubal wall, and spontaneous resolution.
  - The risk associated with expectant management is intraperitoneal hemorrhage, which cannot be predicted. Even women with low and falling β-hCG levels may have significant bleeding. For this reason, expectant management is rarely used.
  - Patients who are Rh negative should receive Rh_o(D) immunoglobulin (RhoGAM), even though the risk of sensitization is low.
- Surgical management:
  - Procedure selection.
  - Surgical options are operative laparoscopy and D&C.
  - In the stable patient, a short waiting time to assemble personnel and equipment and to ensure safety (e.g., allowing time for gastric emptying) may be appropriate.
  - The first choice for surgical management is operative laparoscopy with either salpingostomy or salpingectomy. Laparotomy is reserved for specific indications.
    - Laparoscopic salpingostomy is the procedure of choice in most circumstances (10).
    - Salpingectomy is selected if future fertility is not desired (e.g., ectopic pregnancy after tubal ligation) or if rupture has destroyed the tube. Some authorities argue that salpingectomy is the treatment of choice if the contralateral tube is normal; others reserve salpingectomy only for situations where the tube cannot be salvaged (significant bleeding that cannot be controlled, rupture of the tube, or severely damaged tube).
    - Laparotomy should be performed if laparoscopy is unsatisfactory because of extensive adhesions, if the patient becomes unstable, or if there are medical limitations to laparoscopy. Laparotomy is usually performed via a small Pfannenstiel incision (10).
  - Dilation and curettage is performed only if the pregnancy is undesired or the cervix is widely dilated. If the pregnancy is intrauterine, villi can be identified by floating the uterine contents in saline and searching for characteristic bubble-like structures joined by strands of tissue. Frozen section can also be used to search for villi; however, there are high rates of false-positive and false-negative results with frozen sections, and they may be difficult to obtain in a timely manner.
  - If the clinical presentation is highly suggestive of ectopic pregnancy, laparoscopy should be performed rather than relying on uterine examination unless products of conception are unequivocally seen.
    - When the pregnancy is desired, no instruments should be passed through the cervix until the diagnosis of ectopic pregnancy is verified laparoscopically.
    - After insertion of the laparoscope, peritoneal blood is aspirated with a large-bore aspirator. The pelvis is visualized, with lysis of adhesions if necessary to obtain a

clear view. Both tubes should be carefully examined. The ectopic pregnancy usually appears as a fusiform, hemorrhagic swelling within the tube. Sometimes, tubal abortion has already taken place with the pregnancy partially or completely extruded from the fimbriated end of the tube, and the products of conception may be within the blood and clot that has been aspirated. Salpingotomy is performed by making a 1- to 1.5-cm incision in the antimesenteric aspect of the tube, directly over the most distended part of the tube, using unipolar needlepoint cautery. Hemostasis can be enhanced by injection of a dilute solution of vasopressin into the tube or the mesosalpinx. The pregnancy mass is then gently removed, using traction and fluid dissection between the mass and the tube wall. The trophoblastic site is cauterized for hemostasis using fine point cautery. There is no need to suture the salpingostomy site. If bleeding cannot be controlled, laparoscopic salpingectomy should be performed using cauterization and incision of the mesosalpinx, laparoscopic stapling devices, or endoscopic ligatures (10).

- After conservative surgery (when the tube is not removed), weekly β-hCG levels should be obtained until they are less than negative (values vary by laboratory).
  - Approximately 5% to 10% of women treated with salpingostomy will have persistent trophoblastic activity in the tube, which may result in tubal rupture and/or intra-abdominal hemorrhage.
  - The risk of persistence is increased with larger pregnancies and higher baseline β-hCG levels.
  - If there is concern about the completeness of removal of the pregnancy, postoperative prophylactic methotrexate using the single-dose regimen significantly decreases the rate of persistence.
  - Early detection of trophoblastic persistence is facilitated by persistently elevated or rising β-hCG levels.
- Medical management:
  - Medical management has the advantage of avoiding surgery with its attendant risks. Patients who are clinically stable with a small, unruptured ectopic pregnancy may be offered medical management with systemic methotrexate, a folic acid antagonist that preferentially inhibits rapidly replicating cells such as trophoblast. In properly selected patients, methotrexate is 75% to 85% effective in resolving ectopic pregnancy, with the remaining women requiring surgery.
  - Criteria for medical management include hemodynamic stability, gestational sac less than 3.5 cm in diameter, β-hCG at diagnosis less than 5000 IU, no ultrasound fetal cardiac activity, minimal hemoperitoneum, no underlying liver or renal disease, no blood dyscrasia, not breast-feeding, and ability to have regular follow-up.
  - A D&C should be performed to rule out a nonviable intrauterine pregnancy because medical treatment is ineffective at emptying the uterus.
  - Pretreatment complete blood count and platelet count, β-hCG level, and liver and renal function tests should be obtained.
  - Methotrexate is given in either single-dose or multidose regimens (Table 7-4). The two regimens have been widely studied for treatment of ectopic pregnancy and both are acceptable.
    - The multidose regimen has a lower failure rate; however, the risk of complications including diarrhea, abnormal liver function, and stomatitis is greater with the multidose regimen.
    - The single-dose regimen is slightly less successful, requiring a second dose in up to 20% of women; however, there is a lower incidence of side effects. The failure rate is approximately 15% with the single-dose regimen when the initial β-hCG level is greater than 5000 IU but drops to approximately 4% with lower initial β-hCG levels.
    - The failure rate of either regimen increases when a live embryo, a high initial β-hCG level, or a large adnexal mass is present.

Table 7-4	Methotrexate for Ectopic Pregnancy	
	Single-dose regimen	**Multidose regimen**
Protocol	50 mg/m² IM	1 mg/kg IM days 1, 3, 5, 7 until β-hCG drops Leucovorin 0.1 mg/kg days 2, 4, 6, 8
Follow-up	β-hCG days 4, 7, then weekly	β-hCG each day until >15% drop, then weekly
Success rate	88% 70% single dose 85% two doses	93% 10% single dose 25% two doses 50% ≥4 doses
Side effects	10%–25%	15%–35%

IM, intramuscular; β-hCG, β-human chorionic gonadotropin.

- – Follow-up after methotrexate includes measurement of β-hCG on days 4 and 7 after the single dose.
  - * The day 4 level is usually increased over baseline due to lysis of trophoblast.
  - * The day 7 level should be at least 15% less than the day 4 level or the dose may be repeated.
  - * Repeat dosing may also be required if β-hCG levels increase or plateau.
  - * Levels of β-hCG should be followed weekly until reaching a nonpregnant level (threshold will vary by laboratory) (1).
  - * Transient increase in abdominal pain is common in the days to weeks after methotrexate administration. This is thought to be caused by separation of the trophoblast from the tubal wall with varying amounts of intraperitoneal bleeding. Most separation pain can be managed on an outpatient basis; however, significant pain may require hospitalization and observation to rule out rupture and intraperitoneal hemorrhage.
  - * Surgical intervention is rarely required but may be needed to manage severe pain, hemorrhage, or treatment failure.

Unusual Locations
- Nontubal ectopic pregnancy. More than 95% of ectopic pregnancies occur in the fallopian tube, usually in the distal half. However, pregnancies can implant in a wide variety of sites, including the ovary, intramyometrial portion of the tube or uterine cornua, lower uterine segment or cervix, prior cesarean section scar, and peritoneal cavity (1).
  - These pregnancies are usually diagnosed later than are tubal pregnancies, in part because they tend to grow larger and progress further in gestation before causing symptoms.
  - Catastrophic rupture with hemorrhage and shock is significantly more likely to occur in these nontubal pregnancies.
  - A thorough evaluation including comprehensive transvaginal ultrasound examination is necessary to diagnose these unusual pregnancies.
  - Treatment is individualized, and a combination of medical and surgical therapy is often appropriate.
- Abdominal pregnancy accounts for approximately 0.003% of all pregnancies and 1.4% of all ectopic pregnancies. It arises either from primary implantation in the abdominal cavity or secondary implantation after tubal abortion.
  - Women with abdominal pregnancy often can present with advanced gestation age complaining of abdominal pain, unusual fetal lie, or unusually prominent fetal parts

(11). If partial placental separation has occurred, the patient may present in shock with intra-abdominal hemorrhage.
- Diagnosis may be difficult to make with ultrasound; CT scanning or magnetic resonance imaging may be required.
- Once the diagnosis is established, the patient should be stabilized with fluids, blood typed and cross-matched, and a laparotomy performed. The fetus should be removed, the umbilical cord tied as close as possible to the placenta, and the placenta left in situ. Any attempt to separate the placenta from abdominal organs or the abdominal wall may result in severe blood loss and should therefore be avoided.
- Cervical pregnancy arises from implantation in the cervical epithelium instead of the endometrium and account for less than 1% of ectopic pregnancies.
  - The patient usually presents with heavy vaginal bleeding and a cervical mass. The cervix may be effaced and dilated. It is sometimes difficult to distinguish a cervical implantation from an incomplete abortion with products of conception passing through the cervix.
  - Ultrasound may help distinguish a small uterine fundus above the pregnancy mass.
  - The pregnancy can removed with suction curettage, but bleeding from the implantation site is often very heavy. Paracervical injection with dilute vasopressin may aid with hemostasis. Hysterectomy may be necessary if hemorrhage is severe.
  - Conservative treatment using systemic chemotherapy (typically multiregimen methotrexate) in combination with cervical evacuation and hemostatic techniques (balloon tamponade, uterine artery ligation, cervical sutures) is an option in the stable patient (11).
- Ovarian pregnancy implants within the ovarian stroma. Ovarian pregnancies are rare, and the diagnosis is seldom made preoperatively. Management is cystectomy or wedge resection of the ovary with repair of the ovary or oophorectomy if cystectomy cannot be accomplished.

Long-Term Prognosis
- Women who have had one ectopic pregnancy are at significant risk for future infertility and for recurrent ectopic pregnancies. Regardless of treatment modality, patency of the affected tube can be demonstrated by hysterosalpingogram in approximately 75% of women.
- Women who have had an ectopic pregnancy should be educated about the symptoms associated with ectopic pregnancy and should be counseled to seek care immediately upon diagnosis of a subsequent pregnancy, regardless of symptoms. β-hCG levels should be monitored, and an early ultrasound should be performed.

PATIENT EDUCATION
- Women with known risk factors for ectopic pregnancy should be informed of the risks and symptoms before trying to become pregnant.
- When a woman has a suspected or diagnosed ectopic pregnancy, she should receive detailed counseling about the medical and surgical management options.
- Patients who select medical management with methotrexate must be informed of the need for close, regular follow-up with monitoring of β-hCG levels.

REFERENCES
1. American College of Gynecologists. ACOG Practice Bulletin No. 94: Medical management of ectopic pregnancy. *Obstet Gynecol.* 2008;111:1479–1485.
2. Silva C, Sammel MD, Zhou L, et al. Human chorionic gonadotropin profile for women with ectopic pregnancy. *Obstet Gynecol.* 2006;107:605–610.
3. Ankum WM, Mol BW, Van der Veen F, et al. Risk factors for ectopic pregnancy: a meta-analysis. *Fertil Steril.* 1996;65:1093–1099.

4. Clayton HB, Schieve LA, Peterson HB, et al. Ectopic pregnancy risk with assisted reproductive technology procedures. *Obstet Gynecol.* 2006;107:595–604.

5. Barnhart KT, Sammel MD, Rinaudo PF, et al. Symptomatic patients with an early viable intrauterine pregnancy: HCG curves redefined. *Obstet Gynecol.* 2004;104:50–55.

6. Verhaegen J, Gallos ID, van Mello NM, et al. Accuracy of single progesterone test to predict early pregnancy outcome in women with pain or bleeding: meta-analysis of cohort studies. *BMJ.* 2012;345:e6077.

7. Barnhart K, Mennuti MT, Benjamin I, et al. Prompt diagnosis of ectopic pregnancy in an emergency department setting. *Obstet Gynecol.* 1994;84:1010–1015.

8. Nyberg DA, Laing FC, Filly RA, et al. Ultrasonographic differentiation of the gestational sac of early intrauterine pregnancy from the pseudogestational sac of ectopic pregnancy. *Radiology.* 1983;146:755–759.

9. Shaunik A, Kulp J, Appleby DH, et al. Utility of dilation and curettage in the diagnosis of pregnancy of unknown location. *Am J Obstet Gynecol.* 2011;204:130.e1–e6.

10. Al-Sunaidi M, Tulandi T. Surgical treatment of ectopic pregnancy. *Semin Reprod Med.* 2007;25:117–122.

11. Molinaro TA, Barnhart KT. Ectopic pregnancies in unusual locations. *Semin Reprod Med.* 2007;25:123–130.

8

Spontaneous Preterm Birth

Emily DeFranco and Kristin L. Atkins

INTRODUCTION

- Preterm delivery is one of the most serious problems in obstetrics. Prematurity is the leading cause of neonatal morbidity and mortality in the United States (1). Despite advances in research and medical care, the incidence of prematurity in the United States remains among the highest compared to other industrialized nations.
- The incidence of preterm birth peaked in 2006 and has slightly declined over the last 7 years.
- Spontaneous preterm birth is a multidimensional problem that includes preterm labor, preterm premature rupture of membranes, cervical insufficiency, and short cervix.

PRETERM LABOR

Key Points

- The complex mechanisms leading to preterm labor limit the effectiveness of any single treatment intervention.
- Preterm labor is diagnosed clinically by evidence of regular uterine contractions associated with cervical change.
- Tocolytic medications may prolong pregnancy for a short period of time (48 to 72 hours).
- Antenatal corticosteroids should be administered to women at risk of preterm delivery.
- Progesterone supplementation may reduce the rate of recurrent spontaneous preterm delivery in women with a prior spontaneous preterm birth. It may also reduce preterm birth risk in asymptomatic singleton pregnancies with midtrimester cervical shortening.

Background

Although the causes of preterm labor are not well understood, its clinical impact is clear. Infant prematurity is the leading cause of newborn morbidity, mortality, and health expenditure in the United States. The incidence of serious complications of prematurity increases dramatically as the gestational age at delivery decreases. Neonatal mortality also increases with declining gestational age at delivery (2). The serious complications of prematurity include, but are not limited to, respiratory distress syndrome, intraventricular hemorrhage, necrotizing enterocolitis, sepsis, and patent ductus arteriosus. The costs related to these complications increase exponentially with the degree of prematurity. The economic burden attributed to preterm birth is estimated to be at least 26 billion dollars annually in the United States, with most of that cost incurred in the care of infant survivors of prematurity (3).

Definition
- Preterm labor is defined as regular uterine contractions associated with cervical change occurring from 20 to 36 6/7 weeks of gestational age.

Pathophysiology
- The pathophysiologic mechanisms that lead to the onset of preterm labor are complex and multifactorial. Because of this complexity, the identification of an effective intervention for preterm labor has been elusive.

- In addition to mechanisms as yet unknown, preterm labor likely occurs as a result of the concomitant activation or a cascade of the following events (4,5):
  - Functional progesterone withdrawal
  - Increase in corticotrophin-releasing hormone
  - Premature decidual activation
  - Increased prostaglandin production
  - Oxytocin initiation
  - Increased cytokine production

Etiology

Numerous factors contribute to the high incidence of preterm delivery, including the increase in pregnancies in women over 35 years of age and the increase in the incidence of multiple gestations due to more frequent use of artificial reproductive technologies (6).

There are a multitude of causes of preterm delivery. In general, preterm deliveries can be classified as (a) iatrogenic or indicated due to a significant maternal or fetal complication of pregnancy, (b) spontaneous due to preterm labor, or (c) a result of preterm, premature rupture of membranes (PROM). Spontaneous preterm labor accounts for approximately 50% of preterm deliveries. Iatrogenic prematurity and PROM constitute the remaining 50%, contributing approximately 25% each (7).

This chapter focuses on spontaneous preterm birth, which is divided primarily into two categories: preterm labor with intact membranes and PROM. In addition, we review cervical disorders that predispose a pregnant woman to spontaneous preterm birth: cervical insufficiency and asymptomatic short cervix.

Epidemiology

- The incidence of preterm delivery remains high, with the most recent estimate being 11.5% (8). Preterm delivery occurs more frequently in black women than in white women, especially at the very early gestational ages of less than 28 weeks (9). Of all etiologies of preterm birth, preterm labor is the major contributor.
- Risk factors for preterm labor include (10,11)
  - Prior preterm delivery
  - African American race
  - Low socioeconomic status
  - Lack of prenatal care
  - Intense physical exertion or stress
  - Low body mass index
  - Extremes of maternal age (younger than 18 or older than 40)
  - Tobacco use
  - Substance abuse
  - Prior induced abortion
  - Prior cervical surgery
  - Periodontal disease
  - Uterine overdistension (i.e., multiple gestation or polyhydramnios)
  - Vaginal bleeding during pregnancy
  - Uterine anomaly
  - Anemia
  - Reproductive tract infections
  - Short cervix in the midtrimester of pregnancy
- Numerous risk factor scoring systems have been proposed for the prediction of preterm labor. Unfortunately, these scoring systems have not been proven to reliably predict spontaneous preterm birth, and most lack clinically important reference standards (12).

Evaluation

History and Physical

- Symptoms may or may not be present in women presenting with preterm labor. When present, these symptoms may vary greatly. Some of the most common presenting symptoms of preterm labor are
  - Rhythmic contractions (some women describe this as a feeling of "balling up")
  - Lower abdominal cramping
  - Low back pain
  - Pelvic pressure
  - Increase in vaginal discharge
  - Bloody vaginal discharge (bloody show)
- Cervical examination can be performed by any one or a combination of the following tools:
  - Digital cervical exam:
    - A change in dilation and/or effacement of the cervix in the presence of regular uterine contractions is sufficient for the diagnosis of preterm labor.
    - Alternatively, regular uterine contractions and a cervix greater than 2 cm dilated or ≥80% effaced upon a single examination are sufficient for the diagnosis.
- Visual estimation of cervical dilation and effacement by speculum examination
- Ultrasonography of the cervix to measure cervical length (CL)
  - In some cases where the diagnosis of preterm labor is uncertain, that is, frequent preterm contractions without cervical change or cervical dilation less than 2 cm, a combined approach of cervical length measurement and fFN testing may assist in the diagnosis. This approach has been shown to be reliable for diagnosis of PTL or exclusion of PTL compared to the standard approach of digital cervical exam (13,14).

Laboratory Tests

- Rectovaginal culture for group B streptococcus (GBS) (*Streptococcus agalactiae*) should be obtained.
- Wet mount (swab of vaginal secretions mixed with saline placed on a microscope slide). The presence of "clue cells" indicates bacterial vaginosis. The presence of flagellated microorganisms indicates *Trichomonas vaginalis* infection.
- Urinalysis and culture to evaluate for evidence of urinary tract infection or asymptomatic bacteriuria.
- Fetal fibronectin test from a swab of cervicovaginal secretions. This test
  - Can be especially useful if the diagnosis of preterm labor is in question.
  - Has a high negative predictive value. If negative, the risk of delivering in the upcoming 2 weeks is less than 1% (15).
  - Has a relatively low positive predictive value if used alone. If positive, the risk of delivering in 1 week is 18% (16).
  - Has a relatively high positive predictive value for preterm birth within a short period of time if used in combination with cervical length in symptomatic patients (13).
- Microscope slide of dried vaginal sidewall secretions (do not use a cover slip) to evaluate for evidence of "ferning," which is suggestive of the diagnosis of PROM.
  - This is only necessary if PROM is suspected based on patient's history or exam.
  - Avoid contaminating the slide with saline, which may result in the false appearance of ferning.
  - Cervical mucus may also fern, so close attention should be paid to the collection of the specimen.
  - A new test, AmniSure, may also be used for diagnosis of PROM. It has high screen accuracy for diagnosis of PROM.
- Cervical cultures for *Chlamydia trachomatis* and *Neisseria gonorrhoeae* may be collected as clinically indicated.
- Drug abuse screen, either serum or urine, as clinically indicated.

Ultrasound
- A thorough obstetrical ultrasound is helpful in evaluating the etiology of preterm labor in order to
  - Identify obvious fetal malformations. Some major congenital malformations may be a contraindication to tocolysis, and some may warrant aggressive tocolysis.
  - Identify abnormalities in fetal growth.
  - Identify abnormalities in amniotic fluid volume (oligohydramnios or polyhydramnios).
  - Confirm fetal presentation to aid in planning mode of delivery.
  - Evaluate placenta, identifying its location and noting any abnormalities.
- Ultrasound evaluation of the cervix may help to further refine the risk of preterm delivery (15). Short cervical lengths are associated with an increased risk of preterm delivery.
  - Cervical length of 30 mm or greater is useful to exclude the diagnosis of preterm labor.
  - Short cervical lengths (less than 25 mm or less than 20 mm, depending on gestational age) may assist in confirming the diagnosis of preterm labor, especially when used in combination with positive fFN result (13).

Diagnosis
- Preterm labor is a clinical diagnosis. It should be suspected in any gravida with regular preterm uterine contractions and is confirmed with documented cervical change. The previously mentioned objective criteria may also be useful in establishing the diagnosis (fetal fibronectin and ultrasound measurement of cervical length).

Treatment
Bed Rest and Hydration
- There is no scientific evidence to prove that bed rest, although commonly prescribed, is useful in preventing or treating preterm labor. The American College of Obstetricians and Gynecologists (ACOG) states that "although bed rest and hydration have been recommended to women with symptoms of preterm labor to prevent preterm delivery, these measures have not been shown to be effective for the prevention of preterm birth and should not be routinely recommended. Furthermore, the potential harm, including venous thromboembolism, bone demineralization, and deconditioning, and the negative effects, such as loss of employment, should not be underestimated" (17).
- Hydration, both orally and intravenously, is commonly used in the treatment of preterm labor. Several studies that have evaluated the effect of hydration on preterm labor have demonstrated no benefit (18,19).

Tocolytic Medications
- Women who meet criteria for the diagnosis of preterm labor are candidates for tocolytic therapy. There is no clear "first-line" tocolytic medication (17). Little evidence exists that any tocolytic medication can effectively prolong gestation longer than 2 to 7 days (20). However, this short prolongation is usually sufficient to administer corticosteroids for fetal benefit and to transfer the patient to a tertiary care facility before delivery. These interventions have been shown to improve perinatal outcome.
- Tocolytic medications are, most often, given to women with preterm labor at less than 34 weeks of gestational age. After 34 weeks of gestation, the risk of complications of tocolytic therapy may outweigh the benefits of prolonging the pregnancy for a short period of time. After a determined period of time (48 hours), tocolytic therapy is usually discontinued because prolonged use of tocolysis may increase the maternal–fetal risk without offering a clear benefit (3). Eighty percent of women with presumed preterm labor subsequently deliver at term (15). Therefore, careful consideration should be given before initiating tocolytic therapy.
- There are a number of contraindications to tocolysis including, but not limited to, placental abruption, lethal fetal congenital anomaly, intrauterine infection (chorioamnionitis), severe preeclampsia, and evidence of fetal compromise (3).

- Calcium channel blockers (5,21):
  - The most common calcium channel blocker used for tocolysis is nifedipine.
  - Mechanism of action: decreases the influx of intracellular calcium ions into myometrial cells, promoting relaxation (22).
  - Dosage: 20- to 30-mg loading dose, followed by 10 to 20 mg every 4 to 8 hours orally.
  - Precautions: use with caution in patients with cardiac disease or renal disease and avoid concomitant use with magnesium sulfate.
  - Side effects: flushing, headache, dizziness, hypotension, and peripheral edema.
  - Complications: some side effects can be severe, resulting in the discontinuation of therapy in 2% to 5% of patients. Severe hypotension can occur if used with magnesium sulfate. There are no known adverse fetal effects.
- Magnesium sulfate:
  - Tocolytic agent of choice of many obstetricians and perinatologists in the United States (23).
  - Mechanism of action: inhibits smooth muscle contractions by inhibiting calcium uptake.
  - Dosage: 4 to 6 g as intravenous (IV) bolus over 15 to 30 minutes, followed by 2 to 6 g/h (24). A common clinical approach is to start with a 6-g IV bolus followed by 3 g/h. The hourly rate is titrated until uterine contractions abate or until a serum level of 5 to 8 ng/dL is reached (25). Magnesium sulfate may be discontinued simply by ceasing IV infusion at any time. Weaning the drug is not necessary (26). Serum magnesium levels will slowly decrease as magnesium is cleared by the kidneys.
  - Precautions: magnesium sulfate should be avoided in women with myasthenia gravis, cardiac impairment, renal impairment, or with concomitant use of a calcium channel blocker due to the potential of causing profound hypotension (24,27).
  - Side effects: flushing, nausea, headache, drowsiness, and blurred vision. These are common side effects with therapeutic doses of magnesium and not necessarily evidence of magnesium toxicity.
  - Complications:
    - Monitoring for evidence of magnesium toxicity should be performed at frequent intervals in all patients receiving magnesium tocolysis.
      - Diminished or loss of deep tendon reflexes with serum magnesium levels of greater than 10 ng/dL.
      - Respiratory depression (greater than 15 ng/dL).
      - Cardiac arrest (greater than 18 ng/dL).
      - Magnesium toxicity can be rapidly reversed with 1 g of IV calcium gluconate.
    - Pulmonary edema may occur, especially in women with multiple gestation, multiagent tocolytic therapy, or fluid overload (5).
- β-Sympathomimetics (5,28):
  - Ritodrine is the only medication approved by the Food and Drug Administration (FDA) for tocolysis in the United States. Ritodrine is associated with significant side effects and patient intolerance. Because of these side effects, ritodrine has not been marketed in the United States since 1998.
  - Terbutaline is currently the most commonly used β-sympathomimetic and is β_2 selective. Most studies have shown that it is effective in temporarily arresting preterm labor, but it does not reduce the rate of preterm delivery.
  - Mechanism of action: stimulation of β receptors (some β_2 selective), resulting in uterine smooth muscle relaxation.
  - Dosage:
    - Subcutaneous: 0.25 mg every 20 minutes for 4 to 6 doses. Hold for pulse greater than 120 beats/min.
    - Subcutaneous pump: Although available, this method is not recommended due to increased risk of maternal cardiac toxicity and death. The FDA recommends against its use for more than 48 hours.

- Precautions: avoid or use with caution in patients with cardiac arrhythmias, diabetes, hyperthyroidism, or hypertension.
- Side effects: tachycardia, tremor, decreased appetite, and hypotension.
- Complications: pulmonary edema (especially with multiagent tocolysis), cardiac arrhythmias, hyperglycemia, hypokalemia, neonatal cardiac arrhythmias, and hypoglycemia.
- Prostaglandin synthase inhibitors (5,29):
  - Agents available: aspirin, ibuprofen, indomethacin, sulindac, ketorolac. Indomethacin is the most commonly used agent.
  - Mechanism of action: inhibition of prostaglandin synthetase or cyclooxygenase, blocking prostaglandin production.
  - Dosage: indomethacin can be administered orally, rectally, or vaginally. Common regimens include a 50- to 100-mg loading dose, followed by 25 mg every 6 to 8 hours. Many obstetricians limit the use to 48 to 72 hours to avoid complications (30).
  - Precautions: contraindicated in patients with active peptic ulcer disease, sensitivity to nonsteroidal anti-inflammatory drugs, significant renal or hepatic impairment, or hematologic abnormalities (especially thrombocytopenia).
  - Side effects: nausea and gastrointestinal upset.
  - Complications: indomethacin use has been associated with several fetal and neonatal complications, including premature closure of the fetal ductus arteriosis (especially at gestational ages greater than 32 weeks) (31), pulmonary hypertension, oligohydramnios, intraventricular hemorrhage, and necrotizing enterocolitis. Most of these reported complications occurred in pregnancies with prolonged administration, and these results should be viewed with caution due to multiple potential confounders (32).
- Multiple-agent tocolysis:
  - No clear evidence exists that combining tocolytic drugs improves efficacy. Combining tocolytic agents potentially increases the risk of maternal and neonatal complications (17). Using multiple tocolytic agents simultaneously should be approached with caution.
- Maintenance tocolysis:
  - No clear evidence exists that maintenance tocolysis increases gestational age at birth, increases birth weight, or effectively prolongs pregnancy (33).

Corticosteroids
- Antepartum corticosteroids effectively reduce the incidence of neonatal respiratory distress, intraventricular hemorrhage, necrotizing enterocolitis, and neonatal death in preterm infants. A single course of corticosteroids should be administered to all pregnant women between 24 and 34 weeks of gestation who are at risk of preterm delivery within 7 days (34).
- Either betamethasone or dexamethasone may be used. Neither the National Institutes of Health (NIH) nor the American College of Obstetricians and Gynecologists (ACOG) recommend the use of one over the other (35).
  - Betamethasone, 12 mg intramuscularly (IM) every 24 hours for two doses
  - Dexamethasone, 6 mg IM every 12 hours for four doses
- A single additional dose may be considered if the initial dose was given more than 2 weeks prior and there is additional risk for preterm delivery, as recommended by ACOG. Multiple repeat doses of steroids have not been shown to provide added benefit and may be harmful (35).

Magnesium Sulfate for Neuroprotection
- Several studies have been published to evaluate the use of magnesium prior to delivery of a preterm infant to assess the reduction in risk of neonatal complications (36–40).
- Meta-analyses of these studies have shown that there is a reduction of the incidence of cerebral palsy in these preterm infants when exposed to magnesium sulfate prior to delivery (41,42).

- ACOG Committee on Obstetric Practice has recognized this reduction in the risk of cerebral palsy and has recommended that institutions choosing to use magnesium sulfate for neuroprotection should "develop specific guidelines regarding inclusion criteria, treatment regimens, concurrent tocolysis, and monitoring in accordance with one of the larger trials" (43).

Antibiotics
- There is no evidence that treating women with preterm labor with antibiotics is effective in prolonging pregnancy, and this practice is not recommended (35).
- Antibiotic prophylaxis to prevent GBS sepsis in the newborn is recommended in women with preterm labor (44). The Centers for Disease Control and Prevention recommends GBS culture of all women in preterm labor. If the culture is negative within 4 weeks of delivery, prophylaxis is not recommended.

Prevention
- Progesterone
  - Studies have demonstrated that progesterone given to women with a *history of spontaneous preterm birth* can effectively decrease the incidence of recurrent preterm birth in a subsequent pregnancy (45). The optimal formulation for this indication has not been identified, but the most commonly used agent, based on data from the largest clinical trial, is
    ○ 17-Hydroxyprogesterone caproate.
    ○ Dose: 250 mg IM weekly initiated at 16 to 20 weeks of gestational age and continued until 37.
    ○ Other studies have demonstrated that women with a singleton pregnancy and *asymptomatic cervical shortening in the midtrimester of pregnancy* (less than 20 mm) benefit from vaginal progesterone therapy (45).
    ○ Micronized progesterone 200 mg capsule, one per vagina once daily.
    ○ Progesterone 8% vaginal gel, one applicator daily.

Complications of Preterm Labor
- There are a number of complications that may be either the cause or the result of preterm labor:
  - Placental abruption
  - Intra-amniotic infection (chorioamnionitis)
  - PROM

Patient Education
- Incidence of preterm delivery in patients with preterm labor:
  - Eighty percent of women with presumptive preterm labor go on to deliver at term (15).
- Recurrence of preterm labor in future pregnancies:
  - The incidence of recurrent, spontaneous preterm birth varies greatly in numerous series (from 15% to greater than 50%).
  - The risk increases with multiple factors, including a history of a very early preterm delivery (i.e., less than 28 weeks of gestational age) (46).

PRETERM, PREMATURE RUPTURE OF THE MEMBRANES
Key Points
- PPROM accounts for 25% to 30% of all preterm deliveries.
- The management of preterm PPROM should take into account the risk of pregnancy prolongation (intra-amniotic infection, placental abruption, and fetal compromise) versus the benefits of conservative management (fetal maturation).
- Women with PPROM at greater than 34 weeks' gestation should be delivered.
- Antibiotics have been shown to prolong latency in patients with PROM.
- Corticosteroids decrease neonatal morbidity when given to women with uncomplicated PPROM.

Background

PPROM occurs in approximately 3% of all pregnancies and accounts for 25% to 30% of all preterm deliveries (7,47). PPROM presents a unique management dilemma to obstetricians and perinatologists, who must balance between continued gestation to alleviate the risk of prematurity-related morbidities and the prevention of adverse fetal and maternal outcomes related to membrane rupture.

The interval between membrane rupture and delivery is usually short, but it is inversely proportional to the gestational age at which it occurs (earlier gestational ages have longer latencies). When managed conservatively, more than half of women with PROM before 34 weeks deliver within 1 week (47,48).

Prolonging pregnancy decreases the incidence of neonatal morbidities associated with prematurity, yet longer latencies may increase the likelihood of developing complications of PPROM such as chorioamnionitis, placental abruption, and umbilical cord compression.

Definition

- Preterm rupture of the membranes: rupture of the amniotic membranes before 37 weeks of gestational age.
- Premature rupture of the membranes: rupture of the amniotic membranes before the onset of labor, regardless of gestational age.
- Prolonged rupture of the membranes: rupture of the amniotic membranes for more than 18 hours.
- PPROM: preterm premature rupture of the membranes.
- PPROM indicates the addition of prolonged membrane rupture.

Pathophysiology

- At term, membrane rupture is considered a normal part of parturition and may occur before or after the onset of labor. It occurs due to a combination of physiologic processes that may be exacerbated by uterine contractions (47).
- Preterm rupture of membranes is associated with a higher incidence of intrauterine infection than rupture of membranes at term, especially at very early gestational ages. It is thought that ascending bacteria from the vagina lead to increased cytokine activation and resultant apoptosis in the amniotic membranes, making them more susceptible to rupture (49).
- PROM can also occur as a complication of amniocentesis. This is fairly uncommon and occurs in less than 0.5% of amniocentesis procedures.

Etiology

- Various factors have been associated with PPROM, including
  - Infectious causes (amnionitis, cervicitis, and other vaginoses)
  - Increased uterine volume (polyhydramnios and multiple gestation)
  - Subchorionic hemorrhage
  - Cervical conization or cerclage
  - Fetal anomalies
  - Low socioeconomic status
  - Biochemical structural abnormalities (Ehlers-Danlos syndrome)
  - Maternal trauma
  - Substance abuse, including smoking

Evaluation

History and Physical

- Given the significant adverse effects of PPROM on pregnancy outcome, any patient who presents with a history of leaking fluid from the vagina or has a decreased amniotic fluid volume on US should be carefully evaluated.
- Direct digital cervical exam should be avoided until the diagnosis of PPROM is ruled out or a decision to deliver has been made.

- Sterile speculum exam is used to document rupture of membranes, using the tests described below. The posterior fornix should be examined for evidence of pooling of amniotic fluid. If pooling is not immediately evident, one may visualize fluid coming through the cervix during a Valsalva maneuver or with coughing.

Laboratory Tests
- Fern test
  - The fern test has traditionally been the most common method to determine rupture of membranes.
  - Vaginal secretions from the posterior fornix are collected with a sterile cotton-tipped applicator and smeared thinly on a glass slide. After sufficient time to allow for the sample to air dry, it is examined under the microscope for the presence of an arborized (fernlike) pattern. To prevent false-negative readings, the slide must be completely dry. Any evidence of arborization should be read as a positive test.
  - False-positive tests have been reported with the presence of dried saline and/or cervical mucus.
- AmniSure
  - The AmniSure test is a rapid test for the presence of placental alpha microglobulin-1 (PAMG-1) in the vagina. PAMG-1 is a protein found at high levels within amniotic fluid and extremely low levels within cervical and vaginal fluid.
  - A sterile Dacron swab is used to collect fluid from the vagina. The sterile swab is placed in the vagina no more than 2 to 3 inches deep and left in place for 1 minute. The swab is then rotated in the testing vial for 1 minute. The test strip is then inserted into the vial with solvent. A positive result will be apparent within 10 minutes.
  - A positive test confirms the presence of ruptured membranes. This testing may be better than nitrazine and ferning test in the presence of prolonged time from time of rupture of membranes.
  - This test has a sensitivity of 98.7% to 98.9% and specificity of 87.5% to 100% when compared to the presence of ferning and nitrazine positive (50).
- Nitrazine test
  - The nitrazine test relies on the pH of amniotic fluid (pH 7.0 to 7.5), which is significantly more alkaline than normal vaginal secretions (pH 4.5 to 5.5).
  - A sample of vaginal secretions is smeared onto nitrazine pH paper. A color change to blue-green (pH 6.5) or blue (pH 7.0) is strong evidence for the presence of amniotic fluid.
  - False-positive results may occur with the presence of blood, urine, semen, or antiseptic cleansing agents.
  - Due to quality control concerns, this is becoming a less frequently used test for PROM in labor and delivery units.
- Ultrasound is helpful in confirming PPROM and aiding in management decisions.
  - Amniotic fluid volume by ultrasound helps confirm the diagnosis of PPROM, especially when the fern test or the nitrazine test is equivocal. PPROM is usually associated with a low amniotic fluid volume; however, pockets of fluid larger than 2 × 2 cm are often present.
  - Determination of the fetal presenting part and estimated fetal weight is helpful in the management of women with PPROM. In the case of PPROM, serial ultrasounds for fetal growth should be performed every 3 to 4 weeks as a measure of fetal well-being.
- Amniocentesis
  - Amniocentesis can be used to confirm the diagnosis of PPROM if all other data are inconclusive.
  - One ampule of indigo carmine diluted in 10 to 20 mL of sterile saline is infused into the amniotic sac through an amniocentesis needle. A tampon is placed in the vagina. The tampon is then removed after 30 to 40 minutes. Presence of blue dye on the tampon confirms the diagnosis of PPROM.

- The patient should be warned that if the fetus delivers within several days, the baby may be stained with the dye used for evaluation.
- Methylene blue should not be used because it is associated with fetal hemolytic anemia, hyperbilirubinemia, methemoglobinemia, and fetal staining.
- Amniocentesis may also be used to confirm a diagnosis of intra-amniotic infection. Amniotic fluid glucose concentrations below 16 to 20 mg/dL, a positive Gram stain, or a positive amniotic fluid culture are suggestive of this diagnosis.
- Rectovaginal culture for GBS (*Streptococcus agalactiae*) should be obtained.
- Cervical cultures for *Chlamydia trachomatis* and *Neisseria gonorrhea* may be collected as clinically indicated.
- Amniotic fluid may be sent for fetal lung maturity testing. The sample may be obtained from a vaginal pool or amniocentesis.

Diagnosis
- Clinical evaluation as described above is essential for the diagnosis of PPROM.
- PROM should be suspected when there is a history of leaking fluid from vagina or if a low amniotic fluid volume is detected on ultrasound.

Differential Diagnosis
- Ensure that the fetal kidneys and bladder are present and normal appearing. Oligohydramnios may be the result of renal agenesis, a lethal abnormality. The management of these pregnancies is quite different from those complicated by PPROM.
- Decreased amniotic fluid volume may also be the result of fetal compromise with reduced renal perfusion due to uteroplacental insufficiency.

Clinical Manifestations
- Time from rupture of membranes to delivery is usually brief and is inversely related to gestational age at the time of rupture. However, even with conservative management, 50% of women deliver within 1 week of rupture (47,48). Despite this, these women may benefit from conservative management (51).
- A small percentage of cases of PPROM resolve, and the fluid leakage ceases (2.6% to 13%) (52).

Treatment
- Unless delivery is imminent, the patient should be cared for in a hospital that can provide adequate neonatal care for the infant. This may require transfer to a tertiary care facility.
- Delivery of the fetus may be indicated in the following circumstances:
  - Active labor
  - Chorioamnionitis (maternal fever, uterine tenderness, maternal or fetal tachycardia)
  - Nonreassuring fetal testing
  - Fetal demise
  - Evidence of placental abruption with significant vaginal bleeding
  - Advanced cervical dilation and/or fetal malpresentation with increased concern for umbilical cord prolapse
- In the absence of any of the above concerns, gestational age is the primary factor in the decision to continue conservative management. Prolongation of pregnancy to allow the fetus to mature is of primary concern. Once the fetus is mature or reaches the gestational age where the intensive care unit staff determines it to be relatively mature, the benefit of continued intrauterine growth is outweighed by the risks of continuing the pregnancy.
- *After 34 weeks of gestational age*, conservative management increases the risk for chorioamnionitis, lower umbilical cord gases, and prolonged maternal hospital stay without decreasing perinatal morbidity for the fetus (53). Therefore, these fetuses should be delivered at 34 weeks.

- *Between 32 and 34 weeks,* if fetal lung maturity studies are positive, delaying delivery provides no additional benefit. Conservative management in the setting of mature lung indices has been associated with increase risk of chorioamnionitis (54). If fetal lung maturity is not documented and there are no other complications, conservative management is appropriate.
- *Before 32 weeks,* delivery is associated with significant infant morbidity related to the degree of prematurity. Conservative management is recommended if no other complications exist.
- *When PPROM occurs before the fetus is viable,* different considerations are given to the continuation of the pregnancy. The fetus is at risk for a number of complications, including pulmonary hypoplasia and limb contractures, if the pregnancy is continued to viability. The patient with previable PPROM may be offered conservative management or immediate delivery. In the case of conservative management, the patient may be managed on an outpatient basis until viability is reached. She should then return to the hospital for inpatient management and initiation of fetal surveillance when viability is reached.

Medications
Antibiotics
- One of the best-studied areas in the management of PPROM is the use of antibiotics to prolong gestation. Treatment with antibiotics along with conservative management can potentially
  - Treat or prevent ascending infection
  - Prevent chorioamnionitis
  - Reduce neonatal sepsis
  - Prolong the latency period
- The goal of antibiotic treatment is to provide broad-spectrum antimicrobial coverage, for both gram-positive and gram-negative bacteria (55).
- The antibiotic regimen proven to prolong latency and improve perinatal outcome is as follows:
  - Ampicillin, 2 g, and erythromycin, 250 mg, intravenously every 6 hours the first 48 hours, followed by amoxicillin, 250 mg, and erythromycin, 333 mg, orally every 8 hours for 5 days (56)

Corticosteroids
- Because patients with PPROM are at significant risk of perinatal morbidity, antenatal corticosteroids are administered for fetal benefit. A single course reduces the incidence of neonatal respiratory distress syndrome, intraventricular hemorrhage, and necrotizing enterocolitis (57).
- There is no increase in perinatal infection when steroids are given in the treatment of PROM (58,59).
- Dosing regimens are the same as when used for any other indication:
  - Betamethasone, 12 mg IM every 24 hours for two doses or
  - Dexamethasone, 6 mg IM every 12 hours for four doses

Tocolytic Therapy
- There is no evidence that tocolytic therapy prolongs gestation in the context of ruptured membranes. Despite this lack of evidence, some centers use tocolytics in patients with PPROM in an effort to continue the pregnancy long enough to administer steroids and transport the patient to a tertiary care facility. For details of acute tocolytic therapy, refer to the "Preterm Labor" section in this chapter.

Procedures
- Surveillance of fetal well-being should be performed at least daily (nonstress test and/or biophysical profile).
- Continuous fetal monitoring is preferred if there are signs of umbilical cord compression or other concern for fetal well-being.

- The results of the biophysical profile may be confounded by oligohydramnios or impending labor but are still helpful in management decisions.

Complications
Maternal
- PROM, especially with prolonged membrane rupture, places the pregnancy at risk for chorioamnionitis from ascending bacteria. This risk increases with decreasing gestational age at time of rupture and with increased latency (60,61).
- Postpartum endometritis complicates 2% to 13% of these pregnancies.
- The risk of placental abruption is greater than in the general population and is reported to occur in 4% to 12% of pregnancies complicated by PPROM.

Fetal
- Fetal morbidity after PPROM is predominantly related to the degree of prematurity. The most common complications of prematurity are respiratory distress syndrome, necrotizing enterocolitis, intraventricular hemorrhage, and sepsis.
- Other fetal morbidities are associated with maternal infection, umbilical cord compression, placental abruption, and prolonged fetal compression. These place the fetus at an increased risk of death in utero and at an increased risk of perinatal asphyxia.
- The risk to the fetus is greatly increased if PPROM occurs before the limit of viability. With prolonged oligohydramnios, there is significant risk for maldevelopment of the alveolar tree (pulmonary hypoplasia) as well as fetal compression resulting in malformations similar to those seen in Potter syndrome.
- There is a growing body of literature evaluating the adverse neurologic sequelae of prolonged membrane rupture. At the present time, there is no evidence to discourage conservative management in patients with PPROM if no obvious concomitant complications exist (60).

Patient Education
- Recurrence of PROM in future pregnancies:
  - Patients with PROM are at increased risk of PPROM in subsequent pregnancies.
  - One study found that 32% of patients with a history of PPROM developed recurrent PROM an average of 2 weeks later in their next pregnancy (62).

CERVICAL INSUFFICIENCY
Key Points
- Cervical insufficiency is diagnosed based on a patient's *history of second-trimester pregnancy loss* in a prior pregnancy (or pregnancies), typically described as painless cervical dilation in the absence of uterine contractions.
- Transvaginal ultrasound can be a useful tool in the evaluation and management of cervical insufficiency.
- Cerclage may reduce the risk of midtrimester pregnancy loss and preterm birth in women with a history of cervical insufficiency.
  - *History-indicated cerclage* is usually performed at 13 to 14 weeks of gestation.
  - *Ultrasound-indicated cerclage* is usually performed when the cervix begins to shorten in the midtrimester between 14 and 24 weeks.
  - *Exam indicated or "rescue cerclage"* may be placed when the cervix begins to dilate without labor but is associated with an increased risk of complications.
- By definition, primiparous patients cannot be diagnosed with cervical insufficiency during their first pregnancy.

Background
Definition
- The terms *cervical insufficiency* and *cervical incompetence* have been used to describe the inability of the uterine cervix to retain a pregnancy in the absence of contractions or labor.

- Traditionally, cervical insufficiency has been defined as recurrent second-trimester loss of pregnancy. These losses are characterized by painless dilation and effacement of the cervix, without contractions or blood loss. Often the membranes protrude into the vagina. Membrane rupture is often followed by rapid delivery of the fetus (63).
- Spontaneous preterm labor in the midtrimester of pregnancy (16 to 24 weeks) can present with similar signs and symptoms as cervical insufficiency, and often the two conditions are difficult to definitively distinguish from one another.

Pathophysiology
- The pathophysiology of cervical insufficiency is not well understood.
- Incompetent cervices have less elastin both morphologically and biochemically when compared with normal cervices (64). They also contain a greater amount of smooth muscle than do competent cervices (65,66).
- Cervical insufficiency is also related to the collagen concentration in the cervix. Samples of insufficient cervices during the second trimester had greater collagen extractability and collagenolytic activity (67). Other studies have shown that in the nonpregnant state, clinically insufficient cervices have less collagen (68).

Etiology
- Congenital conditions that predispose women to cervical insufficiency include uterine anomalies and diethylstilbestrol exposure.
- Trauma to the cervix via conization, forceful dilation and curettage, or obstetric lacerations may increase the risk of cervical insufficiency.

Epidemiology
- The incidence of cervical insufficiency varies from 0.05% to 1.8%.

Evaluation

History and Physical
- An obstetric history complicated by the delivery of a fetus at 16 to 24 weeks without the presence of contractions raises the suspicion of cervical insufficiency.
- Digital exam of the cervix was once the only method available to diagnose cervical insufficiency. However, cervical dilation and effacement are often late manifestations of this pregnancy complication and cannot be relied on for early enough diagnosis to provide an operative intervention, that is, cerclage.

Screening and Diagnosis
- Cervical insufficiency can be diagnosed based on (a) *history alone* or (b) *suspicious history plus cervical shortening* found on transvaginal ultrasound.
  - *History alone*: A history of one or more midtrimester loss(es) at 16 to 24 weeks preceded by no symptoms of preterm labor, placental abruption, or PPROM is highly suggestive of cervical insufficiency. Women with cervical insufficiency often present with prolapsed membranes through a dilated cervix and relatively few other symptoms.
  - *Suspicious history plus midtrimester cervical shortening*: Women with a prior term delivery and also a midtrimester loss, or history of only one prior pregnancy complicated by midtrimester loss but with equivocal history (± preterm labor), can present a perplexing management quandary. These women may benefit from midtrimester cervical length screening with cerclage placement when/if the cervix becomes short (69).
- Various diagnostic tools have been evaluated to assess cervical competence, including hysterosalpingography and radiographic evaluation of traction on the cervix with a balloon and assessing the ease with which Hegar or Pratt dilators pass through the cervix to varying diameters (70,71). These tools have not been found to be beneficial.
- Transvaginal ultrasound cervical length (CL) screening is typically reserved to the midtrimester (14 to 24 weeks) in asymptomatic women. The use of CL screening in symptomatic women with uterine contractions at later gestational ages is described in an earlier section of this chapter, preterm labor evaluation (13).

- Cervical length assessments may be useful after 14 weeks of gestation, but not earlier due to the inability to sonographically distinguish the cervix from the lower uterine segment.
- Cervical length of 30 mm or greater assures the physician that the risk of preterm delivery is low and no intervention is necessary.
- Identification of a short cervix (less than 25 mm) in the second trimester in women with a prior preterm birth should alert the examiner to the possibility of cervical insufficiency and increased risk of recurrent spontaneous preterm birth. These women benefit from *ultrasound-indicated cerclage* placement prior to 24 weeks of gestational age (69,72).
- Suggested cervical length screening strategy for women with a history suspicious for cervical insufficiency who elect CL screening rather than history-indicated cerclage:
  o Initiate TV ultrasound cervical lengths at *14 weeks*
    - If CL ≥ 30 mm, repeat every 2 weeks until 23 6/7 weeks.
    - If CL 25 to 29 mm, repeat every 1 week until 23 6/7 weeks.
    - If CL less than 25 mm prior to 24 0/7 weeks, offer cerclage placement.

Treatment

- *History-indicated cerclage* may be offered to women with a clinical history consistent with cervical insufficiency. Prior recommendations suggested that "elective cerclage for purely historical factors generally should be confined to patients with three or more otherwise unexplained second-trimester pregnancy losses or preterm deliveries." In clinical practice, though, many obstetric care providers will counsel patients on the option of history-indicated cerclage based on one or two prior midtrimester losses highly suggestive of CI by recollection of the clinical presentation. This procedure is commonly offered between 13 and 14 weeks, once a living fetus has been documented with ultrasound and no obvious abnormalities are noted on serum screening or ultrasound.
- An alternative approach to history-indicated cerclage placement is serial transvaginal ultrasound cervical length screening with *ultrasound-indicated cerclage* placement if the cervix becomes short (less than 25 mm at less than 24 weeks of gestation).
- Cerclage type
  - Vaginal cerclage is the most common type of cerclage, either McDonald or Shirodkar technique.
    o Typically placed during pregnancy between 12 and 24 weeks of gestation.
    o There is no evidence to suggest superiority of one technique over the other. Because of easier placement and removal, and comparative efficacy, the McDonald cerclage has become the preferred technique (73).
  - Abdominal cerclage is usually reserved for women with a prior failed vaginal cerclage (i.e., midtrimester spontaneous pregnancy loss despite history-indicated cerclage placement). Abdominal cerclage may be placed prior to pregnancy or during early pregnancy.
- Cerclage technique
  - Suture type
    o The most commonly used sutures for vaginal cerclage are Mersilene 5-mm tape and large-caliber nonabsorbable monofilament such as Prolene.
- There is no clear evidence that one suture type has superior efficacy over the other (73). Choice of suture type is left to the preference and experience of the surgeon. The largest clinical trial of ultrasound-indicated cerclage used both suture types, but most patients received Mersilene tape (74).
  - Perioperative antibiotics
- Empiric use of prophylactic antibiotics has not been shown to be useful for *history-indicated cerclage*. Perioperative antibiotics are often used with *ultrasound-indicated* and *exam-indicated cerclage* placement, but there is insufficient evidence to recommend their use routinely (73).

- Prophylactic tocolytic agents
  - There is insufficient evidence to support the routine use of perioperative prophylactic tocolytic agents at the time of cerclage placement (73).
- Cerclage management
  - Transvaginal CL screening following cerclage placement
    - The role of CL screening after intervention has been provided is uncertain.
    - May assist to identify patients at high risk of impending preterm birth (i.e., funneling to the stitch or extremely short CL), who may benefit from corticosteroid therapy.
  - Removal
    - Vaginal cerclage should be removed when there is concern for laceration of the cervix in the event of preterm labor or when the patient reaches 37 weeks of gestation. Abdominal cerclage remains in situ, and cesarean is required when delivery is indicated. The optimal time to remove a cerclage in patients who develop preterm PROM is unclear.

Complications
- Complications of cervical insufficiency include preterm delivery and PROM. A complete description of these pregnancy complications is available in this chapter.
- Cervical cerclage is associated with risk of rupture of membranes, chorioamnionitis, and laceration of the cervix by the suture. Rates of these complications are related to the time at which and the circumstances under which the cerclage was placed. Clinical exam–indicated cerclage is associated with a greater risk of complications.

Patient Education
- Patients with obstetric history consistent with cervical insufficiency or those with a successful vaginal cerclage in a prior pregnancy may benefit from *history-indicated cerclage* placement in the next pregnancy.
- Patients with history of one prior midtrimester loss or later spontaneous preterm birth(s) may benefit from *ultrasound-indicated cerclage* placement if the cervix shortens prior to 24 weeks of pregnancy. They may be offered cervical length screening from 14 to 23 6/7 weeks of gestation.

SHORT CERVIX
Key Points
- A short cervix identified in the midtrimester of pregnancy is associated with a high risk of spontaneous preterm birth.
- Low-risk nulliparous singletons with short cervix noted in the midtrimester of pregnancy (18 to 24 weeks) are at increased risk of preterm birth and benefit from vaginal progesterone therapy. Cerclage is not beneficial in this population.
- High-risk singletons with a prior preterm birth and short cervix noted in the midtrimester of pregnancy (16 to 24 weeks) benefit from ultrasound indicated cerclage placement. They are also offered 17-hydroxyprogesterone acetate based on their history.
- Twin pregnancies (without prior history of preterm birth or midtrimester loss) with midtrimester cervical shortening are at increased risk of preterm birth but do not benefit from cerclage placement. They may benefit from vaginal progesterone therapy.
- Routine midtrimester cervical length screening may be beneficial in all pregnancies at risk of preterm birth and may be considered, but this is not a mandated approach.

Background
A short cervix identified in the midtrimester of pregnancy is associated with a high risk of spontaneous preterm birth in all populations studied. But, despite the strong association between short cervical length and preterm birth, the majority of women with asymptomatic cervical shortening deliver at later than 35 weeks. Therefore, the purpose of cervical

length screening is to identify populations of patients in which interventions have been proven beneficial such as vaginal progesterone, cerclage, and antenatal corticosteroids. An additional goal of cervical length screening should be to avoid unnecessary interventions in women at low risk of preterm birth. Only extremely short cervical lengths in asymptomatic patients in the midtrimester are associated with a significant risk of impending preterm birth within 2 to 4 weeks. Protocols that incorporate universal cervical length screening have demonstrated a reduction in the frequency of preterm birth and have been found to be cost-effective. Universal CL screening in all pregnant women is currently not mandated by ACOG; however, it is considered a reasonable evidence-based practice pattern.

Definition

• There is an inverse relationship between preterm birth risk and cervical length: the shorter the cervical length, the higher the risk of preterm birth.
• Short cervix is commonly defined as a cervical length of less than 25 mm measured by transvaginal ultrasound in the midtrimester of pregnancy, between 14 and 24 weeks of pregnancy.

Pathophysiology

• The complex processes leading to spontaneous preterm birth are not clearly understood. Cervical shortening is thought to be an early manifestation of the parturition process and may precede birth by weeks or months.

Epidemiology

• The prevalence of short cervical length in the midtrimester (20 to 25 weeks) has been reported to be approximately 10% defined as cervical length ≤25 mm and 1.7% CL ≤ 15 mm (75).

Evaluation

• Midtrimester cervical shortening may be discovered incidentally at the time of ultrasound for other indications or may be diagnosed when performing routine transvaginal ultrasound cervical length screening.
• If routine transvaginal ultrasound screening is performed in *low-risk populations*, a single transvaginal cervical length measurement is typically performed at 18 to 24 weeks of gestation at the time of the fetal anatomic survey.
• Cervical length screening in singleton pregnancies with prior history of spontaneous preterm birth at 17 to 34 weeks:
  • Initiate TV ultrasound cervical length measurement at 16 weeks.
    ○ If CL ≥ 30 mm, repeat every 2 weeks until 23 6/7 weeks.
    ○ If CL 25 to 29 mm, repeat every 1 week until 23 6/7 weeks.
    ○ If CL less than 25 mm, offer cerclage placement.
  • No further scheduled CL screening after 23 6/7 weeks.
• Multifetal gestation, uterine malformation, or prior LEEP (screening and treatment similar to *low-risk women*).
  • Single TV US cervical length measurement at 18 to 24 weeks, at time of anatomic survey
    ○ If CL less than 20 mm, consider vaginal progesterone.
    ○ If CL ≥ 20 mm, routine care.
    ○ Cerclage has no role in the treatment of short cervix in these populations and may worsen outcomes in otherwise uncomplicated twin pregnancies.
• For screening recommendations in high-risk pregnancies with prior midtrimester loss, see *Cervical Insufficiency* section.
• Short cervix is a diagnosis based on transvaginal ultrasound measurement. If short cervix is suspected by transabdominal imaging, confirmation by transvaginal ultrasound measurement is recommended.

Diagnosis
- Short cervix is typically defined as cervical length less than 25 mm between 14 and 24 weeks of gestational age. Shortened cervical length at later gestational ages beyond 24 weeks has a weaker correlation with preterm birth risk and prediction, and effective treatments at these later gestational ages have not been studied. Therefore, diagnosis of short cervix is generally limited to measurements obtained less than 24 weeks.

Treatment
- Vaginal progesterone
  - 200 mg micronized progesterone capsules, one capsule inserted vaginally daily from time of diagnosis of short cervix (prior to 24 weeks) until delivery.
  - Efficacious in low-risk singleton pregnancies with short cervix (less than 20 mm) diagnosed less than 24 weeks to reduce preterm birth risk.
  - Unclear if it useful in twins, uterine malformation, or prior LEEP with a short cervix in the midtrimester. May be beneficial and has no known risk.
- Cerclage placement
  - For singleton pregnancies with prior spontaneous preterm birth and cervical shortening noted in the current pregnancy of less than 25 mm at less than 24 weeks of gestational age.

Patient Education
- Women with a prior spontaneous preterm birth may benefit from cervical length screening at 16 and 23 6/7 weeks, with ultrasound-indicated cerclage placement if the cervix shortens less than 25 mm. Weekly 17-OHPC injections are also beneficial to reduce recurrent preterm birth risk in this population. Preconception counseling following a spontaneous preterm birth may be helpful to outline a screening and treatment plan for future pregnancies in these high-risk women.
- Low-risk women in their first pregnancy have as high as 10% likelihood of having a short cervix in the midtrimester. Their risk of preterm birth may be reduced by cervical length screening and initiation of vaginal progesterone if short cervix less than 20 mm is identified. Patient education regarding the benefits of cervical length screening in this low-risk population may help to reduce the burden of preterm birth in the United States.

REFERENCES

1. Mathews TJ, Menacker F, MacDorman MF. Infant mortality statistics from the 2001 period linked birth/infant death data set. *Natl Vital Stat Rep.* 2003;52:1–28.
2. McElrath TF, Robinson JN, Ecker JL, et al. Neonatal outcome of infants born at 23 weeks of gestation. *Obstet Gynecol.* 2001;91:49–52.
3. Institute of Medicine (US) Committee on Understanding Premature Birth and Assuring Healthy Outcomes; Behrman RE, Butler AS, eds. *Preterm birth: causes consequences, and prevention.* Washington, DC: National Academies Press (US), 2007.
4. Castracane VD. Endocrinology of preterm labor. *Clin Obstet Gynecol.* 2000;43:717–726.
5. Goldenberg RL. The management of preterm labor. *Obstet Gynecol.* 2002;100:1020–1037.
6. Wright VC, Schieve LA, Reynolds MA, et al. Assisted reproductive technology surveillance—United States, 2001. *MMWR Surveill Summ.* 2004;53:1–20.
7. Tucker JM, Goldenberg RL, Davis RO, et al. Etiologies of preterm birth in an indigent population: is prevention a logical expectation? *Obstet Gynecol.* 1991;77:343–347.
8. Hamilton B, Martin J, Ventura S. Births: preliminary data for 2012. *Natl Vital Stat Rep.* 2013;62:3.
9. Blakemore-Prince C, Kieke B, Kugaraj KA, et al. Racial differences in the patterns of singleton preterm delivery in the 1988 national maternal and infant health survey. *Matern Child Health J.* 1999;3:189–197.
10. Pschirrer ER, Monga M. Risk factors for preterm labor. *Clin Obstet Gynecol.* 2000;43:727–734.

11. Robinson JN, Regan JA, Norwitz ER. The epidemiology of preterm labor. *Semin Perinatol.* 2001;25:204–214.
12. Honest H, Bachmann LM, Sunduram R, et al. The accuracy of risk scores in predicting preterm birth—a systematic review. *J Obstet Gynaecol.* 2004;24:343–359.
13. DeFranco EA, Lewis DF, Odibo AO. Improving the screening accuracy for preterm labor: is the combination of fetal fibronectin and cervical length in symptomatic patients a useful predictor of preterm birth? A systematic review. *Am J Obstet Gynecol.* 2013;208(3):233.e1-6.
14. Ness A, Visintine J, Ricci E, et al. Does knowledge of cervical length and fetal fibronectin affect management of women with threatened preterm labor? A randomized trial. *Am J Obstet Gynecol.* 2007;197(4):426.e1-7.
15. Peaceman AM, Andrews WW, Thorp JM, et al. Fetal fibronectin as a predictor of preterm birth in patients with symptoms: a multicenter trial. *Am J Obstet Gynecol.* 1997;177:13–18.
16. Iams JD. Preterm birth. In: Gabbe SG, Neibyl JR, Simpson JL, eds. *Obstetrics: normal and problem pregnancies.* 4th ed. Philadelphia: Churchill Livingstone, 2002:755–826.
17. American College of Obstetrics and Gynecology. Practice Bulletin number 127. Management of preterm labor. *Obstet Gynecol.* 2012;119(6):1038–1017.
18. Pircon RA, Strassner HT, Kirz DS, et al. Controlled trial of hydration and bed rest versus bed rest alone in the evaluation of preterm uterine contractions. *Am J Obstet Gynecol.* 1989;161:775–779.
19. Guinn DA, Goepfert AR, Owen J, et al. Management options in women with preterm uterine contractions: a randomized clinical trial. *Am J Obstet Gynecol.* 1997;177:814–818.
20. Gyetvai K, Hannah ME, Hodnett ED, et al. Tocolytics for preterm labor: a systematic review. *Obstet Gynecol.* 1999;94:869–877.
21. Ables AZ, Romero AM, Chauhan SP. Use of calcium channel antagonists for preterm labor. *Clin Obstet Gynecol.* 2005;32:519–525.
22. McDonald TF, Pelzer S, Trautwein W, et al. Regulation and modulation of calcium channels in cardiac, skeletal, and smooth muscle cells. *Physiol Rev.* 1994;74:365–507.
23. Morgan MA, Goldenberg RL, Shulkin J. Obstetrician-gynecologists' screening and management of preterm birth. *Obstet Gynecol.* 2008;112:35–41.
24. Lewis DF. Magnesium sulfate: the first-line tocolytic. *Clin Obstet Gynecol.* 2005;32:485–500.
25. Madden C, Own J, Hauth JC. Magnesium tocolysis: serum levels versus success. *Am J Obstet Gynecol.* 1990;162:1177–1180.
26. Lewis DF, Bergstedt S, Edwards MS, et al. Successful magnesium sulfate tocolysis: is "weaning" the drug necessary? *Am J Obstet Gynecol.* 1997;177:742–745.
27. Anthony J, Johanson RG, Duley L. Role of magnesium sulfate in seizure prevention in patients with eclampsia and pre-eclampsia. *Drug Safety.* 1996;15:188–199.
28. Lam F, Gill P. Beta-agonist therapy. *Clin Obstet Gynecol.* 2005;32:457–484.
29. Vermillion ST, Robinson CJ. Antiprostaglandin drugs. *Clin Obstet Gynecol.* 2005;32:501–517.
30. Niebyl JR, Witter FR. Neonatal outcome after indomethacin treatment for preterm labor. *Am J Obstet Gynecol.* 1986;155(4):747–749.
31. Moise KJ. Effect of advancing gestational age on the frequency of fetal ductal constriction in the association with maternal indomethacin use. *Am J Obstet Gynecol.* 1993;168:1350–1353.
32. Macones GM, Marder SJ, Clothier B, et al. The controversy surrounding indomethacin for tocolysis. *Am J Obstet Gynecol.* 2001;184:264–272.
33. Agency for Healthcare Research and Quality. *Management of preterm labor.* Evidence Report/Technology Assessment no. 18. AHRQ Publication no. 01-E021. Rockville, MD: AHRQ, 2000.
34. Antenatal corticosteroids revisited: repeat courses. NIH Consensus Statement. 2000;17:1–10.
35. American College of Obstetrics and Gynecology. Antenatal corticosteroid therapy for fetal maturation. ACOG Committee Opinion no. 475. *Obstet Gynecol.* 2011;117:422–424.
36. Mittendorf R, Dambrosia J, Pryde PG, et al. Association between the use of antenatal magnesium sulfate in preterm labor and adverse health outcomes in infants. *Am J Obstet Gynecol.* 2002;186:1111–1118.

37. Crowther CA, Hiller JE, Doyle LW, et al. Effect of magnesium sulfate given for neuroprotection before preterm birth: a randomized controlled trial. Australasian Collaborative Trial of Magnesium Sulphate (ACTOMg SO4) Collaborative Group. *JAMA*. 2003;290:2669–2676.
38. Marret S, Marpeau L, Zupan-Simunek V, et al. Magnesium sulphate given before very preterm birth to protect infant brain: the randomized controlled PREMAG trial. PREMAG trial group. *BJOG*. 2007;114:310–318.
39. Rouse DJ, Hirtz DG, Thom E, et al. A randomized, controlled trial of magnesium sulfate for the prevention of cerebral palsy. Eunice Kennedy Shriver NICHD Maternal-Fetal Medicine Units Network. *N Engl J Med*. 2008;359:895–905.
40. Marret S, Marpeau L, Follet-Bouhamed C, et al. Effect of magnesium sulphate on mortality and neurologic morbidity of the very preterm newborn (of less than 33 weeks) with two-year neurological outcome: results of the prospective PREMAG trial. le groupe PREMAG [French]. *Gynecol Obstet Fertil*. 2008;36:278–288.
41. Doyle LW, Crowther CA, Middleton P, et al. Magnesium sulphate for women at risk of preterm birth for neuroprotection of the fetus. *Cochrane Database Syst Rev*. 2009;1:CD004661. doi: 10.1002/14651858.CD004661.pub3.
42. Costantine MM, Weiner SJ. Effects of antenatal exposure to magnesium sulfate on neuroprotection and mortality in preterm infants: a meta-analysis. Eunice Kennedy Shriver National Institute of Child Health and Human Development Maternal-Fetal Medicine Units Network *Obstet Gynecol*. 2009;114:354–364.
43. American College of Obstetricians and Gynecologists. Magnesium sulfate before anticipated preterm birth for neuroprotection. Committee Opinion No. 455. *Obstet Gynecol*. 2010;115:669–671.
44. Scrag S, Gorwitz R, Fultz-Butts K, et al. Prevention of perinatal group B streptococcal disease. Revised guidelines for CDC. *MMWR Recomm Rep*. 2002;51(RR-11):1–22.
45. American College of Obstetricians and Gynecologists. ACOG Practice Bulletin no. 130: prediction and prevention of preterm birth. *Obstet Gynecol*. 2012;120(4):964–973.
46. Mercer BM, Golderberg RL, Moawad AH. The preterm prediction study: effect of gestational age and cause of preterm birth on subsequent obstetric outcome. *Am J Obstet Gynecol*. 1999;181:1216–1221.
47. Mercer BM. Preterm premature rupture of the membranes. *Obstet Gynecol*. 2003;101:178–193.
48. Mercer B, Arheart K. Antimicrobial therapy in expectant management of preterm premature rupture of the membranes. *Lancet*. 1995;346:1271–1279.
49. Naeye RL, Peters EC. Causes and consequences of premature rupture of the fetal membranes. *Lancet*. 1980;1:192–194.
50. Cousins LM, Smok DP, Lovett SM, et al. AmniSure placental alpha microglobulin-1 rapid immunoassay versus standard diagnostic methods for detection of rupture of membranes. *Am J Perinatol*. 2005;22(6):317–320.
51. Mercer BM. Management of premature rupture of membranes before 26 weeks gestation. *Obstet Gynecol Clin North Am*. 1992;19:339–351.
52. Johnson JWC, Egerman RS, Moorhead J. Cases with ruptured membranes that "reseal." *Am J Obstet Gynecol*. 1990;163:1024–1032.
53. Naef RW III, Allbert JR, Ross EL, et al. Premature rupture of membranes at 34 to 37 weeks' gestation: aggressive versus conservative management. *Am J Obstet Gynecol*. 1998;178:126–130.
54. Cox SM, Leveno KJ. Intentional delivery versus expectant management with preterm ruptured membranes at 30–34 weeks' gestation. *Obstet Gynecol*. 1995;86:875–879.
55. Mercer BM, Moretti ML, Prevost RR, et al. Erythromycin therapy in preterm premature rupture of membranes: a prospective randomized trial of 220 patients. *Am J Obstet Gynecol*. 1992;166:794–802.
56. Mercer B, Miodovnik M, Thurnau G, et al. Antibiotic therapy for reduction of infant morbidity after preterm premature rupture of membranes: a randomized controlled trial. *JAMA*. 1997;278:989–995.
57. Harding JE, Pang J, Knight DB, et al. Do antenatal corticosteroids help in the setting of preterm rupture of membranes? *Am J Obstet Gynecol*. 2001;184:131–139.

58. Lewis DF, Brody K, Edwards MS, et al. Preterm premature ruptured membranes: a randomized trial of steroids after treatment with antibiotics. *Obstet Gynecol.* 1996;88:801–805.

59. Pattinson RC, Makin JD, Funk M, et al. The use of dexamethasone in women with preterm premature rupture of membranes: a multicentre, double-blind, placebo controlled, randomised trial. *S Afr Med J.* 1999;89:865–870.

60. Morales WJ. The effect of chorioamnionitis on the developmental outcome of preterm infants at one year. *Obstet Gynecol.* 1987;70:183–186.

61. Hillier SL, Martius J, Krohn M, et al. A case–control study of chorioamnionic infection and histologic chorioamnionitis in prematurity. *N Engl J Med.* 1988;319:972–978.

62. Asrat T, Lewis DF, Garite TJ, et al. Rate of recurrence of preterm PROM in consecutive pregnancies. *Am J Obstet Gynecol.* 1991;165:1111–1115.

63. Bengtsson LP. Cervical insufficiency. *Acta Obstet Gynecol Scand.* 1968;47:9–35.

64. Leppert PC, Yu SK, Keller S, et al. Decreased elastic fibers and desmosine content in the incompetent cervix. *Am J Obstet Gynecol.* 1987;157:1134–1139.

65. Buckingham JC, Buethe RA, Danforth DN. Collagen-muscle ratio in clinically normal and clinically incompetent cervices. *Am J Obstet Gynecol.* 1965;92:232–237.

66. Roddick JW, Buckingham JC, Danforth DN. The muscular cervix—a cause of incompetency in pregnancy. *Obstet Gynecol.* 1961;17:562–565.

67. Rechberger T, Uldbjerg N, Oxlund H. Connective tissue changes in the cervix during normal pregnancy and pregnancy complicated by cervical incompetence. *Obstet Gynecol.* 1988;71:563–567.

68. Petersen LK, Uldbjerg N. Cervical collagen in non-pregnant women with previous cervical incompetence. *Eur J Obstet Gynecol Reprod Biol.* 1996;67:41–45.

69. Berghella V, Mackeen AD. Cervical length screening with ultrasound-indicated cerclage compared with history-indicated cerclage for prevention of preterm birth: a meta-analysis. *Obstet Gynecol.* 2011;118(1):148–155.

70. Rubovits FE, Cooperman NR, Lash AF. Habitual abortion: a radiographic technique to demonstrate the incompetent internal os of the cervix. *Am J Obstet Gynecol.* 1953;66:269–280.

71. Anthony GS, Calder AA, MacNaughton MC. Cervical resistance in patients with previous spontaneous mid-trimester abortion. *Br J Obstet Gynaecol.* 1982;89:1046–1049.

72. Berghella V, Rafael TJ, Szychowski JM, et al. Cerclage for short cervix on ultrasonography in women with singleton gestations and previous preterm birth: a meta-analysis. *Obstet Gynecol.* 2011;117(3):663–671.

73. Berghella V, Ludmir J, Simonazzi G, et al. Transvaginal cervical cerclage: evidence for perioperative management strategies. *Am J Obstet Gynecol.* 2013;209(3):181–192.

74. Owen J, Hankins G, Iams JD, et al. Multicenter randomized trial of cerclage for preterm birth prevention in high-risk women with shortened midtrimester cervical length. *Am J Obstet Gynecol.* 2009;201(4):375.e1-8. doi: 10.1016/j.ajog.2009.08.015.

75. Fonseca EB, Celik E, Parra M, et al.; Fetal Medicine Foundation Second Trimester Screening Group. Progesterone and the risk of preterm birth among women with a short cervix. *N Engl J Med.* 2007;357(5):462–469.

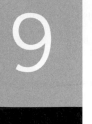

9 Third-Trimester Bleeding

Loralei L. Thornburg and Ruth Anne Queenan

KEY POINTS
- Third-trimester bleeding complicates about 4% of all pregnancies.
- Serious causes include placenta previa, abruption, and vasa previa and can result in significant maternal and/or fetal compromise.
- Availability of blood products and support systems is important for optimal patient management.
- Absence of placenta previa should be confirmed by ultrasound before proceeding with digital examination of the cervix.

VAGINAL BLEEDING
Background
Definition
- Third-trimester bleeding is defined as any episode of vaginal bleeding that occurs after 24 completed weeks of pregnancy.
- Third-trimester bleeding complicates about 4% of all pregnancies.
- Vaginal bleeding during pregnancy is a worrisome symptom to the patient and is usually brought to the attention of her physician at the time that it occurs during pregnancy.

Etiology
- In approximately 50% of cases, vaginal bleeding is secondary to placental abruption or placenta previa. Both of these conditions carry significant risk of maternal and fetal morbidity and mortality and therefore must be expeditiously diagnosed.
- Once these two life-threatening situations are convincingly excluded as a cause of bleeding, attention can be turned to alternate causes of vaginal bleeding in pregnancy.

Evaluation
History
The following information should be obtained:
- Is there a history of trauma?
- What is the amount and the character of the bleeding?
- Is there pain associated with the bleeding?
- Is there a history of bleeding earlier in the pregnancy?

Physical Examination
- Vital sign measurement, including pulse pressure; normal vital signs are reassuring; however, they can be misleading because hypotension and tachycardia are signs of serious hypovolemia, and generally not present until significant blood loss has occurred. Additionally, mild tachycardia can be a normal finding in pregnancy.
- Fetal heart rate and/or category of continuous fetal heart rate tracing.
- Physical examination, initially excluding speculum and digital pelvic examination until after ultrasound is complete.
- Assessment of uterine activity.

- Ultrasound examination of the uterus, placenta, and fetus (transabdominal first and then transvaginal when indicated).
- Speculum and digital pelvic examination once placenta previa has been excluded.

Laboratory Tests
- Hemoglobin and hematocrit determination.
- Coagulation studies when placental abruption is suspected or when there has been significant hemorrhage, including prothrombin time, partial thromboplastin time, platelet count, fibrinogen level, and fibrin split products.
- Red-top tube of blood to perform a bedside clot test.
- Blood type and crossmatch.
- Anti-D immunoglobulin for those who are Rh(D) negative to protect against sensitization.
- Urinalysis for hematuria and proteinuria.
- Apt test may be used to determine maternal or fetal source of bleeding. (Mix vaginal blood with an equal part of 0.25% sodium hydroxide. Fetal blood remains red; maternal blood turns brown.) In general, fetal bleeding will be apparent on fetal heart rate tracing and intervention should not be delayed for Apt testing.
- Kleihauer-Betke (K-B) test is used to quantify fetal to maternal hemorrhage. However, it is positive in only a small proportion of placental abruptions. While the K-B test is helpful to assure adequate anti-D immunoglobulin dosing, it is generally not helpful for diagnosis of abruption (1,2).

PLACENTAL ABRUPTION
Background
Definition
Placental abruption (also known as abruptio placentae) occurs when a normally implanted placenta completely or partially separates from the decidua basalis after the 20th week of gestation and before the third stage of labor.

Incidence
Placental abruption occurs in approximately 1 in 100 deliveries and accounts for 15% of perinatal mortality (3,4).

Classification
Placental abruptions are graded by clinical criteria. Ultrasound is not an accurate or reliable method for diagnosis or classification. Clinically, the classification of abruption can be helpful when deciding on the need for interventions and the need for further monitoring (Fig. 9-1).
- Grade 1, mild (40% of abruptions):
  - Vaginal bleeding is slight or absent (less than 100 mL).
  - Uterine activity may be slightly increased.

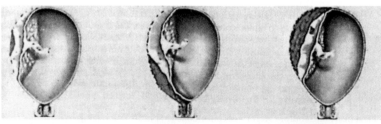

| Partial separation (concealed hemorrhage) | Partial separation (apparent hemorrhage) | Complete separation (concealed hemorrhage) |

Figure 9-1. Types of placental abruption. (From Beckmann CRB, Ling FW. *Obstetrics and gynecology.* 6th ed. Lippincott Williams & Wilkins, 2009).

- Uterine activity often described as having closely spaced, low-intensity contractions—a hyperstimulation-type pattern.
- No fetal heart rate abnormalities are present.
- No evidence of shock or coagulopathy.
- Grade 2, moderate (45%):
  - External bleeding may be absent to moderate (100 to 500 mL).
  - Uterine tone may be increased. Tetanic uterine contractions and uterine tenderness may be present.
  - Fetal heart tones may be absent and, when present, often show evidence of fetal distress.
  - Maternal tachycardia, narrowed pulse pressure, and orthostatic hypotension may be present.
  - Early evidence of coagulopathy may be present (fibrinogen 150 to 250 dL).
- Grade 3, severe (15%):
  - External bleeding may be moderate or excessive (greater than 500 mL) but may be concealed.
  - The uterus is often tetanic and tender to palpation.
  - Fetal death is common.
  - Maternal shock is usually present.
  - Coagulopathy is frequently present.

Etiology

The cause of placental abruption is unknown, but defective placental vasculature has been postulated to be a contributing factor. In the following conditions, the incidence of placental abruption is increased: (3,5)

- Preeclampsia and hypertensive disorders
- History of placental abruption (recurrence rate ~10%)
- High multiparity
- Relatively older maternal age
- Trauma, both direct and indirect uterine traumas
- Cigarette smoking, in a dose-responsive fashion, which is synergistic with hypertension (5)
- Illicit drug use, most notably cocaine use
- Excessive alcohol consumption
- Preterm, premature rupture of the membranes, where the risk increases with length of latency
- Rapid uterine decompression (e.g., after delivery of the first fetus in a twin gestation or rupture of membranes with polyhydramnios)
- Uterine leiomyomas, especially if located retroplacentally, rapidly enlarging, or degenerating

Diagnosis

Clinical Manifestations

- The diagnosis of placental abruption is made by clinical findings, with the symptoms of vaginal bleeding, abdominal pain, uterine tenderness, and uterine contractions.
  - Vaginal bleeding is present in 80% of patients and concealed in 20%.
  - Pain is present in most cases of placental abruption and is usually of sudden onset, constant, and localized to the uterus, low abdomen, and lower back.
  - Localized or generalized uterine tenderness and increased uterine tone are found with the more severe forms of placental abruption.
  - The uterus may increase in size with placental abruption when the bleeding is concealed. This may be monitored by serially measuring abdominal girth and/or fundal height.
  - Amniotic fluid may be bloody.
  - Shock is variably present.
  - Fetal compromise is variably present.
  - Placental abruption may cause rapidly progressive preterm labor and/or preterm premature rupture of membranes.

Laboratory Findings

Laboratory findings that are frequently helpful in the diagnosis include (6)

- Consumptive coagulopathy
  - Placental separation precedes the onset of the consumptive coagulopathy, which in turn progresses until the uterus is evacuated.
  - Coagulation occurs retroplacentally as well as intravascularly, with secondary fibrinolysis.
  - Levels of fibrinogen, prothrombin, factors V and VIII, and platelets are decreased.
  - Fibrin split products are elevated, adding an anticoagulant effect.
  - Hypofibrinogenemia occurs within 8 hours of the initial separation.

Ultrasonography

Ultrasonography is very poorly sensitive in making the diagnosis.

- The three locations of placental hemorrhage are
  - Subchorionic (more common less than 20 weeks)
  - Retroplacental (more common greater than 20 weeks)
  - Preplacental (unusual)
- Symptoms associated with retroplacental hemorrhage are frequently the most severe.
- The sensitivity of ultrasonography in detecting placental abruption is only approximately 25% to 50% at best (7).
- If abruption is visualized on ultrasound, the predictive value is high (88%) (7).

Treatment

Management

- Mild placental abruption
  - Close observation is required to assure maternal stability and reassuring fetal status. The facility should be fully capable of immediate delivery should the condition of the patient or fetus deteriorate.
  - Continuous fetal monitoring should be initiated, although the value of antepartum testing is not established.
  - Maternal hematologic parameters should be monitored and abnormalities corrected.
  - A trial of tocolytics may be carefully undertaken with consideration of an immature fetus. Nifedipine is the tocolytic of choice if the blood pressure will tolerate this therapy.
- Moderate to severe placental abruption
  - Careful maternal and fetal monitoring is essential to minimize long-term complications (3).
  - The vigorous management of shock is outlined in Part V of this manual.
  - Coagulopathy:
    - Fresh whole blood, if available, should be used to replace blood loss because it replaces volume and contains clotting factors. If not, rapid infusion protocols should be followed, which in general advocate starting coagulation factors in a 1:1 (red blood cells [RBC]: fresh frozen plasma [FFP]) ratio after transfusion of four units of packed cells (8).
    - Clotting factors may be replaced using cryoprecipitate or FFP. One unit of FFP increases the fibrinogen level approximately 10 mg/dL. Cryoprecipitate contains approximately 250 mg fibrinogen per unit, with 4 g (15 to 20 U) being an effective dose.
    - Platelet transfusion may be indicated if the platelet count is less than 50,000 per μL, although this is generally reserved for situations with counts of 20,000 to 30,000 per μL or less. One unit of platelets typically raises the platelet count 5000 to 10,000 per μL; 4 to 6 U is the smallest clinically useful dose.
    - Coagulation defects will resolve once delivery occurs, with clotting factors returning to normal within 24 hours and platelets returning to normal within 4 days.
    - Heparin is not indicated.

- Oxygen should be administered.
- Urine output should be monitored with an indwelling bladder catheter.
- Antenatal corticosteroids should be given for any fetus less than 34 weeks.
- For those infants less than 32 weeks, consider magnesium sulfate for neuroprotection during delivery.

Mode and Timing of Delivery
- Delivery should in general be expedited in all but the mildest cases once the mother has stabilized depending on severity and gestational age (2).
  - Nonsevere abruption between 34 and 36 weeks should be monitored carefully and likely will require delivery. Conservative, observational management may be used for selected patients with mild, resolved bleeding, normal laboratory testing, and category 1 fetal testing.
  - Nonsevere abruption less than 34 weeks should be monitored carefully and managed conservatively when possible. Conservative, observational management may be done for selected patients with mild, resolved bleeding, normal laboratory testing, and category 1 fetal testing.
- As long as maternal and fetal surveillance is reassuring, with adequate progress of labor and appropriate volume replacement, the time interval to delivery is less crucial.
- Amniotomy should be performed because it may facilitate delivery and decrease thromboplastin release into the circulation.
- Oxytocin augmentation may be used.
- Vaginal delivery is preferred.
- Cesarean section is indicated in the following cases:
  - Fetal distress without impending vaginal delivery
  - Severe abruption, threatening the life of the mother
  - Failed trial of labor
- For abruption with fetal demise, vaginal delivery remains preferable, but mode of delivery should be chosen to minimize maternal risks. Labor is often rapidly progressive in these cases, and amniotomy will allow visualization of the bleeding and facilitate labor progression.

Complications
- Hemorrhagic shock
- Consumptive coagulopathy
- Couvelaire uterus, or extravasation of blood into the myometrium causing red discoloration of the serosal surface of the uterus, which is found in 8% of patients
- Ischemic necrosis of distant organs, mostly preventable by vigorous volume replacement.
  - Kidney: acute tubular necrosis and cortical necrosis
  - Liver
  - Adrenals
  - Pituitary
  - Lung

Prognosis
Placental abruption is one of the gravest obstetric complications, with perinatal mortality of approximately 30% and morbidity related to both gestational age and degree of asphyxia. Maternal mortality is less than 1% (3,4).

PLACENTA PREVIA
Background
Definition
Placenta previa occurs when any part of the placenta implants in the lower uterine segment in advance of the fetal presenting part. All three types of placenta previa are associated with risk of serious maternal hemorrhage. As pregnancy advances, the degree of placenta previa may change as the uterus elongates, the lower uterine segment develops, and the cervix effaces and dilates (9).

Classification
- Total (complete) placenta previa occurs when the entire internal cervical os is covered by placenta. Central placenta previa is a subtype occurring when the placenta is located concentrically around the internal cervical os.
- Partial (incomplete) placenta previa occurs when part of the internal cervical os is covered by placenta.
- Marginal placenta previa occurs when the placental edge extends to within 2 cm of the internal cervical os (Fig. 9-2).

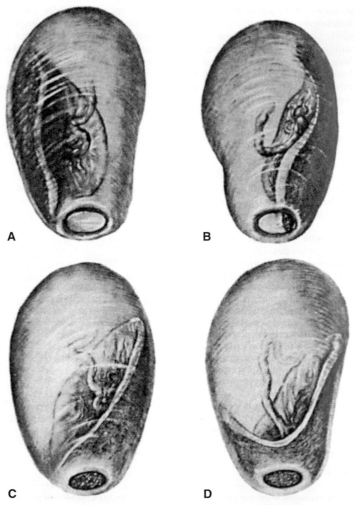

Figure 9-2. Types of placenta previa. **A:** Low-lying placenta. **B:** Marginal placenta previa. **C** and **D:** Varieties of complete placenta previa. (From Beckmann CRB, Ling FW. *Obstetrics and gynecology.* 6th ed. Lippincott Williams & Wilkins, 2009).

Incidence

Placenta previa occurs in approximately 1 in 200 pregnancies. More than 90% of placenta previas diagnosed in the second trimester resolve as pregnancy advances, secondary to differential growth of the placental trophoblastic cells toward the fundus (9).

- The cause of placenta previa is unknown. Endometrial damage from previous pregnancies and defective decidual vascularization have been postulated as possible mechanisms (10).

Associated Conditions

The following are associated with an increased risk of placenta previa: (11)

- Maternal age. Placenta previa is three times more common at age 35 than at age 25.
- Increasing parity.
- Previous uterine scar.
- Prior placenta previa.
- Tobacco use.
- Multiple gestation.
- An increase in the risk of congenital anomalies has been reported, although no single associated anomaly has been identified.

Diagnosis

Clinical Manifestations

- Patients with placenta previa characteristically present with sudden onset of painless vaginal bleeding in the second or third trimester. One-third become symptomatic before 30 weeks and one-third after 36 weeks, with the peak incidence at 34 weeks. Most often, the initial bleeding resolves spontaneously, recurring later in pregnancy.
- One-fourth of patients present with bleeding and uterine contractions without uterine tetany.
- Malpresentation occurs in one-third of cases (11).
- Coagulation disorders are rare in cases of placenta previa but can occur with large amounts of bleeding.

Diagnostic Methodologies

- Sonography is more than 95% accurate in diagnosing placenta previa. Transabdominal ultrasonography should be performed with a full bladder. If placenta previa is suspected, the bladder should be nearly emptied and the scan repeated. Transvaginal ultrasonography is safe and useful in establishing the relationship between the cervix and the placenta, especially in cases of posterior placentation (12).
- Magnetic resonance imaging has been used to confirm the diagnosis of placenta previa and to evaluate for associated placenta accreta. Ultrasonography, however, is likely to remain the more accessible and therefore more useful tool (13).
- Double-setup examination was frequently used in the past for the final step in diagnosing placenta previa. With the improved sensitivity and specificity of ultrasonography, there are fewer indications for this procedure. If the diagnosis remains uncertain or the patient has persistent mild bleeding in labor, the double-setup examination may be undertaken. The procedure should be done in an operating room with blood products and a team available to conduct immediate delivery should hemorrhage occur. Most commonly, double-setup examination is used to determine the existence of marginal placenta previa.

Treatment

Management

Management of placenta previa depends on gestational age and the extent of bleeding.

- Immediate delivery
  - When the pregnancy is ≥36 weeks, the neonate should be delivered by cesarean delivery.
  - Low vertical uterine incision is probably safer in patients with an anterior placenta previa, especially with prior cesarean deliveries or in cases of suspected accreta. If possible, it is best to avoid incisions through the placenta.

- Cesarean delivery should be performed regardless of gestational age if hemorrhage is severe and jeopardizes the mother or fetus.
- Expectant management may be used to address fetal immaturity if the following conditions are met:
  - Bleeding is not excessive.
  - There are significant risks of prematurity to the fetus.
  - The patient is hospitalized or in a location where rapid transportation to the hospital is available.
  - Physical activity is restricted.
  - Intercourse and douching are not permitted.
  - Hemoglobin is maintained at 10 mg/dL or greater.
  - Rh immunoglobulin is administered to Rh-negative, unsensitized patients.
  - Blood products are available.
- Once either fetal lung maturity is documented or the fetus has reached approximately 34 to 36 weeks with documented lung maturity, steps toward prompt delivery should be made. Elective delivery results in less morbidity and lower mortality risk to the mother and fetus than emergent delivery in the context of recurrent bleeding.
- Tocolysis may be used with caution in certain patients. Nifedipine is the agent of choice.
- Some patients are candidates for outpatient management if the following conditions are met:
  - Patient motivation and understanding of the severity of the situation.
  - Home environment allows compliance with restrictions.
  - The bleeding has stopped and not recurred for multiple days.
  - There has not been ≥3 episodes of bleeding.
  - The patient is always attended by a responsible adult with access to ready transport to the hospital.

Complications
- Hemorrhagic shock.
- Complications of cesarean delivery.
- Transfusion-related complications.
- Placenta previa associated with placenta accreta, increta, and percreta; previous uterine scars increase the risk substantially; this complication can lead to excess blood loss and in many cases mandate hysterectomy to control hemorrhage (6).

Prognosis
Maternal mortality from placenta previa should approach zero. Perinatal mortality is less than 10% and is attributed to prematurity.

OTHER CAUSES OF VAGINAL BLEEDING
Of the following causes of late-pregnancy vaginal bleeding, only the rarely encountered vasa previa confers significant immediate risk to the pregnancy and to the fetus in particular. Although the other causes may be serious, they carry much less immediate risk.

Vasa Previa
Vasa previa occurs when fetal blood vessels travel within the membranes, usually as a velamentous insertion, and in so doing, cross the region of the internal cervical os (14).
- When labor or cervical dilation occurs with unrecognized vasa previa, catastrophic fetal bleeding will occur.
- When these vessels rupture, vaginal bleeding is noted, and evidence of fetal distress is universally present.

- An Apt test will indicate fetal blood.
- Emergent cesarean delivery should be performed when the fetus is alive.
- Fetal mortality associated with this condition is greater than 50%.
- Vasa previa is potentially diagnosable by ultrasound. During the course of an ultrasound examination of a marginal previa or low-lying placenta, the placental vessels can be visualized traversing the lower uterine segment and the internal cervical os. Color Doppler allows fairly precise identification of these blood vessels and their locations (14).
- Antenatal diagnosis of vasa previa by ultrasound allows for timing of delivery by cesarean delivery.

Cervical Bleeding
- Cytologic sampling is mandatory.
- Bleeding can be controlled with cauterization or packing.
- Bacterial and viral cultures can be diagnostic.

Cervical Polyps
- Bleeding is usually self-limited.
- Trauma should be avoided.
- Cytologic sampling is mandatory.
- Polypectomy may control bleeding and yield a histologic diagnosis.

Bloody Show
Bloody show is characteristically associated with cervical changes and blood-tinged mucus. Heavy bleeding is rare and should prompt the evaluation for other complications.

Vulvovaginal Trauma
- Patient history frequently elucidates the cause.
- Adequate pelvic examination should be performed, including an examination under anesthesia, if necessary.
- Penetration of the cul-de-sac necessitates exploratory laparotomy.
- Foreign bodies must be removed.
- Wounds should be debrided and closed, if clean.
- Hematomas should be evacuated. Hemostasis should be obtained. Drains as needed should be placed.
- Tetanus prophylaxis is indicated.

Hematuria
Hematuria as a source of vaginal bleeding can be diagnosed by urinalysis.

Management of Hemorrhagic Shock
- Management of the patient in shock requires vigilance (2,15).
  - Vital signs should be monitored.
  - Urine output must be monitored with an indwelling bladder catheter in place and maintained at greater than 30 mL/h.
  - If urine output is not maintained, hemodynamic monitoring should be instituted.
    - A central venous pressure catheter is adequate if left ventricular function appears normal.
    - If left ventricular function is questioned, or urine output is inadequate despite adequate central venous pressure, a Swan-Ganz catheter should be placed.
    - Oxygen should be administered.
- Adequate replacement of blood volume is mandatory. During the wait for blood, colloid or crystalloid (3 mL for every milliliter of blood lost) should be quickly infused. Blood products should be used when available as appropriate. Use of trauma or massive transfusion protocols may be helpful (15).

- Hematocrit is not a sensitive indicator of acute blood loss because hemodilution is only half complete at 8 hours.
- Electrolytes, calcium, oxygenation, and acid–base status should be carefully monitored.
- The underlying event should be identified and treated (16).

PATIENT EDUCATION

- Patients should be informed that vaginal bleeding, particularly in the third trimester, requires urgent attention.
- Patients with placenta previa or vasa previa should be told to avoid intercourse.
- Patients should be educated about the recognition and significance of bloody show as an indicator of early labor.
- Patients who are Rh(D) negative should be made aware of importance of receiving anti-D immunoglobulin to protect against sensitization.

REFERENCES

1. Dhanraj D, Lambers D. The incidences of positive Kleihauer-Betke test in low-risk pregnancies and maternal trauma patients. *Am J Obstet Gynecol.* 2004;190(5):1461.
2. Oyelese Y, Ananth CV. Placental abruption. *Obstet Gynecol.* 2006;108(4):1005.
3. Tikkanen M. Placental abruption: epidemiology, risk factors and consequences. *Acta Obstet Gynecol Scand.* 2011;90(2):140–149.
4. Tikkanen M, Luukkaala T, Gissler M, et al. Decreasing perinatal mortality in placental abruption. *Acta Obstet Gynecol Scand.* 2013;92(3):298–305.
5. Ananth CV, Smulian JC, Demissie K, et al. Placental abruption among singleton and twin births in the United States: risk factor profiles. *Am J Epidemiol.* 2001;153(8):771.
6. de Lloyd L, Bovington R, Kaye A, et al. Standard haemostatic tests following major obstetric haemorrhage. *Int J Obstet Anesth.* 2011;20(2):135–141.
7. Glantz C, Purnell L. Clinical utility of sonography in the diagnosis and treatment of placental abruption. *J Ultrasound Med.* 2002;21(8):837.
8. Duchesne JC, Islam TM, Stuke L, et al. Hemostatic resuscitation during surgery improves survival in patients with traumatic-induced coagulopathy. *J Trauma.* 2009;67(1):33.
9. Dashe JS, McIntire DD, Ramus RM, et al. Persistence of placenta previa according to gestational age at ultrasound detection. *Obstet Gynecol.* 2002;99(5 Pt 1):692.
10. Faiz AS, Ananth CV. Etiology and risk factors for placenta previa: an overview and meta-analysis of observational studies. *J Matern Fetal Neonatal Med.* 2003;13:175–190.
11. Sheiner E, Shoham-Vardi I, Hallak M, et al. Placenta previa: obstetric risk factors and pregnancy outcome. *J Matern Fetal Med.* 2001;10(6):414.
12. Oppenheimer L; Society of Obstetricians and Gynaecologists of Canada. Diagnosis and management of placenta previa. *J Obstet Gynaecol Can.* 2007;29(3):261–273.
13. Warshak CR, Eskander R, Hull AD, et al. Accuracy of ultrasonography and magnetic resonance imaging in the diagnosis of placenta accreta. *Obstet Gynecol.* 2006;108(3 Pt 1):573.
14. Sepulveda W, Rojas I, Robert JA, et al. Prenatal detection of velamentous insertion of the umbilical cord: a prospective color Doppler ultrasound study. *Ultrasound Obstet Gynecol.* 2003;21(6):564.
15. Burtelow M, Riley E, Druzin M, et al. How we treat: management of life-threatening primary postpartum hemorrhage with a standardized massive transfusion protocol. *Transfusion.* 2007;47(9):1564.
16. Thachil J, Toh CH. Disseminated intravascular coagulation in obstetric disorders and its acute haematological management. *Blood Rev.* 2009;23(4):167.

10 Abnormal Labor

Cynthia Bean

KEY POINTS

- Dystocia results from abnormalities during labor with the interplay between the power (uterine contractions and maternal expulsive forces), the passenger (fetal size, presentation, and position), and the passage (maternal bony pelvis and soft tissues).
- Recognition of risk factors and causes of dystocia are critical for proper treatment.
- Appropriate management of dystocia reduces maternal and fetal morbidity and prevents unnecessary cesarean deliveries (CD).

BACKGROUND

Definitions

- Dystocia: difficult labor and childbirth.
- Prolonged latent phase (Table 10-1; Fig. 10-1)
  - Nulliparous patient: greater than 20 hours
  - Multiparous patient: greater than 14 hours
  - It is often difficult to determine the start of the latent phase because of increased uterine activity ("false labor") that may occur days before the onset of spontaneous labor (1).
  - The latent phase is generally considered complete when cervical dilation reaches 3 to 5 cm.
- Protraction disorders—slow progression of labor (Fig. 10-2) (2,3).
  - Protracted active phase dilation:
    o Nulliparous patient: rate of dilation less than 1.2 cm/h
    o Multiparous patient: rate of dilation less than 1.5 cm/h
  - Protracted descent—descent of fetal presenting part during second stage of labor:
    o Nulliparous patient: less than 1 cm/h
    o Multiparous patient: less than 2 cm/h
- Arrest disorders—no progression of labor (Fig. 10-3) (2–4).
  - Secondary arrest of dilation
    o No cervical dilation after 2 hours in active labor with adequate contractions
  - Arrest of descent:
    o No descent of fetal presenting part after 1 hour in the second stage of labor
- Prolonged second stage of labor (4–6)
  - Nulliparous patient without regional analgesia: greater than 2 hours
  - Nulliparous patient with regional analgesia: greater than 3 hours
  - Multiparous patient without regional analgesia: greater than 1 hour
  - Multiparous patient with regional analgesia: greater than 2 hours
- Precipitous labor—rapid labor (7)
  - Delivery of the fetus in less than 3 hours

Epidemiology

- The leading indication for primary CD in the United States is dystocia or "failure to progress" (8,9).
- Approximately 50% to 60% of CD may be attributable to dystocia (9).
- Successful management of abnormal labor and adhering to the appropriate definitions of dystocia will help decrease the CD rate.

Table 10-1	Labor Duration	
Variable	Nulliparous women	Multiparous women
Latent phase		
Mean (h)	6.4	4.8
Upper limit (h)	20.1	13.6
Active phase		
Mean (h)	4.6	2.4
Upper limit (h)	11.7	5.2
Dilation rate	0	
Lower limit (cm/h)	1.2	1.5
Second stage		
Upper limit (h)	2.9	1.1

From Friedman EA. *Labor: clinical evaluation and management.* 2nd ed. New York: Appleton-Century-Crofts, 1978, with permission.

Pathophysiology
- Dystocia results from the abnormal functions and interactions between
  - Uterine contractions and maternal effort: **Power**
  - Fetal size, presentation, and position: **Passenger**
  - Maternal bony pelvis and soft tissues: **Passage**

Etiology
- Associated risk factors for dystocia include (9–15):
  - Advanced maternal age
  - Maternal diabetes mellitus and/or hypertension
  - Short maternal stature
  - Maternal pelvic contractures or tumors (leiomyomas)
  - Infertility or nulligravidity
  - Premature rupture of membranes (PROM) or oligohydramnios
  - Chorioamnionitis
  - High station at complete cervical dilation
  - Fetal malposition
  - Prior perinatal death

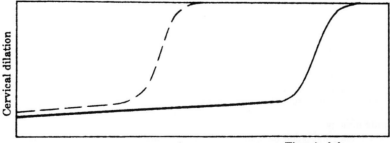

Figure 10-1. Prolonged latent phase pattern (*solid line*). *Broken line* illustrates average dilation curve for nulliparous women. (From Friedman EA. *Labor: clinical evaluation and management.* 2nd ed. New York: Appleton-Century-Crofts, 1978, with permission.)

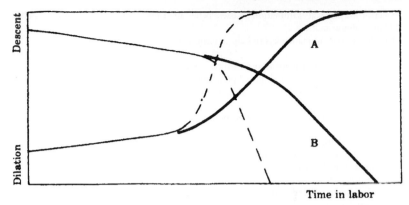

Figure 10-2. Protraction disorders of labor. *A:* Protracted active phase. *B:* Prolonged descent pattern. *Broken lines* illustrate average normal dilation and descent patterns. (From Friedman EA. *Labor: clinical evaluation and management.* 2nd ed. New York: Appleton-Century-Crofts, 1978, with permission.)

- Large for gestational age (LGA)/macrosomia
- Epidural analgesia
- Physician and/or patient anxiety due to prior or current pregnancy complications can result in prematurely labeling the labor as "failure to progress."

EVALUATION

History and Physical
- During antepartum visits:
  - Obtain an accurate history to identify risk factors for dystocia.

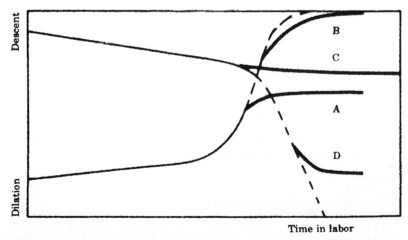

Figure 10-3. Arrest disorders of labor. *A:* Secondary arrest of dilation. *B:* Prolonged deceleration. *C:* Failure of descent. *D:* Arrest of descent. *Broken lines* illustrate normal dilation and descent curves. (From Friedman EA. *Labor: clinical evaluation and management.* 2nd ed. New York: Appleton-Century-Crofts, 1978, with permission.)

- Perform a physical examination to assess pelvic anatomy, which may help predict pelvic outlet abnormalities.
- Perform Leopold maneuvers to help determine fetal presentation.
- During labor:
  - Perform Leopold maneuvers and/or ultrasound to determine fetal presentation.
  - Estimate fetal size with abdominal palpation and/or ultrasound.
  - Perform physical examination to determine:
    ○ Fetal position
    ○ Progress of cervical dilation, effacement, and station

Diagnostic Studies
- Ultrasound evaluation is frequently used to assess
  - Estimated fetal weight (EFW)
  - Amniotic fluid index (AFI)
  - Fetal presentation and position
  - Placental location
  - Uterine anomalies or pelvic tumors
  - Biophysical profile (BPP)

DYSTOCIA—UTERINE FUNCTION
Diagnosis
- The clinician must first distinguish between the latent and active phases of labor before deciding on treatment.

Etiologies
- Causes of uterine dysfunction:
  - Müllerian anomalies (uterine septum or didelphys)
  - Pelvic tumors (leiomyomas or large ovarian tumors)
  - Cervical abnormalities resulting from a loop electrosurgical excision procedure (LEEP), cold knife cone (CKC), cerclage, trauma, or other injuries
  - Uterine overdistension (LGA/macrosomia, multiple gestation, polyhydramnios)

Clinical Manifestations
- Effective contractions are obvious clinically if progression of cervical dilation and effacement occurs.
- External monitoring using either palpation or a displacement transducer provides information about the frequency of uterine contractions.
- Internal monitoring using an intrauterine pressure catheter (IUPC) provides information about the frequency, duration, and intensity of uterine contractions in millimeters of mercury (mm Hg).
  - Montevideo units (MVUs) equal the mean amplitude (mm Hg) of contractions multiplied by the number of contractions in 10 minutes.
  - Two hundred to two hundred and fifty montevideo units are commonly used to define adequate contractions in the active phase of labor (16,17).

Treatment
Medications
- Prolonged latent phase recommendations
  - Augmentation of labor (18–21):
    ○ Oxytocin
    ○ Misoprostol
  - Therapeutic rest (22):
    ○ Nubain, 10 to 15 mg intramuscularly (IM)
    ○ Morphine, 10 to 20 mg IM
    ○ Vistaril, 100 mg orally

- Active management of labor
  - Limited to nulliparous women with (9):
    - Term pregnancies
    - Singleton gestations
    - Cephalic presentation
    - No evidence of fetal compromise
  - The Dublin or O'Driscoll protocol (23):
    - Patient education on signs and symptoms of labor
    - Strict admission criteria—only patients in active labor admitted
    - Amniotomy within 1 hour of admission if unruptured
    - Strict criteria for recognition of abnormal labor patterns
    - Oxytocin infusion if abnormal pattern ascertained:
      - Six milliunits per minute to start
      - Six milliunits per minute increase every 15 minutes
      - Maximum of 40 milliunits per minute or seven contractions in 15 minutes or adequate progress
    - Nurse/patient ratio of 1:1
    - Intermittent or continuous monitoring of contractions and fetal heart tones
    - CD if undelivered 12 hours after admission or if fetal compromise ascertained
    - Protocol resulted in CD rate of 4.8%
      - A second trial in Ireland using the same protocol showed a doubling of the CD rate over the first trial (24).
      - Lopez-Zeno et al. (25) repeated the study in the United States and reported a decrease in the CD rate, length of labor, and febrile morbidity (25).
      - Frigoletto et al. (11) repeated the study and reported no decrease in CD rate but a decrease in labor length and febrile morbidity (11).
      - The American College of Obstetricians and Gynecologists (ACOG) concluded that active management of labor may shorten labor but has not consistently led to a decrease in the CD rate (9).
- Protracted labor and arrest of labor
  - Use O'Driscoll protocol or Seitchik protocol (26).
    - Oxytocin, 5 milliunits per minute with increase every 40 minutes
    - Twenty to forty minutes is needed for plasma levels of oxytocin to reach a steady state.
      - Satin et al. (27) analyzed 1773 cases of augmented labor. Individual patient variables prevented accurate prediction of oxytocin dosage or rate needed to affect adequate labor (27).

Procedures
- Amniotomy (28–31)
  - Benefits
    - Reduction in labor duration
    - Reduction in abnormal 5-minute Apgar score (less than 5)
    - Decreased need for oxytocin
    - No increase in CD rate
  - Risks
    - Increase in abnormal fetal heart rate patterns (without increase in CD rate)
    - Increase in febrile morbidity

Complications
- Treatment of tachysystole: (32,33)
  - Decrease or stop oxytocin.
  - Administer oxygen.
  - Increase intravenous fluid rate (IVF).
  - Administer tocolytics (β2-adrenergic agents such as terbutaline).

- Treatment of fetal heart rate abnormalities (33,34)
  - Discontinue any labor stimulating agent if possible (stop oxytocin, remove prostaglandin insert).
  - Administer oxygen.
  - Change maternal position.
  - Perform cervical exam (check for umbilical cord prolapse, rapid cervical change, or fetal descent).
  - Monitor maternal blood pressure (treat hypotension if present with volume expansion and/or intravenous ephedrine).
  - Assess for uterine tachysystole (treat as above).
  - May perform amnioinfusion (AI) for recurrent variable decelerations.
  - Perform CD if abnormality cannot be corrected.
- Uterine rupture (22,35)
  - Occurs in approximately 1 in 2000 deliveries.
  - Risk factors include prior CD, transfundal uterine surgery, obstructed labor, multiparity, and uterine overdistension.
  - May occur spontaneously without risk factors.
  - Clinical manifestations include abnormal fetal heart rate patterns (most common finding), loss of fetal station, abdominal pain, vaginal bleeding, cessation of uterine contractions, and signs of hemodynamic instability.
  - Can be catastrophic for mother and/or fetus.
  - Immediate CD should be performed once recognized.
- Water intoxication—rare side effect of oxytocin
- Postpartum hemorrhage (see Chapter 4 for management)

DYSTOCIA—FETAL FACTORS
Malpresentations
Diagnosis
Clinical Manifestations
- Asynclitism (36)
  - Fetal sagittal suture is not midway between the maternal symphysis and sacral promontory (lateral deflection of the sagittal suture).
  - Parietal bone is palpated as presenting structure.
- Brow presentation (Fig. 10-4)
  - Partially deflexed cephalic attitude (halfway between full extension and flexion)
  - Diagnosed by palpation (feel brow, orbital ridges, eyes, frontal sutures, anterior fontanelle)
  - Occurs in 0.2% of all deliveries
- Face presentations (Fig. 10-5)
  - Fetal head is hyperextended (fetal occiput in contact with fetal back).
  - Diagnosed by palpation (feel facial features).
  - Reference point for description is the mentum (chin)—mentum anterior (MA) or posterior (MP).
  - Occurs in 0.2% of all deliveries.
- Breech presentations (36,37)
  - Higher incidence of congenital anomalies in breech versus cephalic (6.3% vs. 2.4%)
  - Diagnosed by Leopold maneuvers, vaginal examination, or ultrasound
  - Affects 3% to 4% of all deliveries
  - Conditions that predispose to breech presentation:
    - Prematurity
    - Multiple gestation
    - Abnormal placental implantation (fundal–cornual or previa)
    - Uterine anomalies or pelvic tumors

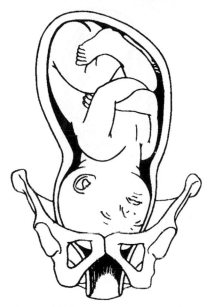

Figure 10-4. Brow presentation. (From Obstetrical presentation and position. Ross Clinical Education Aid 18. Columbus, OH: Ross Laboratories, 1975, with permission.)

- ○ Polyhydramnios or oligohydramnios
- ○ Increased parity
- • Three types of breech presentations (Fig. 10-6)
  - ○ Frank breech—flexion of hips, extension at knees
  - ○ Complete breech—flexion at both hips and knees

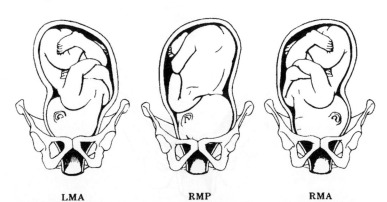

LMA   RMP   RMA

Figure 10-5. Types of face presentation. LMA, left mentum anterior; RMP, right mentum posterior; RMA, right mentum anterior. (From Obstetrical presentation and position. Ross Clinical Education Aid 18. Columbus, OH: Ross Laboratories, 1975, with permission.)

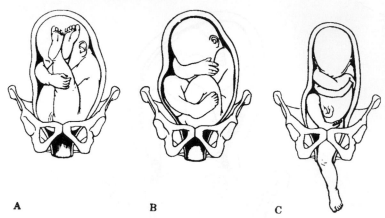

A   **B**   **C**

Figure 10-6. Types of breech presentation. **A:** Frank breech. **B:** Complete breech. **C:** Footling breech. (From Obstetrical presentation and position. Ross Clinical Education Aid 18. Columbus, OH: Ross Laboratories, 1975, with permission.)

- o Incomplete or footling breech—one or both hips deflexed with fetal knee or foot below fetal buttock
- • Transverse lie (Fig. 10-7)
  - o Diagnosed by Leopold maneuvers or ultrasound
  - o Occurs in 0.3% of deliveries
  - o Occurs more commonly in similar situations that predispose to breech presentation (see above)
- • Compound presentation
  - o More than one presenting part—an extremity prolapses beside the presenting part (most common is the head and an upper extremity)
  - o May be delivered vaginally if the vertex precedes the extremity

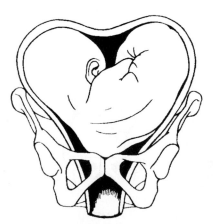

Figure 10-7. Shoulder presentation. (From Obstetrical presentation and position. Ross Clinical Education Aid 18. Columbus, OH: Ross Laboratories, 1975, with permission.)

- Persistent occiput posterior (OP) position
  - Diagnosed by vaginal examination
  - May deliver vaginally (spontaneous, manual rotation, operative vaginal delivery)
  - Occurs in approximately 5% at delivery (38)
- Persistent occiput transverse (OT) position
  - Usually associated with pelvic abnormality (platypelloid or android pelvis)
  - May delivery vaginally (spontaneous, manual, or forceps rotation)
- Fetal anomalies
  - Increases in biparietal diameter (BPD) as in hydrocephalus or other central nervous system anomalies can result in dystocia.
  - Increases in fetal abdominal circumference seen with abdominal tumors, distended bladder, ascites, abdominal organ enlargement, or sacrococcygeal tumors can result in dystocia and fetal malpresentation.
  - Macrosomia can result in dysfunctional labor and shoulder dystocia (see below).
  - With the common availability of ultrasound in the United States, most fetal anomalies are diagnosed antenatally, which facilitates prospective decisions for which fetuses will benefit from CD.

Treatment

- Malpositions
  - OP and OT descend through the pelvis at greater diameters than occiput anterior (OA) and may impede vaginal delivery.
  - Manual rotation
    - First determine the exact orientation of the head.
    - Attempt rotation with effective anesthesia and a skilled operator.
  - Maternal position change aids in turning fetus
    - Knee-to-chest position
    - Side-to-side rotation
  - Forceps rotation
    - Should be attempted only by operators experienced in the procedure.
    - Potential exists for fetal and maternal morbidity.
- Brow and face presentations
  - As a general rule, brow presentations should convert to face or vertex presentations to deliver vaginally. Spontaneous conversion during labor (usually in the second stage) is common. Persistent brow has a poor prognosis for vaginal delivery and usually requires CD.
  - MA face presentation can deliver vaginally in an adequate pelvis.
  - MP cannot be delivered vaginally and must be delivered by CD. Note that conversion from MP to MA may not take place until late in the second stage when pressure from the perineum against the face creates sufficient force to cause the fetus to rotate to MA.
- Breech presentation
  - External cephalic version (ECV) indications (39,40):
    - 35% to 86% success rate (depends on various factors)
    - Gestational age of 37 weeks or later
    - Normal AFI
    - Reactive nonstress test (NST) prior to attempt and after procedure
    - Ultrasound guidance with forward or backward roll
    - Ability to perform emergency CD if needed for fetal distress
  - ECV contraindications (factors that would preclude a vaginal delivery)
    - Absolute contraindications:
      - Placenta previa
      - Oligohydramnios or PROM
      - Certain fetal anomalies (increased risk of fetal injury)
      - Nonreassuring NST or fetal heart rate tracing

- ○ Relative contraindications:
  - − Prior CD
  - − Obesity
  - − LGA/macrosomia
  - − Maternal medical conditions (hypertension, diabetes mellitus, etc.)
- • Breech delivery (41–43)
  - ○ Many centers advocate delivery via CD only.
  - ○ Physician must be experienced in vaginal breech delivery.
  - ○ Must have ability to perform emergent CD.
  - ○ Contraindications:
    - − EFW less than 1500 g
    - − Inadequate pelvis
    - − Incomplete breech
    - − Hyperextended neck
    - − Fetal growth restriction
  - ○ ACOG recommends the decision regarding mode of delivery should depend on the experience of the provider.
- • Techniques for breech delivery
  - ○ **Allow spontaneous delivery to level of umbilicus if possible.**
  - ○ Perform Pinard maneuver if needed (atraumatic delivery of the feet).
  - ○ Support trunk and lower extremities in a moist sterile towel with the sacrum anterior.
  - ○ Place gentle traction on lower extremities until delivery of buttocks.
  - ○ Continue downward traction and slight rotation until scapulas visible.
  - ○ Deliver arms by sweeping each across chest after anterior rotation of the shoulder.
  - ○ Flex fetal head by placing fingers over the maxilla, and with the other hand, use two fingers to hook the fetal neck and grasp the shoulders (Mauriceau-Smellie-Veit maneuver).
  - ○ Apply suprapubic pressure to help deliver head.
  - ○ Perform episiotomy to maximize space if needed.
  - ○ Use modified Prague maneuver if sacrum posterior.
  - ○ Use Piper forceps if needed for the aftercoming head (see "Operative Vaginal Deliveries" below).
- • Transverse lie
  - • ECV may be attempted.
  - • CD required
    - ○ Low transverse hysterotomy for back up transverse lie
    - ○ Vertical (classical) hysterotomy for back down transverse lie

Complications
- • Increased poor outcomes in breech deliveries (41,44).
- • Vaginal breech delivery complications include nuchal arms and head entrapment.
- • Complications associated with ECV include placental abruption, fetal distress, rupture of membranes, fetomaternal hemorrhage, and need for emergent CD.
- • Increase in umbilical cord prolapse with breech presentation and transverse lie.
- • Increased rate of CD for all malpresentations.

DYSTOCIA—MATERNAL PELVIS
Evaluation
Physical Examination
- • Gynecoid pelvis:
  - • Round in shape
  - • Most adapted to normal labor and delivery

- Anthropoid pelvis:
  - Longitudinal oval
  - Also favorable for vaginal delivery
- Android pelvis:
  - Heart shaped
  - More commonly associated with abnormal labor
- Platypelloid pelvis:
  - Transverse oval
  - High incidence of dystocia and malposition of fetus
- Typical pelvis is a combination of forms.
- Severe malnutrition can affect the growth of the bony pelvis.

Diagnostic Studies
- Pelvimetry
  - Measures pelvic inlet or obstetric conjugate
    ○ Anterior–posterior (AP) is distance between symphysis pubis and sacral promontory
    ○ Transverse diameter (T) measured at widest point between lateral margins
  - Measures midpelvic plane
    ○ AP is distance between lower margin of symphysis and sacrum at S4-5.
    ○ T is distance between ischial spines.
- CT has replaced x-ray as the preferred technique for pelvimetry. Although not widely used in current obstetric practice, CT pelvimetry is helpful for assessing adequacy of the pelvis when considering vaginal delivery of a breech fetus or multiple gestation.

Management
- When pelvic abnormalities are suspected, a trial of labor is usually advocated unless obvious deformities are present.

SHOULDER DYSTOCIA
Diagnosis
Clinical Manifestations
- The fetal shoulders fail to deliver after delivery of the fetal head using routine maneuvers.
- Impaction of the anterior fetal shoulder behind the pubic symphysis.
- Turtle sign: the appearance of and then retraction of the fetal head against the perineum.
- The incidence ranges from 0.6% to 1.4% (45).
- Risk factors (45,46):
  - Prior shoulder dystocia
  - Pregestational or gestational diabetes mellitus
  - LGA/macrosomia (and prior history of a macrosomic infant)
  - Maternal obesity
  - Multiparity
  - Postterm pregnancy
  - Prolonged second stage of labor
  - Operative vaginal delivery (midforceps or midvacuum delivery)
- Even though risk factors exist, the majority of shoulder dystocias are unpredictable and unpreventable (45).
- The majority of shoulder dystocias occur in fetuses weighing less than 4000 g and without other risk factors.

Treatment
Procedures
Prompt action is required to avoid fetal and maternal compromise (47):
- Stop maternal pushing and call for HELP—make sure to call for anesthesia and pediatrics.
- Have someone mark the clock to keep track of time.

- Avoid excessive traction on the fetal head.
- *Never* use fundal pressure.
- Cut an episiotomy if needed.
- Begin to perform extra maneuvers:
  - Suprapubic pressure
    - Have assistant apply suprapubic pressure against the fetal shoulder
    - Helps to dislodge the impacted shoulder from under the pubic symphysis
  - McRoberts maneuver
    - Hyperflexion of maternal hips against abdomen.
    - This results in straightening of the lumbosacral angle and anterior rotation of the pubic symphysis.
    - This maneuver alone alleviates 42% of shoulder dystocias (48).
    - Often used in conjunction with suprapubic pressure.
  - Rubin maneuvers (two different maneuvers)
    - First description—Apply force to the maternal abdomen and rotate fetal shoulders from side to side. This helps move fetal shoulders into a more favorable position to allow delivery.
    - Second description—The most accessible fetal shoulder is palpated vaginally, and the shoulder is rotated to the anterior chest (adduction), thus reducing the shoulder–shoulder diameter.
  - Woods maneuver (delivers the posterior shoulder)
    - Palpate the posterior shoulder vaginally and either
      - Apply pressure to the anterior surface of the posterior shoulder (abduction) to rotate into oblique position (Woods maneuver) or
      - Apply pressure to the posterior surface of the posterior shoulder (adduction) to rotate it forward (modified Woods maneuver)
  - Delivery of the posterior arm
    - Physician passes hand beneath the fetal posterior shoulder.
    - Fetal forearm is flexed by applying gentle pressure to the antecubital fossa.
    - Forearm is then grasped and swept across the chest and out.
    - Anterior shoulder delivered using suprapubic pressure and *gentle* downward traction on the fetal head.
    - Some advocate that delivery of the posterior arm should be the next maneuver performed if suprapubic pressure and McRoberts maneuver are unsuccessful (49).
  - Clavicular fracture
    - Performed if other maneuvers are unsuccessful.
    - Break the clavicle by applying upward pressure against the mid portion of the clavicle (upward pressure is used to avoid vascular injury).
    - Reduces shoulder–shoulder diameter.
  - Zavanelli maneuver (cephalic replacement)
    - Use Zavanelli maneuver if all above attempts are unsuccessful.
    - Fetal head rotated to OA position and flexed.
    - Constant, firm pressure maintained on vertex to push fetal head cephalad as far as possible.
    - May need to give uterine relaxants (terbutaline or nitroglycerin).
    - Proceed with immediate CD.

ACOG Recommendations (45)
- Planned CD may be considered for suspected fetal macrosomia with EFWs greater than 5000 g in nondiabetic women and greater than 4500 g in diabetic women.
  - There is not any evidence that one maneuver is superior to another in releasing an impacted fetal shoulder or decreasing the chance of injury. However, starting with McRoberts maneuver is a reasonable approach.

Complications
- Brachial plexus injury (the no. 1 neonatal complication)
- Fracture of the fetal clavicle or humerus
- Fetal anoxia or death from prolonged delivery or compressed umbilical cord
- Increase in perineal trauma (third- and fourth-degree lacerations)
- Maternal femoral nerve injury from overzealous flexion of the maternal hips
- Postpartum hemorrhage

OPERATIVE VAGINAL DELIVERIES
Background
Definitions
- Forceps have four components: the handle, lock, shank, and blades.
- Each blade has two curves:
  - Cephalic curve—fits around the fetal head (the lateral curve)
  - Pelvic curve—corresponds to the axis of the maternal birth canal
- Outlet forceps (50)
  - Fetal scalp visible at introitus without separation of labia.
  - Fetal skull has reached pelvic floor.
  - Rotation less than 45 degrees.
  - Fetal head is at or on perineum.
  - Sagittal suture is in AP diameter or right OA, right OP, left OA, or left OP position.
- Low forceps (50)
  - Leading point of fetal skull is $\geq$+2/5 station and not on pelvic floor.
  - Rotation may be less than or greater than 45 degrees.
  - Any OA or OP position is acceptable.
- Midforceps (50)
  - Fetal head is engaged—BPD has passed through the pelvic inlet.
  - Station is less than +2/5.
- Forceps types (Fig. 10-8) and usage
  - Parallel shank (Simpson, DeLee) used for molded vertex.
  - Overlapping shank (Elliot, Tucker-McLane-Luikart) used for unmolded vertex.
  - Piper forceps are used for the aftercoming head in breech delivery.
  - Barton and Kielland forceps are specifically rotational forceps for rotation of 90 degrees such as in OT to OA.
- Vacuum extraction (51)
  - Most vacuums are plastic or silicone cups that use a hand pump to create suction once the cup is applied to the fetal head.

Treatment
Indications
- Prolonged second stage of labor
- Nonreassuring fetal heart rate tracing
- Shorten the second stage of labor for maternal benefit (certain cardiac, pulmonary, or neuromuscular conditions)
- Maternal exhaustion or poor maternal pushing effort

Contraindications
- Fetal bone demineralization disorder
- Fetal bleeding disorder
- Unengaged fetal head
- For vacuum delivery—pregnancy less than 34 weeks of gestation

Application Principles: Forceps
Prerequisites
- Continuous electronic fetal monitoring throughout the procedure.

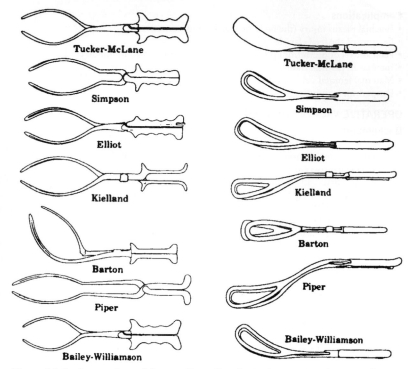

Figure 10-8. Commonly used forceps. (From Douglas R, Stromme W. *Operative obstetrics.* 3rd ed. New York: Appleton-Century-Crofts, 1976, with permission.)

- Fetal head must be engaged.
- Cervix completely dilated and effaced.
- Position, station, and attitude of fetus ascertained.
- Type of maternal pelvis should be ascertained.
- Experienced operator present.
- Adequate anesthesia established.
- Ability to perform an emergent CD.

Technique (52)
- Left blade applied first unless right occiput position.
- Blades inserted into posterior vagina with handle perpendicular to floor.
- Blades swept in an arc from horizontal or oblique angle to midline.
- Shanks should fall together and lock without force if application is correct.
- Sagittal suture palpated equidistant from each blade.
- Posterior fontanelle should be midway between the sides of the blades.
- Posterior fontanelle should be one fingerbreadth above the plane of the shanks.

Application Principles: Vacuum (52)
- Prerequisites listed for forceps delivery should also be present for vacuum application.
- Vacuum is applied to the fetal vertex in the midline avoiding the fontanelles.
- Care should be taken to avoid maternal soft tissues beneath the cup.
- Suction is applied, and pulls by operator occur during contractions.

- Steady traction should be applied in line of the birth canal, avoid torque.
- Maximum of three "pop-offs" is recommended to avoid injury.

Complications
- Fetal
  - Facial nerve or brachial plexus palsies
  - Skull fractures
  - Cephalohematomas or subgaleal hematomas
  - Intracranial or retinal hemorrhage
  - Scalp or facial lacerations
  - Hyperbilirubinemia
  - Asphyxia or death
- Maternal
  - Perineal, vaginal, and cervical lacerations (urinary/fecal incontinence)
  - Pelvic hematomas
  - Hemorrhage
  - Uterine rupture
  - Urinary retention

RETAINED PLACENTA
Background
Definition
- Failure of the placenta to deliver within 30 minutes of infant delivery

Etiology
- Idiopathic
- Abnormal placentation
  - Placenta accreta—abnormal attachment of the placenta to the uterine wall
  - Placenta increta—invasion of the placenta into the myometrium
  - Placenta percreta—penetration of the placenta through the myometrium to or through the uterine serosa

Treatment
Procedures
- Gentle traction on the umbilical cord and external uterine massage usually results in delivery of the placenta.
- Manual extraction of the placenta.
- Sharp curettage under ultrasound guidance if adherent fragments remain.

Complications
- Hemorrhage (see Chapter 4 for treatment)
- Endometrial synechiae from curettage

UTERINE INVERSION
Background
Definition
- Complete inversion: The uterine fundus extends beyond the cervix.
- Incomplete inversion: The inverted fundus does not extend beyond the cervix. This may go unrecognized.

Etiology
- Uterine inversion occurs as result of fundal implantation of the placenta (53).
- Uterine inversion may also result from excessive traction on the umbilical cord.

Epidemiology
• Uterine inversion occurs in approximately 1 in 2500 deliveries.

Diagnosis
Clinical Manifestations
• Postpartum hemorrhage.
• Uterine fundus cannot be palpated postdelivery.
• Beefy, red mass at or protruding through the vaginal introitus.

Treatment
Medications
• Tocolytic drugs such as magnesium sulfate, terbutaline, or nitroglycerin (53,54).
• General anesthesia.
• Resuscitate with intravenous fluids.
• Transfuse with blood products if necessary.

Procedures (55)
• Attempt manual replacement.
  • Place the palm of the hand against the fundus with the fingertips exerting upward pressure circumferentially (keep placenta attached if not already separated to prevent further hemorrhage).
  • Once the uterus is replaced:
    ◦ Manually remove the placenta if needed.
    ◦ Keep hand inside the uterus until the uterus contracts around the hand.
    ◦ Administer a uterotonic to assist with uterine contraction.
• Huntington procedure: laparotomy with serial clamping and upward traction on the round ligaments to allow for elevation of uterus.
• Haultain procedure: laparotomy with incision on the posterior lower uterine segment with both upward traction abdominally and manual replacement vaginally.

CESAREAN DELIVERY
Background
Definitions
• Uterine incision types
  • Low transverse or Kerr incision (LTCS)
    ◦ Most common.
    ◦ Incision made transversely in the lower uterine segment.
    ◦ Least likely to rupture in subsequent pregnancies.
    ◦ Trial of labor acceptable after LTCS (56).
    ◦ Majority of scar separations are incomplete (uterine dehiscence).
  • Low vertical or Kronig incision (LVCS)
    ◦ Incision made vertically in the lower uterine segment.
    ◦ Trial of labor may be acceptable (56).
  • Classical (CCS)
    ◦ Vertical incision into the contractile portion of the uterus
    ◦ Trial of labor not recommended after CCS (56)

Epidemiology
• The rate of CD has increased over last 30 years, with the national rate now at 32% (57).
• Medicolegal concerns influence the CD rate.

Evaluation
Indications
• Protraction and arrest disorders (most common reason for primary CD)

- Nonreassuring fetal heart rate tracings
- Malpresentation
- Placenta previa
- Maternal genital herpes infection
- Prior CD
  - Elective repeat CD should be performed at or beyond 39 weeks of gestation unless fetal lung maturity has been demonstrated.
- Multiple gestation
- Certain maternal comorbidities
- Various fetal anomalies

Complications
Maternal
- Hemorrhage (uterine atony, lacerations, accreta, hematomas)
- Injuries to bladder, bowel, ureters, blood vessels, nerves, and cervix
- Infection (endomyometritis, wound infection, pelvic abscess, necrotizing fasciitis)
  - Antimicrobial prophylaxis is recommended for all CDs (58).
    - ○ Administer antibiotics within 60 minutes of skin incision.
    - ○ Decreases rates of endometritis, wound infection, and febrile morbidity.
- Thromboembolic events
- Anesthesia complications
- Postoperative ileus or bowel obstruction
- Wound complications (infection, separation, dehiscence, evisceration)
- Placenta accreta and/or previa in subsequent pregnancies

Fetal
- Iatrogenic prematurity
- Transient tachypnea of the newborn
- Fetal lacerations

PATIENT EDUCATION

- Widespread availability of medical information has allowed patients to become better informed.
- ACOG pamphlets and other resources provide written explanations of procedure and options.
- Audio–visual tapes allow for viewing of procedures.
- Physicians have the responsibility to discuss all treatment scenarios.
  - Patients identified antenatally at high risk for dystocia should be offered available diagnostic testing that may affect management.
  - Patients with labor dystocia must be informed of risks and benefits of possible treatments and alternatives.
  - Patients with a prior CD should be offered both elective repeat CD and trial of labor after cesarean (TOLAC) options, if medically appropriate, with a detailed discussion of all risks and benefits.
- All discussions with patients and consent forms should be well documented in the patient medical record.

REFERENCES

1. Hendricks CH, Brenner WE, Kraus G. The normal cervical dilation pattern in late pregnancy and labor. *Am J Obstet Gynecol.* 1970;106:1065–1082.
2. Friedman EA. *Labor: clinical evaluation and management.* 2nd ed. New York: Appleton-Century-Crofts, 1978.
3. Friedman EA. Primigravid labor; a graphicostatistical analysis. *Obstet Gynecol.* 1955;6:567.

4. Kilpatrick SJ, Laros RK Jr. Characteristics of normal labor. *Obstet Gynecol*. 1989;74: 85–87.

5. Zhang J, Yancey MK, Klebanoff MA, et al. Does epidural analgesia prolong labor and increase risk of cesarean delivery? A natural experiment. *Am J Obstet Gynecol*. 2001;185:128–134.

6. Alexander JM, Sharma SK, McIntire DD, et al. Epidural analgesia lengthens the Friedman active phase of labor. *Obstet Gynecol*. 2002;100(1):46–50.

7. Hughes EC. *Obstetric-gynecologic terminology*. Philadelphia: Davis, 1972.

8. Gifford DS, Morton SC, Fiske M, et al. Lack of progress in labor as a reason for cesarean. *Obstet Gynecol*. 2000;95:589–595.

9. American College of Obstetricians and Gynecologists. Dystocia and augmentation of labor. *ACOG Pract Bull*. 2003;49.

10. Sheiner E, Levy A, Feinstein U, et al. Obstetric risk factors for failure to progress in the first versus the second stage of labor. *J Matern Fetal Neonatal Med*. 2002;11:409–413.

11. Frigoletto FD Jr, Lieberman E, Lang JM, et al. A clinical trial of active management of labor. *N Engl J Med*. 1995;333:745–750.

12. Howell CJ. Epidural versus non-epidural analgesia for pain relief in labour. *Cochrane Database Syst Rev*. 2003;3:CD003766.

13. Satin AJ, Maberry MC, Leveno KJ, et al. Chorioamnionitis: a harbinger of dystocia. *Obstet Gynecol*. 1992;79:913–915.

14. Piper JM, Bolling DR, Newton ER. The second stage of labor: factors influencing duration. *Am J Obstet Gynecol*. 1991;165:976–979.

15. Fraser WD, Cayer M, Soeder BM, et al. PEOPLE (Pushing Early or Pushing Late with Epidural) Study Group. Risk factors for difficult delivery in nulliparas with epidural analgesia in second stage of labor. *Obstet Gynecol*. 2002;99:409–418.

16. Miller FC. Uterine activity, labor management, and perinatal outcome. *Semin Perinatol*. 1978;2:181–186.

17. Hauth JC, Hankins GV, Gilstrap LC, et al. Uterine contraction pressures with oxytocin induction/augmentation. *Obstet Gynecol*. 1986;68:305–309.

18. Rouse DJ, Weiner SJ, Bloom SL, et al. Failed labor induction: toward an objective diagnosis. *Obstet Gynecol*. 2011;117(2, Part 1):267–272.

19. Hofmeyr GJ. Vaginal misoprostol for cervical ripening and induction of labour. *Cochrane Database Syst Rev*. 1999;2:1–18.

20. Mercer B, Pilgrim P, Sibai B. Labor induction with continuous low dose oxytocin infusion: a randomized trial. *Obstet Gynecol*. 1991;77:659–663.

21. Muller PR, Stubbs TM, Laurent SL. A prospective randomized clinical trial comparing two oxytocin induction protocols. *Am J Obstet Gynecol*. 1992;167:373–381.

22. Gabbe SG, Niebyl JR, Simpson JL, eds. *Obstetrics: normal and problem pregnancies*. 6th ed. Philadelphia: Saunders, 2012.

23. O'Driscoll K, Foley M, MacDonald D. Active management of labor as an alternative to cesarean section for dystocia. *Obstet Gynecol*. 1984;63:485–490.

24. Boylan P, Robson M, McFarland P. Active management of labor 1963–1990. *Am J Obstet Gynecol*. 1993;168:295–300.

25. Lopez-Zeno JA, Peaceman AM, Adashek JA, et al. A controlled trial of a program for the active management of labor. *N Engl J Med*. 1992;326:450–454.

26. Seitchik J, Amico J, Robinson AG, et al. Oxytocin augmentation of dysfunctional labor. IV Oxytocin pharmacokinetics. *Am J Obstet Gynecol*. 1984;150:225–228.

27. Satin AJ, Leveno KJ, Sherman ML, et al. Factors affecting the dose response to oxytocin for labor stimulation. *Am J Obstet Gynecol*. 1992;166:1260–1261.

28. Wei S, Wo BL, Qi HP, et al. Early amniotomy and early oxytocin for prevention of, or therapy for, delay in first stage spontaneous labour compared with routine care. *Cochrane Database Syst Rev*. 2012;9.

29. Garite TJ, Porto M, Carlson NJ, et al. The influence of elective amniotomy on fetal heart rate patterns and the course of labor in term patients: a randomized study. *Am J Obstet Gynecol*. 1993;168:1827–1831.

30. Rouse DJ, McCollogh C, Wren AL, et al. Active phase labor arrest: a randomized trial of chorioamnion management. *Obstet Gynecol.* 1994;88:937–940.
31. Brisson-Carroll G, Fraser W, Breart G, et al. The effect of routine early amniotomy on spontaneous labor: a meta-analysis. *Obstet Gynecol.* 1996;87:891–896.
32. Egarter CH, Husslein PW, Rayburn WF. Uterine hyperstimulation after low-dose prostaglandin E2 therapy: tocolytic treatment in 181 cases. *Am J Obstet Gynecol.* 1990;163: 794–796.
33. American College of Obstetricians and Gynecologists. Intrapartum fetal heart rate monitoring: nomenclature, interpretation and general management principles. *ACOG Prac Bull.* 2009;106.
34. Hofmeyr GJ. Amnioinfusion for potential or suspected umbilical cord compression in labour. *Cochrane Database Syst Rev.* 1998;1:CD000013.
35. American College of Obstetricians and Gynecologists. Vaginal birth after previous cesarean delivery. *ACOG Pract Bull.* 2010;115.
36. Cunningham FG, Leveno KJ, Bloom SL, eds. *Williams obstetrics.* 23rd ed. New York: McGraw Hill, 2010.
37. Creasy RK, Resnik R, Iams JD, eds. *Creasy and Resnik's maternal fetal medicine: principles and practice.* 6th ed. Philadelphia: Saunders, 2009.
38. Gardberg M, Laakkonen E, Salevaara M. Intrapartum sonography and persistent occiput posterior position: a study of 408 deliveries. *Obstet Gynecol.* 1998;91:746–749.
39. American College of Obstetricians and Gynecologists. External cephalic version. *ACOG Pract Bull.* 2000;13.
40. Gilstrap LC, Cunninghman FG, Vandorsten JP, eds. *Operative obstetrics.* 2nd ed. New York: McGraw Hill, 2002.
41. Hannah ME, Hannah WJ, Hewson SA, et al. Planned cesarean section versus planned vaginal birth for breech presentations at term: a randomised multicentre trial. Term Breech Trial Collaborative Group. *Lancet.* 2000;356:1375–1383.
42. Malloy MH, Onstad L, Wright E. National Institutes of Child Health and Human Development Neonatal Research Network: the effect of cesarean delivery on birth outcome in very-low-birthweight infants. *Obstet Gynecol.* 1991;77:498–503.
43. American College of Obstetricians and Gynecologists. ACOG Committee Opinion No. 340. Mode of term singleton breech delivery. 2006;108(1):235–237.
44. Gifford DS, Morton SC, Fiske M, et al. A meta-analysis of infant outcomes after breech delivery. *Obstet Gynecol.* 1995;85:1047–1054.
45. American College of Obstetricians and Gynecologists. Shoulder dystocia. *ACOG Pract Bull.* 2002;40.
46. Baskett TF, Allen AC. Perinatal implications of shoulder dystocia. *Obstet Gynecol.* 1995;86:14–17.
47. Naef RW, Morrison JC. Guidelines for the management of shoulder dystocia. *J Perinatol.* 1994;14:435–441.
48. Gherman RB, Goodwin TM, Souter I, et al. The McRobert's maneuver for the alleviation of shoulder dystocia: how successful is it? *Am J Obstet Gynecol.* 1997;176:656–661.
49. Hoffman MK, Bailit JL, Branch DW, et al. A comparison of obstetric maneuvers for the acute management of shoulder dystocia. *Obstet Gynecol.* 2011;117:1272–1278.
50. American College of Obstetricians and Gynecologists. Operative vaginal delivery. *ACOG Pract Bull.* 2000;17.
51. Bofill JA, Rust OA, Perry KG Jr, et al. Forceps and vacuum delivery: a survey of North American residency programs. *Obstet Gynecol.* 1996;88:622–625.
52. Hale RW, ed. *Dennen's forceps deliveries.* 4th ed. Washington, DC: American College of Obstetricians and Gynecologists, 2001.
53. Watson P, Besch N, Bowes WA Jr. Management of acute and subacute puerperal inversion of the uterus. *Obstet Gynecol.* 1980;55:12–16.
54. Catanzarite VA, Moffitt KD, Baker ML, et al. New approaches to the management of acute puerperal uterine inversion. *Obstet Gynecol.* 1986;68:75–105.

55. American College of Obstetricians and Gynecologists. Postpartum hemorrhage. *ACOG Pract Bull.* 2006;76.

56. American College of Obstetricians and Gynecologists. Vaginal birth after previous cesarean delivery. *ACOG Pract Bull.* 2010;115.

57. U.S. Department of Health and Human Services. Centers for Disease Control and Prevention. National Vital Statistics Report: Births: Final Data for 2010. 2012;61:1–71.

58. American College of Obstetricians and Gynecologists. Use of prophylactic antibiotics in labor and delivery. *ACOG Pract Bull.* 2011;120.

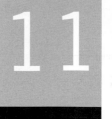

11

Hypertensive Disorders of Pregnancy

John R. Barton and Baha M. Sibai

KEY POINTS

Background

- Hypertensive disorders are the most common medical complication of pregnancy, occurring in approximately 7% to 10% of all pregnancies.
- Hypertensive disorders are associated with significant maternal and perinatal mortality and have a wide spectrum of presentation, ranging from minimal elevation of blood pressure to severe hypertension with multiple organ dysfunction.
- Preeclampsia is a syndrome that only occurs during pregnancy and is defined by hypertension and end-organ manifestations such as proteinuria, thrombocytopenia, and hepatic or cerebral manifestations.

Definitions for Hypertensive Disorder of Pregnancy

- Gestational hypertension
  - The National High Blood Pressure Education Program Working Group has recommended that the term "gestational hypertension" replace the term "pregnancy-induced hypertension" to describe cases in which elevated blood pressure without proteinuria develops in a woman after 20 weeks of gestation and blood pressure levels return to normal postpartum (1).
  - According to the criteria established in pregnant women by the Hypertension in Pregnancy Task Force sponsored by the ACOG, gestational hypertension is defined as a persistent systolic blood pressure level of 140 mm Hg or greater or a diastolic blood pressure level of 90 mm Hg or greater that occurs on two occasions 4 hours apart after 20 weeks of gestation in a woman with previously normal blood pressure (2).
- Preeclampsia
  - A syndrome of gestational hypertension plus end-organ manifestations including proteinuria with proteinuria defined as urinary excretion of 0.3 g protein or more in a 24-hour urine specimen or a protein/creatinine ratio ≥0.3 mg/dL. In the absence of proteinuria, new-onset hypertension with thrombocytopenia (less than 100,000 platelets/mL) or renal insufficiency (serum creatinine concentration greater than 1.1 mg/dL) or impaired liver functions (transaminases twice the upper limits of normal concentration) constitute diagnostic criteria of preeclampsia (2).
  - The previous definition of preeclampsia as hypertension of more than 30 mm Hg systolic or 15 mm Hg diastolic above the patient's baseline blood pressure is no longer used.
- Eclampsia
  - The development of convulsions or coma in patients with signs and symptoms of preeclampsia in the absence of other causes of convulsions
- Chronic hypertension
  - Patients with a persistent elevation of blood pressure to at least 140/90 mm Hg on two occasions before 20 weeks' gestation, and patients with hypertension that persists for more than 6 weeks postpartum
- Superimposed preeclampsia or eclampsia
  - The development of either preeclampsia or eclampsia in patients with previously diagnosed chronic hypertension

PREECLAMPSIA

Background

Definition
- Preeclampsia is a syndrome of gestational hypertension as defined above.
- There are only two types of preeclampsia: mild and severe.

Etiology
Preeclampsia is a disorder of unknown etiology that is peculiar to human pregnancy. Many theories regarding its etiology have been suggested, including
- Abnormal placentation
- Immunologic phenomena
- Coagulation abnormalities
- Abnormal cardiovascular adaptation
- Dietary factors
- Genetic factors
- Angiogenesis factors
- Vascular endothelial damage
- Abnormal prostaglandin metabolism

Epidemiology
- Preeclampsia is principally a disease of young, nulliparous women.
- The incidence of gestational hypertension is 6% to 17% for healthy nulliparous women and 2% to 4% for multiparous women.
- The incidence of mild preeclampsia is 2% to 7% in healthy nulliparous women and 14% in twin gestations.
- Seventy-five percent of patients with preeclampsia develop the disorder at ≥37 weeks of gestation.

Risk Factors
Although geographic and racial differences in incidence have been reported, several risk factors have been identified as predisposing to the development of preeclampsia:
- Nulliparity
- Multiple gestation
- Previous pregnancy with preeclampsia
- Family history of preeclampsia or eclampsia
- Preexisting hypertension or renal disease
- Pregestational diabetes
- Use of donor oocytes
- Nonimmune hydrops fetalis
- Molar pregnancy
- Obesity

Diagnosis

Clinical Manifestations
- Preeclampsia traditionally has been described as hypertension and proteinuria. It may, however, present as a spectrum of clinical signs and symptoms, alone or in combination, often making diagnosis difficult.
  - Hypertension
    - Abnormally elevated blood pressure is the traditional hallmark for the diagnosis of preeclampsia. The blood pressure criteria for gestational hypertension and preeclampsia are presented earlier in the chapter.
  - Proteinuria
    - Protein excretion in the urine increases in normal pregnancy from approximately 5 mg per 100 mL in the first and second trimesters to 15 mg per 100 mL in the third trimester.

○ Significant proteinuria should be defined as greater than 300 mg per 24-hour urine sample or protein/creatinine ratio ≥0.3 mg/dL.
○ When making a diagnosis of severe preeclampsia, the criterion of proteinuria of greater than 5 g excreted in a 24-hour urine has been discontinued (2).

- Early recognition of the development of preeclampsia can allow for more timely intervention to improve maternal and perinatal outcome. This reinforces the reason for frequent antenatal visits late in pregnancy to allow early detection of disease.
- Some preeclamptic pregnancies, particularly those with more severe disease, can be associated with reduced uteroplacental blood flow, which may be manifested as poor fetal growth. This can be the primary initial manifestation of preeclampsia and can be seen in both mild and severe forms of the disease.

Management
- Figure 11-1 shows a sample algorithm for the management of a normotensive patient who may be developing subtle signs and symptoms of preeclampsia.
- Once the diagnosis of preeclampsia has been made, definitive therapy in the form of delivery is the desired goal because it is the only cure for the disease.
- The ultimate goals of the therapy must always be first the safety of the mother and then the delivery of a mature newborn that will not require intensive and prolonged neonatal care.
- The decision between expectant management and immediate delivery usually depends on one or more of the following factors:
  - Severity of the disease process
  - Fetal condition
  - Maternal condition
  - Fetal gestational age
  - Presence of labor or rupture of membranes

MILD PREECLAMPSIA
Evaluation
- At the time of diagnosis, all patients with preeclampsia should be evaluated regarding maternal/fetal condition.

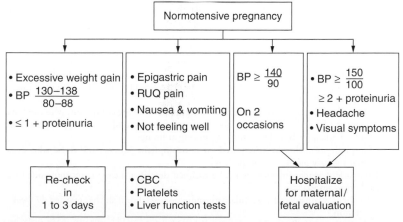

Figure 11-1. A sample algorithm for the management of a normotensive patient who may be developing subtle signs of preeclampsia.

Maternal Evaluation

History

Markers for possible severe preeclampsia:
- Persistent occipital or frontal headaches
- Visual disturbances
- Right upper quadrant abdominal or epigastric pain

Physical Evaluation
- Blood pressure assessment at diagnosis, then twice weekly by the health care provider.
- Urine protein assessment at diagnosis. If significant proteinuria is identified, subsequent proteinuria evaluation is not necessary as the amount or change in the amount of proteinuria will not influence the need for delivery (2).
- Weight daily.

Laboratory Evaluation
- Hematocrit and platelet count once per week
- Liver function tests once per week
- Twenty-four–hour urine collection at diagnosis for total protein excretion and creatinine clearance or a protein/creatinine ratio to confirm the diagnosis

Fetal Evaluation
- Daily fetal movement assessment (kick counts)
- Nonstress test (NST) twice weekly
- Biophysical profile if nonreactive NST
- Amniotic fluid volume assessment weekly
- Ultrasound evaluation of fetal growth every 3 weeks

Management

- Women with mild disease who achieve a gestational age of 37 weeks should undergo delivery.
  - Even if conditions for induction of labor are unfavorable, the pregnancy should not continue (beyond 37 weeks' gestation) because uteroplacental blood flow is suboptimal.
  - The optimal management of mild preeclampsia remote from term is controversial. In general, there is considerable controversy regarding the need for hospitalization versus outpatient management. The use of antihypertensive drugs is not recommended nor is the use of sedatives and anticonvulsive prophylaxis.
  - For a patient who has mild preeclampsia with an immature fetus, the goal of therapy should be to
    o Retard the hypertensive process so as not to endanger the mother or the fetus
    o Allow time for the fetus to mature and increase the potential for neonatal survival
  - Therapy for patients with mild disease can be conducted by either outpatient management or hospitalization.
    o Outpatient management is acceptable for patients who are compliant, who can have frequent office visits including laboratory assessments, and who can perform some form of adequate blood pressure monitoring at home.
    o Hospitalization should be required for noncompliant patients and those who show unsatisfactory progress as outpatients.
  - If outpatient management is used, the regimen described below is recommended for mild preeclampsia.
    o A patient is considered a candidate for induction of labor if she has reached 37 weeks' gestation.
    o She is also a candidate for induction if her blood pressure continues to rise despite conservative management.
    o Figure 11-2 shows a sample algorithm for the management of a patient with mild preeclampsia.

Mild GHTH – Preeclampsia

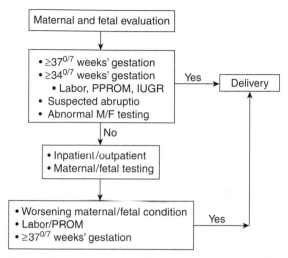

Figure 11-2. A sample algorithm for the management of a patient with mild preeclampsia.

◦ After 34 weeks' gestation, rupture of membranes, the spontaneous onset of labor or the development of intrauterine growth retardation with an estimated fetal weight less than 5th percentile, are indications for delivery.

PATIENT EDUCATION
- Close communication between the patient and physician is obligatory for successful outpatient management of mild gestational hypertension and preeclampsia. Patients are instructed to contact their managing physician for one for more of the following symptoms specific to preeclampsia:
  - Blood pressure above a chosen target level
  - A severe, long-lasting headache
  - Epigastric or right upper quadrant abdominal pain
  - Visual disturbances
  - Nausea and vomiting
- The patient should also be instructed to notify her physician for the following complications of pregnancy, regardless of preeclampsia:
  - Vaginal bleeding
  - Leakage of fluid from the vagina
  - Regular preterm uterine contractions
  - Decreased fetal movement
- Patients should be provided a contact telephone number for the physicians' call service and the hospital at which they intend to deliver. Patients are instructed that if they are unable to contact their physician and their condition worsens, they should come to their physician's office or hospital for further evaluation.

SEVERE PREECLAMPSIA
Background
- The clinical course of severe preeclampsia is usually characterized by progressive deterioration in both maternal and fetal status.

- These pregnancies are usually associated with increased rates of perinatal mortality and morbidity.
- Most of the fetal or neonatal complications are related to intrauterine fetal growth retardation, placenta abruption, or prematurity.

Diagnosis

- The criteria for the diagnosis of severe preeclampsia are (adapted from *ACOG Practice Bulletin* No. 33, 2002)(3).
  - Blood pressure $\geq$160 mm Hg systolic or $\geq$110 mm Hg diastolic on two occasions at least 4 hours apart with the patient on bed rest.
  - Cerebral or visual disturbances.
  - Severe and persistent epigastric or right upper quadrant abdominal pain.
  - Pulmonary edema or cyanosis.
  - Thrombocytopenia.
  - Fetal growth restriction.
  - Of note, the previous criteria for severe disease based on proteinuria ($\geq$5 g) are no longer utilized (2).

Management

- Because the only cure for severe preeclampsia is delivery, there is unanimous agreement that all patients should be delivered if severe disease develops beyond 34 weeks 0 days' gestation or if there is evidence of fetal jeopardy before that time. In this situation, appropriate management should include (4,5)
  - Parenteral magnesium sulfate to prevent convulsions
  - Control of maternal blood pressure within a safe range
  - Initiating delivery
- Management of patients with severe disease remote from term (less than 34 weeks 0 days) is controversial.
  - Some institutions consider delivery as the definitive therapy for all cases, regardless of gestational age.
  - Others recommend prolonging pregnancy in all patients remote from term until one or more of the following is achieved:
    - Fetal lung maturity
    - Fetal jeopardy
    - Maternal jeopardy
    - Achievement of 34 weeks 0 days' gestation
- All patients with severe preeclampsia should be admitted to the labor and delivery area for close observation of maternal and fetal condition and provided steroids for lung maturity if less than 34 weeks' gestation during initial evaluation and with the decision for delivery.
- All patients should receive intravenous magnesium sulfate to prevent convulsions (Fig. 11-3).

SEVERE PREECLAMPSIA IN MIDTRIMESTER

- Occasionally, a patient may develop severe preeclampsia at or before 28 weeks' gestation.
- These pregnancies are associated with high maternal and perinatal mortality and pose a difficult management decision for every obstetrician.
- Immediate delivery will result in extremely high perinatal morbidity and mortality, whereas an aggressive attempt to delay delivery may cause severe maternal morbidity. As a consequence, in the circumstance of a potentially viable fetus, these pregnancies should be managed in a tertiary care center (5).

Severe preeclampsia <$34^{0/7}$ weeks

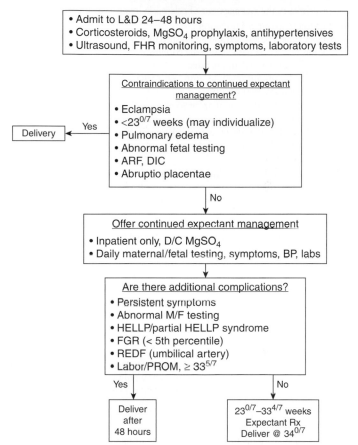

Figure 11-3. A sample algorithm for the management of a patient with severe preeclampsia.

ECLAMPSIA

Background

Definition

- Eclampsia is the development of convulsions or coma unrelated to other cerebral conditions during pregnancy or in the postpartum period in patients with signs and symptoms of preeclampsia.

Epidemiology

- The hazards of convulsions in pregnancy have been documented for centuries.
- The reported incidence ranges from 1 in 100 to 1 in 3448 pregnancies.
- The incidence is increased among nonwhite, nulliparous women of low socioeconomic status.
- For patients obtaining prenatal care, the incidence is about 1 in 800 patients.
- Eclamptic convulsions constitute a life-threatening emergency.

Treatment

Management

The basic principles in the management of eclampsia involve the following measures (6).

Support of Cardiorespiratory Functions

- Airway patency should be assessed and established to ensure adequate maternal oxygenation.
- Suction should be used as needed and the patient protected from injury by making sure the bed side-rails are elevated and padded.
- Oxygen should be administered to improve maternal oxygen concentration and to increase oxygen delivery to the fetus.

Control of Convulsions and Prevention of Recurrent Convulsions

- The natural tendency for those caring for an eclamptic patient is to provide therapy to immediately abolish the seizure activity; however, this may increase maternal risk of aspiration and acute change in blood pressure.

Magnesium Sulfate Therapy

- Parenteral magnesium sulfate is the drug of choice for convulsions resulting from eclampsia (7).
- Its major advantages include relative maternal and fetal safety when properly used. The mother is awake and alert most of the time, and laryngeal reflexes are intact, which helps protect against aspiration problems.
- There are several regimens of magnesium sulfate used to prevent convulsions. The most commonly used is an intravenous regimen popularized by Sibai.
  - An intravenous loading dose of 6 g of magnesium sulfate ($MgSO_4 \cdot 7H_2O$) prepared as 6 g diluted in 150 mL D5W or lactated Ringer solution is administered via infusion pump over 20 to 30 minutes.
  - If the patient develops recurrent convulsions after the initial infusion of magnesium sulfate, a further dose of 2 g can be infused over 5 to 10 minutes.
  - On completion of the magnesium sulfate loading infusion, a maintenance infusion of 2 to 3 g/h is used.
  - The infusion rate of magnesium sulfate should be adjusted on the basis of physical examination and maternal urine output. Serial serum magnesium levels need not be followed except in situations with increased serum creatinine or decreased urine output.
- Patients receiving magnesium sulfate therapy must be monitored for evidence of drug toxicity.
- Clinical findings associated with increased maternal plasma levels of magnesium are listed in Table 11-1.
- Magnesium is excreted by the kidneys, and renal dysfunction may cause toxic accumulation. Magnesium toxicity can be avoided by
  - Confirming adequate renal function with hourly urinary output assessment
  - Serial evaluation for the presence of patellar deep tendon reflexes
  - Closely observing respiratory rate
  - Monitoring serial serum magnesium levels when toxicity is suspected

Table 11-1	Clinical Findings Associated with Increased Maternal Plasma Magnesium Levels	
Serum magnesium level (mg/dL)	**Clinical findings**	
1.5–2.5	Normal pregnancy level	
4–8	Therapeutic range for seizure prophylaxis	
9–12	Loss of patellar reflex	
15–17	Muscular paralysis, respiratory arrest	
30–35	Cardiac arrest	

From Barton JR, Bronstein SJ, Sibai BM. Management of the eclamptic patient. *J Matern Fetal Med* 1992;1:313–319. Ref. (8)

- If magnesium toxicity is suspected, the following steps should be taken:
  - The magnesium sulfate infusion should be discontinued.
  - Supplemental oxygen should be administered.
  - A serum magnesium level should be assessed.
- If magnesium toxicity is recognized, 10 mL of 10% calcium gluconate is administered (1 g total) intravenously.
  - This medication must be given slowly (i.e., 2 to 5 mL/min) to avoid hypotension, bradycardia, and vomiting.
  - Calcium competitively inhibits magnesium at the neuromuscular junction, but its effect is only transient because the serum concentration is unchanged. Symptoms of magnesium toxicity can recur following calcium gluconate administration if the magnesium level remains elevated.
- If respiratory arrest occurs, prompt resuscitative measures including intubation and assisted ventilation are indicated.

Correction of Maternal Hypoxemia and Acidemia
- Maternal hypoxemia and acidemia may result from
  - Repeated convulsions
  - Respiratory depression from the use of multiple anticonvulsant agents
  - Aspiration
  - A combination of these factors
- Supplemental oxygen may be administered by face mask or face mask with an oxygen reservoir at 8 to 10 L/min.
  - At 10 L O_2 per minute, the oxygen concentration delivered approaches 100% using a face mask with an oxygen reservoir.
- Maternal oxygenation can be monitored noninvasively by transcutaneous pulse oximetry, whereas acid–base status may be assessed by arterial blood gas analysis

Control of Severe Hypertension
- The objective of treating severe hypertension is to prevent maternal cerebrovascular accidents and congestive heart failure without compromising cerebral perfusion or jeopardizing uteroplacental blood flow, which is already reduced in eclampsia.
- Although the underlying causative factors are not completely delineated, hypertension in preeclampsia is clearly a consequence of a generalized arterial vasoconstriction.
- Desirable antihypertensive agent properties for the use in hypertensive emergencies in pregnancy include a rapid onset of action following administration and short duration of action in the event of overtitration. See Table 12-2 for specific hypertensive agents.
- Labetalol
  - Labetalol is a competitive antagonist at both postsynaptic α_1-adrenergic and β-adrenergic receptors.
  - Labetalol is available in oral and intravenous forms.
  - Parenteral labetalol has a rapid onset of action and produces a smooth reduction in blood pressure with rare overshoot hypotension.
  - Labetalol is contraindicated in patients with a greater than first-degree heart block.
  - Labetalol is administered in intermittent intravenous boluses of 20 to 80 mg.
- Hydralazine
  - Hydralazine is a direct arteriolar vasodilator.
  - Intravenous hydralazine has an onset of action of 10 to 20 minutes, with a peak effect in 60 minutes, and a duration of action of 4 to 6 hours.
  - Hydralazine is administered in intermittent bolus injections with an initial dose of 5 mg. Blood pressure should be recorded every 5 minutes.
  - If an adequate reduction in blood pressure is not achieved 20 to 30 minutes after the initial dose, then a repeat dose of 5 mg or a dose increased to 10 mg in increments of every 20 to 30 minutes should be given for a maximum of 25 mg/h.

- Nifedipine
  - Nifedipine is a calcium channel antagonist.
  - Nifedipine improves renal function with a beneficial effect on urine output when treating preeclampsia in the postpartum period.
  - Nifedipine is administered 10 to 20 mg orally every 4 hours.
  - Profound reductions in blood pressure with nifedipine can be partially reversed by the slow intravenous administration of calcium gluconate.
- Sodium nitroprusside
  - Sodium nitroprusside relaxes arteriolar and venous smooth muscle by interfering with both influx and the intercellular activation of calcium.
  - Onset of action is immediate, and duration of action is very short (1 to 10 minutes).
  - Because preeclamptic patients have a propensity for depleted intravascular volume, they are especially sensitive to its effects. The initial infusion dose should therefore be 0.2 μg/kg/min, rather than 0.5 μg/kg/min as is standard in nonpregnant patients.
  - Cyanide and thiocyanate are products of metabolism of this drug with potential deleterious effects for the fetus.

Initiation of the Process for Delivery
- Because evacuation of the uterus is the definitive treatment of preeclampsia and eclampsia, patients are evaluated for delivery once they have been stabilized.
- Vaginal delivery, unless obstetrically contraindicated, is the preferred method of delivery.
  - An oxytocin infusion for induction or augmentation of labor may be administered simultaneously with the magnesium sulfate infusion.
  - Total fluid intake is limited to 100 mL/h.
  - The protocol for oxytocin infusion for preeclampsia or eclampsia is the same as for routine patients; yet, because of fluid restrictions, oxytocin may need to be more concentrated and dosages per minute accordingly adjusted.
  - Continuous fetal monitoring should be performed.
- At delivery, neonatal side effects of maternal administration of magnesium sulfate include
  - Hypotension
  - Hypotonia
  - Respiratory depression
  - Lethargy
  - Decreased suck reflex
- The pediatrician and newborn nursery should be informed of patients receiving magnesium sulfate. Calcium gluconate may also be administered to the newborn if magnesium toxicity is suspected.
- Following delivery, the patient should be monitored in the recovery room or on the labor and delivery unit under close observation for a minimum of 24 hours. During this time, magnesium sulfate should be continued and maternal vital signs and intake–output should be monitored hourly.
- Some of these patients may require intensive and invasive hemodynamic monitoring because they are at increased risk of developing pulmonary edema from fluid overload, fluid mobilization, and compromised renal function.
- Magnesium sulfate administration should continue until improvements in blood pressure, urine output, and sensorium are noted.

Complications of Eclampsia
- Maternal complications with eclampsia convulsions including
  - Abruptio placentae
  - Pulmonary edema
  - Acute renal failure
  - Aspiration pneumonia

- Intracerebral hemorrhage
- Retinal detachment
- Ruptured subcapsular liver hematoma

POSTPARTUM ECLAMPSIA

- Approximately 30% of eclampsia cases will occur during the postpartum period, with one-half within the first 48 hours from delivery.
- Late-onset postpartum eclampsia is defined as convulsions occurring more than 48 hours after delivery in patients with signs and symptoms of preeclampsia (8).
- If postpartum eclampsia is confirmed, the management is as previously noted for antepartum convulsions.
- More vigorous control of blood pressure is possible postpartum, however, because there is no longer a concern about compromising the uteroplacental circulation.
- Magnesium sulfate therapy should be continued for 24 to 48 hours from seizure onset.
- Fortunately, most of the complications resolve after delivery with proper management.

HELLP SYNDROME

Background

- Hemolysis, abnormal liver function tests, and thrombocytopenia have long been recognized as complications of preeclampsia and eclampsia.
- In 1982, Weinstein (9) described 29 cases of severe preeclampsia and eclampsia complicated by these abnormalities. He suggested that this collection of signs and symptoms constituted an entity separate from severe preeclampsia and coined the term HELLP syndrome:
  - *H* for hemolysis
  - *EL* for elevated liver enzymes
  - *LP* for low platelet count
- There is considerable controversy regarding the time of onset and the type and degree of laboratory abnormalities used to make the diagnosis of HELLP syndrome.
- In an attempt to standardize the diagnosis of HELLP syndrome, investigators at the University of Tennessee at Memphis published criteria using cutoff values of more than 2 standard deviations above the mean to indicate abnormality. Their criteria for the diagnosis of HELLP syndrome are summarized in Table 11-2.
- The incidence of severe preeclampsia or eclampsia complicated by HELLP syndrome has been reported to range from 2% to 12%.
- Patients with HELLP syndrome may present with a variety of signs and symptoms, including

Table 11-2	Criteria for the Diagnosis of HELLP Syndrome
Hemolysis	
Abnormal peripheral smear	
Total bilirubin >1.2 mg/dL	
Lactic dehydrogenase >600 U/L	
Elevated liver functions	
Serum aspirate aminotransferase >70 U/L	
Lactic dehydrogenase >600 U/L	
Low platelets	
Platelet count <100,000/mm^3	

From Sibai BM. The HELLP syndrome (hemolysis, elevated liver enzymes, and low platelets): much ado about nothing? *Am J Obstet Gynecol.* 1990;162:311–316. Ref. (18)

- Epigastric or right upper-quadrant abdominal pain
- Nausea or vomiting
- Nonspecific viral syndrome–like symptoms
- History of malaise for the past few days before presentation
- It is important to appreciate that severe hypertension (systolic blood pressure greater than 160 mm Hg, diastolic blood pressure greater than 110 mm Hg) is not a constant or even a frequent finding in HELLP syndrome.
  - In Weinstein's initial report of 29 patients, less than half (13 patients) had an admission blood pressure greater than 160/100 mm Hg.
- As a result, these patients are often misdiagnosed as having various medical and surgical disorders including appendicitis, gastroenteritis, pyelonephritis, or viral hepatitis.

Treatment
Management of HELLP Syndrome
- Patients with HELLP syndrome who are remote from term should be referred to a tertiary care center, and initial management should be as for any patient with severe preeclampsia (11).
- Following is an outline of the management of antepartum HELLP syndrome:
  - Maternal condition is assessed and stabilized.
    - If disseminated intravascular coagulopathy (DIC) present, coagulopathy is corrected.
    - Antiseizure prophylaxis is given with magnesium sulfate.
    - Treatment of severe hypertension is begun.
    - Computed tomography or ultrasound of the abdomen is done if a subcapsular hematoma of the liver is suspected.
  - Fetal well-being is evaluated.
    - NST
    - Biophysical profile
    - Ultrasonographic biometry
- If the patient is less than 34 weeks' gestation, fetal lung immaturity is assumed. Without laboratory evidence of DIC in a stable patient, steroids can be given to accelerate fetal lung maturity, and delivery should then be done 48 hours later. Maternal and fetal conditions should, however, be assessed continuously during this time. If the syndrome develops at or beyond 34 weeks' gestation, or fetal or maternal jeopardy before that time, then delivery is the definitive therapy.

Treatment
Prevention of Preeclampsia
- There are numerous reports and clinical trials describing the use of various methods to prevent or reduce the incidence of preeclampsia (12,13).
- Methods used have included
  - Salt restriction or prophylactic diuretic therapy
  - Low-dose aspirin (14,15)
  - Calcium supplementation (16)
  - Administration of fish oil or evening primrose oil
  - Antioxidant therapy (17)
- Because the etiology of the disease is unknown, the reported methods have been used in an attempt to correct the pathophysiologic abnormalities of preeclampsia in the hope of preventing the disease or ameliorating its course.
- Several multicenter studies have been completed and have demonstrated a failure of antioxidant therapy and fish oil to prevent preeclampsia. Also not effective and not recommended are dietary salt restriction and antihypertensive therapy to prevent preeclampsia. Per the Cochrane Collaboration, antiplatelet agents (low-dose aspirin) have been shown to provide small reductions in recurrence of preeclampsia (17%) (15).

REFERENCES

1. Report of the National High Blood Pressure Education Program Working Group on High Blood Pressure in Pregnancy. *Am J Obstet Gynecol.* 2000;183:S1–S22.
2. American College of Obstetricians and Gynecologists. Report of Hypertension in Pregnancy Task Force. *Obstet Gynecol.* 2013 (in press).
3. American College of Obstetricians and Gynecologists. Diagnosis and management of preeclampsia and eclampsia. *ACOG Pract Bull.* 2002;33.
4. Sibai BM, Barton JR. Expectant management of severe preeclampsia remote from term: patient selection, treatment and delivery indications. *Am J Obstet Gynecol.* 2007;196:514. e1–e9.
5. Sibai BM. Evaluation and management of severe preeclampsia before 34 weeks' gestation. Publications Committee, Society for Maternal-Fetal Medicine. *Am J Obstet Gynecol* 2011;205(3):191–198.
6. Sibai BM. Diagnosis, prevention and management of eclampsia. *Obstet Gynecol.* 2005;105:402–410.
7. Sibai BM. Magnesium sulfate is the ideal anticonvulsant in preeclampsia-eclampsia. *Am J Obstet Gynecol.* 1990;162:1141–1145.
8. Lubarsky SL, Sibai BM, Mercer BM, et al. Late postpartum eclampsia revisited. *Obstet Gynecol.* 1994;83:502–505.
9. Weinstein L. Syndrome of hemolysis, elevated liver enzymes, and low platelet count: a severe consequence of hypertension in pregnancy. *Am J Obstet Gynecol.* 1982;142:159–167.
10. Barton JR, Bronstein SJ, Sibai BM. Management of the eclamptic patient. *J Matern Fetal Med.* 1992;(1):313–319.
11. Sibai BM. Diagnosis, controversies, management of the syndrome of hemolysis, elevated liver enzymes and low platelets. *Obstet Gynecol.* 2004;103:981–991.
12. Barton JR, Sibai BM. Prediction and prevention of recurrent preeclampsia. *Obstet Gynecol.* 2008;112.359–372.
13. Caritis S, Sibai B, Hauth J, et al. Predictors of preeclampsia in women at high risk. *Am J Obstet Gynecol.* 1998;179:946–951.
14. Caritis S, Sibai B, Hauth J, et al. Low-dose aspirin to prevent preeclampsia in women at high risk. *N Engl J Med.* 1998;338:701–705.
15. Duley L, Henderson-Smart DJ, Meher S, King JF. Antiplatelet agents for preventing preeclampsia and its complications. *Cochrane Database Syst Rev.* 2007; (2):CD004659.
16. Levine RJ, Hauth JC, Curet LB, et al. Trial of calcium to prevent preeclampsia. *N Engl J Med.* 1997;337:69–76.
17. Poston L, Briley AL, Seed PT, et al. Vitamin C and vitamin E in pregnant women at risk for preeclampsia (VIP trial): randomized placebo-controlled trial. *Lancet.* 2006;367:1145–1154.
18. Sibai BM. The HELLP syndrome (hemolysis, elevated liver enzymes and low platelets): much ado about nothing? *Am J Obstet Gynecol.* 1990;162:311–316.

PART III

Maternal Complications

Cardiovascular Disease and Chronic Hypertension

Samuel Parry

CARDIOVASCULAR COMPLICATIONS AND CHRONIC HYPERTENSION

Cardiovascular Complications

Key Points
- Women with heart disease are at risk for cardiovascular complications during pregnancy and have a higher incidence of neonatal complications.
- Knowledge of the hemodynamics of the woman's condition and the normal cardiovascular/hemodynamic changes of pregnancy, and how they are likely to interact, is essential to adequate counseling.

Background
Antenatal Cardiovascular Changes
- Blood volume
  - Blood volume increases on average by 40% to 60% during gestation, but there is significant individual variation. Blood volume begins to increase early in the first trimester and reaches a maximum in the early third trimester.
  - The expansion in plasma volume is greater than the expansion of red cell mass, causing the physiologic anemia of pregnancy.
  - With multiple fetuses, the increase in blood volume will be greater still: on average 500 mL more than in a singleton gestation.
- Cardiac output
  - Cardiac output increases on average by 40% to 50% during gestation, beginning early in the first trimester and peaking at 20 to 24 weeks.
  - In early pregnancy, most of this change results from an increase in stroke volume, whereas later in pregnancy, it also reflects an increase in heart rate.
  - Conversely, as pregnancy progresses, supine positioning will decrease cardiac output by 25% to 30% because of compression of the vena cava by the gravid uterus.
- Blood pressure
  - Due in part to the smooth muscle relaxing effects of progesterone, systemic vascular resistance decreases during pregnancy, causing a decrease in diastolic blood pressure beginning in the first trimester and becoming maximal in the second trimester. There is also a modest decrease in systolic blood pressure in the second trimester.
  - Blood pressure returns to prepregnancy levels in the third trimester.

- Heart size
  - With the volume expansion of pregnancy, the heart adapts, as to any chronic volume overload state, by undergoing eccentric hypertrophy. Ventricular chamber size is increased with wall thickness maintained.
  - Systolic function (i.e., ejection fraction) is unchanged.

Intrapartum Cardiovascular Changes
- First-stage labor
  - With each contraction, there is an increase in circulating blood volume of 300 to 500 mL as blood is expelled from the uteroplacental circulation. This, in turn, increases venous return, maternal cardiac output, and blood pressure.
  - The magnitude of the cardiovascular effects of labor is dependent on maternal position and pain management. With the woman in a supine position, the baseline cardiac output between contractions will rise progressively to a maximum increase of 15%. If she remains in a lateral position, the increase will be less (~5%).
  - Most of the increase in baseline cardiac output between contractions during labor is caused by maternal pain and anxiety and, therefore, can be minimized by adequate anesthesia.
- Second-stage labor
  - With bearing-down efforts to expel the fetus, there will be diminished venous return, causing decreased stroke volume and increased heart rate in an attempt to maintain cardiac output. If these efforts are very frequent, then cardiac output may not return to baseline between contractions.
  - Shortening of the second stage by operative vaginal delivery is, therefore, frequently advised for patients with significant cardiac disease.
- Postpartum
  - Immediately postpartum, the shunt provided by the uteroplacental circulation is lost. This creates an increase in circulating blood volume and increases in venous return and cardiac output.
  - In the days that follow, there is mobilization of extravascular fluid into the vascular system, which further increases circulating blood volume.
  - The postpartum period can be a particularly hazardous time for the cardiac patient sensitive to an increase in preload.

Evaluation
Physical Examination
- Cardiac physical examination
  - There is an increase in intensity of the first heart sound with exaggerated splitting. A third heart sound is not commonly heard, but the presence of a fourth heart sound should not be attributed to pregnancy.
  - Systolic ejection flow murmurs are commonly heard, but diastolic murmurs are rare and should prompt further evaluation.

Diagnostic Evaluation
- Diagnostic evaluation should proceed as necessary during pregnancy. A thorough evaluation of functional status greatly aids counseling regarding maternal prognosis. This evaluation should include a thorough history, physical examination, and diagnostic tests as indicated.
- Functional classification using the New York Heart Association (NYHA) guidelines and the Cardiac Disease in Pregnancy (CARPREG) Investigators (Tables 12-1 and 12-2) has been used to assess the risk of morbidity for the pregnant cardiac patient (1).
- This assessment relies strongly on subjective symptoms; therefore, it is important to substantiate findings with objective testing.
  - Chest x-ray films may be obtained safely with abdominal shielding; however, other tests such as echocardiogram probably provide more information.
  - Radionuclide perfusion tests such as the thallium scan pose little risk with a fetal exposure of approximately 0.8 rad. Such tests should not be withheld if indicated.

Table 12-1	New York Heart Association Functional Classification of Heart Disease
Class	**Description**
I	Asymptomatic
II	Symptoms with normal activity
III	Symptoms with less than normal activity
IV	Symptoms at rest

- Right-sided heart catheterization may be performed for the usual indications without concern for increased risks to the mother or fetus.
- Left-sided heart catheterization should be reserved for cases that clearly cannot be evaluated by other means because the use of fluoroscopy represents a potential risk to the developing fetus.
- There are some differences in physical findings and common studies that may be attributed to pregnancy.
  - *Chest x-ray.* The lordotic posture of pregnancy can create straightening of the left upper cardiac border, mimicking left atrial enlargement. Elevation of the diaphragm by the enlarging uterus causes a more horizontal position of the heart, creating an increase in the cardiac shadow. The pulmonary vasculature frequently appears more prominent.
  - *Electrocardiogram.* The horizontal positioning of the heart due to the elevated diaphragm may result in a left shift of the QRS axis. Minor ST-segment and T-wave changes are commonly seen in lead 3 and aVF lead.
  - *Echocardiogram.* An increase in end-diastolic and end-systolic ventricular measurements is seen with no increase in wall thickness. Ventricular systolic function (i.e., ejection fraction) is unchanged. Mild tricuspid regurgitation is common and is believed to be secondary to increased blood volume.
  - *Pulmonary artery catheterization.* The information regarding hemodynamic measurements by pulmonary artery catheterization in pregnancy is limited to the study of a small number of normal women. Pulmonary capillary wedge pressure, central venous pressure, and mean pulmonary artery pressures appear to be unchanged in pregnancy (2).

Table 12-2	CARPREG Risk Score: Predictors of Maternal Cardiovascular Events

NYHA functional class >II
Cyanosis (room air saturation <90%)
Prior cardiovascular event
Systemic ventricular ejection fraction <40%
Left heart obstruction (e.g., mitral valve area <2 cm^2 or aortic valve area <1.5 cm^2, or left ventricular [LV] outflow gradient of >30 mm Hg)

CARPREG Points	**Risk of Cardiovascular Maternal Complications**
0	5%
1	27%
≥2	75%

From Siu SC, Sermer M, Colman JM, et al.; Cardiac Disease in Pregnancy (CARPREG) Investigators. Prospective multicenter study of pregnancy outcomes in women with heart disease. *Circulation.* 2001;104:515–521.

Treatment

General Antepartum Management

- Activity level
  - During pregnancy, this is individualized to the patient's level of tolerance as in the nonpregnant cardiac patient. With the increased demands of pregnancy, this may mean restricting activity in cases in which there are significant functional limitations.
- Diet
  - It is generally recommended that the pregnant cardiac patient avoid excessive weight gain and excessive salt intake.
- Rapid treatment of stressors
  - Additional stressors may lead to rapid decompensation; therefore, it is important to screen for other abnormalities, including anemia, thyroid disease, and asymptomatic infections such as bacteriuria.
  - It is important to respond rapidly if abnormalities are found to prevent potential complications.
- Subacute bacterial endocarditis (SBE) prophylaxis
  - The rate of bacteremia with vaginal or cesarean delivery is low, and routine SBE prophylaxis is not recommended for most pregnant cardiac patients by the American Heart Association or American Dental Association.
  - SBE prophylaxis is recommended at delivery in patients with prosthetic valves, a history of bacterial endocarditis, complex cyanotic congenital heart disease, or surgically constructed systemic pulmonary shunts.
  - High-risk procedures that require SBE prophylaxis in pregnant cardiac patients include some types of dental work and some respiratory, gastrointestinal, and genitourinary procedures.

Medications

- Most medications used in cardiac patients may be continued during pregnancy without causing fetal harm. The known exceptions are
  - Warfarin (Coumadin), which may cause an embryopathy (nasal hypoplasia, mental retardation, optic atrophy)
  - Angiotensin-converting enzyme (ACE) inhibitors or angiotensin II receptor blockers (ARBs), which may cause fetal death or intractable neonatal renal failure
- In women with mechanical prosthetic heart valves
  - Warfarin appears to be superior to heparin (which has no fetal risks) for preventing thromboembolic complications (2).
  - There is some evidence that low molecular weight heparin may be more effective than unfractionated heparin in pregnant women with mechanical valves, but all heparin formulations can result in heparin-induced thrombocytopenia (3).

General Intrapartum Management

- Maternal position.
  - Avoidance of supine positioning is critical for mother and fetus.
  - In the supine position, there will be obstruction of venous return by the gravid uterus, which will result in decreased cardiac output during contractions and a rebound effect resulting in a higher baseline cardiac output between contractions. The decreased placental perfusion during contractions may result in fetal compromise, and the increased baseline cardiac output may result in maternal compromise.
- Anesthesia should be used liberally because stress and pain in labor will greatly increase cardiac demand.
  - Epidural anesthesia is the agent of choice in most cases.
  - In cases such as aortic stenosis, in which a decrease in afterload may result in maternal decompensation, slow infusion of epidural anesthetics should be used to minimize peripheral vasodilatation.

- The second stage of labor may be shortened.
  - For cardiac patients, maternal exhaustion and frequent Valsalva maneuvers may result in maternal decompensation.
  - The choice of forceps or vacuum extraction to expedite delivery should be based on the usual obstetric criteria.
- Cesarean section should be reserved for normal obstetric indications.
  - Delivery by cesarean section does not avoid the hemodynamic alterations that occur with vaginal delivery, so trial of labor may be pursued in most cases by following the principles outlined previously.
- Hemodynamic monitoring.
  - Use of a pulmonary artery catheter may be advisable in patients with NYHA Class III–IV disease or CARPREG score ≥ 2 as an aid to avoid major hemodynamic fluxes during labor and delivery.

SPECIFIC CARDIAC LESIONS IN PREGNANCY
Congenital Heart Disease
Background
- There has been a marked increase in the incidence of pregnancies complicated by congenital heart disease because patients who previously would have died in childhood before the availability of modern medical and surgical techniques are surviving to reproductive age.
- Fetal risks include
  - Growth restriction due to maternal cyanosis (i.e., tetralogy of Fallot, Eisenmenger syndrome) or decreased uterine blood flow (i.e., coarctation of the aorta, aortic stenosis)
  - Inheritance of congenital heart disease (between 5% and 20% risk for most lesions)

Atrial Septal Defect (ASD)
Background
- ASD is the most common heart lesion complicating pregnancy.
- Hemodynamic effects.
  - Most patients are asymptomatic, and the lesion is discovered by auscultation of a murmur.
  - The left-to-right shunting will cause an increase in pulmonary blood flow, but pulmonary hypertension is a relatively late finding.
- Effect of pregnancy.
  - In the absence of pulmonary hypertension, this lesion is well tolerated in pregnancy and should not threaten maternal health. In fact, peripheral vasodilation may reduce left-to-right shunting during pregnancy.
  - If the patient has experienced pulmonary hypertension, then she is at risk for Eisenmenger syndrome (see below), a diagnosis that carries a maternal mortality of 50%.
  - When counseling the patient with an ASD, it is critical to evaluate her for pulmonary hypertension either by noninvasive testing such as an echocardiogram or by right-sided heart catheterization.
Treatment
- In the absence of pulmonary hypertension, there are no special requirements during pregnancy.
- With pulmonary hypertension, the management should be as for any patient at risk for Eisenmenger syndrome.
- A small percentage of patients with ASD have atrial fibrillation or flutter, which may be managed conservatively with antiarrhythmic agents such as digoxin.

Ventricular Septal Defect (VSD)

Background
- Hemodynamic effects
  - The size of the defect frequently determines the degree of disability.
  - A small lesion is hemodynamically insignificant and is well tolerated.
  - With a large defect with significant left-to-right shunting, the initial abnormality would be left ventricular hypertrophy to compensate for the decrease in forward flow, followed by the development of pulmonary hypertension caused by the increased pressures delivered to the pulmonary vasculature, and, finally, biventricular hypertrophy with the right side pumping against a significant afterload.
- Effect of pregnancy
  - The impact of pregnancy will depend on the hemodynamic abnormalities of the individual patient.
  - Without pulmonary hypertension, the decrease in systemic vascular resistance caused by pregnancy may be beneficial, causing an increase in forward flow. However, the increase in blood volume may lead to congestive heart failure in the patient with long-standing left ventricular hypertrophy.
  - When there is preexisting pulmonary hypertension, Eisenmenger syndrome may develop, a diagnosis that carries a risk of maternal morbidity of 50% (see below).
  - The patient with an uncomplicated, repaired VSD is not at risk during pregnancy.

Treatment
- In the absence of pulmonary hypertension, there are no special requirements during pregnancy.
- With pulmonary hypertension, the management should be as for any patient at risk for Eisenmenger syndrome.

Patent Ductus Arteriosus

Background
- Historically, patent ductus arteriosus (PDA) was one of the more common congenital cardiac lesions complicating pregnancy. It is rare today as a result of early detection and surgical repair.
- Hemodynamic effects and consequences are similar to those described for VSD.
- Effect of pregnancy.
  - With a small lesion, pregnancy is well tolerated.
  - With pulmonary hypertension, there is significant risk for Eisenmenger syndrome, with its attendant risks (see below).
  - With a corrected PDA, there is no additional risk as a result of pregnancy.

Treatment
- In the absence of pulmonary hypertension, there are no special requirements during pregnancy.
- With pulmonary hypertension, the management should be as for any patient at risk for Eisenmenger syndrome.

Coarctation of the Aorta

Background
- Coarctation is frequently associated with other cardiovascular abnormalities such as bicuspid aortic valve and congenital berry aneurysm of the circle of Willis.
- Hemodynamic effects.
  - Upper extremity hypertension is common secondary to the obstruction to outflow, and there is compensatory left ventricular hypertrophy.
  - Visible and palpable collateral arteries in the scapular region and lower extremity hypotension are found commonly.

- Effect of pregnancy.
  - With uncomplicated coarctation of the aorta, pregnancy is usually well tolerated.
  - A minority of cases will be complicated by congestive heart failure secondary to long-standing left ventricular hypertrophy and dysfunction.
  - There may be an increased risk for aortic dissection during pregnancy secondary to the effect of maternal hormones on the blood vessel wall architecture.

Treatment
- Hypertension should be controlled to decrease the risk for aortic dissection and rupture. However, aggressive treatment in women with significant coarctation (i.e., gradient of greater than 20 mm Hg) should be pursued with caution to prevent placental hypoperfusion.

Tetralogy of Fallot
Background
- This is the most common cyanotic lesion complicating pregnancy.
- It is a syndrome of pulmonary stenosis, right ventricular hypertrophy, large VSD, and dextroposition of the aorta that overrides the right ventricle.
- The vast majority of pregnant women will have already had full or partial surgical repair because the disease is otherwise usually fatal in childhood or early adulthood.
- Hemodynamic effects.
  - There is right outflow obstruction with resultant right-to-left shunting. This delivers blood with decreased oxygen saturation to the systemic circulation.
  - Right ventricular hypertrophy will develop as a result of the right outflow obstruction.
- Effect of pregnancy.
  - Patients with a full surgical repair before pregnancy are not at increased risk during pregnancy.
  - Pregnancy is poorly tolerated in patients who have not had surgical repair, because the decrease in systemic vascular resistance will cause an increase in right-to-left shunting with further desaturation of blood flowing to the systemic circulation. Patients believed to have an especially poor prognosis in pregnancy are those with
    - A baseline hematocrit greater than 60%,
    - Arterial oxygen saturation less than 80%,
    - A history of syncopal episodes, and
    - Significant right ventricular hypertension
  - Patients with palliative (partial) repairs such as the Blalock-Taussig (anastomosis of the subclavian artery to the right pulmonary artery), Potts (anastomosis of the descending aorta to the left pulmonary artery), or Waterston-Cooley (anastomosis of the ascending aorta to the right pulmonary artery) may be minimally symptomatic before pregnancy and yet may be at risk for decompensation during pregnancy.
  - Therefore, it is important to evaluate functional status by the parameters described above in the Cardiovascular Complications, Diagnostic Evaluation section.

Treatment
- It is essential to avoid hypovolemia and decreased venous return so as not to increase right-to-left shunting.
  - Pressure-graded elastic support hose are recommended.
  - Supplemental oxygen should be used as necessary.

Aortic Stenosis
Background
- May result from congenital or acquired heart disease
  - The most common congenital lesion is a bicuspid valve, and frequently, there are other associated cardiovascular anomalies. The lesion may not be stenotic at birth but may become progressively stenotic with aging.

- Hemodynamic effects
  - When the valve reaches critical narrowing with an area of less than 1 cm^2, there is obstruction to left ventricular outflow with development of left ventricular hypertrophy. This, in turn, may result in a fixed stroke volume and ischemia as a result of poor perfusion of the coronary blood vessels.
  - Decompensation may occur with additional stress, progressing to left ventricular dilation and failure.
- Effect of pregnancy
  - Pregnancy is poorly tolerated in the patient with critical aortic stenosis.
  - The patient has a fixed stroke volume and is able to increase cardiac output to meet the increased demands of pregnancy only by increasing heart rate. An increase in heart rate will decrease relatively the diastolic portion of the cardiac cycle, and this will result in decreased time for coronary perfusion and ventricular filling. In addition, the decreased systemic vascular resistance is also detrimental because the heart may be unable to fill a dilated vascular bed. This may result in syncope and hypotension.
  - The risk of maternal mortality with critical aortic stenosis is approximately 15%; therefore, it is important to discuss options and offer termination of pregnancy with severe aortic stenosis.

Treatment
- In a patient with critical aortic stenosis, strict limitation of activity is essential to minimize the need for cardiac output augmentation during pregnancy.
- Avoid situations that will further impede venous return such as hypovolemia.
- Use of support hose may help to maintain venous return.
- Left-sided heart failure should be treated as in the nonpregnant patient.

Pulmonary Stenosis
Background
- Unlike aortic stenosis, this lesion usually is not progressive.
- Hemodynamic effects.
  - Mild degrees of pulmonary stenosis usually cause no symptoms or hemodynamic compromise.
  - With severe stenosis, there will be obstruction to right ventricular outflow, causing the development of right ventricular hypertrophy. The patient with severe stenosis may be unable to augment cardiac output, leading to symptoms of exertional dyspnea and fatigue.
- Effect of pregnancy.
  - Most patients with pulmonary stenosis tolerate pregnancy well.
  - The patient with severe stenosis may be unable to meet the demands for augmented cardiac output and may not tolerate the volume expansion of pregnancy, leading to right-sided heart failure.

Treatment
- Hypervolemia and hypovolemia should be avoided.
- Right-sided heart failure should be treated as in the nonpregnant patient.
- If medical therapy fails, a transvenous balloon valvuloplasty may be performed safely during pregnancy.

Marfan Syndrome
Background
- This genetic disorder affects the structure of connective tissue, causing myxomatous degeneration of the mitral and aortic valves and cystic medial necrosis of the aorta, resulting in dissecting aneurysms.
- The genetic defect result from mutations in the fibrillin gene on chromosome 15, and Marfan syndrome is inherited as an autosomal dominant trait with variable expressivity.

- Hemodynamic effects.
  - Mitral valve prolapse with mitral regurgitation is common. During systole, there will be regurgitation of blood from the left ventricle into the left atrium, resulting in left atrial enlargement and compensatory left ventricular hypertrophy.
  - With long-standing disease, the left ventricle will deteriorate with the potential for development of left-sided heart failure.
  - Chronic left atrial enlargement is associated with the risk of atrial fibrillation and thrombus formation.
  - Aortic involvement can occur with dilation of the aortic root. Aortic regurgitation then occurs, allowing regurgitant flow of blood during diastole from the aorta into the left ventricle, leading to left ventricular dilatation from chronic overload. With extreme dilatation of the aortic root, there is risk of aortic dissection and rupture.
- Effect of pregnancy.
  - Regurgitant lesions are generally well tolerated during pregnancy because the decrease in systemic vascular resistance will increase forward flow.
    - Severe regurgitation is the exception because the increased blood volume of pregnancy could result in decompensation and left-sided heart failure.
  - The risk of aortic rupture is increased in pregnancy, possibly because of hormonal changes affecting blood vessel wall architecture and the relatively hyperdynamic state (4).
  - In patients with an aortic root measuring greater than 4 cm in diameter, the risk of maternal death has been estimated to be as high as 50%, mostly secondary to aortic rupture (5).

Treatment
- Activity restrictions are recommended to prevent hypertensive complications.
- Long-acting β-blockers are recommended during pregnancy to decrease the pulsatile force on the aorta, thereby minimizing the risk of aortic rupture.
- Once the aortic root diameter reaches 5 cm, most authorities recommend valve and root replacement due to the high risk of aortic dissection.

Eisenmenger Syndrome
Background
- This is a syndrome describing reversal of flow when there is an anatomic defect, allowing communication between the right and left circulations.
- This syndrome is associated, in descending order of frequency, with a large VSD, a large PDA, ASD, Tetralogy of Fallot, and other complex cyanotic congenital heart diseases.
- Hemodynamic effects.
  - The underlying anatomic defect initially creates a left-to-right shunt secondary to higher pressures in the left side of the heart.
  - Prolonged exposure of the pulmonary circulation to increased pressures from the left ventricle results in pulmonary hypertension.
    - When pulmonary pressures equal systemic pressures, the shunt will become bidirectional.
    - Eisenmenger syndrome develops when pulmonary pressures exceed systemic pressures, and the shunt becomes predominately right to left with delivery of desaturated blood to the systemic circulation.
  - With a predominant right-to-left shunt, compensatory polycythemia develops, increasing the risk for thromboembolic phenomenon.
- Effect of pregnancy.
  - Pregnancy is hazardous in patients with preexisting Eisenmenger syndrome, as well as in patients with pulmonary hypertension and an anatomic shunt because of their risk for Eisenmenger syndrome.
  - Several cardiovascular changes predispose to shunt reversal or increasing a preexisting right-to-left shunt. These include the normal decrease in systemic vascular resistance,

the hypercoagulable state with risk for thromboembolic phenomena and consequent increased pulmonary vascular resistance, and hypovolemia (from obstetric causes such as bleeding) resulting in an acute decrease in systemic vascular resistance.
- Maternal–fetal mortality is nearly 50% in patients with Eisenmenger syndrome as a result of intractable hypoxia.
  - The time of greatest risk is during the intrapartum and immediate postpartum periods, as a result of the major fluid shifts occurring at these times.
  - The woman at greatest risk for death is the one with advanced, fixed pulmonary hypertension unresponsive to oxygen therapy.

Treatment
- Termination of pregnancy should be strongly encouraged, although medical management of termination procedures for these patients is also complicated.
- Patients who choose not to terminate must be carefully monitored throughout pregnancy.
- Prolonged bed rest is advised with an existing right-to-left shunt to limit the need for increased oxygen consumption.
- Prevention of hypovolemia is essential to avoid either the development of right-to-left shunting in those at risk or increasing a preexisting right-to-left shunt.
- It is also important to avoid conditions such as hypoxia, acidosis, and hypercarbia, which will increase pulmonary vascular resistance.
- Prophylactic heparin has been recommended by some to decrease the risk of thromboembolic phenomenon, which would acutely increase pulmonary pressures. However, the few studies addressing the use of prophylactic heparin in this setting have not shown an improvement in maternal mortality.
- Vaginal delivery is preferred to cesarean section because the risk for maternal mortality has been reported to be as high as 75% with cesarean delivery. The validity of this statistic has been questioned because confounding factors leading to a decision for a rapid delivery may be responsible for a significant portion of the risk.
- It is crucial to watch for signs of shunt reversal or a worsening right-to-left shunt and to treat this development aggressively.
- The intrapartum period confers the greatest risk. Recommendations are for
  - Invasive monitoring with arterial and pulmonary artery catheters
  - Oxygen therapy
  - Strict attention to preload and systemic vascular resistance
  - Vasoconstrictor agents as needed to maintain systemic pressures
  - A shortened second stage of labor

ACQUIRED HEART DISEASE
Rheumatic Heart Disease—Mitral Stenosis
Background
- Although the incidence of rheumatic heart disease has declined substantially in developed countries, there are many young women who emigrate to the Western world who have sequelae of this disease.
- The mitral valve is most commonly affected with stenosis or, less frequently, a regurgitant component. Less commonly, the aortic valve is involved, predominantly with stenosis but sometimes with a regurgitant component.
  - Hemodynamic effects.
    - With a stenotic valve, there is obstruction to flow, leading to left atrial enlargement and increased pulmonary venous pressures. With long-standing disease, this can lead to the development of pulmonary hypertension.
    - When the valve is critically narrowed (less than 1 cm^2), stroke volume is fixed, and cardiac output can be augmented only by increasing heart rate. With an increase in heart rate, diastolic time will decrease relatively more than systolic time, decreasing

the time available for ventricular filling. This leads to further left atrial enlargement and an increase in left atrial pressures, pulmonary congestion, and pulmonary edema.

  o With marked atrial enlargement, atrial fibrillation is common, further decreasing the ability to fill the left ventricle and with the attendant risk of thrombus formation.
- Effect of pregnancy.
  - The increase in heart rate and blood volume in pregnancy may be poorly tolerated in a patient with severe stenosis.
  - A patient without myocardial damage but with severe stenosis may be asymptomatic before pregnancy. Therefore, prepregnancy functional status is of limited usefulness in predicting ability to tolerate the cardiovascular demands of pregnancy. Valve orifice area, as measured by echocardiography, is generally a better predictor.
  - Left atrial irritability is increased in pregnancy, increasing the risk for atrial fibrillation, further compromising cardiac output.
  - Maternal mortality is less than 1% with mild mitral stenosis but may be as high as 10% to 15% with severe disease and new-onset atrial fibrillation.

Treatment
- As with other cardiac diseases complicating pregnancy, activity should be curtailed as necessary, and stresses should be avoided.
- Prophylactic digoxin is recommended in patients with Class III and IV disease to slow heart rate and to prevent a rapid ventricular response if atrial fibrillation develops.
  - Alternative therapy is a β-blocker.
- If atrial fibrillation does develop, therapeutic anticoagulation with heparin to prevent thrombus formation is recommended.
- If heart failure develops, treatment is the same as in nongravid patients. If medical therapy fails, percutaneous balloon valvuloplasty can be performed safely during pregnancy.
- During labor, it is important to avoid maternal tachycardia and to avoid major changes in volume status. For patients with Class III or Class IV disease, this may most easily be accomplished with the aid of invasive monitoring.

Idiopathic Hypertrophic Cardiomyopathy
Background
- This class of cardiomyopathy is characterized by hypertrophy of the ventricular myocardium that is often localized. Myocardial function is normal or hyperdynamic.
- The most common type is asymmetric septal hypertrophy, a localized thickening of the interventricular septum.
- It is usually inherited as an autosomal dominant trait with variable penetrance.
- Hemodynamic effects.
  - With ventricular contraction, the thickened myocardial walls approach one another and may cause obstruction to outflow.
  - Factors influencing the degree of obstruction include the preload, the force of the contraction, and the afterload by maintaining some degree of ventricular distension at the end of systole.
- Effect of pregnancy.
  - The increase in blood volume during pregnancy usually offsets the potentially detrimental effect of decreased systemic vascular resistance.
  - Myocardial contractility is most likely unchanged during pregnancy.

Treatment
- Hypovolemia should be avoided.
- The use of β-adrenergic agonists to treat preterm labor or other positive inotropic agents is absolutely contraindicated.

Dilated Cardiomyopathy
Background
- This class of cardiomyopathy is characterized by enlarged heart chambers, systolic and diastolic dysfunction, and a predisposition to thromboembolism.
- Peripartum cardiomyopathy is a form of dilated cardiomyopathy that occurs in the last month of pregnancy or the first few months after delivery in women with no previous cardiac disease.
  - The cause of peripartum cardiomyopathy is unknown.
  - The risk of maternal mortality is approximately 20%, with the cause of death usually intractable heart failure, an embolic event, or an arrhythmia.
  - The recurrence risk in subsequent pregnancies may be as high as 50%.
- Hemodynamic effects.
  - Pump failure occurs, leading to pulmonary edema and other congestive symptoms.
- Effect of pregnancy.
  - The increased blood volume of pregnancy is poorly tolerated. The patient with limited reserve is unable to meet the demands for augmented cardiac output required by pregnancy.

Treatment
- Efforts such as prolonged bed rest that minimize the need for augmentation of cardiac output are warranted.
- Treatment of heart failure is the same as that for nongravid patients, and afterload reduction may be beneficial.
- Prophylactic heparinization is recommended in some cases.
- The use of immunosuppressive agents such as prednisone or intravenous immune globulin has been recommended by some, presuming an inflammatory cause. This hypothesis has not been well tested, and clinical trials are lacking.
- Because this disease may recur, future pregnancies are inadvisable.

Primary Pulmonary Hypertension
Background
- The primary abnormality with this disease is a thickening of the media of the muscular pulmonary arteries and development of muscle in the pulmonary arterioles with resulting pulmonary hypertension.
- The disease is progressive and commonly is asymptomatic until relatively late in its course.
- Hemodynamic effects.
  - Pulmonary hypertension causes right ventricular hypertrophy. With progression, right-sided heart failure occurs.
  - Arrhythmias and thromboembolic complications are common.
- Effect of pregnancy.
  - The increased cardiac demands of pregnancy and the increase in blood volume may cause an asymptomatic patient to decompensate.
  - Maternal mortality during pregnancy has been reported to be as high as 50%.
  - There have been some reports suggesting that pregnancy may accelerate the course of this disease.

Treatment
- With the high risk for maternal mortality, termination of pregnancy should be strongly encouraged.
- Heart failure should be treated as in nongravid patients.
- Prophylactic heparinization to therapeutic levels is recommended.
- Efforts to minimize the need for augmentation of cardiac output, such as prolonged bed rest, are warranted.

Coronary Artery Disease
Background
- Although the occurrence of coronary artery disease during pregnancy is rare, the incidence is rising with delayed childbearing and presumably will rise further with new assisted reproductive techniques.
- Effect of pregnancy.
  - The increase in myocardial oxygen consumption related to the increase in cardiac output seen in pregnancy may cause significant decompensation.
  - The increase in heart rate will be particularly detrimental because the relative decrease in diastolic filling time will decrease coronary perfusion.

Treatment
- The major effort must be directed toward decreasing the need for augmentation of cardiac output.
- Physical activity should be limited, and strict bed rest may be required.
- Therapy of angina should be the same as for nongravid patients.
- β-Adrenergic blocking agents may be beneficial to limit the increase in heart rate seen in normal pregnancy.
- Calcium channel blockers and nitrates may be used as required.
- Labor should be managed so as to minimize stress and pain, and a regional anesthetic is indicated.

Patient Education
- Women with cardiovascular disease should seek preconceptional consultation with a maternal–fetal medicine specialist before considering pregnancy.
- A thorough discussion about the impact and risks of pregnancy should be held with the patient, including the management options for future pregnancies.
- The goal is to give the woman adequate information to allow her to make well-informed decisions about future pregnancies.

Chronic Hypertension
Key Points
- Hypertensive disorders complicate approximately 10% to 20% of pregnancies in the United States and are responsible for approximately 15% of maternal deaths (6).
- Maternal hypertension is an important cause of perinatal morbidity and mortality resulting from direct fetal effects (growth restriction, oligohydramnios, stillbirth, etc.) and iatrogenic preterm delivery performed for maternal or fetal indications.
- Chronic hypertension predisposes women to pregnancy-related hypertensive complications, yet the physiology and management of these two conditions are different.

Gestational Hypertension (see Chapter 11, Hypertensive Disorders of Pregnancy)
Background
Definitions
- **Gestational hypertension** is the new onset of hypertension after 20 weeks' gestation that returns to normal postpartum.
- **Hypertension** is defined as sustained (for at least 6 hours) blood pressure readings greater than 140/90 mm Hg (7).
  - Clinical subsets of gestational hypertension are defined according to the presence of end-organ damage.
- **Mild preeclampsia:** renal involvement with proteinuria (≥0.3 g in a 24-hour urine specimen or ≥1+ on two random urine samples).
- **Severe preeclampsia:** blood pressure exceeding 160 mm Hg systolic or 110 mm Hg diastolic, or evidence of end-organ manifestations (proteinuria ≥5 g in 24 hours or ≥3+ on two random urine samples, oliguria less than 500 mL in 24 hours, pulmonary

edema, thrombocytopenia, hepatocellular dysfunction, epigastric pain, cerebral or visual disturbances, or fetal growth restriction) in women with preeclampsia.
- **Eclampsia:** central nervous system involvement with the occurrence of seizures.
- **HELLP syndrome:** hematologic and hepatic involvement resulting in **H**emolysis, **E**levated **L**iver enzymes, and **L**ow **P**latelets. Approximately 20% of women with preeclampsia develop HELLP syndrome (8), although 10% to 20% of women with HELLP syndrome are normotensive (8).
- **Chronic hypertension:**
  - Hypertension preceding pregnancy, developing before 20 weeks' gestation, or persisting beyond the postpartum period (12 weeks) (7).
  - Preeclampsia is superimposed upon chronic hypertension when there is a sustained increase in the blood pressure after 20 weeks' gestation in association with the appearance of proteinuria, an increase in proteinuria if already present in early gestation, or the development of HELLP syndrome.

Chronic Hypertension
Background
- **Chronic hypertension** is present either prior to onset of pregnancy or diagnosed before the 20th week of pregnancy (9).
  - Mild: blood pressure greater than 140 to 159/90 to 109 mm Hg.
  - Severe: blood pressure greater than 160/110 mm Hg.
  - Elevated blood pressure must be documented on more than one occasion, at least 4 to 6 hours apart.

Evaluation
- **History and Physical**
  - Renal function:
  - A baseline 24-hour urine should be collected to measure creatinine clearance and total protein. Alternatively, a spot urine for protein/creatinine ratio may be performed.
  - Baseline BUN, creatinine, and uric acid should be determined.
  - If these tests are normal, no repeat testing is needed unless the patient exhibits signs of superimposed preeclampsia.
  - Funduscopic examination should be performed to diagnose retinal changes associated with long-standing hypertension.
  - Women in whom severe hypertension is diagnosed for the first time in early pregnancy may benefit from further evaluation for potentially reversible causes of secondary hypertension, including pheochromocytoma, Cushing syndrome, and renal artery stenosis (9).

Screening
- Electrocardiogram and chest x-ray may be indicated in patients with long-standing hypertension. Echocardiogram should be considered in women with abnormal electrocardiogram or chest x-ray findings.
- Fetal ultrasound should be obtained to confirm gestational dating for later comparison should the patient develop superimposed preeclampsia or fetal growth restriction.

Treatment
Counseling
- Possible adverse outcomes of hypertension should be reviewed with the patient at her initial prenatal visit.
  - Specifically, the risks of superimposed preeclampsia, intrauterine growth restriction, iatrogenic preterm delivery, and perinatal mortality should be reviewed.
  - The risk of adverse outcome is related to the severity of disease and the presence of renal insufficiency.
  - In the highest risk group, total perinatal survival of 75% is reported with optimal management (10).

- Behavioral modification.
  - Nutritional requirements and sodium intake should be reviewed.
  - Women should be cautioned that smoking, illegal drugs, caffeine, and anxiety may have a negative impact on maternal blood pressure and perinatal outcome.
- Compliance with prescribed medication and frequently scheduled prenatal visits should be stressed.

Medications

- For the patient with mild hypertension, the use of antihypertensive agents shows no significant benefit (7,11).
  - In this group, therapy does not reduce the rate of superimposed preeclampsia, fetal growth restriction, placental abruption, or perinatal morbidity.
  - While the majority of antihypertensive agents are believed to be safe during pregnancy, with the exception of α-methyldopa, experience is limited. Therefore, with the threat of unknown adverse fetal effects and an inability to document benefit, the most prudent course is to defer therapy of mild hypertension during pregnancy unless the maternal blood pressure is greater than 150/100 mm Hg or the patient has other complicating factors (e.g., cardiovascular or renal disease) (9).
- In patients with severe hypertension (diastolic blood pressure greater than 110 mm Hg), antihypertensive therapy should be initiated to decrease the incidence of cardiovascular events and cerebrovascular accidents.
- The most commonly used antihypertensive agents are
  - α-Methyldopa—a central alpha$_2$-receptor agonist
    - This is the agent most commonly used to treat hypertension during pregnancy, because methyldopa is the only agent whose long-term safety for the mother and the fetus has been adequately assessed.
    - The usual starting dose is 250 mg tid, with a maximum total dose of 2 g/d.
    - A study by Cockburn et al. (12) extended to a 7-year follow-up of two cohorts of children delivered by women with moderate hypertension. Mothers were randomly assigned to α-methyldopa course versus no therapy. At birth and at 6 months, head circumference was smaller in the treated group. On further analysis this was associated with entry into the trial at 16 to 20 weeks' gestation. This difference persisted at 7 years only in this subset of male children. This difference was probably a statistical artifact and of no clinical significance. More importantly, no differences in growth, development, or behavior were reported.
  - β-Adrenergic antagonists (atenolol)
    - Atenolol may be dosed once daily; the usual starting dose is 50 mg, and the maximum dose is 100 mg.
    - All β-adrenergic antagonists should be used with caution in women with heart failure or asthma.
    - β-Adrenergic antagonists have been reported to be associated with increased rates of small-for-gestational-age (SGA) newborns in women with mild chronic hypertension, probably due to decreased uteroplacental blood flow (13,14). However, the failure to adjust therapy in response to an excessive fall in maternal blood pressure may contribute to the observed increased rate of SGA newborns delivered by women treated with β-adrenergic antagonists (15). Therefore, the target blood pressure for all pregnant women treated with antihypertensive agents should be 140/90 mm Hg.
  - Labetalol
    - This is a combined α- and β-adrenergic antagonist that may be used as an acceptable alternative to α-methyldopa during pregnancy.
    - The usual starting dose is 100 mg bid, with a maximum total dose of 2400 mg/d.
    - Labetalol does not significantly decrease maternal cardiac output or uteroplacental blood flow. In one study comparing labetalol with α-methyldopa use during pregnancy, the authors found no differences in outcomes between the two medications (16).

- Calcium channel blockers (nifedipine)
  - These are potent vasodilators that may cause reflex tachycardia and flushing.
  - Nifedipine may be prescribed in extended-release formulations at doses that range from 30 to 120 mg/d.
  - A theoretical concern regarding potential interactions between magnesium sulfate and calcium channel blockers, resulting in severe hypotension or respiratory failure, has been proposed, but these interactions have not been observed in pregnant women who do not have concomitant cardiovascular disease (17).
- ACE inhibitors (i.e., captopril, enalapril, and lisinopril) and ARBs (i.e., losartan)
  - These drugs are contraindicated during the second and third trimesters of pregnancy. Several fetal and neonatal complications have been reported, including neonatal hypotension, underdeveloped calvarial bone, fetal growth restriction, oligohydramnios, and renal failure (18).
  - The use of ACE inhibitors during the first trimester also has been associated with an increase in congenital malformations (i.e., cardiovascular and central nervous system malformations) (19). In some women with chronic hypertension, these medications provide long-term benefits, so careful counseling about family planning is recommended.
- Thiazide diuretics
  - These drugs may interfere with physiologic maternal volume expansion during pregnancy (20).
  - However, if diuretics are indicated during pregnancy, they are safe and may potentiate the response to other antihypertensive agents. Diuretics are not contraindicated except in settings in which uteroplacental perfusion may already be reduced (i.e., preeclampsia, fetal growth restriction) (7).
- Antihypertension agents suitable for treating hypertensive emergencies are listed in Table 12-3.

Fetal Surveillance
- Fetal surveillance should include testing for acute and chronic signs of uteroplacental insufficiency.
- Serial fetal nonstress testing and amniotic fluid assessment should be initiated at 32 weeks' gestation.
- Serial ultrasound examinations should be performed if there is clinical suspicion of intrauterine growth restriction or evidence of superimposed preeclampsia.

Induction of Labor
- Induction of labor at 39 to 40 weeks' gestation should be considered with the presence of severe chronic hypertension, because of the associated increased perinatal morbidity.
- The patient with mild, uncomplicated hypertension (not requiring medication) may be allowed to continue pregnancy until 41 to 42 weeks with reassuring fetal surveillance.

Table 12-3	Antihypertensive Agents for Use in Hypertensive Emergencies During Pregnancy		
Medication	**Initial dose**	**Maximum effect**	**Duration**
Direct vasodilators			
Hydralazine	5 mg	20 min	2–6 h
Nitroglycerin	10–25 µg/min	2 min	2–5 min
Nitroprusside	0.25 µg/kg/min	2 min	3–5 min
Sympatholytic vasodilators			
Labetalol	20 mg	10 min	2–8 h
Clonidine	0.2 mg	2–4 h	6–12 h

Table 12-4	Therapeutic and Toxic Effects of Magnesium Sulfate	
Effect	mEq/L	mg/dL
Antiseizure	4–7	4.8–8.4
Loss of deep tendon reflexes	10	12
Respiratory arrest	15	18
General anesthesia	15	18
Cardiac arrest	>30	>36

Complications

Maternal Complications
- Superimposed preeclampsia.
  - This develops in 10% to 50% of women with chronic hypertension.
  - This diagnosis may be difficult to confirm in women with underlying renal disease.
    - Serum uric acid levels may be helpful because this value is usually normal with uncomplicated chronic hypertension and will rise (greater than 5 mg/dL) with superimposed preeclampsia.
  - When preeclampsia superimposes, it frequently occurs in the late second or early third trimester and necessitates delivery. When this occurs, magnesium sulfate is generally required for seizure prophylaxis. Table 12-4 lists the therapeutic benefits and toxic effects for this drug.
- Progression of maternal end-organ disease is not accelerated by pregnancy. End-organ complications associated with chronic hypertension, including nephropathy, ventricular hypertrophy, and retinal changes, are not more likely to occur or worsen during pregnancy.

Fetal Complications
- Intrauterine growth restriction probably results from placental vascular disease and decreased uteroplacental perfusion.
  - In women with mild, uncomplicated (no superimposed preeclampsia) chronic hypertension, the incidence of fetal growth restriction is similar to normotensive pregnancies.
  - With superimposed preeclampsia, the incidence rises to 30% to 40% (10).
- Prematurity is increased over the general population.
  - In one series, 70% of newborns born to mothers with severe chronic hypertension (diastolic blood pressure greater than 110 mm Hg) were delivered preterm (10).
  - Much of this increase can be accounted for by patients with superimposed preeclampsia.
- Perinatal mortality.
  - Perinatal mortality is not increased in patients with mild, uncomplicated chronic hypertension.
  - Perinatal mortality approaches 25% in women with severe chronic hypertension, despite intensive fetal surveillance and careful control of maternal blood pressure (10).

Patient Education
- Additional patient information may be found at the following Web sites:
  - http://www.obgyn.net
  - http://www.mayoclinic.com

REFERENCES

1. Siu SC, Sermer M, Colman JM, et al.; Cardiac Disease in Pregnancy (CARPREG) Investigators. Prospective multicenter study of pregnancy outcomes in women with heart disease. *Circulation.* 2001;104:515–521.
2. Clark SL, Cotton DB, Lee W, et al. Central hemodynamic assessment of normal term pregnancy. *Am J Obstet Gynecol.* 1989;161:1439–1442.

3. McLintock C. Anticoagulant choices in pregnant women with mechanical heart valves: balancing maternal and fetal risks—the difference the dose makes. *Thromb Res.* 2013;131:S8–S10.
4. Elkayam U, Ostrzega E, Shotan A, et al. Cardiovascular problems in pregnant women with the Marfan syndrome. *Ann Intern Med.* 1995;123:117–122.
5. Pyeritz RE. Maternal and fetal complications of pregnancy in the Marfan syndrome. *Am J Med.* 1981;71:784–790.
6. ACOG Committee on Practice Bulletins—Obstetrics. ACOG practice bulletin. Diagnosis and management of preeclampsia and eclampsia. Number 33, January 2002. *Obstet Gynecol.* 2002;99(1):159–167.
7. Report of the National High Blood Pressure Education Program Working Group on High Blood Pressure in Pregnancy. *Am J Obstet Gynecol.* 2000;183:S1–S22.
8. Sibai BM, Ramadan MK, Usta I, et al. Maternal morbidity and mortality in 442 pregnancies with hemolysis, elevated liver enzymes, and low platelets (HELLP syndrome). *Am J Obstet Gynecol.* 1993;169:1000–1006.
9. American College of Obstetricians and Gynecologists. ACOG Practice Bulletin No. 125: Chronic hypertension in pregnancy. *Obstet Gynecol.* 2012;119(2 Pt 1):396–407.
10. Sibai BM, Anderson GD. Pregnancy outcome of intensive therapy in severe hypertension in first trimester. *Obstet Gynecol.* 1986;67:517–522.
11. Sibai BM. Treatment of hypertension in pregnant women. *N Engl J Med.* 1996;335:257–265.
12. Cockburn J, Moar VA, Ounsted M, et al. Final report of study on hypertension during pregnancy: the effects of specific treatment on the growth and development of the children. *Lancet.* 1982;1:647–649.
13. Magee LA, Elran E, Bull SB, et al. Risks and benefits of beta-receptor blockers for pregnancy hypertension: overview of the randomized trials. *Eur J Obstet Gynecol Reprod Biol.* 2000;88:15–26.
14. von Dadelszen P, Ornstein MP, Bull SB, et al. Fall in mean arterial pressure and fetal growth restriction in pregnancy hypertension: a meta-analysis. *Lancet.* 2000;355:87–92.
15. Easterling TR, Carr DB, Brateng D, et al. Treatment of hypertension in pregnancy: effect of atenolol on maternal disease, preterm delivery, and fetal growth. *Obstet Gynecol.* 2001;98:427–433.
16. Sibai BM, Mabie WC, Shamsa F, et al. A comparison of no medication versus methyldopa or labetalol in chronic hypertension during pregnancy. *Am J Obstet Gynecol.* 1990;162:960–966; discussion 966–967.
17. Magee LA, Miremandi S, Li J, et al. Therapy with both magnesium sulfate and nifedipine does not increase the risk of serious magnesium-related maternal side effects in women with preeclampsia. *Am J Obstet Gynecol.* 2005;193:153–163.
18. Buttar HS. An overview of the influence of ACE inhibitors on fetal-placental circulation and perinatal development. *Mol Cell Biochem.* 1997;176:61–71.
19. Cooper WO, Hernandez-Diaz S, Arbogast PG, et al. Major congenital malformations after first-trimester exposure to ACE inhibitors. *N Engl J Med.* 2006;354:2443–2451.
20. Sibai BM, Grossman RA, Grossman HG. Effects of diuretics on plasma volume in pregnancies with long-term hypertension. *Am J Obstet Gynecol.* 1984;150:831–835.

Renal Complications
Kimberly W. Hickey and Joseph V. Collea

KEY POINTS
- Understand the basic physiologic changes accompanying pregnancy in the genitourinary system.
- Recognize and manage basic genitourinary diseases in the pregnant patient.
- Understand the complex and multidisciplinary approach needed to manage chronic renal disease in pregnancy.

ALTERATIONS OF NORMAL RENAL FUNCTION
Background
- Pregnancy induces anatomic and physiologic changes in the genitourinary system. The alterations affect function, thus changing baseline and normative values in pregnancy as compared to the nonpregnant state.
- Changes begin in the first 5 to 7 weeks' gestation and resolve between 6 and 12 weeks postpartum (1).

Pathophysiology
Anatomic Alterations
- Renal size increases approximately 1 to 1.5 cm. These changes are secondary to
  - Increase in renal vascular volume
  - Increase in capacity of the collecting system
  - Glomerular hypertrophy
- Renal volume increases 30% (1).
- Ureteral dilation:
  - Changes begin in the first trimester.
  - Normal pregnancy measurement:
    - Up to 2 cm
    - Right side affected to a greater extent than the left
  - Dilation may be due to
    - Smooth muscle relaxation due to progesterone effects that is supported by:
      - Maternal ureteral dilation prior to 14 weeks' gestation
      - Dilation of the fetal ureter as seen on sonogram
    - Inhibition of ureteral peristalsis due to prostaglandin E2
    - Mechanical obstruction:
      - Due to enlarging uterus
      - Right ureteral dilation greater than left ureteral dilation may be due to
        * Dextrorotation of the uterus
        * Compression of the right ovarian vein complex as it crosses over the right ureter
        * Cushioning of the left ureter by the sigmoid colon
  - Physiologic dilation does not extend below the pelvic brim.
    - Dilation below the pelvic brim is pathologic.
  - Resolves by 3 to 4 months postpartum.
- Renal pelvicalyceal dilation:
  - Changes begin in the first trimester

214

- Dilation may be due to
  - Decreased ureteral peristalsis
  - Hormonal influences of estrogen and progesterone
  - Mechanical obstruction due to enlarging uterus
- Resolves by 3 to 4 months postpartum.

Physiologic Changes
- Renal blood flow (RBF) may increase up to 75% due to (2,3)
- Increase in cardiac output (CO) of 30% to 40%
- Decrease in peripheral vascular resistance (PVR)
  - Normal blood pressures decreases 10 mm Hg.
- Increase in blood volume of 50% (1,3,4)
  - Plasma and red cell volume begin to increase in the first trimester.
  - Plasma volume is increased due to decreased PVR and stimulation of sodium retention that leads to an increase of total body water.
- RBF begins to decrease at 34 weeks and may drop by 25%.
- Glomerular filtration rate (GFR) is increased by approximately 50% due to the increased RBF, which is seen by 16 weeks' gestation.
  - GFR remains elevated until 36 weeks, and then declines to prepregnancy values several weeks postpartum (1).
  - Increased GFR and renal tubular adaptation leads to (4)
    - Serum creatinine decreasing from an average of 0.8 mg/dL to 0.5 mg/dL.
      - *If persistently greater than 0.9 mg/dL, then underlying renal disease must be suspected*
    - Blood urea nitrogen decreasing from 13 mg/dL to 9 mg/dL.
    - Creatinine clearance increases from 120 mL/min in nonpregnant states to 150 to 200 mL/min in pregnancy.
    - Uric acid levels decrease from 5 mg/dL to 2.4 mg/dL but will increase in late pregnancy due to decreases in RBF.
    - Glucosuria can be a normal finding.
      - Ninety percent of women with normal blood glucose levels spill 1 to 10 g of glucose per day.
    - Proteinuria and aminoaciduria are increased, but proteinuria should not exceed 300 mg/24 hours in the normal pregnant patient.
  - GFR remains stable while RBF decreases (1,2).
- Resetting of vasopressin osmoreceptor with lowered thirst threshold combined with unimpaired water clearance leads to (5)
- Decrease in plasma osmolality of approximately 10 mOsm per kg H_2O
- Decrease in serum sodium to 135 mEq/L
  - *Sodium of 140 mEq/L or greater is indicative of hemoconcentration.*
- Potassium is retained to support fetal–placental development.
  - May unmask potassium excretion defects associated with
    - Sickle cell disease
    - Diabetes mellitus
    - Renal insufficiency
  - May lead to hyperkalemia, arrhythmia, and death.
- Renal compensation for progesterone stimulation of the respiratory center and subsequent respiratory alkalosis occurs by (1)
- Decrease in PCO_2 by 10 mm Hg.
- Increase in pH to an average of 7.44.
- Increased excretion of serum bicarb to 18 to 20 mEq/L to compensate for alkalosis.
- Note that these changes place the mother and fetus at increased risk of exposure to acidemia in times of infection or stress.

Evaluation
Initial Laboratory Evaluation
- Urinalysis, urine culture, and blood pressure are an initial screen for underlying renal disease.
- Abnormalities will prompt further evaluation with a basic metabolic panel and a 24-hour urine collection for protein and creatinine.
- Creatinine excretion is approximately 15 to 20 mg/24 h/kg and will yield information regarding the compliance with collection of the 24-hour urine sample.
- Hematuria or proteinuria should trigger further workup for renal disease.
- Hypertension prior to 20 weeks' gestation should also raise suspicion of underlying renal disease.

URINARY TRACT INFECTIONS
Background
Definition
- Asymptomatic bacteriuria (ASB): Minimum of 10^5 per mL of a single organism on *two consecutive, clean-catch urine specimens* or $\geq 10^2$ per mL of a single organism in a *single catheterized specimen* (6).
- Urinary tract infection (UTI): Minimum of 10^3 per mL of a single organism in the presence of symptoms (2).
- Uncomplicated UTI: Infection of the lower tract in women who do not have structural or functional lesions in the genitourinary system.
- Complicated UTI: UTI with pyelonephritis or where the patient is predisposed to reduced efficacy of treatment due to functional or structural abnormalities. *By definition, all UTIs in pregnancy fall into this category* (7).
- Pyelonephritis: Characterized by fever of greater than 38°C, chills, flank pain, costovertebral angle tenderness, nausea, emesis, anorexia, and either 20 bacteria per high-power field or pyuria (8).

Pathophysiology
- Untreated ASB progresses to a symptomatic UTI in 30% to 40% of patients.
- Vesicoureteral reflux, slowed emptying, and dilated renal collecting system due to hormonal factors and pressure from the gravid uterus predispose patients to upper and lower UTIs.
- Aminoaciduria and glucosuria may promote bacterial growth.
- Increased incidence in women who are older, higher parity, of lower socioeconomic status, history of UTI, anatomic or functional abnormality, and affected by diabetes mellitus or sickle cell trait or disease (9).

Etiology
- Normal vaginal flora
- Most common organisms
  - *Escherichia coli* is isolated in 70% of cases.
  - *Klebsiella* is isolated in 3% of cases.
  - *Proteus* is isolated in 2% of cases.
  - Gram-positive cocci such as group B streptococcus are implicated in 10% of cases.

Epidemiology
- ASB occurs in 2% to 13% of pregnancies (9).
- Symptomatic UTIs complicate 1% to 2% of pregnancies.
  - Incidence of UTI is unchanged if prior ASB is recognized and treated.
- Recurrent UTIs: Two or more bladder infections in 1 year (9).
  - Consider evaluation for underlying renal anomaly.
- Pyelonephritis complicates an additional 1% to 2% of pregnancies (6).

- Most common nonobstetric etiology for hospitalization.
- Ninety percent of cases may be avoided by treatment of ASB.
- May be associated with a reversible decrease in GFR.
- Ninety percent of cases occur in the second and third trimesters.

Evaluation
Laboratory Tests
- **ASB or UTI**
  - Urinalysis and urine culture.
  - Follow up culture 2 weeks after treatment to assess for eradication.
- **Pyelonephritis**
  - Urinalysis, urine culture, blood cultures, basic metabolic panel to assess creatinine, and electrolytes

Treatment
Procedures
- **ASB or UTI**
  - Treat with oral antibiotics for 3 to 7 days.
  - Thirty percent recurrent infection rate regardless of treatment regimen.
  - Recurrent infections require 10 days of oral antibiotic therapy.
- **Complicated UTI or recurrent UTIs**
  - Treat with oral antibiotics for 10 days.
  - Daily suppressive therapy for the remainder of pregnancy for history of recurrent UTIs or recurrent infections complicating the antenatal course.
- **Pyelonephritis**
  - Admission for inpatient treatment
  - Antibiotics for 24 hours after resolution of flank pain and fever
  - Combined IV and oral course for 10 to 14 days after clinical improvement
  - Daily suppressive therapy for the remainder of pregnancy

Medications
- **Adjust antibiotics based on culture/sensitivity results.**
- **ASB or UTI**
  - Macrobid 100 mg PO bid
    - Avoid if past medical history of G6PD deficiency to avoid hemolytic crisis.
  - Bactrim DS one tab PO bid
    - Avoid in first trimester as trimethoprim is an antifolate agent with theoretical risk of neural tube defects.
    - Avoid in the third trimester due to risk of kernicterus.
  - Amoxicillin 500 mg PO tid
  - Ampicillin 250 mg PO qid
  - Keflex 500 mg PO qid
- **Pyelonephritis**
  - Intravenous antibiotics
    - Ampicillin 2 g every 6 hours plus gentamicin with dose dependent on selection of daily versus three times daily dosing regimen
    - Cefazolin 2 g every 8 hours
    - Ceftriaxone 1 g every 24 hours
  - Oral antibiotics to complete course of treatment
    - Selection based on sensitivities.
    - Avoid nitrofurantoin (Macrobid) for completion of antibiotic regimen due to poor tissue penetration.
  - Antibiotic suppression with Macrobid 100 mg PO qd for remainder of pregnancy to prevent recurrent UTIs or pyelonephritis (10)

Complications

- Pyelonephritis (2,11)
  - Sepsis requiring intensive care unit (ICU) admission
  - Perinephric abscess
  - Adult respiratory distress syndrome
  - Preterm labor
  - Preterm delivery
  - Recurrent infections

URINARY CALCULI

Background

Definition
- Urolithiasis: Presence of calculi in the urinary tract (12)

Epidemiology
- Incidence (0.03%) is the same in pregnant and nonpregnant women.
- Occurs three times more often in multiparous than primiparous women although when corrected for age, the prevalence is the same.
- The majority (80% to 90%) of symptomatic calculi present in the second and third trimester.
- Calculi occur in equal frequency on the left and right sides.
- Ureteric calculi occur twice as often as renal calculi.
- Diagnosis of urolithiasis missed in up to 28% of patients (12,13).

Evaluation

Laboratory Tests
- Urinalysis to screen for infection and hematuria
  - Microscopic hematuria is present in 75% of specimens.
  - Gross hematuria is present in 15% of specimens.
- Urine culture to screen for infection

Imaging
- Renal ultrasound to assess for ureteral dilation. Detection ranges from 29% to 95% (13).
  - Dilation below the pelvic brim is highly suspicious of renal pathology.
- X-ray for visualization of calculi.
  - May be difficult due to displacement of ureters by enlarging uterus and fetal skeleton obscuring calculi.
  - Plain films combined with ultrasound will lead to diagnosis in 95% of cases.
- Computed tomography (CT) intravenous pyelogram (IVP) to assess for hydroureter and hydronephrosis with possible visualization of calculi.
- Ideally, low-dose CT offers sensitivity and specificity greater than 98% for identification of renal calculi in the pregnant patient (14).

Diagnosis

- Characterized by flank pain, abdominal pain, nausea, emesis, and microscopic or gross hematuria

Differential Diagnosis
- Pyelonephritis
- Appendicitis
- Diverticulitis
- Ovarian torsion
- Cholecystitis
- Abruptio placentae

Treatment
Procedures
- Conservative treatment with oral hydration and narcotic analgesia results in spontaneous passage of calculi in 70% to 80% of patients.
- Surgical intervention is indicated in patients with (14)
  - Infected hydronephrosis
  - Sepsis
  - Intractable pain
  - Ureteral obstruction
  - Failure of conservative management
- Ureteral stents to relieve obstruction with recommendation for changing stents every 4 weeks to prevent encrustation.
- Percutaneous nephrostomy tubes (PCN).
  - Rapid drainage and decompression of urinary collecting system
  - Successful in greater than 90% of cases
- Ureteroscopy for stone fragmentation and removal.
- Open surgical removal.
- Lithotripsy remains contraindicated in pregnancy, although in a small series of pregnant women with exposure in the first trimester due to unknown pregnancy, there were no spontaneous abortions, malformations, or complications of pregnancy (15).

Medications
- Conservative therapy
  - Narcotics for pain management
  - Antibiotics if concern for concomitant UTI

Referrals/Counseling
- Urology for all active management

Complications (13)
- Preterm premature rupture of membranes
- Preterm labor
- Preterm delivery
- Ureteral perforation
- Failure of procedure

CHRONIC RENAL DISEASE
Background
- Obstetrical outcome depends largely on early, aggressive control of hypertension, on the absence of severe, prolonged nephrotic syndrome, and on preservation of renal function rather than the specific underlying disease.

Definition
- Mild renal insufficiency is defined by a serum creatinine of 1.3 mg/dL or less.
- Moderate renal insufficiency is defined by a serum creatinine of 1.3 to 1.9 mg/dL.
- Severe renal insufficiency is defined by a serum creatinine of 1.9 mg/dL or greater.
- Chronic renal failure is characterized by oliguria or anuria requiring dialysis (2,16).

Pathophysiology
- Impairment of acid–base regulation predisposes the fetus to acidemia.
- Inadequate blood pressure control is associated with a dismal obstetric prognosis.
- Hypertension secondary to renal disease places the fetus at risk due to
  - Uteroplacental insufficiency
  - Decreased perfusion
  - Decreased oxygen availability

Etiology
- The etiologic causes of renal insufficiency or renal failure are numerous.
  - Most common causes are
    - Diabetes mellitus—33%
    - Hypertension—24%
    - Glomerulonephritis—17%
    - Polycystic kidney disease—5%
- The etiologies that have been associated with worsening of renal disease in pregnancy are
  - Membranoproliferative glomerulonephritis
  - Reflux nephropathy
  - Immunoglobulin A nephropathy
  - Focal sclerosis

Epidemiology
- Fertility is substantially decreased in women with GFRs less than 50%.
- Eighty-five percent of women with mild renal disease will have a surviving infant.
- Worsening renal function is directly correlated with prepregnancy creatinine.
- One-third of women with preexisting moderate to severe renal insufficiency will develop end-stage renal disease within 1 year of delivery (16,17).
- Uncontrolled hypertension is the single most important indicator of poor pregnancy outcome (2).
- Of women with renal disease requiring dialysis, 2% with hemodialysis will conceive over a 4-year period versus 1% of women treated with peritoneal dialysis.

Evaluation
- Baseline 24-hour urine collection for protein and creatinine clearance should be obtained and repeated monthly (16).
  - Nephrotic-range proteinuria is most commonly due to preeclampsia in women with underlying renal disease.
  - The appearance of worsening proteinuria is common but does not necessarily portend worsening of renal function.
- Baseline serum creatinine with repeated assessment at regular intervals.
- Baseline blood pressure with home monitoring.
- Prenatal visits at least twice monthly.
- Targeted ultrasound at 18 to 20 weeks followed by monthly sonograms to assess for fetal growth restriction.
- Antepartum fetal testing twice weekly starting at 32 weeks' gestation or earlier if severe hypertension, preeclampsia, or other specific complications occur (see Chapter 32, Fetal Monitoring and Testing).

Treatment
Procedures
- Medical management of comorbidities of renal insufficiency should be addressed.
  - Hypertension and anemia
- Delivery for
  - Uncontrollable hypertension
  - Preeclampsia
  - Decreasing renal function once viability is reached
  - Standard fetal indications

Medications
- Hypertension (see Chapter 12, Cardiovascular Disease and Chronic Hypertension)
  - β-Blockers, calcium channel blockers, and hydralazine

- Anemia
  - Maintain hematocrit at 25% or greater with (in order of preference)
  - Ferrous sulfate, erythropoietin, and/or transfusion

Referrals/Counseling
- Nephrology consultation for comanagement

Complications (2,16,17)
- Deterioration of renal function
- Renal failure requiring dialysis
  - Fetal compromise due to hypotension associated with dialysis
  - Decreased fertility and increased spontaneous abortion associated with renal failure
- Worsening hypertension
- Superimposed preeclampsia
- Abruption
- Fetal loss as spontaneous abortion or intrauterine fetal demise
- Fetal growth restriction
- Preterm labor and/or indicated preterm delivery
- Rate of fetal complications rises with worsening baseline creatinine

Patient Education
- Patients must be educated regarding
  - The risk of pregnancy and worsening renal function or resultant end-stage renal disease within 1 year of delivery
  - Recommendation for termination if renal function and blood pressure acutely worsen in the first trimester
  - The need for intensive monitoring throughout the pregnancy to optimize maternal and fetal outcomes

SYSTEMIC LUPUS ERYTHEMATOSUS (SLE): RENAL COMPLICATIONS (SEE CHAPTER 20, IMMUNOLOGIC DISEASES)
Background
- Autoimmune disorder occurring primarily in women.
- Patients with hypertension and active renal disease frequently have maternal and fetal complications (18).
- Specifically, women with active lupus disease, hypertension, and nephropathy have increased rates of fetal loss, fetal growth restriction, and preterm delivery.
- Renal disease complicates 50% of cases of SLE.
- Patients who have been in remission for at least 6 months prior to conception with mild renal insufficiency tend to have successful pregnancy outcomes.

Definition
- Lupus glomerulonephritis is characterized by hematuria, proteinuria, thrombocytopenia, hyperuricemia, and hypocomplementemia.

Evaluation
Laboratory Tests
- Patients should be screened at initial visit with baseline 24-hour urine collections for total protein and creatinine clearance and then at least every trimester if both blood pressure and disease status remain stable.
  - Proteinuria may increase without exacerbation of renal disease.
  - New-onset proteinuria or hematuria is a definite sign of active disease.
- Serum creatinine should be obtained at initiation of prenatal care and then every month or more frequently if there is concern for progression of disease.

- Complement levels (C3, C4) should be drawn when attempting to distinguish super-imposed preeclampsia from activation of SLE, since hypocomplementemia is associated with active SLE (18).

Treatment
- A team approach should be utilized for management of this complex disease and its complications in pregnancy.
- Management by a rheumatologist with nephrology consultation as needed for concomitant renal disease.
- Patients should be seen in the office at least every 2 weeks.

Complications
- Hypertension is increased (2.9%) in comparison to 0.4% found in otherwise healthy pregnant women (18).
- Preeclampsia is increased fourfold over baseline.
- Impairment of renal function.

DIABETIC NEPHROPATHY
Background
- Diabetes is the most common cause of end-stage renal disease in the United States.
- The incidence of renal failure is correlated to disease duration.
- No evidence that pregnancy worsens the course of renal disease in pregnancies complicated by insulin-dependent diabetes (5).

Definition
- Total protein 500 mg/d or greater or persistent positive albuminuria in the absence of infection (5).

Pathophysiology
- Increased capillary pressure leads to glomerular hyperfiltration, which results in structural damage and renal disease.
- Factors associated with development of nephropathy (5):
  - Glycemic control
  - Hypertension
  - Dietary protein intake

Epidemiology
- Renal failure eventually occurs in 30% to 40% of patients with insulin-dependent diabetes.
- Renal failure accounts for one-half of the deaths of patients less than 40 years old with diabetes and is the most common cause of death of diabetic patients in their 20s and 30s.

Evaluation
- Prenatal visits weekly for assessment of glycemic control and hypertension

Laboratory Tests
- Baseline 24-hour urine collection for protein, albumin, and creatinine clearance. Followed by collections every trimester or sooner as needed for evaluation of disease status.
- Urine analysis at each office visit to assess for proteinuria and hematuria.
- Baseline serum creatinine with follow-up at least every trimester.
- Baseline hemoglobin A1C value.

Treatment
- The mainstays of treatment in the pregnancy complicated by diabetes and nephropathy are glycemic control and control of hypertension.

Referrals/Counseling
- Consider referral to a maternal–fetal medicine subspecialist for obstetric management.
- Consider comanagement with a nephrologist for assistance with renal disease.

Complications
- Urinary tract infections
- Renal papillary necrosis
- Hypertension
- Preeclampsia
- Decline in renal function

SICKLE CELL ANEMIA: RENAL COMPLICATIONS (SEE CHAPTER 19, HEMATOLOGIC COMPLICATIONS)

Background
Definition
- Genetic disorder resulting in abnormal hemoglobin molecules: hemoglobin S.
- Sickle cell trait is characterized by one normal hemoglobin gene and one hemoglobin S gene (heterozygous).
- Sickle cell disease is characterized by two hemoglobin S genes (homozygous).

Pathophysiology
- Sickle cell disease is characterized by sickling deformity of red blood cells, which leads to occlusion of vessels and infarction of affected tissue.
- Infarction is manifested by painful "crises" or aplastic crises resulting in anemia.
- Sickle cell disease also leads to chronic anemia due to decreased life of the affected red blood cells.

Etiology
- Initially, there is hyperfiltration due to increased GFR and increased RBF.
- Subsequently with disease progression, RBF decreases leading to ischemia, papillary renal necrosis, and infarction (19).

Epidemiology
- Approximately 10% of African Americans have sickle cell trait.
- Sickle cell disease is estimated to affect 1 in 500 African Americans.
- UTIs are twice as likely to occur in individuals with sickle cell trait as in unaffected pregnant women.

Evaluation
Laboratory Tests
- Complete blood count to assess for anemia
- Monthly urine analysis and culture to assess for infection, nephropathy, or papillary necrosis

Treatment
Procedures
- Prenatal visits with urine analysis and culture at each visit
- Transfusions with packed red blood cells
- Treatment of underlying predisposing factor

Medications
- Daily suppressive antibiotic therapy to prevent UTIs

Referrals/Counseling
- Consider referral to a nephrologist for concerns of nephropathy or papillary renal necrosis.

Complications
- Urinary tract infections
- Gross hematuria
- Papillary renal necrosis

ACUTE RENAL FAILURE
Background
- There is a higher incidence of acute renal failure (ARF) in older patients with underlying hypertensive renal disease.
- Renal function associated with acute tubular necrosis resolves more quickly in pregnant than nonpregnant women.

Definition
- Impairment of renal function characterized by progressive azotemia accompanied by oliguria developing over hours to days (20).
- Oliguria is defined as production of 400 mL or less of urine in 24 hours.

Pathophysiology
- ARF is the end point of a common pathway developing after renal ischemia.
- Acute tubular necrosis is a subset of ARF characterized by prolonged ischemia, which is reversible since the glomeruli are not damaged.
- Acute cortical necrosis is also a subset of ARF, but it is associated with severe ischemia resulting in irreversible damage of the glomeruli (21).
  - Renal cortical necrosis is characterized by oliguria for greater than 1 week or by the presence of anuria.
  - Hematuria is frequently present.

Etiology
- Abruptio placentae—due to hemorrhage leading to hypotension and hypovolemia.
- Placenta previa—if associated with hemorrhage may lead to hypotension and hypovolemia.
- Septic abortion—due to hypotension or hemorrhage after evacuation of the uterus.
  - *Clostridium welchii* or *Streptococcus pyogenes* are the causative organisms.
  - Thirty percent mortality rate.
- Hyperemesis gravidarum—due to profound volume depletion and electrolyte imbalances.
- Preeclampsia—due to diffuse endothelial swelling, which may result in ischemia.
  - Proteinuria is attributed to decreased RBF with hypofiltration and loss of glomerular permeability leading to the spilling of protein.
  - ARF incidence of 1% to 2% in preeclampsia.
  - ARF incidence up to 7% in HELLP.
    ○ Dialysis required in one-third of cases.
    ○ Renal function and blood pressures return to prepregnancy baseline in healthy women with resolution of disease.
- Acute fatty liver of pregnancy is frequently accompanied by renal failure.
  - Prognosis is determined largely by the liver disease rather than the renal disease.
- Amniotic fluid embolism.
- Idiopathic postpartum renal failure known as postpartum hemolytic uremic syndrome.
  - May occur days to months after delivery
  - History of a preceding viral illness
  - Attributed to circulating toxins
- Retained fetus.
- Obstructive uropathy due to compression of the ureters by
  - Leiomyomata
  - Polyhydramnios

- Multiple gestation
- Presence of a solitary kidney
- Presence of congenital renal abnormalities
- Medications.
  - Specifically NSAIDs

Epidemiology
- Complicates 1 in 10,000 pregnancies.
- Normal urine output will be maintained in 20% of cases.

Evaluation
History and Physical
- Targeted history and physical looking for underlying etiology of ARF

Laboratory Tests
- Urinalysis to assess for elevated specific gravity (due to dehydration), ketonuria (which may be a marker of dehydration and hyperemesis), and cells and casts (which may point toward a specific etiology)
- Urine culture to exclude infection
- Complete blood count to assess for anemia or infection
- Peripheral smear for schistocytes and burr cells associated with postpartum hemolytic uremic syndrome
- Blood cultures if there is concern for sepsis or infection
- Chemistry panel to evaluate renal function and to assess for electrolyte abnormalities
- Liver function tests to assess for acute fatty liver of pregnancy and HELLP
- Renal biopsy for worsening function or no improvement in function with unclear etiology
  - Glomerular thromboses, fibrin deposition, and fibrinoid necrosis within arterioles are associated with renal cortical necrosis.

Imaging
- Renal arteriogram with findings of patchy blood flow or an absent nephrogram support the diagnosis of renal cortical necrosis.

Diagnosis
- Made by findings of azotemia (increasing creatinine and decreased clearance electrolytes) with decreasing urine output

Treatment
- Treatment is largely supportive.
- Oral fluid restriction.
- Hydration with normal saline to maintain sodium and to correct hypovolemia of hyperemesis gravidarum.
- Serial chemistry panels to assess and manage acute electrolyte abnormalities.
- Antibiotics as needed for sepsis.
- Transfusions and volume replacement for ARF associated with profound anemia.
- Delivery in cases associated with preeclampsia, HELLP, and acute fatty liver of pregnancy.
- *Medications cleared by the kidneys should be dosed to compensate for renal insufficiency to avoid further complications and toxicities.*

Procedures
- Dialysis for hemolytic uremic syndrome to remove endotoxins
- Dialysis for progressive hypernatremia or hyperkalemia, severe acidosis, volume overload, and worsening uremia

Referrals/Counseling
- Consult nephrology to comanage ARF and for determination and initiation of dialysis.

RENAL TRANSPLANT PATIENTS

Background

- Renal transplantation is associated with restored fertility in women after 1 to 20 months following successful transplant.
- Incidence of pregnancy in reproductive-age women after transplant is approximately 2%.
- Prognosis of pregnancy is best when the allograft comes from a living donor (2,22).

Epidemiology

- Spontaneous abortion occurs in 13% of women after transplant, which is the same rate of women with no underlying disease.
- Hypertension and preeclampsia occur in 30% of women.
- Acute graft rejection occurs in 9% of patients, which is similar to nonpregnant transplant recipients (22).

Evaluation

Laboratory Tests

- Baseline 24-hour urine collections to assess for proteinuria and creatinine clearance, which are subsequently repeated monthly or with signs of worsening renal function.
  - Proteinuria may increase during course of pregnancy, but if the creatinine remains stable, the proteinuria will return to baseline after delivery.
- Baseline serum creatinine and electrolytes, which are repeated monthly or with signs of worsening renal function (22).
  - If the serum creatinine is abnormal, then obtain serial estimations of GFR to follow renal function.
  - If there is a decline in GFR, then a search for the etiology must be undertaken:
    - Acute rejection
    - Cyclosporine toxicity
    - Preeclampsia
    - Urinary tract obstruction
- Frequent urinalysis to detect ASB or UTIs.

Treatment

- Prompt treatment of infection.
- Suppressive antibiotic therapy for recurrent ASB or UTIs.
- Continue antirejection medication regimen.
- Limit cesarean section for obstetric indications.

Referrals/Counseling

- Consultation with nephrology or transplant service for comanagement of renal issues during pregnancy

Complications

- Preterm delivery occurs in 45% to 60% of pregnancies.
- Fetal growth restriction occurs in 20% to 30% of pregnancies (22).

Patient Education

- Pregnancy can be safely considered after the following criteria are met (23):
  - Good health for 2 years after transplant
  - Stable allograft function
  - No recent episodes or ongoing episodes of rejection
  - Minimal or absent proteinuria
  - Absence of pelvicalyceal dilation
  - Normal blood pressure with or without antihypertensive agents
  - Immunosuppressive regimens that are acceptable in pregnancy

- ○ Prednisone less than 15 mg/d
- ○ Azathioprine equal to or less than 2 mg/d
- ○ Cyclosporine at therapeutic levels
- ○ Tacrolimus at therapeutic levels
- Cessation of mycophenolate mofetil or sirolimus 6 weeks prior to conception

REFERENCES

1. Chesnutt AN. Physiology of normal pregnancy. *Crit Care Clin.* 2004;20:609–615.
2. Davison JM. Renal disorders in pregnancy. *Curr Opin Obstet Gynecol.* 2001;13:109–114.
3. Brown MA, Gallery ED, Ross MR, et al. Sodium excretion in normal and hypertensive pregnancy: a prospective study. *Am J Obstet Gynecol.* 1988;159:297–307.
4. Yeomans ER, Gilstrap LC. Physiologic changes in pregnancy and their impact on critical care. *Crit Care Med.* 2005;33:256–258.
5. Miodovnik M, Rosenn B, Khoury JC, et al. Does pregnancy increase the risk development and progression of diabetic nephropathy? *Am J Obstet Gynecol.* 1996;174:1180–1189.
6. Nicolle LE, Bradley S, Colgan R, et al. Infectious Diseases Society of America guidelines for the diagnosis and treatment of asymptomatic bacteriuria in adults. *Clin Infect Dis.* 2005;40(5):643.
7. Rubenstein JN, Schaeffer AJ. Managing complicated urinary tract infections: the urologic view. *Infect Dis Clin North Am.* 2003;17:333–351.
8. Gilstrap LC III, Cunningham FG, Whalley PJ. Acute pyelonephritis in pregnancy: an anterospective study. *Obstet Gynecol.* 1981;57:409–413.
9. Dwyer PL, O'Reilly M. Recurrent urinary tract infection in the female. *Curr Opin Obstet Gynecol.* 2002;14:537–543.
10. Lenke RR, VanDorsten JP, Schifrin BS. Pyelonephritis in pregnancy: a prospective randomized trial to prevent recurrent disease evaluating suppressive therapy with nitrofurantoin and close surveillance. *Am J Obstet Gynecol.* 1983;146:953–957.
11. Hill JR, Sheffield JS, McIntire DD, et al. Acute pyelonephritis in pregnancy. *Obstet Gynecol.* 2005;105:18–23.
12. Burgess K, Gettman M, Rangel L, et al. Diagnosis of urolithiasis and rate of spontaneous passage during pregnancy. *J Urol.* 2011;186(6):2280–2284.
13. Lewis DF, Robichaus AG, Jaekle RK, et al. Urolithiasis in pregnancy. Diagnosis, management, and pregnancy outcome. *J Reprod Med.* 2003;48:28–32.
14. McAleer SJ, Loughlin KR. Nephrolithiasis and pregnancy. *Curr Opin Urol.* 2004;14:123–127.
15. White W, Zite N, Gash J, et al. Low-dose computed tomography for the evaluation of flank pain in the pregnant population. *J Endourol.* 2007;21(11):1255–1260.
16. Fischer M. Chronic kidney disease and pregnancy: maternal and fetal outcomes. *Adv Chronic Kidney Dis.* 2007;14(2):132–145.
17. Katz AL, Davison JM, Hayslett JP, et al. Effect of pregnancy on the natural history of kidney disease. *Contrib Nephrol.* 1981;25:56–60.
18. Meng C, Lockshin M. Pregnancy in lupus. *Curr Opin Rheumatol.* 1999;11:348–351.
19. Pham PT, Pham PC, Wilkinson AH, et al. Renal abnormalities in sickle cell disease. *Kidney Int.* 2000;57:1–8.
20. Lindheimer M, Grunfeld J, Davison J. Renal disorders. In: Barron W, Lindheimer M, Davison M, eds. *Medical disorders during pregnancy.* 2nd ed. St. Louis: Mosby, 1995:37–62.
21. Grunfeld JP, Ganeval D, Bournerias F. Acute renal failure in pregnancy. *Kidney Int.* 1980;18:179–191.
22. Crowe AV, Rustom R, Gradden C, et al. Pregnancy does not adversely affect renal transplant. *Q J Med.* 1999;92:631–635.
23. Levidiotis V, Chang S, McDonald S. Pregnancy and maternal outcomes among kidney transplant recipients. *J Am Soc Nephrol.* 2009;20:2433–2440.

Respiratory Complications

Nicole A. Smith, Errol R. Norwitz
and Julian N. Robinson

RESPIRATORY COMPLICATIONS
Key Points
- Pregnancy does not predispose to pre-existing pulmonary disorders but may intensify the pathophysiologic alterations in lung function, thus increasing the risks of medical complications.
- Poor lung function can adversely affect not only maternal but also fetal oxygenation.
- Most routine diagnostic tests and treatment algorithms are generally considered safe during pregnancy.
- Evaluation and optimization of chronic pulmonary conditions before conception should be considered in order to improve perinatal outcomes.

Background
Physiologic Adaptations of the Respiratory System
- During pregnancy, the diaphragm rises by 4 cm, the transverse diameter of the thoracic cage increases by 2 cm, and the subcostal angles increase from 68 to 103 degrees at term.
- Increased oxygen demands of pregnancy are met by deeper ventilation rather than more frequent respiration. The minute ventilation increases 40% due to an increase in tidal volume (the amount of air inspired and expired in a normal breath) from 500 to 700 mL. The respiratory rate and the total lung capacity are unchanged (1).
- Progesterone stimulates hyperventilation, which results in a compensatory mild respiratory alkalosis with arterial pH of 7.45, and decreased $PaCO_2$ (28 to 32 mm Hg) and bicarbonate (18 to 31 mEq/L). The normal PaO_2 range is 104 to 108 mm Hg.
- Because the fetal hemoglobin has a higher O_2 affinity compared to maternal hemoglobin, fetal O_2 delivery is not reduced until the maternal PaO_2 drops to 65 mm Hg, corresponding to a maternal O_2 Sat of less than 90%.

Diagnostic Modalities
Spirometry
- Forced vital capacity (FVC) and forced expiratory volume in 1 second (FEV_1) are unchanged during pregnancy.

Radiologic Imaging
- The chest x-ray (two views) and chest CT are acceptable for use in pregnancy with proper shielding of the maternal abdomen as they expose the fetus to 0.02 to 0.07 mrad and less than 1 rad, respectively (2).
- Risks of fetal anomalies, growth restriction, or abortions are not increased with radiation exposure of less than 5 rad. Cumulative dosimetry should be calculated if multiple x-rays are anticipated.
- One to two rad of fetal radiation exposure may increase the risk of leukemia from the background rate of 1 in 3000 to 1 in 2000 children.

ASTHMA

Background

- Asthma affects approximately 10% of reproductive-age women in the United States (3).
- Severity is unchanged in 50%, improved in 29%, and worse in 22% (4). In general, women with poorly controlled or severe asthma are more likely to worsen during pregnancy.

Definition

Asthma is a chronic inflammatory disease of the airways that causes exaggerated bronchial smooth muscle contraction, mucus hypersecretion and edema, and airway wall remodeling. Bronchoconstriction results from IgE-dependent release of histamine, tryptase, leukotrienes, and prostaglandins from the mast cells. Atopy is the strongest identifiable predisposing factor.

Evaluation

History of Precipitating Factors

- Inhalant allergens: Animal allergens, house-dust mites, cockroach allergens, indoor molds, outdoor allergens
- Occupational exposures
- Irritants: Tobacco smoke, pollution, and irritants
- Others: Rhinitis/sinusitis, gastroesophageal reflux, aspirin, other nonsteroidal anti-inflammatory drugs, sulfites (a common preservative for processed food), topical and systemic nonselective β-blockers, and viral respiratory infections

Physical Evaluation

- Physical findings: Poor air entry, expiratory wheezing, prolonged phase of forced exhalation, use of accessory muscles, nasal secretion, mucosal swelling, nasal polyp, and atopic dermatitis/eczema.
- Spirometry: Decreased FEV_1 and FEV_1/FVC measurements, as well as an increase of 12% or greater and 200 mL in FEV_1 after inhaling a short-acting bronchodilator.
- Peak expiratory flow (PEF) measurements show diurnal variations of 20% or greater.
- Arterial blood gases (performed with severe exacerbation or poor response to initial treatment) show hypoxemia associated with an elevated $PaCO_2$. This should be interpreted as a sign of severe respiratory compromise.

Treatment

Antepartum Management

- Monitor asthma with spirometry or PEF measurements.
- Monitor fetal growth with ultrasound examinations if asthma is suboptimally controlled.
- Reduce exposure to allergens.
- Pharmacotherapy (Table 14-1) is managed in a stepwise approach (5).
- There is no evidence of teratogenic effects in humans from $β_2$-agonists, theophylline, cromolyn, and inhaled corticosteroids. There is conflicting evidence suggesting an increased risk of isolated cleft lip from 0.1% in the general population to 0.3% in women using systemic steroids during the first trimester (6). There are minimal data available on the fetal effects of leukotriene modifiers.
- Theophylline levels should be monitored (serum concentration of 5 to 12 µg/mL) due to its decreased clearance in the last trimester.
- Treatment of exacerbating factors is paramount:
  - Intranasal corticosteroids are the most effective medications for chronic rhinitis.
  - Loratadine and cetirizine are the preferred nonsedating antihistamines.
- Influenza vaccination is recommended annually during influenza season (October to May) regardless of gestational age (7).
- Asthma is an indication for pneumococcal vaccine during pregnancy (8).

Table 14-1	Stepwise Approach to Pharmacotherapy of Asthma		
Step	**Symptoms**	**PEF or FEV$_1$**	**Daily medications**
4 Severe persistent	Continual (day) or frequent (night)	<60%	High-dose inhaled corticosteroid and long-acting inhaled β$_2$-agonist (and if needed, corticosteroid tablets) Alternative: High-dose inhaled corticosteroid and theophylline
3 Moderate persistent	Daily or >1 night/week	60% to 80%	Low-dose inhaled corticosteroid and long-acting inhaled β$_2$-agonist or medium-dose inhaled corticosteroid (and long-acting inhaled β$_2$-agonist if recurring severe exacerbations) Alternatives: Low-dose inhaled corticosteroid and either theophylline or leukotriene receptor antagonist
2 Mild persistent	>2 d/wk but less than daily or >2 nights/month	>80%	Low-dose inhaled corticosteroid Alternative: Cromolyn, leukotriene receptor antagonist, theophylline
1 Mild intermittent	2 or fewer days/week or 2 or fewer nights/month	>80%	No long-term medications A course of systemic corticosteroid for severe exacerbations

From NAEPP Working Group Report on Managing Asthma During Pregnancy. Recommendations for Pharmacologic Treatment: Update 2004. NIH Publication No. 05-3279. Bethesda, MD.

Acute Exacerbation
- Obtain history, physical examination, pulse oximetry, FEV$_1$ or PEF, arterial blood gas, and chest x-ray if pneumonia suspected.
- Administer oxygen by face mask to achieve O$_2$ Sat greater than 95%.
- Start intravenous hydration and nebulizer treatment with:
  - Albuterol 2.5 to 5.0 mg every 20 minutes for three doses, then 2.5 to 10 mg every 1 to 4 hours as needed.
- Add ipratropium if there is a severe exacerbation.
- Add systemic corticosteroids if refractory to above regimen.
  - Oral "burst" of prednisone 60 to 80 mg/d for 3 to 10 days in outpatient management.
  - Intravenous prednisone or methylprednisolone 120 to 180 mg/d in three or four divided doses for 48 hours, then 60 to 80 mg/d until PEF reaches 70% of predicted or personal best in inpatient management.
- Consider admission to the intensive care unit if poor response (FEV$_1$ or PEF less than 50%, PaCO$_2$ greater than 42 mm Hg, mental status changes) or signs of impending respiratory arrest.
- Provide continuous electronic fetal monitoring if fetal viability (≥23 weeks) is present.

Labor Management
- Continue prenatal asthma medications.
- Inhaled β-agonists do not delay the onset or slow the progress of labor.
- Both prostaglandins and ergometrine (methergine) can cause bronchospasm and therefore should be avoided if possible. Hemabate, a $PGF_2 \alpha$, should be avoided while local dinoprostone, a PGE_2 analog, and misoprostol, a PGE_1 analog, can be used safely.

Complications
- Poorly controlled asthma is associated with increased risks of preeclampsia, prematurity, and low birth weight (9).
- Pregnancy does not alter the diagnostic tests for or the treatment of asthma.
- Inadequate control of asthma can cause more harmful fetal effects than the medications.

INFLUENZA
Background
Influenza A and B are the two types of influenza that can cause epidemic human illness during the winter months (October to May). Influenza is airborne with an incubation period of 1 to 4 days. It is usually a self-limited respiratory illness lasting a few days, but women in the third trimester have an increased risk of complications.

Evaluation
- Signs and symptoms include fever, myalgia, headache, malaise, cough, sore throat, and rhinitis (10).

Treatment
- Immunoprophylaxis is associated with reductions in influenza-related respiratory illness, physician visits, hospitalization, and death.
- *Inactivated influenza vaccine* is preferred and may be given in any trimester (11), postpartum, and during breast-feeding. Postpartum vaccination can protect infants from influenza as children under 6 months of age cannot be vaccinated.
- No data or evidence exists of any harm caused by the low level of mercury exposure that might occur from influenza vaccination (11).
- Influenza and pneumococcal polysaccharide vaccines can be given concurrently.
- The *intranasal live attenuated influenza vaccine*, marketed as FluMist, should not be used during pregnancy.
- The influenza antiviral agent oseltamivir (FDA Category C) can be used in pregnancy when potential benefit justifies the potential fetal risk (10).

Complications
- Exacerbation of underlying medical conditions (e.g., pulmonary or cardiac disease)
- Secondary bacterial pneumonia
- Coinfection with other viral or bacterial pathogens

PERTUSSIS
Background
The incidence of pertussis is increasing in the United States. In an effort to decrease the burden of disease in infants, the CDC has updated pertussis immunization guidelines.

Recommendations
- Women should receive the tetanus toxoid, reduced diphtheria toxoid, and acellular pertussis vaccine (Tdap) in every pregnancy, ideally in the third trimester (12).

PNEUMONIA
Background
Pregnancy does not predispose to pneumonia. The pathogens in pregnancy are the same as those affecting nonpregnant women of reproductive age:
- Bacterial: *Streptococcus pneumoniae, Haemophilus influenzae,* Legionella
- Viral: Influenza A, varicella
- *Mycoplasma*

Diagnosis
- Typical symptoms are cough, dyspnea, sputum production, and pleuritic chest pain.
- Signs include fever, tachypnea, rales, dullness to percussion, and bronchial breath.
- Chest x-ray may reveal single lobar infiltrate typical of bacterial pneumonias or patchy multilobular infiltrates typical of *Mycoplasma* or viral infections.
- Routine sputum cultures, serological testing, cold agglutinin, and bacterial antigen testing are not recommended.

Treatment
- Hospitalization for intravenous hydration, oxygen supplementation, and empirical antibiotic treatment is indicated.
- Erythromycin monotherapy is effective in most community-acquired pneumonias (13). Cefotaxime or ceftriaxone should be added for
  - Staphylococcal or *Haemophilus* pneumonia (suspected or documented)
  - Coexisting chronic conditions
  - Respiratory rate of 30 per minute or faster, hypotension, pulse of 125 bpm or faster, temperature of less than 35°C or greater than 40°C, altered mental status
  - Extrapulmonary disease, sepsis, coagulopathy, or anemia
  - White blood cell less than 4000 per μL or greater than 30,000 per μL
  - PaO_2 of 60 mm Hg or less and/or CO_2 retention
  - Elevated serum creatinine
  - Multilobar involvement, cavitation, or pleural effusion
- Penicillin can be used if pneumococcal disease is strongly suspected (13).
- Strains of *S. pneumoniae* resistant to penicillin and erythromycin are increasingly common.
- Pneumococcal polysaccharide vaccine (PPV-23) is not recommended in healthy pregnant women. However, PPV-23 should be given to pregnant women with immunosuppression, asthma, diabetes mellitus, asplenia, tobacco use, and renal and cardiopulmonary diseases (8).

Complications
- Women hospitalized for pneumonia may have higher rates of low birth weight, preterm birth, and preeclampsia (14).

AMNIOTIC FLUID EMBOLISM SYNDROME
Background
- Also known as anaphylactoid syndrome of pregnancy, the amniotic fluid embolism syndrome (AFES) occurs in approximately 1 in 20,000 to 30,000 deliveries.
- AFES is characterized by unpredictable and unpreventable sudden hypoxemia, cardiovascular collapse, and disseminated intravascular coagulopathy during labor or immediately postpartum resulting in hemorrhage. Seizure activity can be present. Extensive ventilation/perfusion mismatch causes early, significant hypoxemia. Left ventricular dysfunction causes cardiovascular decompensation.
- The prevailing theory is that AFES is a profound adverse allergic reaction to the presence of amniotic fluid in the maternal circulation.

Diagnosis
- AFES is primarily a clinical diagnosis.
- The presence of amniotic fluid contents in the lungs on pathologic examination is not diagnostic of AFES.
- Air or pulmonary embolism (PE), anesthetic complications, anaphylaxis, sepsis, hemorrhage, aspiration, and myocardial infarction must be excluded.

Treatment
- Prompt supportive care with judicious intravascular resuscitation, vasopressors, and mechanical ventilation is essential. Central monitoring may be considered.
- Continuous external fetal monitoring is indicated when the fetus is viable.
- The risk of recurrent AFES is unknown; however, there are a few case reports describing uncomplicated subsequent pregnancies.

Complications
- AFES results in substantial morbidity and mortality. Many survivors suffer persistent neurologic impairment.
- Neonatal complications such as hypoxic ischemic encephalopathy and stillbirth are also common (15).

PULMONARY EDEMA
Background
Pulmonary edema in pregnancy is usually secondary to
- Preeclampsia
- Tocolytic therapy
- Massive fluid resuscitation
- Amniotic fluid embolism
- Sepsis
- Cardiac disease (peripartum cardiomyopathy, structural disease, myocardial infarction)

Diagnosis
- Symptoms of dyspnea and orthopnea.
- Respiratory examination may reveal rales and crackles. There is evidence of hypoxemia.
- Chest x-ray reveals fluffy infiltrates or Kerley B lines.

Treatment
Basic principles of management of pulmonary edema should be similar to that in non-pregnant women:
- Identification and reversal of underlying cause.
- LMNOP: *l*asix (diuresis), *m*orphine (to dilate airways), Na^{2+} and water restriction, *o*xygen, and *p*osition patient upright.
- Consider management in an intensive care unit setting.
- Antibiotics and inotropic support if indicated.

TUBERCULOSIS
Background
- Tuberculosis case rates in the United States continue to decline, with an estimated 2012 rate of 3.2 per 100,000 population (16).
- The majority of cases occur in foreign-born persons. Mexico, Philippines, Vietnam, India, and China are the top countries of origin (16).
- Adults aged 15 to 64 years accounted for 73% of reported TB cases (16).
- The acid–fast bacillus *Mycobacterium tuberculosis* is transmitted from person to person through an airborne route. Infectivity is associated with cavitary pulmonary disease,

sputum AFB smear positivity, and frequency of cough. Of note, patients with sputum AFB smear–negative pulmonary TB can also transmit the infection.

Diagnosis
- The Mantoux tuberculin skin test (0.1 mL of purified protein derivative, PPD) is a safe and valid screening test at any stage of pregnancy. The degree of induration (not redness) that constitutes a positive PPD in pregnancy varies with risk factors (e.g., ≥5 mm if HIV positive, ≥10 mm if intravenous drug user, and ≥15 mm if low risk).
- A chest x-ray may be used to rule out the possibility of pulmonary TB in a person with a positive skin test (including patients previously vaccinated with *bacilli Calmette-Guérin, BCG*).
- Asymptomatic individuals with a positive skin test and a negative chest x-ray have latent tuberculosis infection (LTBI). They have been exposed to TB at some point in the past. These individuals are not contagious but may progress to TB upon bacterial activation. The risk of progression to active disease is highest in the 2 years after seroconversion to positive PPD.
- Neither a chest x-ray nor a sputum test for acid–fast bacilli smear can confirm a diagnosis of TB. Only a positive culture for *M. tuberculosis* can provide a definite diagnosis of TB.
- Drug susceptibility should always be obtained from the initial isolates because multi-drug-resistant TB is common.

Treatment
- Treatment should be initiated before the culture results are available whenever the probability of active TB is moderate to high.
- The first-line regimen consists of isoniazid (INH), rifampin (RIF), and ethambutol daily for 2 months, followed by INH and RIF daily or twice weekly for 7 additional months. Streptomycin should be avoided due to possible fetal ototoxicity. The fetal risks of using pyrazinamide are unknown; however, the benefits of including pyrazinamide in the treatment of women with HIV or multidrug-resistant tuberculosis outweigh potential fetal risks (16). Such women should also be managed in a laminar flow room with contact and respiratory precautions.
- LTBI is treated with daily INH 300 mg for 9 months after the first trimester (12 months if HIV infected). INH therapy can be started during pregnancy (16).
- INH should be supplemented with pyridoxine (vitamin B_6), daily tablets of 50 mg, to decrease neurotoxicity.
- Because pregnancy itself does not increase the risk of LTB1 progression to active TB, some experts recommend delaying treatment in pregnant women without risk factors until 6 weeks postpartum because of an increased risk for hepatotoxicity during the puerperium.
- Antituberculosis medications are not contraindicated during breast-feeding.
- Routine vaccination with *BCG* is not recommended due to low risk of infection, variable effectiveness against adult pulmonary TB, and potential interference with tuberculin skin test reactivity (16).

Complications
- Perinatal complications include low birth weight and, rarely, neonatal tuberculosis.
- Congenital infection may occur via hematogenous spread or at the time of delivery.

CYSTIC FIBROSIS
Background
- Cystic fibrosis (CF) is an autosomal recessive condition caused by a mutation of the gene encoding for the cAMP-regulated chloride ion channel, known as the cystic fibrosis transmembrane conductance regulator (CFTR). To date, over 1700 mutations in this single-copy gene have been described.

- The defective CFTR protein produces thickened secretions throughout the respiratory and alimentary tracts, sweat ducts, and the reproductive organs leading to
  - Undernutrition, due to pancreatic insufficiency, and malabsorption
  - Respiratory failure due to chronic infection, bronchiectasis, and progressive lung destruction
  - Diabetes mellitus and cirrhosis due to pancreatic and biliary injury
  - Reduced fertility:
    o In females this is contributed to by the increased tenacity of the cervical mucus plug.
    o Male infertility (98%) results from abnormalities of the vas deferens.

Treatment
- Counseling should be undertaken before conception to address the maternal risks based on the mother's disease status as well as the risk for having a child with CF.
- Genetic counseling in women with CF:
  - All infants will be obligate carriers of one of their mother's CFTR alleles.
  - The father's carrier status will determine the risk of having an affected child.
  - The CF carrier detection rates of the standard screening panel of the more common 23 mutations differ among ethnic groups (see Table 14-2); therefore, a negative screen result will reduce but not eliminate the risk of having a fetus affected with CF. For couples where both are carriers, or one is affected by CF, genetic counseling should be offered to assess the value of expanded screening or gene sequencing (17). Genotype and phenotype are poorly correlated.
- Routine CF screening:
  - The American College of Obstetricians and Gynecologists (ACOG) currently recommends that all women, regardless of ethnicity, be offered CF screening either prior to or during pregnancy for a panel that includes at least the most common 23 CFTR gene mutations.
  - If the woman screens negative, no further testing is necessary.
  - If the woman screens positive, then the father of the baby should be tested and genetic counseling recommended.
- Management of women with CF should include
  - Nutritional counseling and early screening for diabetes mellitus
  - Pulmonary function monitoring with spirometric tests before, during, and after pregnancy
  - Aggressive antibiotic therapy. *Pseudomonas aeruginosa* is the most common pathogen associated with recurrent infections and chronic airway inflammation. Fluoroquinolones should be avoided due to potential adverse effects on fetal cartilage

Table 14-2	Cystic Fibrosis Detection and Carrier Rates Before and After Testing		
Ethnic group	Detection rate	Carrier rate before testing	Carrier rate after negative test result
Ashkenazi Jewish	94%	1/24	1/380
Non-Hispanic white	88%	1/25	1/200
Hispanic white	72%	1/58	1/200
African American	64%	1/61	1/170
Asian American	49%	1/94	1/180

From American College of Obstetricians and Gynecologists. Update on Carrier Screening for Cystic Fibrosis. Committee Opinion No. 486, April 2011.

Complications

- Perinatal complications include poor maternal weight gain, irreversible deterioration of pulmonary function, congestive heart failure, prematurity, and perinatal death.
- Pulmonary function is the best predictor of maternal long-term survival, and poor lung function increases the risk of preterm delivery (18).
- Pulmonary hypertension and cor pulmonale from chronic lung disease are contraindications to pregnancy.
- Adequate pancreatic function is associated with a better overall outcome.

PULMONARY EMBOLISM (SEE CHAPTER 22, THROMBOEMBOLIC DISORDERS)

Background

Venous thromboembolic disease (pulmonary embolism [PE] and deep vein thrombosis [DVT]) is a leading obstetric cause of maternal mortality.

Etiology

- Pregnancy is a thrombogenic state. Thromboembolic events are fivefold more common in pregnant women than in nonpregnant women.
- Other predisposing factors include trauma (surgery), infection, obesity, and underlying thrombophilia.

Treatment

- Some authorities recommend low molecular weight heparin (LMWH) as the treatment of choice for acute thromboembolism (19). Because of its long half-life and resistance to reversal by protamine sulfate, many authorities recommend converting LMWH to unfractionated heparin at 36 weeks, prior to the onset of labor.
- Unfractionated heparin must be given intravenously or subcutaneously to maintain a therapeutic aPTT (activated partial thromboplastin time). Target aPTT ranges are laboratory specific but correspond to an anti-Xa level of 0.3 to 0.7 U (19). Heparin does not cross the placenta and, as such, is not teratogenic. Adverse effects include hemorrhage, thrombocytopenia, and osteoporosis. In the setting of acute hemorrhage, protamine sulfate can be given to reverse heparin action.
- Treatment should be continued for the duration of pregnancy and for at least 6 weeks postpartum. After delivery, anticoagulation can be restarted 6 hours after vaginal delivery and 12 hours after cesarean delivery. Treatment can be transitioned to oral warfarin (which is teratogenic and should therefore be avoided in pregnancy), and women on warfarin can breast-feed.
- Alternative therapies (fibrinolytic agents, surgical intervention) are associated with a high incidence of complications in pregnancy and, as such, are best avoided.

Prophylaxis

- Women with prior unexplained DVT have an increased risk of recurrence in a subsequent pregnancy. In women with a documented thrombophilic disorder, antepartum *prophylactic* heparin is indicated (5000 to 10,000 units SQ bid). PTT should not increase. The management of women with a prior thrombosis but no thrombophilic disorder is controversial. In the United Kingdom, such women are generally given prophylactic anticoagulation in the postpartum period for at least 6 weeks. The practice in the United States favors *prophylactic* anticoagulation throughout pregnancy and postpartum (19).

Complications

Venous thrombotic events are more common in pregnancy and the puerperium, with further increased risk after cesarean delivery. If untreated, 15% to 25% of patients with DVT will have a PE as compared with 4% to 5% of treated patients.

Patient Education

- Asthma http://www.nhlbi.nih.gov/health/dci/Diseases/Asthma/Asthma_WhatIs.html
- Influenza, pneumonia, and tuberculosis http://www.cdc.gov
- Immunizations http://www.cdc.gov/vaccines
- Cystic fibrosis www.cff.org

REFERENCES

1. De Swiet M. The respiratory system. In: Hytten F, Chambergain G, eds. *Clinical physiology in obstetrics*. 2nd ed. London, UK: Blackwell, 1991:83.
2. Cunningham FG, Leveno KJ, Bloom SL, et al. General considerations and maternal evaluation. In: *Williams obstetrics*. 23rd ed. New York: McGraw-Hill, 2009:912–925.
3. Centers for Disease Control and Prevention. National Center for Health Statistics. Health data interactive. Available at: http://www.cdc.gov/nchs/hdi.htm Accessed April 9, 2013.
4. Turner ES, Greenberger PA, Patterson R. Management of the pregnant asthmatic patient. *Ann Intern Med* 1980;93:905.
5. NAEPP Working Group Report on Managing Asthma During Pregnancy: recommendations for Pharmacologic Treatment. *Update 2004. NIH Publication No. 05–3279*. Bethesda, MD: U.S. Department of Health and Human Services; National Institute of Health; National Heart, Lung, and Blood Institute, 2004.
6. Park-Wyllie L, Mazzotta P, Pastuszak A, et al. Birth defect after maternal exposure to corticosteroids: prospective cohort study and meta-analysis of epidemiological studies. *Teratology* 2000;62(6):385–392.
7. Centers for Disease Control and Prevention (CDC). Prevention and Control of Influenza: recommendations of the Advisory Committee on Immunization Practices (ACIP). *MMWR Morb Mortal Wkly Rep*. 2004;53(RR06):1–40.
8. Centers for Disease Control and Prevention (CDC). Updated recommendations for prevention of invasive pneumococcal disease among adults using the 23-Valent pneumococcal polysaccharide vaccine (PPSV23), *MMWR Morb Mortal Wkly Rep*. 2010;59(34):1102–1106.
9. Mendola P, Laughon K, Mannisto TI, et al. Obstetric complications among US women with asthma. *Am J Obstet Gynecol*. 2013;208:127 e1–e8.
10. Centers for Disease Control and Prevention, National Center for Immunization and Respiratory Diseases. http://cdc.gov/flu. Accessed April 9, 2013.
11. American College of Obstetricians and Gynecologists. Influenza vaccination and treatment during pregnancy. ACOG committee opinion no. 468. *Obstet Gynecol*. 2010;116:1006–1007.
12. Lutffiyya MN, Henley E, Chang LF, et al. Diagnosis and treatment of community-acquired pneumonia. *Am Fam Physician*. 2006;73(3):442–450.
13. Centers for Disease Control and Prevention (CDC). Updated recommendations for Use of Tetanus Toxoid, reduced diphtheria toxoid, and acellular pertussis vaccine (Tdap) in pregnant women- Advisory Committee on Immunization Practices (ACIP), 2012. *MMWR Morb Mortal Wkly Rep*. 2013;62(7):131–135.
14. Chen YH, Keller J, Wang IT, et al. Pneumonia and pregnancy outcomes: a nationwide population-based study. *Am J Obstet Gynecol*. 2012;207(4):288.e1–e7.
15. Dedhia JD, Mushambi MC. Amniotic fluid embolism. *Contin Educ Anaesth Crit Care Pain*. 2007;7(5):152–156.
16. Centers for Disease Control and Prevention (CDC). Reported tuberculosis in the United States, 2012. Atlanta, GA: U.S. Department of Health and Human Services, September 2013.
17. American College of Obstetricians and Gynecologists. Update on Carrier Screening for Cystic Fibrosis. Committee Opinion No. 486, April 2011.
18. Thorpe-Beeston JG, Madge S, Gyi K, et al. The outcome of pregnancies in women with cystic fibrosis—single centre experience 1998–2011. *BJOG* 2013;120(3):354–361.
19. Bates SM, Greer IA, Middeldorp S, et al. VTE, thrombophilia, antithrombotic therapy, and pregnancy: Antithrombotic Therapy and Prevention of Thrombosis, 9th ed: American College of Chest Physicians Evidence-Based Clinical Practice Guidelines. *Chest* 2012;141:e691S.

Hepatobiliary Complications

R. Moss Hampton

KEY POINTS
- Distinguishing between pregnancy-induced liver problems and liver problems related to maternal disease is crucial and often challenging.
- Pregnancy-induced liver disease presents significant risks for maternal and fetal morbidity and mortality.
- Pregnancy should not adversely affect mild to moderate maternal liver disease.
- Pregnancy in patients with portal hypertension and esophageal varices carries a high risk of life-threatening hemorrhage.

BACKGROUND

It is necessary to understand the characteristic alterations of hepatic function common to pregnancy in order to differentiate normal physiologic changes from abnormalities attributable to disease states.

Pathophysiology
- There is no change in the size of the liver during pregnancy.
- There is no change in blood flow during pregnancy.
- Biochemical changes (see Table 15-1)
  - Serum albumin decreases due to increasing plasma volume.
  - Increase in alkaline phosphatase level due to increased placental production and increased bone turnover.
  - Increased production of clotting factors.

EVALUATION
History and Physical
- Common complaints with hepatic dysfunction
  - Right upper quadrant pain
  - Nausea and vomiting
  - Pruritus
- Common physical findings with hepatic dysfunction
  - Jaundice.
  - Hepatomegaly or splenomegaly.
  - Palmar erythema and spider angiomata do not correlate with liver disease in pregnancy.

Laboratory Tests
- Liver function tests: a broad range of serum chemistries that typically includes aspartate transaminase (AST), alanine transaminase (ALT), alkaline phosphatase, gamma glutamyl transpeptidase (GGT), 5′-nucleotidase, serum bilirubin, serum albumin, and bile acids
- Coagulation studies
- Sonography

Table 15-1	Pregnancy-Related Changes in Laboratory Measures of Hepatic Function

Laboratory measure of hepatic function	Pregnancy-related change
Albumin	Approximately 20% decrease
Alkaline phosphatase	Twice normal
Bilirubin	No change
Ceruloplasmin	Elevated (twice normal)
Cholesterol	Elevated (twice normal)
Globulins (α, β)	Slight increase
Globulins (γ)	Slight increase
γ-Glutamyl transpeptidase	No change or slight increase
Haptoglobins	No change
Serum transaminases	No change
Total protein	No change or slight decrease (dilutional)
Transferrin	Slight increase
Triglycerides	Gradual rise to term
Clotting factors	
Fibrinogen (I)	20% elevation at term
Prothrombin (II)	Minimal increase
Factor V	50% elevation
Factor VII	25% elevation
Factor VIII	Twofold elevation
Factor IX	30% elevation

PREGNANCY-RELATED HEPATIC DISEASE STATES

Intrahepatic Cholestasis of Pregnancy

Background
- Intrahepatic cholestasis of pregnancy (ICP) is a liver disorder in pregnancy occurring in about 1 in 500 pregnancies. It is the second most common cause of jaundice in pregnancy.

Definition
- Pruritus of the trunk and extremities (palms and soles of the feet) beginning in the third trimester is the hallmark of this disease. The itching is often intense and unrelenting.

Pathophysiology
- Pruritus is thought to result from deposition of bile salts in the subcutaneous tissue and skin.

Etiology
The exact etiology is unknown but theories include
- A defect in biliary transport of bile secretion(1)
- Receptor changes affecting detoxification of bile acids (2)
- A possible link to maternal estrogen and progesterone levels (3)

Epidemiology
- The incidence is increased in Scandinavians and Chilean Indians.
- The disease is rare in African Americans.
- Seasonal variations have been noted, with more cases seen in the fall (November).

Evaluation
History and Physical
- Pruritus usually begins after 26 weeks (third trimester) and becomes more intense as pregnancy advances.
- It is not associated with a rash, but excoriations may be present.
- Distribution is typically across the trunk, extremities, palms, and soles.

- Pruritus resolves with delivery.
- Frequently, a history exists of ICP in a previous pregnancy, another family member, or similar symptoms with oral contraceptive pill use.

Jaundice
- Usually mild
- Develops in 10% to 25% of patients with ICP (4)
- Usually begins 1 to 4 weeks after the onset of pruritus

Laboratory Tests
- Serum bile acid levels are increased (4).
- Increase in serum bilirubin (predominately conjugated) may be up to six times greater than the upper limit of normal (5).
- Transaminases may be elevated 2 to 10 times greater than the upper limit of normal.

Genetics
- Possibly an autosomal dominant trait

Diagnosis
Differential Diagnosis
- Viral hepatitis
- Gallbladder disease

Clinical Manifestations
- In addition to severe pruritus, the patient may have anorexia, steatorrhea, and dark urine.

Treatment
- Treatment is used primarily to relieve symptoms until the fetus is mature enough for delivery.

Medications
- Ursodeoxycholic acid (UDCA) is the treatment of choice (10 to 15 mg/kg/d) (3).
- Antihistamines for symptomatic relief of pruritus.
- Corticosteroids—dexamethasone 12 mg/d.
- Cholestyramines—8 to 16 g/d in divided doses.

Procedures
- Begin antenatal fetal assessment (biophysical profile or nonstress testing) at the time of diagnosis.
- Delivery at 37 weeks of gestation (6).

Risk Management
- No test reliably predicts fetal demise (7).
- Majority of fetal deaths occur after 37 weeks (6).
- Mother should begin supplemental vitamin K at the time of diagnosis.

Complications
Long-term maternal complications are not seen with ICP, but there are several pregnancy-related complications:
- Increased perinatal mortality
- May be related to maternal serum bile acid level
  - Fetal mortality rate of 11% to 20% when untreated (6).
  - Fetal testing is not always predictive of imminent fetal death.
- Preterm delivery
- Meconium-stained amniotic fluid
- Postpartum hemorrhage

Patient Education
The pregnant patient should be counselled regarding
- The increased risks of preterm labor and delivery
- The signs and symptoms of preterm labor

- The increased risk of intrauterine fetal demise (IUFD) and regular fetal movement counts
- A 45% to 70% risk of ICP recurring in subsequent pregnancies (4)

Hemolysis, Elevated Liver Enzymes, and Low Platelets (HELLP) Syndrome and Preeclampsia (see Chapter 11, Preeclampsia)
Background
Preeclampsia affects 5% to 7% of all pregnancies and is characterized by new-onset hypertension and proteinuria. It often has significant hepatic effects including reduced perfusion, abnormal liver function, and edema of the hepatic parenchyma and capsule. A variant of severe preeclampsia is the syndrome of hemolysis, elevated liver enzymes, and low platelets (HELLP) syndrome. HELLP syndrome affects 5% to 10% of patients diagnosed with preeclampsia and is associated with several significant complications (8).

Pathophysiology
The manifestations of preeclampsia and HELLP syndrome are thought to be the results of
- Placental hypoperfusion
- Endothelial cell dysfunction
- Alteration of vasomotor tone
- Activation of coagulation cascade
- Release of proinflammatory mediators
Liver biopsy reveals
- Periportal hemorrhage and parenchymal necrosis
- Fibrin deposition in sinusoids
- Steatosis

Etiology
- Exact etiology is unknown; see Chapter 11, Preeclampsia for details.

Epidemiology
- Usually seen in older, multiparous Caucasian patients.
- Generally occurs in late second or third trimester, although 30% of cases occur postpartum.
- HELLP syndrome affects 5% to 10% of pregnancies with severe preeclampsia (8).

Evaluation
Physical Exam
Presenting signs and symptoms can be vague and variable. The most common symptoms are
- Epigastric or right upper quadrant pain
- Nausea and vomiting
- Malaise
- Nondependent edema

The physical exam is often consistent with preeclampsia:
- Hypertension is usually present but may not be in the severe range.
- Significant peripheral edema and sudden weight gain often occur.
- Hyperreflexia is typically present.

Laboratory Tests
The diagnosis of HELLP syndrome requires evidence of
- Hemolytic anemia
  - Abnormal peripheral smear
  - Elevated serum bilirubin (greater than 1.2 mg/dL) (9)
  - Low serum haptoglobin
  - Elevated lactate dehydrogenase (LDH, greater than 600 U/L) (9)
  - Significant drop in hemoglobin
- Elevated liver enzymes

- Abnormal transaminases (greater than 70 units/L or greater than two times upper limit of normal) (9)
- Abnormal bilirubin level
- Low platelets
  - Must be less than 100,000 (9).
  - Severity of low platelets appears to predict the severity of the disease (10).

Diagnosis
Differential Diagnosis
- Pancreatitis
- Idiopathic thrombocytopenia purpura
- Cholecystitis
- Appendicitis
- Pyelonephritis
- Acute fatty liver of pregnancy (AFLP)
  - Signs and symptoms are similar to HELLP.
  - AFLP often lacks hypertension and proteinuria.
  - Liver function tests are not as intensely abnormal.
- Hemolytic uremic syndrome (HUS)
  - Usually seen in children.
  - There is typically more renal involvement.
  - In pregnancy, HUS most often occurs postpartum.
- Thrombotic thrombocytopenic purpura (TTP)
  - Neurologic symptoms
  - Fever

Clinical Manifestations
The diagnosis of HELLP should be considered in any patient with preeclampsia or who presents in the late second or third trimester with nausea, vomiting, and abdominal pain, especially if the pain is in the right upper quadrant of the abdomen.

Treatment
Management
Management of HELLP is the same as that for severe preeclampsia.
- Seizure prophylaxis, usually with magnesium sulfate ($MgSO_4$)
- Control of blood pressure
- Corticosteroids to enhance fetal lung maturity if indicated
- Delivery

Counseling
- Risk of recurrence with subsequent pregnancies is 2% to 20% (9).

Complications
HELLP syndrome has a high rate of significant maternal complications:
- Disseminated intravascular coagulopathy (DIC).
- Acute renal failure.
- Eclampsia.
- Abruptio placentae.
- Pulmonary edema.
- Intracranial hemorrhage.
- Postpartum hemorrhage.
- Hepatic rupture.
  - Maternal and fetal mortality is more than 50% when there is rupture of the liver or rupture of a subcapsular liver hematoma (9).
  - Usually occurs in the anterior aspect of the right lobe of the liver (9).
  - Surgical emergency.

- Fetal morbidity and mortality are related to the degree of prematurity and presence of intrauterine growth restriction.
- Maternal mortality rate may be as high as 50% (4).

Acute Fatty Liver of Pregnancy
Background
AFLP is a rare complication of pregnancy affecting approximately 1 in 10,000 pregnancies. It usually presents after 30 weeks' gestation and may be associated with significant maternal and fetal morbidity and mortality if not treated aggressively or if it goes unrecognized.

Pathophysiology
With AFLP, there is centrilobular, microvesicular fatty infiltration of the hepatocytes. This leads to mitochondrial disruption and widespread hepatic necrosis. Fulminant hepatic failure results if treatment (i.e., delivery) is delayed.

Etiology
- The exact etiology is unknown.
- Recent studies suggest an abnormality in the maternal and fetal metabolism of long-chain fatty acids (LCFA). In 31% to 79% of pregnancies with AFLP, there was a deficiency in fetus had long-chain three-hydroxyacyl coenzyme A dehydrogenase (LCHAD) (11).
- LCHAD functions in the mitochondrial trifunctional complex, which is responsible for oxidation of fatty acids (12). With LCHAD deficiency, the fetus is unable to metabolize LCFAs, and excessive LCFA metabolites accumulate in the maternal liver where they are hepatotoxic (2).

Epidemiology
- AFLP is more common in
  - Patients with multiple gestation
  - Nulliparous patients
  - Male fetus (3:1 male-to-female ratio)
- Preeclampsia is present in about 50% of the cases.

Evaluation
History and Physical
- Presents in the third trimester of pregnancy (usually greater than 30 weeks' gestation).
- Nausea and vomiting are the most common presenting symptoms (75% of patients) (13).
- Abdominal pain is present in 51% of patients (13).
- Jaundice is common.
- Twenty percent to forty percent of patients will have signs or symptoms of preeclampsia.

Laboratory Results
- Liver transaminases are elevated 3 to 10 times normal but usually less than 1000 international units/L.
- Bilirubin is often greater than 10 mg/dL.
- Serum ammonia is elevated.
- Hypoglycemia (a poor prognostic sign).
- Alkaline phosphate is elevated 5 to 10 times normal.
- Lactic acidosis.
- Coagulation profile is often affected.
- Hypofibrinogenemia (vitamin K–dependent factors [II, VII, IX, X] are decreased).
- Thrombocytopenia (less than 100,000 per µL).
- Prolonged prothrombin time (PT) and partial thromboplastin time (PTT).

Genetics
- Thought to be an autosomal recessive disorder
- G1548C mutation of LCHAD associated with AFLP (14)

Diagnosis
Diagnosis is one of exclusion and is usually made based on laboratory findings, patient symptoms, and clinical exam. Ultrasound, computerized tomography (CT) scan, and magnetic resonance imaging (MRI) scans may be suggestive. Liver biopsy may also be helpful. Decisive action is needed to avoid significant maternal and fetal morbidity and mortality.

Differential Diagnosis
• Severe preeclampsia
• HELLP syndrome
• Hemolytic–uremic syndrome
• Thrombotic thrombocytopenia purpura

Clinical Manifestations
• Distinguish from severe preeclampsia and HELLP syndrome
• Risk for fulminant hepatic failure
• Severe maternal hypoglycemia
• DIC

Treatment
• The definitive treatment of AFLP is delivery.
• Management prior to delivery is dependent on the presence or absence of other related problems:
  • Preeclampsia/eclampsia
  • Maternal metabolic abnormalities
  • Hemostatic disorders
  • Renal failure
  • Sepsis
  • Fetal distress
• Once the patient is stabilized, delivery should be accomplished. Vaginal delivery may be attempted if both the mother and fetus are stable. Otherwise, cesarean section is used if either is unstable or if delivery must be performed expeditiously.

Procedures
Liver transplant may be necessary if patient has extensive liver necrosis.

Counseling
• The risk of recurrence with subsequent pregnancies is uncertain.
• If there is a family history for AFLP, the patient should consider genetic consultation to evaluate for possible LCHAD abnormalities (15).

Complications
• Maternal mortality is 1% to 4% and is often due to
  • Cerebral edema
  • Gastrointestinal hemorrhage
  • Renal failure
  • Sepsis
• Fetal mortality is 10% to 20% (7).
• DIC occurs in 75% of cases.
• Postpartum hemorrhage risk is increased.
• After delivery and initial postpartum recovery, expect the liver function to return to normal. There are no long-term sequelae.

Patient Education
Patients should be evaluated for genetic predisposition to LCHAD disorders.
• If patient is in an "at-risk" group with future pregnancies, she should
  • Maintain high-carbohydrate, low-fat diet
  • Avoid fasting
  • Avoid nonsteroidal anti-inflammatory drugs, tetracycline, and valproic acid (16)

- Possible risks to the newborn
  - Child should be screened for fatty acid oxidation (FAO) disorder
  - Reye syndrome

Concurrent Maternal Hepatic Disease and Pregnancy

In general, severe maternal hepatic disease precludes pregnancy because these patients are usually amenorrheic. Pregnancy does not seem to adversely impact mild to moderate hepatic disease and vice versa.

Viral Hepatitis

Viral hepatitis is the most common cause of hepatitis in pregnancy. The course of the disease is usually unaffected by pregnancy. Diagnosis and treatment are generally the same as for the nonpregnant patient. Multiple viruses are involved, and while the symptoms and presentation may be similar, the outcomes, complications, and long-term sequelae vary significantly.

Hepatitis A Virus (HAV)

Background
Etiology
- Single-stranded RNA enterovirus
- Usually spread by fecal–oral transmission
- Short incubation period of 4 weeks

Epidemiology
- Endemic in Africa, Asia, and Central America
- Sporadic outbreaks in the United States, usually food borne

Evaluation
History and Physical
- The patient will present with a flu-like illness including
  - Malaise and fatigue
  - Headache and arthralgias
  - Fever
  - Pruritus

Physical Findings
- Hepatosplenomegaly
- Dark urine
- Jaundice

Laboratory Tests
- Transaminases are elevated.
- IgM antibodies to *hepatitis A virus (HAV)* are diagnostic.

Differential Diagnosis
- Hepatitis due to other viruses
  - B, C, D, or E
  - Cytomegalovirus (CMV)
  - Herpes simplex virus (HSV)
  - Epstein-Barr Virus (EBV)
- Chemical hepatitis
- Jaundice due to other types of hepatic dysfunction
- Increased production of bilirubin
- Intrahepatic cholestasis of pregnancy

Treatment
Treatment for HAV is supportive as this is usually a self-limited infection. Postexposure prophylaxis with hepatitis immune globulin is effective 80% of the time if given within

2 weeks of exposure. Immunization of pregnant women in endemic areas should be encouraged. There does not appear to be vertical transmission to the fetus. However, if active infection is present at the time of delivery, prophylaxis with immunoglobulin is recommended for the fetus.

Complications
• Hepatic failure is reported but rare.

Patient Education
• Patients should be vaccinated if they live in endemic areas.
• Stress good hand washing.

Hepatitis B Virus (HBV)
Background
Etiology
• Double-stranded DNA virus in the core particle
• Long incubation period (up to 180 days)

Epidemiology
• Endemic in Southeast Asia and China.
• In the United States, hepatitis B virus (HBV) is transmitted by contaminated needles, blood products, or direct mucosal contact with contaminated body fluids.
• Chronic carrier state and chronic infection can occur.

Evaluation
History and Physical
The acute infection may be asymptomatic and anicteric. When obtaining a history, look for risk factors that include
• Intravenous (IV) drug use
• Multiple sexual partners
• History of multiple blood transfusions
• Partner with HBV
• History of human immunodeficiency virus (HIV) infection

Physical Exam
Physical Exam may reveal
• Urticarial rash.
• Arthralgias and arthritis.
• Myalgias.
• Hepatomegaly and/or right upper quadrant tenderness.
• Jaundice is less common.

Laboratory Tests
• All pregnant patients should be screened for HBV infection.
• Transaminases are elevated with acute infection.
• Tests for the presence of antigen/antibodies to the following:
  • Viral surface components
    ○ Hepatitis B surface antigen (HBsAg)
  • Core DNA
    ○ Hepatitis B core antigen (HBcAg)
  • Enzymatic components of viral core ("C" antigens)
    ○ Usually present with acute infection
    ○ Indicative of high infectivity if present
  • E antigen
    ○ HBeAg is a marker for infectivity.
• Specific antigens and antibodies associated with hepatitis B infection vary over the course of the disease.

Diagnosis
Differential Diagnosis
- Hepatitis due to other viruses
  - A, C, D, or E
  - CMV
  - HSV
  - EBV
- Chemical hepatitis
- Jaundice due to other types of hepatic dysfunction
- Increased production of bilirubin
- Intrahepatic cholestasis of pregnancy

Treatment
Active treatment for an acute infection is not indicated unless the patient has fulminant hepatic necrosis and acute liver failure. For patients acquiring HBV infection during pregnancy, passive immunization with hepatitis B immunoglobulin (HBIG) may be given up to 48 hours after exposure. Vaccination with anti-HBV vaccines is safe to give during pregnancy (17).

Risk Management
- Preventing vertical transmission to the fetus
  - Ninety-five percent of perinatal transmission occurs intrapartum (5).
  - Risk of transmission to fetus is highest (80% to 90%) when the mother is infected in third trimester (14) or is HBeAg positive at delivery.
  - Newborns should receive HBIG within 12 hours of delivery if mother is HBsAg positive. (18) HBV vaccination should be given in the first 6 months.
  - Cesarean section does not prevent transmission from mother to fetus but does lessen the risk (13).
  - Breast-feeding is not contraindicated in the immunized newborn (17).
  - Lamivudine may be given to patients with high levels of HBV DNA during the last month of pregnancy to decrease the risk of vertical transmission (19).

Complications
- Chronic active hepatitis with eventual cirrhosis
- Chronic HBV infection
- Increased risks for hepatocellular carcinoma
- Acute liver failure

Hepatitis C Virus (HCV)
Background
Etiology
- Single-stranded RNA virus with an envelope
- Blood borne
- Percutaneous transmission
- Incubation time about 50 days (ranges from 15 to 160 days)

Epidemiology
- Most common chronic blood-borne infection in the United States (20). Hepatitis C virus (HCV) affects 1% to 2.5% of the pregnant population in the United States with a higher rate in developing countries.
- The risk factors are the same as for hepatitis B although many HCV-positive women have no known risks factors (21).
- HCV is a common cause of cirrhosis.
- Twenty to fifty percent of symptomatic patients will spontaneously clear the virus.
- Asymptomatic patients have a higher rate of chronic infection.

Evaluation

History and Physical

The acute infection of hepatitis C is very mild. Patients are often asymptomatic and anicteric, although some may have a history of a recent flu-like illness. The history should focus on identifying risk factors; physical exam should look for signs of cirrhosis.

• Palmar erythema and spider angioma can be seen in normal pregnancy.
• Splenomegaly may be suggestive of cirrhosis.

Laboratory Tests

• Hepatitis C IgM and IgG antibodies.
• Hepatitis C RNA levels.
  • Evaluate viral load
• Thrombocytopenia and leukopenia may be suggestive of cirrhosis.
• Elevations in transaminase levels are variable.

Differential Diagnosis

• Hepatitis due to other viruses
  • A, B, D, or E
  • CMV
  • HSV
  • EBV
• Chemical hepatitis
• Jaundice due to other types of hepatic dysfunction
• Increased production of bilirubin
• Intrahepatic cholestasis of pregnancy

Treatment

Hepatitis C infection does not affect the pregnancy and does not require active treatment. If the patient has cirrhosis and/or portal hypertension, procedures to diagnose and treat esophageal varices may be indicated. Use of interferon or ribavirin is contraindicated in pregnancy. Patients who are HCV RNA positive after pregnancy should be actively treated. Universal screening of pregnant patients for hepatitis C is not currently felt to be cost-effective, but debate is ongoing (22).

Complications

Vertical transmission is the common route of HCV infection.

• Transmission rates range from 1% to 5% (4).
• Transmission risk is higher if the mother is HCV RNA positive, HIV positive, or viremic at time of delivery (23).
• Higher rate of transmission occur with higher viral loads (greater than 1 million copies per mL) (24).
• Prolonged rupture of membranes (greater than 6 hours) increases the transmission rate (5).
• Mode of delivery and breast-feeding do not affect the transmission rate.
• Fetus passively acquires immunization from mother that may persist up to 12 months (24).

Chronic maternal disease after hepatitis C.

• Chronic hepatitis.
• Hepatocellular carcinoma and/or cirrhosis develops in 20% to 30% of patients (25).
• Fulminant hepatitis is rare.

Hepatitis E Virus (HEV)

Background

This disease is seen primarily in underdeveloped countries of the world. It is the leading cause of acute viral hepatitis worldwide and the most prevalent viral cause of acute liver failure in pregnancy (26).

Etiology

• Single-stranded RNA virus
• Incubation time from 15 to 60 days

Epidemiology
- Fecal/oral spread similar to HAV.
- Parenteral and vertical transmission is implicated.
- Endemic to underdeveloped countries in the Far East.
- Seasonal variation exists, being more common during monsoon conditions.
- Usually self-limited if patient is not pregnant.

Evaluation
History and Physical
This infection often presents as jaundice in the third trimester. Fever and dark urine are common.

Laboratory Tests
- Presence of IgM anti-hepatitis E virus (HEV) antibody and HEV-RNA
- Abnormal liver function tests

Differential Diagnosis
- Hepatitis due to other viruses
  - A, B, C, or D
  - CMV
  - HSV
  - EBV
- Chemical hepatitis
- Jaundice due to other types of hepatic dysfunction
- Increased production of bilirubin
- Intrahepatic cholestasis of pregnancy

Clinical Manifestations
Onset of jaundice is usually in the third trimester in patients without a history of chronic liver disease.

Treatment
There is no active treatment for this disease. Fulminant liver failure is common (greater than 50% of cases), and pregnancy seems to increase the severity of the disease. Maternal mortality rates as high as 41% to 54% have been reported (27). An effective vaccine may be available in the near future (29).

Complications
Increased rates of
- Preterm labor
- Premature rupture of membranes
- Intrauterine growth restriction
- Fetal mortality rate up to 69% has been reported (29)

Vertical transmission
- Occurs in up to 50% of HEV-RNA–positive mothers (12).
- There is significant perinatal morbidity/mortality.

Hepatitis G Virus (HGV) and GB Agents
Background
These represent a poorly understood group of viruses and virus-like agents that are responsible for transfusion-related hepatitis.

Etiology
- Single-stranded RNA virus similar to HCV.
- Coinfection with hepatitis A, B, C, and HIV common.
- GB group are viral agents of flavi-like viruses.

Epidemiology
- Thought to be transfusion-associated hepatitis
- Same risk groups as HBV and HCV
- Thought to cause 10% of non-A, non-B hepatitis

Evaluation
History and Physical
- Symptoms of hepatitis G virus (HGV) are mild and nonspecific.
- Physical exam may reveal mild right upper quadrant tenderness.
- Clinical significance of infection is uncertain (30).

Laboratory Tests
- Polymerase chain reaction (PCR) can detect hepatitis G nucleic acid.
- Enzyme-linked immunosorbent assay (ELISA) can detect viral envelope protein.

Treatment
- Symptomatic
- May cause chronic hepatitis as well as acute disease

Complications
- Acute infection is not thought to alter or affect pregnancy.
- Vertical and sexual transmission is more common than was previously suspected (32).

Cytomegalovirus (CMV) Hepatitis
Background
- CMV infection is not uncommon in pregnancy, but hepatitis is rare, except in immuno-suppressed patients.

Etiology
- DNA herpes virus

Epidemiology
- CMV is endemic to most populations, and its prevalence increases with age.

Evaluation
History
- CMV infection presents with a flu-like illness
  - Malaise
  - Fever
  - Arthralgias
  - Nausea/vomiting

Physical
- Intermittent fever
- Sore throat
- Cervical adenopathy
- Splenomegaly
- Jaundice

Laboratory Tests
- IgM antibody to CMV
- Positive viral culture from serum or urine

Diagnosis
Differential Diagnosis
- Hepatitis due to other viruses
  - A, B, C, D, or E
  - HSV
  - EBV
- Chemical hepatitis.

- Jaundice due to other types of hepatic dysfunction.
- Increased production of bilirubin.
- Intrahepatic cholestasis of pregnancy.
- Thirty-three to forty-four percent of patients with acquired immunodeficiency syndrome (AIDS) have CMV hepatitis (33).

Treatment
The disease is self-limited with a favorable prognosis. Fulminant hepatitis is rare.

Complications
- CMV is the most common in utero viral fetal infection.
- Ten percent of infected fetuses are severely affected, resulting in
  - Intrauterine growth restriction
  - Ventriculomegaly
  - Microcephaly
- Fetal risks are greatest if infection occurs when less than 22 weeks' gestation.
- There is a long-term risk of developmental problem.

Epstein-Barr Virus (EBV) Hepatitis
Background
Etiology
- DNA herpes virus responsible for mononucleosis

Evaluation
Presenting Symptoms Suggest Mononucleosis
- Intermittent fever
- Malaise
- Headache
- Sore throat

Physical Exam
- Cervical and axillary adenopathy
- Splenomegaly present in 75% of cases
- Hepatomegaly present in 17% of cases
- Jaundice present in 11% of cases

Laboratory Tests
- IgM antibodies specific to EBV
- IgM antibody specific to EBV nuclear antigen
- Rising IgG antibody to EBV

Differential Diagnosis
- CMV infection with hepatitis

Treatment
- Supportive care
- Not associated with known fetal morbidity
- Reports of acute liver failure with pregnancy

Herpes Simplex Virus (HSV) Hepatitis
Background
- While 0.5% to 1.0% of all pregnant women may have an overt herpetic infection during pregnancy, HSV hepatitis is very rare.

Etiology
- Double-stranded DNA virus

Epidemiology
- HSV is found in all populations.
- Spread is by intimate contact.

- Once infected, the herpes virus can be found in a dormant state in the neural ganglia.
- Reactivation of the virus is common.
- Hepatitis is only seen in immunosuppressed patients.

Evaluation
History and Physical
- Patients may or may not have a previous history of HSV infection.
- History of immunosuppression or immune deficiency diseases.
- May have painful, ulcerative lesion, often in the genital tract.
- Usually presents in the third trimester of pregnancy.
- May present with hepatic failure, pneumonia, and encephalitis (33).

Laboratory Tests
- PCR assays are very sensitive.
- Viral culture of lesion if one is present.
- IgG and IgM antibodies for HSV 1 and 2.
- HIV testing if status is unknown.
- Serum transaminases are usually markedly elevated.
- PTT may be prolonged along with thrombocytopenia and normal bilirubin (35).
- Liver biopsy should show presence of viral inclusion bodies.

Differential Diagnosis
- Hepatitis due to other viruses
  - Hepatitis A, B, C, D, or E
  - CMV
  - EBV
- Chemical hepatitis
- Intrahepatic cholestasis of pregnancy
- AFLP
- HELLP

Treatment
- Antiviral drugs, such as acyclovir, are the mainstay of therapy (33).
- Supportive care, as these patients are usually critically ill.

Complications
- Hepatic failure
- Maternal and fetal death

Hepatic Cirrhosis
Background
- Hepatic cirrhosis is the result of a wide variety of insults to the liver resulting in chronic hepatic dysfunction and eventually chronic liver failure. Infection, metabolic disease, inherited disease, and toxic exposures (commonly alcohol or medications) can lead to microarchitectural change with areas of fibrosis and nodular regeneration replacing normal hepatic tissue.
- Pregnancy appears to have little effect on hepatic function of patients with mild liver dysfunction.
- Severe hepatic dysfunction is usually associated with infertility.
- Pregnancy-associated maternal morbidity correlates with the prepregnancy disease state and the presence of portal hypertension.

Pathophysiology of Cirrhosis and Pregnancy
- Changes in maternal hemodynamics during pregnancy
  - Increased blood volume
  - Changes in venous return
  - Increased cardiac output
  - Decreased systemic blood pressure

Portal Hypertension
- Initiated by increased resistance within the portal venous bed.
- Pregnancy may also increase portal pressure due to
  - Increased blood volume
  - Increased cardiac output
  - Mesenteric vasodilation
  - Increased pressure on the inferior vena cava by the enlarging uterus
- Varices develop from portosystemic collateral circulation.

Etiology
- Inherited diseases
  - Wilson disease
  - Hemochromatosis
- Infectious diseases
  - Hepatitis B and C
- Chronic cholestasis
  - Primary biliary cirrhosis
- Autoimmune hepatitis
- Toxins
  - Alcohol (ETOH) consumption
  - Hepatotoxic drugs (see Table 15-2)

Epidemiology
Inherited Disease
- Wilson disease
  - Autosomal recessive disorder
  - Involves abnormal copper metabolism in the liver
- Hemochromatosis
  - Autosomal recessive disorder
  - Excessive absorption of iron, which leads to increased storage in the liver
  - More common in males (8:1 male:female ratio)

Table 15-2	Common Hepatotoxic Medications

Mimic viral hepatitis
Halothane
Isoniazid
Methyldopa
Phenytoin
Sulfonamides

Cholestasis
Anabolic steroids
Androgens (17α)

Fatty liver
Alcoholic hepatitis
Corticosteroids
Tetracyclines
Valproic acid

Other liver disease
Acetaminophen
Aspirin
Carbon tetrachloride

Infectious Disease
- Hepatitis B—see previous discussion
- Hepatitis C—see previous discussion

Chronic Cholestasis
- Primary biliary cirrhosis
  - Bile duct destruction of unknown etiology resulting in cholestasis.
  - Autoimmune basis of disease is suspected as 90% of patients have elevated antimitochondrial antibodies present in their serum.
  - This usually affects older patients and is rare in pregnancy.

Autoimmune Hepatitis (AIH)
Background
- Self-perpetuating hepatocellular inflammation of unknown etiology (35).
- More common in females than in males.
- Commonly seen in younger age groups.
- Thirty percent of patients present with cirrhosis (36).
- Patients may also have the diagnosis of Sjögren syndrome or ulcerative colitis (36).

Evaluation
History
Cirrhosis is a result of long-standing insult to the liver. Therefore, there should be a history of antecedent disease or problems. Patients may complain of malaise, fatigue, weakness, and/or anorexia. Pruritus is often present.

Physical
- Jaundice
- Ascites
- Ecchymoses or excessive bruising
- Hepatomegaly and splenomegaly
- Right upper quadrant pain and tenderness
- Hyperpigmentation of the skin
- Kayser-Fleischer rings on the cornea of patients with Wilson disease

Laboratory Tests
- Liver function tests will be abnormal.
  - Elevated bilirubin and transaminase levels
  - Elevated alkaline phosphatase and GGT
  - Abnormal coagulation studies
    - Prolonged PT and PTT
    - Prolonged bleeding time
    - Thrombocytopenia

Tests for Other Etiologies of Hepatitis
- Test for serum ceruloplasmin levels (less than 20 mg/dL) and urinary copper levels (greater than 100 µg) if Wilson disease is suspected.
- Antimitochondrial antibodies to evaluate for primary biliary cirrhosis.
- Serum iron levels if hemochromatosis is suspected.
- Increases in circulating antibodies, hypergammaglobulinemia, and serum transaminases are seen with autoimmune hepatitis (AIH).

Differential Diagnosis
- Diffuse liver disease
- Viral hepatitis
- AFLP
- HELLP

- Metastatic or multifocal cancer of the liver
- Vascular congestion of the liver
- ICP
- Cholelithiasis
- Disorders of bilirubin metabolism

Clinical Manifestations

Patient presentation ranges from asymptomatic liver disease to acute liver failure. With long-standing disease, an acute gastrointestinal bleed may signify esophageal varices. Hepatic encephalopathy is seen with liver failure.

Treatment

Medications

- Depends on cause of cirrhosis.
- Polyethylene glycol (PEG) alpha-interferon and ribavirin are used to treat hepatitis C but are contraindicated in pregnancy.
- Lamivudine is used to treat active HBV infection after 36 weeks of pregnancy.
- UDCA is used to treat patients with biliary cirrhosis.
- Prednisone and azathioprine are used to treat AIH and should be continued as needed during pregnancy.
- *D*-penicillamine or trientiral chelation therapy is the mainstay of therapy for Wilson disease and should be continued at lower doses during pregnancy as long as the disease process is controlled.
- Propranolol lowers portal pressures in patients with esophageal varices. Its use in pregnancy has been associated with fetal bradycardia and intrauterine growth restriction.
- Spironolactone and furosemide are used for ascites.
- Vitamin K.

Procedures

- Endoscopy
  - All pregnant patients with cirrhosis should have endoscopy, preferably prior to pregnancy, to evaluate for esophageal varices. Variceal banding, sclerotherapy, or balloon tamponade may be used in pregnancy for bleeding varices.
- Transjugular intrahepatic portosystemic stent shunting (TIPSS) may also be attempted to control bleeding varices (37).
- Abdominal sonography should be done early in pregnancy to screen patients for splenic artery aneurysms.
- Liver transplant is possible in pregnancy.

Complications of Maternal Portal Hypertension

- Complications occur in 30% to 50% of pregnant women with portal hypertension (5).
- Includes variceal hemorrhage, hepatic encephalopathy, hepatic failure, and splenic artery aneurysm.
- Bleeding occurs in 20% to 25% of patients with varices, especially if the patient has a history of a prior hemorrhage (4).
- Bleeding from esophageal varices occurs most commonly in the second trimester (5).
- Maternal straining should be limited in the second stage of labor if varices are present.

Hepatic Failure

- Occurs when there has been extensive hemorrhage and hypotension.
- Rupture of splenic artery aneurysm.
  - Sixty-nine percent rupture in the third trimester (5).
  - Presents with sudden pain and hypovolemic shock.
  - Historically, maternal and fetal mortality rates have been very high.
- Spontaneous bacterial peritonitis occurs rarely.

- Postpartum hemorrhage
  - Occurs in 7% to 26% of patients
  - Usually a result of a coagulopathy and thrombocytopenia

Patient Education
- There is a high rate of fetal wastage and spontaneous abortion (up to 33%).
- Risk of vertical transmission if hepatitis virus is involved.

Hepatic Vein Thrombosis (Budd-Chiari Syndrome)
Background
Definition
- Obstruction of the large hepatic veins causing congestion and necrosis of centrilobular areas of the liver

Etiology
- Myeloproliferative disorders are the most prevalent underlying condition (38).
- Hypercoagulable states have been associated with this process.
- Underlying acquired or inherited thrombophilia, especially factor V Leiden mutation (38).
- Oral contraceptive pill use and pregnancy are also common findings.
- Occasionally seen as part of HELLP syndrome.

Epidemiology
- Hepatic vein thrombosis is primarily seen in women.
- Survival rate of 87% was documented in a recent study (38).

Evaluation
History
- Right upper quadrant pain
- Sudden abdominal distention
- Pregnant or immediate postpartum period
- History of thrombophilia

Physical
- Sudden onset of painless ascites
- Hepatomegaly

Laboratory Tests
- Elevated alkaline phosphatase, aminotransferases, and bilirubin levels.
- Ultrasonographic pulsed-wave Doppler images of the liver is the best imaging modality.
- Liver biopsy is not specific.
- Abnormal coagulation studies.
- Percutaneous hepatic vein catheterization is diagnostic.
- Bone marrow evaluation is indicated if polycythemia is suspected.

Differential Diagnosis
- Thrombosis of the high inferior vena cava
- Venoocclusive disease
- Peliosis hepatitis
- Myeloproliferative disorders

Treatment
- Begin thrombolytics and diuretics.
- Medical management of ascites is difficult but should be attempted.
- Evaluate for thrombophilias and treat if necessary.
- Surgical shunting is possible but associated with high maternal morbidity and mortality rates.
- Successful liver transplant has been reported.
- Fetal outcomes are dependent on maternal outcomes.

Liver Transplant and Pregnancy
- Liver transplant is becoming more frequent and more successful. Increasing numbers of patients are becoming pregnant.
- Graft function is not affected by pregnancy.
- Pregnancy should be delayed 1 to 2 years after transplant so that immunosuppressive regimens can be stabilized (39).
- Risks associated with pregnancy in liver transplant patients:
  - Preterm labor and premature rupture of membranes
  - CMV infection
  - Worsening hypertension and preeclampsia
  - Rupture of splenic artery aneurysm
  - First-trimester abortion
  - Gestational diabetes
  - Higher cesarean section rate
- Liver transplant during pregnancy should be considered for patients with acute liver failure and otherwise poor survival.
  - Transplant surgery during pregnancy is complicated by increased risks of hemorrhage, infection, renal failure, and respiratory distress syndrome.
  - Most immunosuppressive drugs are relatively safe to use during pregnancy.

Gallbladder Disease
Key Points
- Gallbladder disease and its related problems are common in pregnancy and the postpartum period.
- Evaluation and treatment for the pregnant patient with gallbladder disease is essentially the same as for the nonpregnant patient.

Background
Gallbladder disease is a common problem in the adult population, and more common in females than in males. Pregnancy seems to be responsible for alterations in gallbladder function that may predispose the pregnant patient to the formation of gallstones. Gallbladder disease is the second most common indication for surgery during pregnancy (40).

Pathophysiology
- Increase in gallbladder volume and decrease in gallbladder emptying time mirror changes in maternal progesterone levels.
- Incomplete emptying of gallbladder during pregnancy increases risk of gallstone formation and biliary sludge.
- Hormonal effects of pregnancy (i.e., estrogen and progesterone) cause increased saturation of bile with cholesterol making it more lithogenic.
- Gallstones form when the concentration of cholesterol exceeds the ability of bile to keep it in solution (41).
- High rate of spontaneous resolution of gallstones during the postpartum period.

Etiology
Most authorities feel that the increasing levels of estrogen and progesterone during pregnancy are the basis for these problems.

Epidemiology
- Incidence of biliary tract disease is 0.05% to 0.3% during pregnancy (42).
- Asymptomatic gallstones are present on routine sonography of gallbladder in 3% to 11% of pregnant females (43).
- Gallstones are more common in multiparous patients.

Evaluation
- Sonography is the imaging modality of choice for diagnosing cholelithiasis in pregnancy.
- Abnormal liver function tests are also suggestive of disease.

Acute Cholecystitis

Background
- Pregnancy appears to be a predisposing factor to the development to cholelithiasis, and cholecystitis is becoming more common.
- Incidence of acute cholecystitis in pregnancy is increased and may be due to
  - Increasing prevalence of obesity
  - Marked dietary changes
  - Changes in ethnicity of population

Definition
- Inflammation of the gallbladder occurring acutely, often secondary to previously asymptomatic gallstones

Pathophysiology
- Occlusion of the biliary tract, most often due to cholelithiasis, with secondary inflammation and infection

Epidemiology
- Affects 5 to 8 patients per 10,000 births (44).
- More than 50% of patients will have a history of biliary colic (45).
- May present in any trimester.
- More common in American Indians and Mexican Americans.

Evaluation
History
- Sudden onset of nausea, vomiting, and colicky or stabbing pain in the right upper quadrant of the abdomen.
- Pain may be localized to the right flank, scapula, or shoulder.
- Intolerance to, or exacerbation of, symptoms with fatty food intake.

Physical
- The patient appears ill.
- Presence of Murphy sign (inspiratory arrest elicited when palpating right upper quadrant while asking the patient for deep inhalation) may be less common in pregnancy.
- Fever, tachycardia, and tachypnea may be present.
- May have guarding and/or rebound tenderness on abdominal exam.
- Jaundice may be severe.

Laboratory Tests
- Hyperbilirubinemia
- Elevated serum transaminases
- Elevated white blood cell count
- Cholelithiasis in the gallbladder, thickening of the gallbladder wall, or dilatation of the biliary tract on sonography

Differential Diagnosis
- Any cause of cholestatic jaundice
- Pyelonephritis
- Pancreatitis
- Appendicitis
- Peptic ulcer disease
- Ascending cholangitis
- Acute hepatitis
- Pneumonia

- Myocardial infarction
- Herpes zoster

Treatment
Medical Management
- Bowel rest
- Nasogastric suction in more severe cases
- Adequate pain relief
- Hydration with IV fluids
- Broad-spectrum antibiotics
- High rate of relapse in the pregnant patient who is treated medically

Procedures
- Cholecystectomy
  - Second most common surgical procedure during pregnancy.
  - Ideally should be performed in the second trimester.
  - Laparoscopic approach is safe during pregnancy.
- Percutaneous cholecystostomy may be used if surgery is contraindicated.
- Endoscopic retrograde cholecystopancreatography (ERCP)
  - Appears to be safe during pregnancy.
  - Fetal radiation exposure reported to be 310 mrads (±164 mrads) in one study (46).
  - Sphincterotomies, stent passage, and stone extraction have been done safely in pregnancy *but not without risks* (37).

Complications
- Gallstone pancreatitis
- Gallbladder perforation
- Sepsis
- Peritonitis
- Preterm labor
- Intrauterine fetal demise

Disease of the Pancreas
Key Points
- Pancreatitis in pregnancy is rare but deserves prompt evaluation and treatment.

Background
Basic pancreatic physiology is unchanged by pregnancy. The exocrine function of the gland is, however, increased. Insulin and glucagon secretion is increased to offset the diabetogenic effects of pregnancy. Serum amylase and lipid levels increase with gestational age.

Acute Pancreatitis
Background
- Affects 1 in 1000 to 1 in 10,000 deliveries (47).
- Incidence increases with gestational age.
  - Most common in late third trimester or postpartum.
- In pregnancy, there is a strong correlation with the presence of gallstones.
- Acute, severe pancreatitis in pregnancy has approximately a 25% mortality rate (45).

Definition
- An inflammatory, autodigestive process of the pancreas

Pathophysiology
- Inflammation of the pancreas due to release of pancreatic enzymes
  - Damages vascular endothelium, ductal and acinar cells.
  - Microcirculatory changes lead to increased vascular permeability and edema.
  - Inflammatory response can lead to necrosis and hemorrhage.

- May be acute or chronic.
- Symptoms may be mild or severe.
- Inflammatory process may involve surrounding tissue and/or organs.
- May become secondarily infected and form an abscess or develop a pseudocyst.

Etiology
- In pregnancy, 70% of pancreatitis is due to occlusion of the biliary tract by gallstones (48)
  - Possible damage from bile refluxing into pancreatic ducts
  - Possible damage from increased pressure within the ducts causing release of pancreatic enzymes
- Familial hypertriglyceridemia
  - Types I, IV, and V
  - Causes 4% to 5% of pancreatitis in pregnancy (49)
- ETOH abuse, although this is less frequent during pregnancy
- Hypercalcemia
- Medications
  - Diuretics
    - Thiazide
    - Furosemide
  - Salicylates
  - AIDS therapy
  - Drugs for inflammatory bowel disease
    - Azathioprine
    - Valproic acid

Evaluation
History
- Nausea and vomiting present in more than 70% of patients.
- Pain is located in midepigastric region and radiates to the back.
- Pain usually presents suddenly and is constant and severe.

Physical Exam
- The patient appears ill.
- Signs and symptoms of an acute abdomen.
- Signs of retroperitoneal hemorrhage in the area of the flank (Turner sign) or in the periumbilical area (Cullen sign) are present with hemorrhagic pancreatitis.
- Occasionally the patient may be jaundiced.
- Fever.

Laboratory Tests
- Elevated serum amylase and lipase levels
  - Amylase-to-creatinine clearance ratio may be more helpful in pregnancy.
  - Values do not necessarily reflect the severity of the disease in pregnancy (50).
- Leukocytosis
- Cholelithiasis on gallbladder sonography
- Inflammatory changes of the pancreas on CT scan or MRI
- Evidence of hypertriglyceridemia
  - Pancreatitis occurs when triglycerides greater than 2000 mg/dL (50).

Differential Diagnosis
- Peptic ulcer disease with or without perforation
- Cholelithiasis
- Acute cholecystitis
- Intestinal obstruction
- Renal colic
- Pyelonephritis

- Pancreatic neoplasm
- Appendicitis
- Aortic aneurysm

Clinical Manifestations

These patients can be critically ill and will often need to be cared for in an intensive care setting. Assisted ventilation and hyperalimentation are often needed before the patient recovers. Fetal well-being will depend on the acuity of the mother's illness and how well she responds to treatment, as well as the gestational age of the fetus.

Treatment

Medical Management

- Bowel rest.
- Adequate hydration with IV fluids to prevent hypovolemia.
- Monitor for metabolic changes.
  - Decreased calcium and magnesium levels
  - Hyperglycemia
  - Electrolyte abnormalities
- Total parenteral nutrition may be necessary in severe cases.
- Antibiotics if secondary infection is present.
- Adequate pain management.
- Ventilatory support may be necessary in severe cases.
- For treating hypertriglyceridemia, gemfibrozil has been reported to be safe and effective in pregnancy (51).

Procedure

- ERCP
- Cholecystectomy and common bile duct exploration if secondary to gallstones
- Endoscopic or percutaneous drainage of pseudocyst if greater than 5 cm (51)
- Induction of labor if patient is greater than 34 weeks' gestation may be considered.

Complications

- Hemorrhagic pancreatitis may lead to shock, pleural effusion, acute respiratory distress syndrome, ascites, and ileus.
- Hypocalcemia.
- Hypovolemia and shock.
- Hyperglycemia and subsequent nonketotic coma.
- Preterm labor.
- Recurrent pancreatitis.
- Formation of pancreatic pseudocysts.
- Maternal and/or fetal death.

Patient Education

- Patients with active or chronic liver, gallbladder, or pancreatic disease should receive appropriate assessment and counseling before conception.
- These patients need specific education that, except in selected conditions, hepatobiliary disease is rarely a contraindication to pregnancy.

REFERENCES

1. Stieger B, Geier A. Genetic variation of bile salt transporters as predisposing factors for drug induced cholestasis, intrahepatic cholestasis of pregnancy, and therapeutic response of viral hepatitis. *Expert Opin Drug Metab Toxicol.* 2011;7(4):411–425.
2. Benjaminov FS, Heathcote J. Liver disease in pregnancy. *Am J Gastroenterol.* 2004;99:2479–2488.
3. Pathak B, Sheibani L, Lee RH. Cholestasis of pregnancy. *Obstet Gynecol Clin N Am.* 2010;37:269–282.

4. Hay JE. Liver disease in pregnancy. *Hepatology.* 2008;47(3):1067–1076.

5. Sandhu BS, Sanyal AJ. Pregnancy and liver disease. *Gastroenterol Clin N Am.* 2003;32:407–436.

6. Williamson C, Hems CM, Goulis DG, et al. Clinical outcome in a series of obstetric cholestasis identified via a patient support group. *BJOG.* 2004;111:676.

7. Lee RH, Incerpi MH, Miller DA, et al. Sudden fetal death in intrahepatic cholestasis of pregnancy. *Obstet Gynecol.* 2009;113:528.

8. Martin JN, Rose CH, Briery CM. Understanding and managing HELLP syndrome: the integral role of aggressive glucocorticosteriods for mother and child. *Am J Obstet Gynecol.* 2006;195:914–934.

9. Barton JR, Sibai BM. Diagnosis and management of hemolysis, elevated liver enzymes, and low platelets syndrome. *Clin Perinatol.* 2004;31:807–833.

10. Martin JN, Rinehart B, May WL, et al. The spectrum of severe preeclampsia: comparative analysis by HELLP syndrome classification. *Am J Obstet Gynecol.* 1999;180:1373–1384.

11. Jamerson PA. The association between acute fatty liver of pregnancy and fatty acid oxidation disorders. *J Obstet Neonatal Nurs.* 2005;34:87–92.

12. Ibdah JA, Bennett MJ, Rivaldo P, et al. A fetal fatty acid oxidation disorder as a cause of liver disease in pregnant women. *N Engl J Med.* 1999;340:1723–1731.

13. Rajasri AG, Srestha R, Mitchell J. Acute fatty liver of pregnancy (AFLP)—an overview. *J Obstet Gynaecol.* 2007;27:237.

14. Steingrub JS. Pregnancy associated severe liver dysfunction. *Crit Care Clin.* 2004;20:763–776.

15. Tran TT. Hepatitis B: treatment to prevent perinatal transmission. *Clin Obstet Gynecol.* 2012;55(2):541–549.

16. Sorrell MF, Belongia EA, Costa J, et al. National Institutes of Health consensus development conference statement: management of hepatitis B. *Hepatology.* 2009;49:S4–S12.

17. Van Nunen AB, deMan RA, Heijtinh RA, et al. Lamivudine in the last 4 weeks of pregnancy to prevent perinatal transmission in highly viremic chronic hepatitis B patients. *J Hepatol.* 2000;32:1040–1041.

18. National Institute of Health (NIH). Management of hepatitis C [Review]. NIH consensus. *NIH Consens State Sci Statements.* 2002;19(3):1–46.

19. Su GL. Hepatitis C in pregnancy. *Curr Gastroenterol Rep.* 2005;7:45–49.

20. Plunkett BA, Grobman WA. Routine hepatitis C virus screening in pregnancy: a cost effective analysis. *Am J Obstet Gynecol.* 2005;192:1153–1161.

21. Polis CB, Shah SN, Johnson KE, et al. Impact of maternal HIV co-infection on the vertical transmission of hepatitis C virus: a meta-analysis. *Clin Infect Dis.* 2007;44(8):1123–1131.

22. Mast EE, Hwang LY, Sito DS, et al. Risk factors for perinatal transmission of hepatitis C virus (HCV) and the natural history of HCV infection acquired in infancy. *J Infect Dis.* 2005;192(11):1880–1889.

23. Centers for Disease Control and Prevention. Recommendation for prevention and control of hepatitis C virus (HCV) and HCV-related chronic disease. *MMWR Recomm Rep.* 1998;47(RR-19):1–39.

24. Castello G, Scala S, Palmieri G, et al. HCV related hepatocellular carcinoma: from chronic inflammation to cancer. *Clin Immunol.* 2010;134(3):237–250.

25. Mushawhar IK. Hepatitis E virus: molecular virology, clinical features, diagnosis, transmission, epidemiology, and prevention. *J Med Virol.* 2008;80:646–658.

26. Kumar A, Beniwal M, Kar P, et al. Hepatitis E in pregnancy. *Int J Gynecol Obstet.* 2004;85:240–244.

27. Labrique AB, Shigufta SS, Krain LJ. Hepatitis E, a vaccine preventable cause of maternal death. *Emerg Infect Dis.* 2012;9(18):1401–1403.

28. Khuroo MS, Kanrili S. Aetiology, clinical course and outcome of sporadic acute viral hepatitis in pregnancy. *J Viral Hepat.* 2003 Jan;10(1):61–69.

29. Fischler B, Lara C, Chen M, et al. Genetic evidence for mother to infant transmission of hepatitis G virus. *J Infect Dis.* 1997;176(1):281–285.

30. Paternoster D, Serena A, Santin M, et al. GB virus C infection in pregnancy: maternal and perinatal importance of the infection. *Eur J Obstet Gynecol Reprod Biol.* 2009;144(2):115–118.
31. Creasy RK, Resnik R, eds. *Maternal-Fetal Medicine: Principles and Practice.* 4th ed. Philadelphia: W.B. Saunders, 1999:1055–1056.
32. Cohen J, Powderly WG. *Infectious diseases.* 2nd ed. St Louis: Mosby, 2004:1169–1171.
33. Deepah J, James A, Quaglia A, et al. Liver disease in pregnancy. *Lancet.* 2010;375:594–605.
34. Feldman M. *Sleisenger and Fordtran's Gastrointestinal and Liver disease.* 7th ed. Philadelphia: Saunders, 2002:1462–1464.
35. Lee WM. Pregnancy in patients with chronic liver disease. *Gastroenterol Clin North Am.* 1992;21:889–903.
36. Khan S, Tudur Smith C, Williamson P, et al. Portosystemic shunts versus endoscopic therapy for variceal rebleeding in patients with cirrhosis. *Cochrane Database Syst Rev.* 2006;4:CD000553.
37. Murad SD, Plessier A, Hernandez-Guerra M, et al. Etiology, management, and outcome of the Budd-Chiari syndrome. *Ann Intern Med.* 2009;151(3):167–175.
38. Gandhi H, Davies N. Liver transplant and obstetrics. *J Obstet Gynaecol.* 2004;24:771–773.
39. Jabbour N, Brenner M, Gagandeep S, et al. Major hepatobiliary surgery during pregnancy: safety and timing. *Am Surg.* 2005;71:354–358.
40. Johnston DE, Kaplan MN. Medical progress: pathogenesis and treatment of gallstones. *N Engl J Med.* 1993;328(6):412–421.
41. Lu EJ, Curet MJ, Yasser Y, et al. Medical versus surgical management of biliary tract disease in pregnancy. *Am J Surg.* 2004;188:755–759.
42. Ko CW, Beresford SA, Schulte SJ, et al. Incidence, natural history, and risk factors for biliary sludge and stones during pregnancy. *Hepatology.* 2005;41:359–365.
43. Ramin KD, Ramsey PS. Disease of the gallbladder and pancreas in pregnancy. *Obstet Gynecol Clin North Am.* 2001;28:571–580.
44. Cunningham FG, Leveno KJ, Bloom SJ, et al., eds. *Hepatic, gallbladder, and pancreatic disorders. Williams obstetrics.* 23rd ed. USA: McGraw-Hill, 2010:1073.
45. Tham TCK, Vandervoot J, Wang RCK, et al. Safety of ERCP during pregnancy. *Am J Gastroenterol.* 2003;98:308–311.
46. Hernandez A, Petrov MS, Brooks DL, et al. Acute pancreatitis and pregnancy: a 10 year single center experience. *J Gastrointest Surg.* 2007;11:1623–1627.
47. Ramin K, Richey S, Ramin S, et al. Acute pancreatitis in pregnancy. *Am J Obstet Gynecol.* 1995;173(1):187–191.
48. Neill AM, Hackett GA, Overton C, et al. Active management of acute hyperlipidaemic pancreatitis in pregnancy. *J Obstet Gynaecol.* 1998;18:174–175.
49. Sharp HT. The acute abdomen during pregnancy. *Clin Obstet Gynecol.* 2002;45:405–413.
50. Saadi JF. Kurlander DJ, Erkins JM, et al. Severe hypertriglyceridemia and acute pancreatitis during pregnancy: treatment with gemfibrozil. *Endocr Pract.* 1999;5:33–36.
51. Eddy JJ, Lynch GE, Treacy DE. Pancreatic pseudocysts in pregnancy: a case report and review of the literature. *J Perinatol.* 2003;23:69–72.

16 Gastrointestinal Complications

Nicolette P. Holliday and David F. Lewis

KEY POINTS

- Most pregnant women have gastrointestinal (GI) complaints during pregnancy.
- The majority of pregnant women experience nausea, vomiting, and constipation.
- Many pregnant women experience symptoms of gastroesophageal reflux.
- Others have more serious GI problems.
- Health care providers must become familiar with treatment options for the minor complaints and be able to diagnose patients with serious pathologic conditions in order to optimize maternal and perinatal outcomes.

Nausea and Vomiting

Background

Most patients complain of mild to severe nausea and vomiting during the first and early second trimesters of pregnancy. Although the etiology remains unclear, rapidly rising human chorionic gonadotropin (hCG) and estrogen levels have been implicated.

Epidemiology

As many as 85% of pregnancies are accompanied by nausea and vomiting. The majority of these cases are self-limited and resolve spontaneously.

Evaluation

Physical assessment should include a complete abdominal examination.

Laboratory Tests

- Urinalysis will check for degree of dehydration (ketones, elevated specific gravity) and signs of a urinary tract infection (nitrite, leukocyte esterase).
- A chemistry panel is needed to detect and correct any electrolyte imbalances. The potassium concentration is especially important to note.
- Thyroid function tests (Free T_3, Free T_4, and TSH), while typically abnormal when there is nausea and vomiting of pregnancy, may be considered if a patient exhibits signs or symptoms of thyroid disease.
- Liver function tests along with amylase and lipase may also be abnormally elevated with nausea and vomiting of pregnancy. A hepatitis panel can be considered in refractory cases or with markedly elevated transaminases in order to rule out some infectious etiologies.
- Human chorionic gonadotropin is ordered to screen for possible molar pregnancy.
- Ultrasound is ordered to determine whether a molar or partial molar pregnancy exists and to assess for presence of multifetal gestation.

Diagnosis

Differential Diagnosis

Numerous illnesses present with nausea and vomiting (see Table 16-1).

Clinical Manifestations

In severe or refractory cases, it is extremely important to rule out possible pathologic processes.

Table 16-1	Differential Diagnosis for Nausea and Vomiting in Pregnancy
Acute appendicitis	
Bowel obstruction	
Food poisoning	
Hepatitis	
Hiatal hernia	
Hyperthyroidism	
Molar pregnancy	
Pancreatitis	
Peptic ulcer disease	
Pyelonephritis	
Renal colic	

Treatment

Diet

Encourage patients to eat frequent, small meals that are rich in simple carbohydrates (e.g., dry toast, crackers).

Medications

Results from the Cochrane database (1) concluded that most drugs used for treating nausea and vomiting during pregnancy are more effective than is placebo.

- Bendectin contains both vitamin B_6 (FDA class A) and doxylamine (FDA class A). Although it is not available in the United States due to medical–legal concerns, evidence indicates that both drug components appear safe and effective.
- Promethazine (Phenergan, FDA class C) and prochlorperazine (Compazine, FDA class C): Oral or rectal use has become very popular in the United States. Initial treatment favors rectal suppositories due to limited gastric absorption caused by emesis (2).
- Droperidol (Inapsine, FDA class C) represents a dopamine antagonist that is unresponsive to first-line therapy. Continuous infusion seems more effective in refractory cases (3).
- Meclizine (Antivert, FDA class B) and cyclizine (Marezine, FDA class B): These antihistamines are effective when given alone or in combination with vitamin B_6 in 80% to 90% of patients.
- The promoting agent metoclopramide (Reglan, FDA class B) accelerates gastric emptying.

Alternative Therapies

- Ginger (FDA class C): Some evidence suggests that ginger decreases nausea. No adverse effects have been reported (4).
- Acupressure: Pressure stimulates the PC-6 site. Large studies have failed to confirm the efficacy of acupressure.
- Sensory afferent stimulation: Transcutaneous nerve stimulation (TENS) of P6 on the wrist has been effective (5).

Complications

- Electrolyte imbalance, especially hypokalemia, may induce cardiac arrhythmias.
- Hypovolemia (severe) may lead to uteroplacental insufficiency.
- Weight loss accompanied by negative nitrogen balance can result in ketone production.

HYPEREMESIS GRAVIDARUM

Background

This manifests as severe nausea and vomiting with significant metabolic disturbances (6).

Etiology

Although the specific etiology is uncertain, hCG, estrogen, psychological factors, and certain personality traits are associated with hyperemesis gravidarum. Other suggested etiologies include thyrotoxicosis, serotonin anomalies, nutritional dysfunction, and *Helicobacter pylori* infections (7).

Epidemiology

The incidence of hyperemesis gravidarum is 1 in 200 pregnancies (0.5%). Women with a female fetus are more likely to have hyperemesis gravidarum, heavy ketonuria, and higher number of hospital admissions (8,9).

Evaluation

Laboratory

- Urinalysis: Specific gravity, urine ketones, and bilirubin evaluation. The specific gravity assesses hydration status of the patient, and bilirubin is used to evaluate for hepatitis and hemolysis.
- Serum electrolytes: Potassium and creatinine are especially pertinent.
- Hepatic functions: These tests evaluate for severe dehydration, and they are also elevated with hepatitis.
- Thyroid function tests in patients with signs or symptoms of hyperthyroidism may help rule out thyrotoxicosis (TSH is commonly suppressed in hyperemesis gravidarum).
- Fetal ultrasound: This is used to exclude molar or partial molar pregnancy and to assess for multifetal gestation.

Diagnosis

Differential Diagnosis

- Please see Table 16-2.

Clinical Manifestations

Hyperemesis gravidarum usually manifests between 4 and 10 weeks of gestation and is resolved by 20 weeks of gestation. It is usually well tolerated at its inception but leads to weight loss, dehydration, electrolyte abnormalities, and ketosis.

Treatment

If hospitalization is required, patients should remain NPO for 24 to 48 hours and have intravenous replacement of isotonic fluids containing dextrose. Electrolytes can be replaced intravenously as clinically indicated. After 48 hours, their diet can be slowly advanced from clear liquids to abundant undersized meals rich in simple carbohydrates, such as dry toast and crackers.

Medications

Data from the Cochrane database (1) indicated that most drugs used for treating nausea and vomiting during pregnancy were more effective than placebo.

- Bendectin is a combination of vitamin B_6 (FDA class A) and doxylamine (FDA class A). Although it is not available in the United States due to medical–legal concerns, evidence indicates that it is safe and effective.
- Promethazine (Phenergan, FDA class C) and prochlorperazine (Compazine, FDA class C) are used orally or rectally and are very popular in the United States. Rectal suppositories are recommended for initial treatment because of the lack of gastric absorption resulting from emesis.
- Droperidol (Inapsine, FDA class C) represents a dopamine antagonist that is unresponsive as first-line therapy. However, continuous infusion is effective for refractory cases.
- Theclizine (Antivert, FDA class B) and cyclinine (Marezine, FDA class B) are antihistamines that are effective alone or in combination with vitamin B_6 in 80% to 90% of patients.

Table 16-2	Commonly Used Antiemetics in Pregnancy			
Class	Generic name	Proprietary name	FDA rating	Dose
Piperazine antihistamine Derivatives	Buclizine	Bucladin	C[a]	50 mg PO q12h
	Cyclizine	Marezine	B	IM only: 50 mg q6h, prn
	Meclizine	Antivert	B[a]	25–50 mg PO q24h
Phenothiazine antihistamine derivatives	Chlorpromazine	Thorazine	C	PO: 10–25 mg q6h IM: 25 mg q4–6h Suppository: 50–100 mg q8h
	Prochlorperazine	Compazine	C	PO: 5–10 mg q8h IM: 5–10 mg q4h, max 40 mg/24 h Suppository: 25 mg q12h
	Promethazine	Phenergan	C[b]	PO: 25 mg q6h
Antihistamine	Diphenhydramine	Benadryl	B[b]	PO: 25–50 mg q6h
	Dolasetron	Anzemt	B	12.5 mg IV
SHT3 Antagonistic	Ondansetron	Zofran	B	PO: 8 mg PO b.i.d.–t.i.d. IV: 4–8 mg IV q8h
	Doxylamine	Unisom	A	Manufacturer recommends against use in pregnancy
Benzoquinolizine antihistamine	Benzoquinamide	Emete-con		Manufacturer recommends against use in pregnancy
Dopamine antagonist	Metoclopramide	Reglan	B[b]	PO: 10–15 mg q6h IM: 10 mg q6h IV: 10 mg q6h, given slowly over 1–2 min
Apomorphine antagonist	Droperidol	Inapsine	C[b]	IM or slow IV: 2.5–5 mg; use in intractable vomiting

[a]Manufacturer recommends against use in early pregnancy. See Chapter 24 for details of FDA rating categories.
[b]Manufacturer recommends use only if potential benefit justifies potential risk to fetus.
FDA, Food and Drug Administration.

- Promoting agents: Metoclopramide (Reglan, FDA class B) accelerates gastric emptying.
- Alternative therapies
  - Ginger (FDA class C): Some evidence suggests that ginger decreases nausea. Adverse associations have not been reported.
  - Acupressure: This treatment stimulates the PC-6 site with pressure, but numerous studies have not confirmed its efficacy.
  - Sensory afferent stimulation: TENS of P6 on the wrist has been effective (5).
- Ondansetron (Zofran, FDA class B): This agent is effective for refractory cases.
- Steroids: In some trials, limited courses of methylprednisolone have been effective.
  - This therapy remains controversial (6).
- Glycopyrrolate (Robinul, FDA class B): This agent is acceptable for patients with ptyalism.

Additional Therapy for Refractory Cases
- Enteral feedings: This option should be considered for patients with significant weight loss and inability to keep down food for 1 to 2 weeks or longer. It enables normal function of the intestines.
- Hyperalimentation: This may be necessary in certain cases to help maintain volume requirements and allow weight gain. This treatment requires placement of a central venous line, which increases the risk of systemic infection and other serious complications. Due to associated risks in pregnancy, this option is generally reserved for cases in which enteral feedings have been unsuccessful.
- Vitamins: Intravenous thiamine and multivitamin should be considered in patients unable to tolerate oral intake for 1 to 2 weeks or longer.

Complications
- Mallory-Weiss tear of esophagus.
- Diaphragmatic tear (10).
- Vitamin deficiency, including Wernicke encephalopathy (vitamin B deficiency).
- Renal damage resulting from hypovolemia.
- Intrauterine growth restriction, prematurity, and fetal death have been associated with these disorders (8).

GASTROESOPHAGEAL REFLUX DISEASE
Background
Definition
Reflux esophagitis or dyspepsia results in reflux of gastric contents into the esophagus.

Pathophysiology and Etiology
Relaxation of the esophageal sphincter due to elevated progesterone levels and increased intra-abdominal pressure from the expanding uterus are reasons that this condition complicates a large percentage of pregnancies.

Epidemiology
As many as 80% of Caucasian and 10% of African American women experience symptoms of gastroesophageal reflux at some point during pregnancy. The incidence of gastroesophageal reflux disease (GERD) is similar across all trimesters of pregnancy (11). There is a correlation with prepregnancy body mass index and GERD symptoms (12).

Evaluation
A history and physical should include careful examination of the chest and the abdomen. Symptoms include classical substernal or epigastric burning or pain that usually occurs after meals or when supine.

Diagnosis
Differential diagnosis includes cardiovascular pain (angina), pulmonary causes (pneumonia or pleuritic chest pain), and other etiologies of abdominal pain (cholecystitis, appendicitis, or other intra-abdominal processes). In the second and third trimesters, hemolysis, elevated liver enzymes, and low platelets (HELLP) syndrome or hepatic hematoma must also be considered.

Treatment
Medications
- Oral antacids such as Maalox or Mylanta decrease gastric acid levels and may be effective in mild cases.
- Histamine-2 (H-2) receptor antagonist (FDA class B drugs).
  - Cimetidine (Tagamet, FDA class B) has antiandrogenic activity, and it is recommended that other H-2 blockers be used initially.

- Ranitidine (Zantac, FDA class B). A dose of 150 mg twice a day appears to be effective.
- Famotidine (Pepcid, FDA class B). The dosage for GERD is 20 to 40 mg twice a day.
- Nizatidine (Axid, FDA class B). The usual dose is 150 mg b.i.d.
- Proton pump inhibitors (PPIs) (Omeprazole, FDA class C, Lansoprazole, FDA class B): These drugs control gastric secretions and are excreted in human milk. If used postpartum, breast-feeding should be avoided. Reserve the use of PPIs for cases refractory to H2 blockers because carcinogenic and adverse fetal effects have been reported in animal studies.

PEPTIC ULCER DISEASE (PUD)

Background

Definition

A peptic ulcer is an ulcerative area in the gastric lining. Evidence suggests that the incidence of peptic ulcer disease (PUD) is lower during pregnancy because of decreased gastric acid output and increased protective mucus production resulting from elevated progesterone levels. The incidence of PUD in pregnancy is quite low—this disorder complicates 1 in every 4000 pregnancies. The incidence may be actually higher because the diagnosis is difficult during pregnancy (13). Pregnancy is considered to be protective against PUD.

Pathophysiology

Excess acid production and the failure of mucus to protect the underlying mucosa are considered the primary causes. Risk factors include genetic predisposition, older age, smoking, excessive alcohol intake, and use of nonsteroidal anti-inflammatory drugs (NSAIDs) or aspirin. *H. pylori* has been also implicated as a causative agent, and it is present in 85% to 100% of duodenal ulcers (14).

Evaluation

History and Physical

Patients usually have long-term GERD. Symptoms suggestive of gastric ulcers include dull, epigastric pain that radiates to the back. Pain improves with eating or antacids. Duodenal ulcers result in sharp or burning epigastric pain.

Tests

During pregnancy, direct endoscopic evaluation is the most effective method to confirm PUD. If possible, radiographic evaluations should be avoided because of radiation exposure during an upper GI series.

Treatment

Medications

- Oral antacids such as Maalox or Mylanta decrease stomach acid with minimal GI absorption and are safe during pregnancy. Both of these drugs are magnesium-based antacids and are superior to the aluminum-based antacids that predispose patients to constipation. The dosage is 15 to 30 mL taken after each meal and at bedtime.
- H2 receptor antagonist (FDA class B drugs). Long-term safety has not been clearly established; however, these agents are commonly used in pregnancy. All four medications are labeled as probably safe in lactation as there is limited information in animals and/or humans demonstrating no risk/minimal risk of adverse effects to infant/breast milk production.
  - Cimetidine (Tagamet, FDA class B): Use other H2 blockers initially because cimetidine exerts antiandrogenic activity in some animal models.
  - Ranitidine (Zantac, FDA class B): A dosage of 150 mg b.i.d. appears to be effective.
  - Famotidine (Pepcid, FDA class B): The dosage for PUD is 40 mg/d.
  - Nizatidine (Axid, FDA class B): The usual dose is 150 mg b.i.d.

- Proton pump inhibitors (PPIs, FDA class C): Reserve the use of these for cases refractory to H2 blockers. These drugs control the gastric secretions. They have theoretical risks of carcinogenesis risk to the fetus based on animal studies. They should be reserved for cases in which the risk/benefit balance justifies their use.
- Sucralfate (Carafate, FDA class B): Inhibits acid adhering to mucosal ulceration. It may also stimulate local production of bicarbonate and inhibit the action of pepsin. This drug causes constipation and should be reserved for difficult cases.
- Antibiotic therapy: The combination of bismuth subsulfate and paired antibiotics has been proven to be efficacious in treating peptic ulcers with evidence of *H. pylori* infection. This treatment is recommended after delivery because the therapy has not been evaluated for safety in pregnancy.

Complications
Most patients with PUD during pregnancy improve. Complications are rare; however, bleeding, perforation, and obstruction can arise during pregnancy and must be considered. The risk of fetal loss is increased if these complications do occur. There is also an increased risk for low birth weight, small for gestational age infants, and preterm delivery (15). If significant ongoing bleeding from a gastric ulcer occurs, surgical treatment should be considered because of the risk of fetal mortality and maternal morbidity (16).

BOWEL DISEASE IN PREGNANCY
Gastroenteritis
Background
Definition
- Acute onset of diarrhea

Etiology
- Both viral and bacterial infections can cause this condition (see Table 16-3).

Evaluation
Signs and Symptoms
Symptoms include diarrhea associated with fever, abdominal pain and cramping, and bloody or mucoid stooling. During pregnancy, dehydration poses the greatest risk to the fetus.

Laboratory Tests
If diarrhea persists for more than 24 to 48 hours, consider workup, unless concerned about *Clostridium difficile*, and then initiation of testing should begin immediately.

Table 16-3	Acute Gastroenteritis
Variable	**Organism**
Bacterial infections	*Campylobacter jejuni*, *Escherichia coli*, *Listeria*, Salmonella species, Shigella species, *Yersinia enterocolitica*, *Vibrio parahaemolyticus*
Bacterial toxins	*Bacillus cereus*, *C. difficile*, *V. cholerae*, *E. coli*, *Staphylococcus aureus*
Protozoans	*Entamoeba histolytica*, *Giardia lamblia*, malaria species, *Toxoplasma gondii*
Helminths	Cestodes (hydatid, *Taenia*), nematodes (*Ancylostoma, Ascaris, Enterobius, Strongyloides*), Trematodes (*Schistosoma*)
Viruses	Cytomegalovirus, herpes, polio, others

- The absence of leukocytes in a stool smear suggests that a bacterial infection is unlikely.
- Stool culture for *Campylobacter*, *Salmonella*, *Shigella*, and enterotoxigenic *Escherichia coli*.
- A stool smear should be obtained to test for enteric parasites such as *Giardia* and *Amoeba*.

SPECIFIC BACTERIAL INFECTIONS

Campylobacter jejuni

This usually presents with bloody diarrhea, fever, abdominal pain, and tenesmus. These symptoms usually resolve within 5 days; however, they may persist for up to 4 weeks.

- Therapy: Hydration is the most important therapy. The symptoms usually spontaneously resolve, although erythromycin may shorten the duration of illness.

Vibrio cholerae

This is caused by drinking contaminated water.

- Therapy: The symptoms usually spontaneously resolve. Chloramphenicol therapy may be considered for severe cases. This drug is FDA category C. It crosses the placenta and has been associated with gray baby syndrome when used late in pregnancy.

Clostridium difficile

Background

Clostridium difficile colitis is usually due to an enterotoxin produced from overgrowth of the organism after antibiotic therapy and leads to pseudomembranous colitis. The symptoms normally present 4 to 10 days after antibiotic therapy but may persist for as many as 6 weeks after therapy.

Evaluation
Clinical Presentation
Watery diarrhea containing leukocytes and sometimes blood.

Diagnosis
Clostridium difficile enterotoxins can be detected in stool studies. The toxins can also be detected via PCR (highly sensitive and specific), EIA (enzyme immunoassay) for GDH (*C. difficile* gluatamate dehydrogenase), EIA for *C. difficile* toxins A and B, cell culture cytotoxicity assay (the gold standard), and selective anaerobic culture. The selective anaerobic culture is the most sensitive but does not differentiate between the toxin and nontoxin strains. Diagnosis can also be made by endoscopic or histologic findings of pseudomembranous colitis (17)

Treatment
Therapy
Vancomycin (FDA class B) is the drug of choice; alternative therapy includes metronidazole (FDA class B).

Escherichia coli

Results from consuming fecal-contaminated food or water. Two types of *E. coli* are detected: the first type is caused by endotoxins (Montezuma's revenge), whereas the second type results from local invasion of bowel mucosa.

- Therapy: Enterotoxin-derived infection does not require antibiotic therapy. Severe infection responds to aminoglycoside.

Salmonella

Salmonella is caused by consuming contaminated food. Typhoid fever is rare in the United States. Intra-amniotic and fetal infections are uncommon but have been reported with pregnancy loss.

Diagnosis
The usual presentation involves rash, fever, and leukopenia with bradycardia.

Therapy
Antibiotics such as chloramphenicol (FDA class C), ampicillin (FDA class B), trimethoprim–sulfamethoxazole (FDA class C), or ceftriaxone (FDA class B) should be reserved for severe cases. Chloramphenicol has been associated with "gray baby syndrome," which is rare (1 in 30,000 patients). This condition, though its existence is controversial, results from use of the drug at term, and the newborns have cardiovascular collapse. Most authorities recommend using chloramphenicol only as a last resort because of this risk.

Shigella

Caused by bacterial dysentery manifested by bloody, mucoid diarrhea.
• Therapy: Health care providers should avoid prescribing medications that inhibit bowel function. Consider using ampicillin (FDA class B) for severe infections, while recognizing that resistance frequently occurs. Consequently, treatment with chloramphenicol or trimethoprim–sulfamethoxazole may be necessary in the most severe cases.

Staphylococcus

Caused by consuming unrefrigerated dairy products. Usually self-limited and presents as explosive diarrhea accompanied by nausea and vomiting. Dehydration can be a significant problem in these patients.

INFLAMMATORY BOWEL SYNDROME

Inflammatory bowel disease (IBD) includes Crohn disease and ulcerative colitis. The incidence is 1 in 1000 pregnancies. This syndrome usually develops during the peak reproductive span of 15 to 35 years of age (18–21).

Both diseases are associated with rectal bleeding and diarrhea. Fertility does not appear impaired in patients suffering from IBD. Similarly, once pregnant, IBD patients do not appear to suffer increased pregnancy complications (premature birth, miscarriage, or congenital anomalies). Patients have a 30% chance of experiencing recurrent disease some time during pregnancy. This rate is comparable to that observed among nonpregnant populations. The effects of IBD on pregnancy are controversial. Some investigators (22,23) have found increased rates of preterm delivery in ulcerative colitis, whereas others (24–27) found no significantly increased perinatal morbidity. If an exacerbation of IBD complicates a pregnancy, there is an increased likelihood of miscarriage or preterm labor (28). Patients with active disease at conception tend to continue with symptoms during pregnancy while those who conceive while in remission tend to undergo a normal pregnancy course (29).

Crohn Disease (Regional Enterocolitis)

Background
Pathology
Pathologically, it is expressed by transmural involvement that encompasses the colon, small bowel, and rectum. Fistula formation is common, and the bowel usually has "skip" lesions (intermittent affected areas).

Etiology

The exact etiology of Crohn disease remains unknown; autoimmune, familial, and infections have been implicated.

Evaluation
Initial Presentation

Lower abdominal pain, low-grade fever, weight loss, and diarrhea are common findings, and there are often bloody stools. The clinical picture can be easily confused with appendicitis.

Diagnosis

The diagnosis can be difficult during pregnancy. The mainstay for diagnosis in a non-pregnant state is radiographic evaluation (lower GI series or sigmoidoscopy with direct biopsy). However, radiographic evaluations should be restricted during pregnancy, and sigmoidoscopy requires sedation and may be technically difficult to perform with uterine enlargement.

Treatment

Optimal treatment varies depending on disease severity. Mild disease can be treated medically with both antidiarrheal drugs and nutritional support. Severe disease requires the use of either steroids or immunosuppressive drugs, such as azathioprine or 6-mercaptopurine. The latter drugs should be reserved for the most severe cases. Augmentin is the preferred antibiotic if there are complications that require the use of antibiotics (29).

Complications

Preexisting Crohn disease does not alter perinatal outcome. However, new-onset disease during pregnancy may be associated with increased perinatal mortality. Vaginal delivery is not recommended if perineal fistula(s) is present. There is also a higher risk of antepartum hemorrhage—highest risk among those without a flare (30). Thus, careful prenatal evaluation should be completed in these patients in order to plan an appropriate delivery option.

Ulcerative Colitis
Background

Ulcerative colitis involves the large bowel and is more superficial than is Crohn disease. These ulcers are usually present in the descending colon, sigmoid, and rectum; they do not skip among segments like Crohn disease.

Etiology

The etiology of ulcerative colitis remains unclear; autoimmune, familial genetic predisposition and infection have all been implicated.

Evaluation
Clinical Presentation

Patients with ulcerative colitis usually present with abdominal pain, fever, cramping, bloody diarrhea, weight loss, and tenesmus.

Diagnosis

The diagnosis can be difficult during pregnancy. The mainstay for diagnosis in a non-pregnant state is radiographic evaluation (lower GI series) or sigmoidoscopy with direct biopsy. However, radiographic evaluations should be restricted during pregnancy, and sigmoidoscopy requires sedation and may be technically difficult to perform with uterine enlargement.

Treatment

Treatment includes antidiarrheal drugs, steroids, and sulfasalazine (FDA class B) in select cases. There also has been documented safe use of allopurinol therapy in pregnancy (31). Occasionally, proctocolectomy may be necessary for severe disease or complications.

Management

Inflammatory bowel disease is managed similarly in both pregnant and nonpregnant patients. However, special consideration should be given to the medications used because of their limited safety data for the fetus.

• Evaluate the causes of diarrhea and rectal bleeding.
• Rest the GI tract by maintaining strict NPO (excluding medications) for several days.
• If symptoms persist, initiate corticosteroid therapy. Steroids administered by retention enemas followed by oral prednisone are commonly employed. Rule out infections (both bacterial and parasitic) as an etiology before starting steroids. Sulfasalazine (FDA class B) can be given, if necessary. In acute exacerbations during pregnancy, both corticosteroids and sulfasalazine are given in high doses. These drugs appear safe to the fetus. Start intravenous hydration with isotonic solutions containing dextrose.
• Parenteral hyperalimentation may be needed in severe cases of IBD. Risk of severe complications of this therapy in pregnancy have been reported and should be considered.
• Occasionally, surgery is indicated in patients with IBD. However, advancing gestational age increases the technical difficulty of bowel surgery in pregnancy, especially the last trimester.

Medications

• Sulfasalazine (Azulfidine, FDA class B). The drug is metabolized to 5-aminosalicylic acid and sulfapyridine. Three to four gram dosages administered three to six times daily are commonly given. Sulfasalazine should be taken with meals, and extra folate supplementation should be initiated (29).
• 5-Aminosalicylic acid (mesalamine, FDA class B or olsalazine, FDA class C) can be given by itself. Usually, these drugs are better tolerated than sulfasalazine (class B). It may be used as initial treatment in mild to moderate disease or to prevent relapse. Specifically, in disease confined to the rectosigmoid areas, topical preparations are recommended (32).
• Infliximab (Remicade, FDA class B) can be used as well; however, it is usually discontinued at 30 weeks in quiescent patients to limit neonatal exposure (33).
• Corticosteroids appear to be safe during pregnancy, but higher doses more than 15 mg/d have been associated with increased risk of infection and premature delivery (29).
• Metronidazole (Flagyl, FDA class B) is used for the treatment of pouchitis (29)

Other immunosuppressive drugs such as cyclosporine, azathioprine, or 6-mercaptopurine are sometimes needed in severe cases of IBD (29). Both drugs may potentially cause problems during pregnancy; low birth weight and congenital anomalies have been reported in animal models. However, recent results from a small human study have failed to confirm these animal findings. The decision to use this drug should be made in consultation with the patient while explaining the potential risks and the absence of long-term follow-up data. Methotrexate and thalidomide are contraindicated in pregnancy (29).

Complications

Complications include toxic megacolon, strictures, and perforations. This disease does not alter the incidences of perinatal morbidity and mortality, and its clinical course is not affected by pregnancy. The risk of venous thromboembolism is increased in these patients (30).

PROTOZOAL ENTERITIS

Giardia lamblia

Caused by drinking contaminated or untreated water or fecal–oral transmission. This is the most commonly diagnosed protozoal infection in the United States.

- Symptoms: Can cause acute symptoms or chronic carrier state. The carrier state manifests itself by flatulence, epigastric pain, and loose stools.
- Diagnosis: Stool evaluations for cysts or trophozoites.
- Therapy: Metronidazole (Flaygl, FDA class B) is the drug of choice. The dosage is either 2 g/d for 3 days or 750 mg/d for 5 days. Metronidazole should be avoided in the first trimester due to possible teratogenicity.

Entamoeba histolytica

This protozoa causes amebiasis. Carriers include cats, dogs, rats, and humans, and infections are acquired by direct contact. Infections have a range of presentations from benign carrier state, severe diarrhea, and severe infection such as hepatic abscess or pulmonary involvement caused by violent strains usually from foreign countries.

- Diagnosis: Fresh stool examination for a cyst or trophozoites. Serologic examinations are also available.
- Therapy: Metronidazole (FDA class B) is the drug of choice. The usual dosage is 750 mg t.i.d. for 5 to 10 days. Chloramphenicol (FDA class C) is an alternative for resistant strains.

HELMINTHIC INFECTIONS

The most common infection and treatments are

Cestodes (Tapeworms)
- *Diphyllobothrium latum*—niclosamide, praziquantel, or paromomycin
- Echinococcus species—mebendazole
- Taenia saginata or Taenia solium—niclosamide

Nematodes (Roundworms)
- *Ascaris lumbricoides*—mebendazole
- *Ancylostoma duodenale* (hookworms)—mebendazole
- *Enterobius vermicularis*—pyrvinium pamoate, mebendazole
- Filaria species—mebendazole
- *Necator americanus* (hookworm)—mebendazole
- *Trichinella spiralis, Trichinella trichura*—mebendazole
- Trematoda (flatworms)—praziquantel

OTHER GASTROINTESTINAL PROBLEMS
Bariatric Surgery

Surgical procedures for alleviating morbid obesity are now relatively common. Pregnancy may occur following these procedures, and those pregnancy outcomes are comparable to those without bariatric surgery (34). Inadequate nutritional intake or absorption of iron, folate, calcium, vitamins A, B_{12}, and K may occur in these patients. Thus, proper supplemental nutritional and vitamin therapy are needed. These patients should not be given large glucose loads for gestational diabetes screening (glucose challenge test or glucose tolerance test). Fasting and 2-hour postprandial finger stick glucose monitoring may be an alternative screening approach for diabetes in these patients. After the Roux-en-Y procedure, there are reports of increased rates of cesarean section, preterm delivery, and neonatal death compared to pregnancy following laparoscopic adjustable gastric banding (35). Clinicians should maintain clinical suspicion for postoperative complications from this procedure including bowel obstruction and internal hernias (36,37).

Irritable Bowel Syndrome

Irritable bowel syndrome (IBS) is the most commonly diagnosed GI condition and is characterized by altered bowel habits and abdominal discomfort without organic disease. IBS is associated with an increased risk of miscarriage and ectopic pregnancy but not association with preeclampsia or intrauterine fetal demise (38).

Lactose Intolerance

Some adults are intolerant to lactose. This condition occasionally results in nutritional problems during pregnancy due to decreased calcium intake. Oral calcium supplementation is recommended at a dosage of 1200 mg/d. Lactose intolerance presents as abdominal cramps accompanied by watery diarrhea. Patients complain of pain and clinically have increased intestinal peristalsis.

Gluten Allergy/Sensitivity

Celiac disease is an autoimmune disorder associated with production of antiendomysium which is an antibody against human tissue tranglutaminase. Women with celiac disease have a shorter reproductive period with later menarche and earlier menopause (39). With undiagnosed celiac disease, women have an increased risk for miscarriage, intrauterine growth restriction, low birth weight babies, preterm birth, and cesarean section compared to patients who receive treatment for celiac disease (39–41). On the other hand, there has been no link to increased neural tube defects, preeclampsia, ectopic pregnancy, and postpartum hemorrhage (39). Of note, the severity of the celiac disease does not relate to the outcome of pregnancy, and the risks can be reduced after diagnosis and treatment (41,42).

Constipation

Constipation is a common problem during pregnancy. Similar to nonpregnant patients, increased fiber and fluid ingestion are important in the prevention and treatment of this common complaint. If necessary, the use of osmotic laxatives, which mobilize fluid into the intestines, is very effective. Examples include Miralax™ and milk of magnesia. Other medications such as the stool softeners Surfak and Colace are also effective.

PATIENT EDUCATION

- GI disorders are very common. Patients with these disorders should be identified, counseled, and treated appropriately prior to pregnancy if possible.
- Patients can be counseled that most GI disorders do not worsen during pregnancy with the exception of IBD.
- Particular attention should be given to proper management of nutrition, which requires patient education and continuous reinforcement.
- By promoting compliance with treatment and thus control of the underlying disease, patient education helps achieve optimal perinatal outcomes for these pregnancies.

REFERENCES

1. Jewell D, Young G. Interventions for nausea and vomiting in early pregnancy (Review). *Cochrane Database Syst Rev.* 2003;(4):CD 000145.
2. Hansen WF, Yankowitz J. Pharmacologic therapy for medical disorders during pregnancy. *Clin Obstet Gynecol.* 2002;45:136–151.
3. Nageotte MP, Briggs GG, Towers CV, et al. Droperidol and diphenhydramine in the management of hyperemesis gravidarum. *Am J Obstet Gynecol.* 1996;174:1801–1806.
4. Borrelli F, Capasso R, Aviello G, et al. Effectiveness and safety of ginger in the treatment of pregnancy-induced nausea and vomiting. *Obstet Gynecol.* 2005;105:849–856.
5. Evans AT, Samuels SN, Bertolucci LE. Suppression of pregnancy-induced nausea and vomiting with sensory afferent stimulation. *J Reprod Med.* 1993;38:603–606.

6. Eliakim R, Abulafia O, Sherer DM. Hyperemesis gravidarum: a current review. *Am J Perinatol.* 2000;17:207–218.

7. Davis M. Nausea and vomiting of pregnancy: an evidence-based review. *J Perinat Neonat Nurs.* 2004;18:312–328.

8. Veenendaal MV, van Abeelen AF, Painter RC, et al. Consequences of hyperemesis gravidarum for offspring: a systematic review and meta-analysis. *BJOG.* 2011;118(11):1302–1313.

9. Rashid M, Rashid MH, Malik F, et al. Hyperemesis gravidarum and fetal gender: a retrospective study. *J Obstet Gynaecol.* 2012;32(5):475–478.

10. Chen X, Yang X, Cheng W. Diaphragmatic tear in pregnancy induced by intractable vomiting: a case report and review of the literature. *J Matern Fetal Neonatal Med.* 2012;25(9):1822–1824.

11. Rey E, Rodriguez-Artalejo F, Herraiz MA, et al. Gastroesophageal reflux symptoms during and after pregnancy: a longitudinal study. *Am J Gastroenterol.* 2007;102(11):2395–2400.

12. Habr F, Raker C, Lin CL, et al. Predictors of gastroesophageal reflux symptoms in pregnant women screened for sleep disordered breathing: a secondary analysis. *Clin Res Hepatol Gastroenterol.* 2013;37(1)93–99.

13. Michaletz-Onody PA. Peptic ulcer disease in pregnancy. In: Gastrointestinal and liver problems in pregnancy. *Gastroenterol Clin North Am.* 1992;21:817–826.

14. Peterson WL. *Helicobacter pylori* and peptic ulcer disease. *N Engl J Med.* 1991;324: 1043–1048.

15. Chen YH, Lin HC, Lou HY. Increased risk of low birthweight, infants small for gestational age, and preterm delivery for women with peptic ulcer. *Am J Obstet Gynecol.* 2010;202(2):164. e1–e8.

16. Jones RF, McEwan AB, Bernard RM. Hemorrhage and perforation complicating peptic ulcer in pregnancy. *Lancet.* 1969;2:350–352.

17. LaMont JT, Calderwood SB, Baron EL. *Clostridium difficile* in adults: clinical manifestations and diagnosis. In: Basow DS, ed. *UpToDate.* Waltham, MA: UpToDate, 2013.

18. Korelitz BI. Inflammatory bowel disease in pregnancy. Gastrointestinal and liver problems in pregnancy. *Gastroenterol Clin North Am.* 1992;21:827–836.

19. Korelitz BI. Inflammatory bowel disease in pregnancy. Pregnancy and gastrointestinal disorders. *Gastroenterol Clin North Am.* 1998;27:213–223.

20. Botoman VA, Bonner GF, Botoman DA. Management of inflammatory bowel disease. *Am Fam Physician.* 1998;57:57–68.

21. Katz JA. Pregnancy and inflammatory bowel disease. *Curr Opin Gastroenterol.* 2004;20: 328–332.

22. Baird DD, Narendranathan M, Sandler RS. Increased risk of preterm birth for women with inflammatory bowel disease. *Gastroenterology.* 1990;99:987–994.

23. Fedor Kow KM, Persaud D, Nimrod CA. Inflammatory bowel disease: a controlled study of late pregnancy outcome. *Am J Obstet Gynecol.* 1989;160:998–1001.

24. Baiocco RJ, Korelitz BI. The influence of inflammatory bowel disease and its treatment on pregnancy and fetal outcome. *J Clin Gastroenterol.* 1984;6:211–216.

25. Nielsen OH, Andreasson B, Bordesen S, et al. Pregnancy in ulcerative colitis. *Scand J Gastroenterol.* 1983;18:735–742.

26. Porter RJ, Stirrat GM. The effects of inflammatory bowel disease on pregnancy: a case-controlled retrospective analysis. *Br J Obstet Gynaecol.* 1986;93:1124–1131.

27. Katz JA, Pore G. Inflammatory bowel disease and pregnancy. *Inflamm Bowel Dis.* 2001;7:146–157.

28. Hanan IM, Kirsner JB. Inflammatory bowel disease in the pregnant woman. *Clin Perinatol.* 1985;12:669–682.

29. Vermeire S, Carbonnel F, Coulie PG, et al. Management of inflammatory bowel disease in pregnancy. *J Crohns Colitis.* 2012;6(8):811–823.

30. Broms G, Granath F, Linder M, et al. Complications from inflammatory bowel disease during pregnancy and delivery. *Clin Gastroenterol Hepatol.* 2012;10(11):1246–1252.

31. Seinen ML, de Boer NK, von Hoorn ME, et al. Safe use of allopurinol and low-dose mercaptopurine therapy during pregnancy in an ulcerative colitis patient. *Inflamm Bowel Dis.* 2013;19(3):E37. doi: 10. 1002/ibd.22945.

32. Richter JM, Kushkuley S, Barrett JA, et al. Treatment of new-onset ulcerative colitis and ulcerative proctitis: a retrospective study. *Aliment Pharmacol Ther.* 2012;36(3):248–256.

33. Zelinkova Z, van der Ent C, Bruin KF, et al.; Dutch Delta Group. Effects of discontinuing anti-tumor necrosis factor therapy during pregnancy on the course of inflammatory bowel disease and neonatal exposure. *Clin Gastroenterol Hepatol.* 2013;11(30):318–321.

34. Sheiner E, Balaban E, Dreiher J, et al. Pregnancy outcome in patients following different types of bariatric surgeries. *Obes Surg.* 2009;19(9):1286–1292.

35. Dalfra MG, Busetto L, Chilelli NC, et al. Pregnancy and foetal outcome after bariatric surgery: a review of recent studies. *J Matern Fetal Neonatal Med.* 2012;25(9):1537–1543.

36. Wax JR, Pinette MG, Cartin A. Roux-en-Y gastric bypass-associated bowel obstruction complicating pregnancy-an obstetrician's map to the clinical minefield. *Am J Obstet Gynecol.* 2013;208(4):265–271.

37. Leal-Gonzalez R, De la Garza-ramos R, Guajardo-Perez H, et al. Internal hernias in pregnant women with history of gastric bypass surgery: case series and review of literature. *Int J Surg Case Rep.* 2013;4(1):44–47.

38. Khashan AS, Quigley EM, McNamee R, et al. Increased risk of miscarriage and ectopic pregnancy among women with irritable bowel syndrome. *Clin Gastroenterol Hepatol.* 2012;10(8):902–909.

39. Tata LJ, Card TR, Logan RFA, et al. Fertility and pregnancy-related events in women with celiac disease: a population-based cohort study. *Gastroenterology.* 2005;128:849–855.

40. Martinelli P, Troncone R, Paparo F, et al. Coeliac disease and unfavourable outcome of pregnancy. *Gut.* 2000;46:332–335.

41. Ludvigsson JF, Montgomery SC, Ekbom A. Celiac disease and risk of adverse fetal outcome: a population-based cohort study. *Gastroenterology.* 2005;129:454–463.

42. Ciacci C, Cirillo M, Auriemma G, et al. Celiac disease and pregnancy outcome. *Obstet Gynecol Surv.* 1996;51(11):643–644.

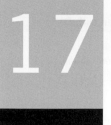

17 Endocrine Disorders: Diabetes

Margarita de Veciana, Arthur T. Evans and Nancy C. Lintner

KEY POINTS

- Screening for gestational diabetes mellitus (GDM) should be undertaken at 24 to 28 weeks' gestation. Patients at high risk for GDM (e.g., obesity, prior history of GDM or glucose intolerance, fetal macrosomia, history of polycystic ovarian syndrome, presence of glycosuria, strong family history of type 2 diabetes) should be screened at the first prenatal visit.
- Pregnant women with diabetes may experience periods of hyperglycemia, which can result in fetal hyperglycemia and hyperinsulinemia that is associated with excessive fetal growth and other morbidities.
- Poor glycemic control during early pregnancy (organogenesis) is associated with an increased risk for miscarriage. Congenital malformations occur two to four times more frequently in infants born to women with pregestational diabetes. Cardiac, central nervous system (CNS), and skeletal malformations are most common, but there are no malformations that are pathognomonic for diabetes.
- Preconceptional counseling and medical management should be offered to all patients with pregestational diabetes or glucose intolerance in order to optimize perinatal outcome with pregnancy.
- Women with diabetes complicated by vascular disease (especially nephropathy and retinopathy) are at greatest risk for poor perinatal outcome with an increased risk for preeclampsia, preterm delivery, and fetal growth restriction (FGR).

Background

Diabetes mellitus (DM) is the most common medical complication of pregnancy. It is a metabolic disorder characterized by hyperglycemia resulting from relative deficiency of pancreatic insulin production, limited insulin release in response to a carbohydrate (CHO) challenge, or impaired effect of insulin at the cellular level. Clinically, it manifests as hyperglycemia and increased fat and protein catabolism. This may result in ketosis, which progresses to ketoacidosis. Epidemiologic studies have shown that the prevalence of DM diagnosed among women of childbearing age has increased dramatically in the United States and that a substantial proportion of the population has undiagnosed DM, abnormal fasting glucose levels, or impaired glucose tolerance (1). The cause is multifactorial and includes genetic and environmental contributing factors.

White Classification of DM during Pregnancy

- The White classification was first proposed by Priscilla White, M.D. in 1932. This classification is only used during pregnancy and is based on the duration of diabetes and the secondary vascular and other end-organ complications (2). Although it is somewhat descriptive of risk and health status, it does not differentiate by underlying pathophysiology (Table 17-1).
- The American Diabetes Association Expert Committee categorizes patients by underlying pathogenesis (insulin-deficient type 1, insulin-resistant type 2, and GDM) (3).

Table 17-1	White Classification for Pregnant Women with DM

Class	Criteria
A_1	Gestational diabetes (GDM) not requiring insulin or oral agents
A_2	Gestational diabetes requiring insulin or oral agents
B	Onset at ≥ 20 y of age or duration of <10 y
C	Onset at 10–19 y of age or duration of 10–19 y
	No vascular disease
D	Onset at <10 y of age or duration of ≥ 20 y or any onset/duration but with background retinopathy or hypertension
F	Nephropathy (≥ 500 mg proteinuria per day at <20 wk of pregnancy)
H	Arteriosclerotic heart disease, clinically evident
R	Proliferative retinopathy or vitreous hemorrhage
T	Prior renal transplantation

- American Diabetes Association Classification (3)
  - **Type 1 diabetes** results from pancreatic β-cell destruction, usually leading to absolute insulin deficiency (previously known as insulin-dependent DM or juvenile-onset DM). These patients are prone to ketosis.
  - **Type 2 diabetes** may be variably expressed as
    - Insulin resistance with relative insulin deficiency or
    - An insulin secretory defect with insulin resistance (previously known as non–insulin-dependent DM or adult-onset DM)
    - Ketosis is unlikely except with severe illness.
    - Obesity, family history, and prior history of GDM are common clinical risk factors.
  - **Other specific types**
    - Genetic defects of the β-cell (e.g., maturity-onset DM of the young, MODY)
    - Defects in insulin action
    - Diseases of the pancreas
  - **Gestational diabetes** is any degree of glucose intolerance with onset or first recognition during pregnancy. The diagnosis is established by glucose tolerance testing.

Pathophysiology

Normal Maternal Glucose Regulation (2)

- **Maternal tendency to fasting hypoglycemia** between meals and overnight while fasting because the fetus continues to draw glucose from maternal bloodstream across the placenta. Peak postprandial blood glucose values rarely exceed 120 mg/dL at any time in normal pregnancy.
- **Relative insulin sensitivity** improves in the first half of pregnancy. This results in a 50% reduction from prepregnancy insulin requirements and results in increased insulin sensitivity.
- **Peripheral resistance to maternal insulin** increases due to placental hormones and cytokines (e.g., human placental lactogen, progesterone, prolactin, cortisol, and TNF-α), which progressively increase throughout the second and third trimesters. These cause changes in metabolism and blunt the effectiveness of insulin to lower blood glucose levels (4). This explains why gestationally induced DM is usually not clinically apparent until 24 to 30 weeks of gestation.
- **Increased pancreatic insulin release** (up to 50% greater by the end of pregnancy) results from maternal insulin resistance.

Fetal Metabolism

- The fetus depends on maternal glucose transported across the placenta as its primary energy source.
- Glucose is continuously transported across the placenta from mother to fetus by facilitated diffusion, whereas insulin does not cross the placenta in significant amounts in either direction (2).

- Fetal glucose levels are approximately 10 to 20 mg/dL lower than maternal (4). By 10 to 12 weeks of gestation, the fetal pancreas is able to produce and secrete both insulin and glucagon (5).
- When postprandial maternal glucose levels surge excessively, the consequent fetal hyperglycemia leads to episodic stimulation of the fetal pancreatic β-cells to produce excess amounts of insulin (fetal hyperinsulinemia).
- Fetal hyperinsulinemia may promote storage of excess nutrients and fetal macrosomia.
- Fetal hyperglycemia and hyperinsulinemia may have detrimental effects on fetal growth and well-being and are probably responsible for most of the complications incurred by infants of diabetic mothers (IDMs).

Maternal Risks

- With current DM management capabilities, avoidance of pregnancy is rarely recommended in women with pregestational diabetes who have achieved good glycemic control. There has been concern that pregnancy may accelerate the progression of diabetic vascular complications. The relative risk of these complications is directly related to the duration and severity of disease as well as to the degree of metabolic control. With aggressive management of DM, this risk, although increased, is acceptable and possibly no greater than that which would occur over the same 9- to 12-month period (2,6–9).
- Pregnancy may be relatively contraindicated in women with
  - Severe cardiovascular complications such as symptomatic coronary artery disease (50% maternal mortality rate) or uncontrolled chronic hypertension
  - Severe vascular complications from DM, for example, untreated proliferative diabetic retinopathy or significant renal impairment (serum creatinine greater than 3 mg/dL or creatinine clearance less than 50 mL/min)
  - Significant autonomic neuropathy, for example, intractable gastropathy
- Diabetic pregnancies are also at increased risk for various maternal obstetric complications such as
  - Accelerated chronic hypertension or preeclampsia
  - Preterm delivery
  - Maternal birth trauma with vaginal delivery or increased risk for cesarean delivery
  - Infectious morbidity (genitourinary tract, endometritis, wound infections)

Fetal Risks

- **Diabetic embryopathy** (spontaneous abortions and birth defects) occurs in the first 7 weeks of gestation.
- Etiology is probably multifactorial (10).
- Hyperglycemia in early pregnancy increases risk for spontaneous abortions (11,12). Women with tight glycemic control and normal glycosylated hemoglobin (HbA_{1c}) values in early pregnancy have a risk for miscarriage equivalent to that of patients without diabetes (2).
- Other potential teratogens synergistic with hyperglycemia include ketones, inhibitors of somatomedin activity, deficiency of myoinositol, accumulation of sorbitol, and reduced levels of arachidonic acid with overproduction of oxygen free radicals that leads to abnormalities in prostaglandin metabolism. This may result in embryopathy by disrupting the vascularization of developing tissues (13).
- Among the general population, the risk in pregnancy of a major birth defect is 1% to 2%. Among women with overt diabetes before conception, the risk of a fetal structural anomaly is increased up to eightfold. Congenital anomalies account for approximately 50% of the perinatal deaths in IDMs, but there is no anomaly that is pathognomonic for fetal exposure to maternal diabetes (14).
  - Two-thirds of anomalies involve cardiovascular (8.5 per 100 live births) or CNS (5.3 per 100 live births).
  - Anencephaly and spina bifida occur 13 to 20 times more frequently among IDMs compared to infants born to pregnancies not complicated by diabetes.

- ○ Genitourinary, gastrointestinal, and skeletal defect rates are also increased.
- ○ Small left colon syndrome (transient inability to pass meconium, which resolves spontaneously) is unique to IDMs.
- ○ The majority of cases of caudal regression syndrome (sacral agenesis) occur in IDMs. This syndrome consists of a spectrum of structural defects of the caudal region including incomplete development of the sacrum and to a lesser degree, the lumbar vertebrae (2).
- **Diabetic fetopathy** (predominantly growth and metabolic abnormalities) occurs in the second and third trimesters.
- **Fetal growth abnormalities:**
  - ○ **Fetal macrosomia** (fetal obesity, large for gestational age) is increased threefold in IDMs compared to controls. The fetal macrosomia occurring with DM is believed to be secondary to hyperglycemia (which results in fetal hyperinsulinemia) and various growth factors. Increased subcutaneous fat deposition and organomegaly (liver and spleen primarily) occur, whereas the head and brain remain normal in size. The disproportion in size of the fetal head and the body can result in a traumatic vaginal delivery complicated by shoulder dystocia and attendant risks (e.g., brachial plexus injury, clavicle/humerus fractures). Approximately 70% of fetal growth occurs in the third trimester. These complications may be associated with significant neonatal morbidity.
  - ○ **Fetal growth restriction** (FGR) and small for gestational age (SGA) may occur especially in women with underlying vasculopathy (retinal, renal, or hypertension) and may result from compromised uteroplacental blood flow. Concurrent hypertension and fetal structural anomalies may contribute to FGR/SGA.
- **Polyhydramnios** occurs presumably as a result of fetal osmotic diuresis associated with hyperglycemia.
- **Intrauterine death** risk may be related to fetal hypoxia, acidosis, or fetal cardiac arrhythmia particularly in the setting of diabetic ketoacidosis (DKA).
- **Neonatal metabolic abnormalities** are more likely with poor glycemic control (15).
  - ○ **Neonatal hypoglycemia** can lead to neonatal seizures, coma, and brain damage if unrecognized.
  - ○ **Polycythemia** is due to increased erythropoietin production and red blood cell hyperplasia. Polycythemia can lead to poor circulation and postnatal **hyperbilirubinemia.**
  - ○ **Hypocalcemia** is secondary to a functional hypoparathyroidism with unclear etiology.
- **Hypertrophic and congestive cardiomyopathies** may also occur and are thought to be secondary to fetal hyperinsulinemia. Episodic fetal hypoxia stimulated by hyperglycemia may lead to an outpouring of adrenal catecholamines and may result in fetal hypertension, cardiac remodeling, and hypertrophy (2).
- **Respiratory distress syndrome** or delayed fetal pulmonary maturity may also occur in pregnancies with poor glycemic control.
- **Childhood obesity** and **glucose intolerance** may occur later in life (16,17).

EVALUATION

Pregestational Diabetes and GDM Diagnosed Prior to 20 Weeks
Maternal Evaluation
- The history and physical should be comprehensive.
  - Refer to an ophthalmologist for retinal assessment if this has not been completed in the past 6 to 12 months.
- Initial laboratory tests/studies should include
  - Routine prenatal blood tests.
  - Complete metabolic panel (CMP) with baseline preeclampsia labs including liver function studies (some pregestational patients may have underlying fatty liver changes), BUN, creatinine, and uric acid.

- Thyroid function tests (thyroid-stimulating hormone [TSH], free T_4, and free T_3 if indicated) are indicated as up to 20% of patients with pregestational diabetes may have thyroid dysfunction. More recent data suggest that trimester-specific TSH cutoffs should be used to identify thyroid dysfunction during pregnancy (TSH >2.5 mIU/L in the first trimester, TSH >3.0 mIU/L in the second and third trimesters).
- Glycosylated hemoglobin (HbA_{1c}).
- Urine tests: urinalysis and culture, 24-hour urine collection for total protein and creatinine clearance. A microalbumin dip <30 mg or 24-hour total protein less than 300 mg and/or creatinine clearance greater than 60 mL/min are normal.
- EKG for women with pregestational DM >10 years' duration, >35 years of age, or for any patient with history or clinical symptoms of cardiovascular disease (including hypertension).
- Subsequent laboratory tests to consider include
  - Prenatal genetic screening options as otherwise indicated. This includes first-trimester early aneuploidy screening (11 to 14 weeks), Tetra marker analyte screening (15 to 20 weeks), and maternal blood–free fetal DNA screening. Maternal serum α-fetoprotein (MSAFP), unconjugated estriol (uE3), and inhibin A that are components of some second-trimester Down syndrome screening tests are significantly reduced in women with diabetes such that the MoM values must be adjusted. Maternal DM does not increase the risk for fetal aneuploidy.
  - Serial HbA_{1c} assessments every 4 to 8 weeks.
  - Repeat 24-hour urine collection in the second and third trimester if abnormal on initial evaluation (e.g., if the 24-hour total protein is greater than 300 mg or creatinine clearance is less than 50 mL/min) or if increased proteinuria is noted on urine dipstick evaluations.
- Common maternal complications to monitor on follow-up visits include
  - Hypertension (greater than 140/90 mm Hg)
    - Chronic if identified in the first 20 weeks' gestation
    - Possibly preeclampsia if identified in the latter part of pregnancy
  - Discovery of nephropathy, retinopathy, gastropathy, or neuropathy
  - Preterm labor +/– polyhydramnios
  - Increased risk for hypoglycemia and DKA

Fetal Evaluation
- **Growth and Development:**
  - Dating ultrasound to confirm gestational age as soon as possible.
  - Ultrasound at 11 to 14 weeks' gestation for nuchal translucency (if indicated).
  - Ultrasound at 18 to 20 weeks' gestation to evaluate fetal morphology.
  - Fetal echocardiogram at 22 to 23 weeks' gestation to exclude congenital heart disease.
  - Ultrasound at 28 to 32 weeks' gestation to assess fetal growth (macrosomia or FGR) and to assess amniotic fluid volume (polyhydramnios or oligohydramnios).
  - Ultrasound prior to delivery (38 weeks' gestation) for estimated fetal weight (EFW) may be helpful in delivery planning.
- **Fetal Well-Being:**
  - **Antenatal fetal testing** is recommended as surveillance for potential uteroplacental insufficiency and fetal compromise in diabetic pregnancies requiring insulin or oral agent therapy for glycemic control.
  - Fetal kick counts starting at 26 to 28 weeks' gestation.
  - Fetal testing options are contraction stress test (CST), nonstress test (NST), biophysical score (BPS), and modified biophysical profile (MBPP = BPS + amniotic fluid volume).
  - Testing should start no later than 32 to 34 weeks' gestation and should continue until delivery.
    - Fetal testing should be individualized. Patients with vasculopathy (e.g., class F, R, H, T) or who develop complications during pregnancy (e.g., hypertension, very poor glycemic control, or FGR) may benefit from fetal testing earlier in pregnancy (26 to 32 weeks).

- The following testing schemes are acceptable:
  - **CST** alternating with **MBPP** every 3 to 4 days (i.e., on a Monday/Thursday or Tuesday/Friday schedule) has been shown to be an effective method of fetal surveillance for diabetic pregnancies specifically. When CST is contraindicated, is not readily available, or yields an equivocal result, then BPS is an appropriate backup test.
  - **CST and BPS** alternating every 3 to 4 days.
  - **NST and BPS** alternating every 3 to 4 days.
  - **MBPP** alone every 3 to 4 days.
  - Note that the testing schemes of alternating NST/BPS or MBPP alone are most commonly used for class A_1, A_2, B, and C DM (e.g., diabetes without vascular complications).

Pregestational Diabetes
Maternal Evaluation
- A comprehensive history and physical should be performed.
- Initial laboratory tests should include
  - Routine prenatal blood tests.
  - HbA_{1c} should be considered if there is any question that DM may be long-standing and undiagnosed.
  - Twenty-four-hour urine collection for total protein and creatinine clearance.
  - Thyroid function tests (TSH and free T_4, plus free T_3 if indicated).
    - Baseline preeclampsia labs if patient has concurrent chronic hypertension.
- Subsequent laboratory tests to consider:
  - Serial HbA_{1c} assessments every 4 to 8 weeks can be helpful if compliance with dietary recommendations and self-monitoring of blood glucose (SMBG) is questionable.
  - CMP including liver function studies. This is of particular importance when using oral agent therapy in order to rule out underlying liver abnormalities.
- Serial prenatal assessments for
  - Preeclampsia
  - Preterm labor
  - Fetal growth disorders
  - Polyhydramnios

Fetal Evaluation
- **Growth and Development:**
  - Ultrasound at 28 to 32 weeks to assess fetal growth (LGA/macrosomia or SGA/FGR) and to assess amniotic fluid volume (polyhydramnios and oligohydramnios).
  - Ultrasound prior to the onset of labor for EFW may be helpful in delivery planning. However, EFW values have a variance of ±15% generally and potentially even greater for a macrosomic fetus.
- Antenatal fetal surveillance (using a similar testing scheme as outlined above):
  - GDM A_1 not requiring insulin or oral agents does not require testing prior to 40 weeks' gestation unless hypertension, polyhydramnios, or fetal macrosomia is present.
  - GDM A_2 requiring insulin or oral agents requires testing starting at 32 to 34 weeks' gestation.
  - Fetal kick counts should be encouraged starting at 26 to 28 weeks' gestation.

DIAGNOSIS
Overt Diabetes
- It is not unusual for undetected, pregestational diabetes to be diagnosed during pregnancy. Any woman with suspected DM when prenatal care begins should be tested immediately to establish the diagnosis. Glycosuria is common but not diagnostic nor necessary for the diagnosis.
- The IADPSG (International Association of Diabetes in Pregnancy Study Group) Guidelines states that any one of the following criteria establishes the diagnosis of pregestational DM during the first trimester (Table 17-2):

Table 17-2	Diagnosing Preexisting Diabetes during Pregnancy
Measure of glycemic control	**Consensus threshold (IADSPG)**
FPG	126 mg/dL ($\geq$7.0 mmol/L)
HbA$_{1c}$	$\geq$6.5% (DCCT/UKPDS standardized)
Random plasma glucose	200 mg/dL (>11.1 mmol/L) plus confirmation by FPG or Hb$_{A1c}$

Adapted from The International Association of Diabetes and Pregnancy Study Group (18).

- An early HbA$_{1c}$ of 5.7% to 6.5% or an FPG >92 mg/dL and <126 mg/dL is highly suspicious for "prediabetes" and should, preferably, have confirmation by two-step screening or managed as GDM.
- GDM diagnosed at less than 20 weeks' gestation should be managed as if there was known pregestational DM.
- The American College of Obstetricians and Gynecologists (ACOG) and the National Institutes of Health (NIH) Consensus Panel currently recommend the use of two-step screening and diagnostic criteria. Neither organization endorses the use of the one-step screening and diagnostic criteria recommended by the American Diabetes Association (ADA) and IADPSG.

Gestational Diabetes Mellitus (GDM)
- GDM, defined as "carbohydrate intolerance of varying degree of severity with onset or first recognition during pregnancy" (19), affects 1% to 10% of all pregnancies and accounts for about 90% of all patients with DM during pregnancy. Specific ethnic groups (Hispanic, African American, Native American, South or East Asian, or Pacific Island ancestry) are at significantly greater risk for GDM. The prevalence of GDM is increasing and varies in direct proportion to the prevalence of obesity and type 2 DM in any given population (19). The definition of GDM applies regardless of whether or not insulin is used for treatment. Importantly, the definition does not exclude the possibility that unrecognized glucose intolerance may have antedated pregnancy.

Screening and Diagnosis for GDM
- Screening for GDM is based on either universal or selective criteria.
- The cost-effectiveness of universal screening of all pregnant women for GDM has been widely debated.
- Selective screening based on historical risk factors alone may identify only 50% of all women with GDM depending on the prevalence of disease in the screened population.
- Selective screening for GDM is accomplished by screening only pregnant women at higher risk for GDM by the following characteristics (19):
  - Age greater than 25 years
  - Member of a racial or ethnic group with high prevalence of GDM
  - Body mass index greater than 25 kg/m^2
  - History of abnormal glucose tolerance
  - Previous history of adverse pregnancy outcomes usually associated with GDM
  - Known diabetes in first-degree relatives
- Two different protocols are presently advocated for the screening and diagnosis of GDM:
  - **The one-step diagnostic protocol** has been proposed by the World Health Organization (WHO) and IADPSG (18).
    - A 2-hour 75-g oral glucose tolerance test (OGTT) is performed with measurement of plasma glucose values at 1- and 2-hour postglucose challenge (unless FBG exceeds 92 mg/dL since this is diagnostic of GDM).
    - This protocol has the advantage of a single set of criteria for screening and diagnosis. However, the cost-effectiveness of this protocol has not been confirmed.

○ The patient should perform the test after fasting overnight for at least 8 hours. The current guidelines do not have any requirement for specific dietary preparation prior to the 2-hour 75-g OGTT.

○ The test is considered abnormal and diagnostic for GDM if any single serum glucose value meets or exceeds the following cutoffs (NIH 20, ADA 21):

Fasting plasma glucose (FPG) ≥92 mg/dL (5.1 mmol/L)
One-hour postchallenge ≥180 mg/dL (10.0 mmol/L)
Two-hour postchallenge ≥153 mg/dL (8.5 mmol/L)

○ The cutoff values are based on the Hyperglycemia and Adverse Pregnancy Outcomes (HAPO) study identifying a 1.75-fold increase for selected adverse neonatal outcomes (22). The HAPO study found associations between maternal hyperglycemia and increasing rates of LGA neonates, fetal hyperinsulinemia, neonatal hypoglycemia, and cesarean delivery. Single-step screening using the above cutoff values proposed by the IADPSG may identify a group of patients with "milder" glucose intolerance than those identified with the two-step protocol. It is important to note that the NIH Consensus Panel (2013) determined that there is insufficient evidence-based research to support using this protocol for routine screening at this time (20).

• **Two-step diagnosis protocol** is commonly used in North America and is endorsed by the American College of Obstetricians and Gynecologists (19) and the NIH Development Conference Statement (20). Note that the two-step approach was not developed to diagnose diabetes in pregnancy per se, but rather, to identify women "at risk" for developing diabetes later in life.

○ An initial 1-hour 50-g OGTT is performed.

○ No specific dietary preparation or fasting is needed, but it is advisable to instruct the patient to eat at least 3 hours prior to test administration to avoid false-positive results.

○ A universally agreed upon cutoff value for the 1-hour 50-g OGTT has NOT been established. Values of 135 and 140 mg/dL are most commonly used:

‒ A cutoff of 140 mg/dL has an 80% sensitivity, with 10% to 15% of patients requiring a 3-hour 100-g OGTT.

‒ A cutoff of 135 mg/dL has greater than 90% sensitivity, with 20% of patients requiring a 3-hour 100-g OGTT (2).

○ A 3-hour 100-g OGTT is recommended when the 1-hour 50-g OGTT is abnormal. In preparation for this test, the patient should be instructed to eat more than 150 g of CHO per day for 3 days and to fast for at least 8 hours prior to the test. The test is diagnostic for GDM if any two or more plasma glucose values meet or exceed the following thresholds (19,23):

Fasting plasma glucose ≥95 mg/dL (5.3 mmol/L)
One-hour postchallenge ≥180 mg/dL (10.0 mmol/L)
Two-hour postchallenge ≥155 mg/dL (8.6 mmol/L)
Three-hour postchallenge ≥140 mg/dL (7.8 mmol/L)

○ If the 1-hour 50-g OGTT is ≥190 mg/dL, there is limited value to proceeding with the 3-hour 100-g OGTT because more than 95% will be abnormal and a presumptive diagnosis of GDM should be made. Further testing is not required except to exclude a significantly elevated fasting glucose and possible immediate need for insulin therapy. The degree of abnormality on the initial 1-hour 50-g OGTT correlates directly with the risk of having an abnormal 3-hour 100-g OGTT (22).

○ For patients who cannot tolerate the OGTT, an alternative glucose load may be substituted (e.g., 18 Brach's jelly beans, 400 kcal mixed-meal tolerance test, or Polycose meal tolerance test). Patients with a history of gastric bypass surgery (Roux-en-Y)

are not always candidates for testing by OGTT as ingesting glucose may result in dumping syndrome. Alternatively, these patients should be evaluated by several days of glycemic profiling (pre- and postprandial glucose values) by SMBG values. GDM will be diagnosed by persistent hyperglycemia (greater than 30% or more if glucose values exceed target ranges).
  - Plasma glucose values should be obtained by venipuncture. The glucose meters that are currently available are quite accurate, but the validity of using capillary glucose values for screening and diagnosis has not been confirmed.
  - A patient should be classified as having GDM A_1 if euglycemia is achieved with nutrition therapy alone, as indicated by greater than 70% to 80% of SMBG values being within normal range. Requirement for additional therapy with insulin or oral agents is indicative of GDM A_2.

TREATMENT
Antepartum Management
Patient Counseling and Education
- Patients with DM, classes B to T, should be counseled regarding maternal–fetal risks. Referral to genetics for counseling should be considered for a significantly elevated first-trimester glycosylated hemoglobin (HbA$_{1c}$ ≥ 10%), exposure to potential teratogens (e.g., oral hypoglycemics, angiotensin-converting enzyme [ACE] inhibitors, angiotensin receptive blockers [ARBS], and cholesterol-lowering statins), or other usual obstetrical and medical indications.
- Team management goals should be reviewed:
  - Identification and roles of team members
  - Time commitments regarding appointments
  - Maternal–fetal testing required
  - Self-monitoring of blood glucose (SMBG)
  - Medication management
  - Nutrition management
  - Physical activity/exercise
  - Stress management
  - Communication with health care providers (contact person for emergencies)

Medical Nutrition Therapy (MNT)
- Medical nutrition therapy (MNT) is the mainstay of therapy for all patients with DM. Nutrition therapy will successfully optimize glycemic control in approximately 80% to 90% of patients with GDM. Unfortunately, there is limited evidence-based research to endorse one dietary plan versus another in the management of DM during pregnancy, and some have questioned the need for "low-carbohydrate diet" in the treatment of GDM (25). A registered dietitian (RD) should initiate MNT within 1 week of diagnosis and monitor the patient's progress.
- Meal plans should be individualized and adjusted by an RD experienced with diabetes and pregnancy depending on glycemic control documented by SMBG. Patients with unusual/erratic work hours should be encouraged to change to more predictable schedules if possible. Alternatively, insulin therapy (if applicable) and meal times should be customized to the woman's schedule. The importance of compliance with a repetitive daily schedule for meals and snacks cannot be overemphasized.
- Recommended daily intake (RDI) of calories ranges from 1800 to 2000 calculated as 30 to 35 cal/kg/d (ideal body weight, IBW). This should be divided into three groups as 40% to 45% carbohydrates, 20% to 30% protein, and 30% fat.
- Total caloric intake should be divided into three meals and three snacks per day spaced 2 to 3 hours apart. Midmorning, midafternoon, and bedtime snacks containing protein and carbohydrate (CHO) are essential to blunt the glucose surge that may occur after

meals. The adequacy of calories and CHO intake may be assessed by using daily prepran-dial urinary ketone levels if needed as well as by monitoring the patient's weight gain. Note that fasting ketonuria is common in pregnancy even in women without diabetes.

- A CHO counting meal plan for pregnancy is commonly utilized with at least 175 g/d.
- Concentrated sweets and added sugar should be eliminated from the meal plan. Foods with low glycemic index (e.g., complex carbohydrates with high fiber content) are prefer-able because this results in a slower rise in glucose levels after ingestion.
- Avoiding cereal with milk and fruit/fruit juice for breakfast and before lunch lowers post-prandial glycemic excursions and helps optimize morning and afternoon glycemic control.
- Avoiding foods with high fat content is advisable given that fat can lead to postprandial hyperglycemia by altering insulin sensitivity for several hours after a meal (25).
- Adding protein to all meals and snacks generally helps stabilize glycemic control.
- Weight management should be individualized in conjunction with an RD.
- Encouraged patients to keep a journal to record daily dietary intake.

Physical Activity/Exercise Recommendations
- Physical activity is a major determinant of glycemic control and insulin requirement.
- Regular daily activity (preferably 30 to 60 minutes after meals) can decrease insu-lin requirement by as much as 50%. Radical changes in daily activity levels should be avoided because this can adversely affect glucose control.
- During hospitalization, routine daily activity levels should be maintained if possible.

Glucose Monitoring
- Assessment of HbA$_{1c}$ levels every 4 to 8 weeks or at least each trimester during pregnancy may be helpful in evaluating overall glycemic control.
- SMBG is the standard of care for managing diabetes complicating pregnancy (2).
- Timing of SMBG must be individualized, but postprandial values have the strongest cor-relation with fetal growth (26–28). Women with GDM will often develop postprandial hyperglycemia before a rise occurs in fasting levels. Moreover, there is usually greater insulin resistance in the morning hours, and postbreakfast glucose levels are generally the first to exceed target range.
- Frequency of monitoring:
  - GDM:
    - Patients should test at least seven times per day initially: fasting and 1 or 2 hours after the start of breakfast, lunch, and dinner and prior to the evening snack. Most pregnant women will have a peak glucose at 1 to 2 hours after a meal, and this may vary by meal time and content. Recommendations for timing of postprandial glu-cose measurement are for either 1 or 2 hours after the start of the meal. One-hour postprandial measurement is frequently used because it is pragmatically difficult for many women to remember to perform SMBG 2 hours after a meal.
    - If glycemic control is achieved for more than 80% of the values with nutrition ther-apy alone, the frequency of SMBG may be decreased to every other day with con-tinuation of nutrition therapy for the remainder of pregnancy. Patients with more than 30% of recorded glucose values exceeding target values will require additional therapy with oral agent(s) or insulin to achieve euglycemia (see below).
  - Pregestational DM or GDM requiring medication therapy:
    - Daily SMBG by glucose values at fasting, preprandial, 1 to 2 hours after the start of each meal, and before the bedtime snack.
    - Preprandial glucose monitoring enables use of supplemental premeal insulin therapy to cover preprandial hyperglycemia and, at the same time, address excessive post-prandial glycemic excursions (see below).
    - For patients using intermediate or long-acting insulin, or oral agent(s), there is value in occasionally obtaining glucose values between 3:00 AM to 4:00 AM to assess for subclinical nocturnal hypoglycemia and resultant rebound fasting hyperglycemia (Somogyi effect).

- Target goals for glycemic control with SMBG should be established in order to optimize perinatal outcome. Although some controversy exists regarding appropriate target glucose values, most investigators supporting intensified monitoring during pregnancy recommend (2):
  - Fasting or preprandial and overnight glucose values of 60 to 99 mg/dL.
  - Peak postprandial glucose values of 100 to 129 mg/dL.
  - Mean daily glucose less than 110 mg/dL.
  - HbA_{1c} less than 6.0%.
  - Glucose levels in the 50 to 60 mg/dL range are acceptable for pregnancy, and values as low as 40 to 50 mg/dL are generally well tolerated in pregnant women with well-controlled DM. However, the long-term effects of recurrent hypoglycemic episodes have not been defined.
  - Target glucose levels may need to be less stringent for patients with unstable or poorly controlled diabetes, particularly those prone to persistent hypoglycemia or hypoglycemic unawareness.
- Women should keep a record of all glucose values (or utilize a memory-based glucose meter), the insulin or oral agent regimen, and information on other factors (e.g., dietary intake, physical activity, and illness) in a logbook. These data are necessary to optimize glycemic control and teach the patient recognition of factors that affect glycemic patterns.

Medications
Oral Agents
- The safety and effectiveness of oral agent therapy as an alternative to insulin in women with GDM failing nutrition therapy have not yet been confirmed; however, these agents are widely used in clinical practice.
- Oral agents should NOT be used during the first trimester of pregnancy for glucose control.
- At less than 20 weeks' gestation, insulin therapy is the standard management for DM whether preexisting or newly diagnosed. However, in the special circumstance of mild or intermittent hyperglycemia between 13 and 20 weeks' gestation, oral agents may be used to decrease the risk of hypoglycemia. A significant advantage of oral agent therapy is that it may improve patient compliance (see Table 17-3).
- Optimization of dietary intake is absolutely essential for the successful treatment with oral agents particularly with antihyperglycemic agents.
- Single or combined oral agent therapy is currently offered at several perinatal centers, and preliminary published reports are encouraging (2,29,31,32). Overall, women with GDM failing nutritional therapy have at least an 80% chance of achieving glycemic control with oral agent therapy.

Insulin
- Pregnant patients requiring insulin are treated with either multiple-dose injection (MDI) therapy or continuous subcutaneous insulin infusion (CSII) pump. For MDIs, either a split-dose insulin regimen or basal–bolus insulin regimen is selected combining rapid-acting analog insulin (lispro/Humalog or aspart/NovoLog) with intermediate-acting (Humulin N/Novolin N) or long-acting insulin (detemir/Levemir). CSII pump therapy uses only rapid-acting insulin (see Table 17-4).
- Insulin initiation dosage calculation for class A_2 GDM or class B diabetes entering pregnancy on oral hypoglycemics:
  - All patients taking oral hypoglycemic agents should immediately be transitioned to insulin therapy, preferably before conception. (A possible exception is Glucophage use in patients with PCOS and infertility.)
  - To calculate the initial 24-hour total daily dose (TDD) insulin requirement, the health care provider should use the patient's current weight and the number of weeks of gestation.

Table 17-3	Oral Agent Therapy			
Drug	Mode of Action	Usual starting dose (mg)	Maximum dose	Timing of dose
Glyburide	Sulfonylurea, hypoglycemic, increases insulin supply	2.5 mg qd or bid	20 mg/d, no more than 7.5 mg at one time	30–60 min before breakfast, after 10 PM
Acarbose	Antihyperglycemic, slows down carbohydrate absorption	25 mg po tid	300 mg/d	With first bite of a main meal
Glucophage	Insulin sensitizer, reduces gluconeogenesis	500 mg po bid or tid	2,550 mg/d	Take with meals

The insulin regimen is individualized based on the type of DM, glucose control, and gestational age. Insulin absorption is most effective when injected into the subcutaneous tissue in the **abdomen**. Table 17-5 includes dosing recommendations for women with DM1, DM2, and GDM A$_2$. If the patient is beginning insulin on an outpatient basis, consider reducing the starting dose by 10% (0.1 unit/kg).

After calculating the TDD, divide by 1/3; two-thirds of the insulin for the AM dose and one-third for the PM dose. For example, 60 units (TDD) = 40 units AM and 20 units PM. Two-thirds of the AM dose = 27 units of NPH (intermediate-acting) insulin and one-third of the AM dose = 13 units of Humalog/NovoLog (rapid-acting) insulin. Half of the PM dose = 10 units of Humalog/NovoLog with dinner and 10 units of Humulin N/Novolin N at bedtime.

SPLIT-DOSE INSULIN REGIMEN (TABLE 17-6)

BASAL–BOLUS INSULIN REGIMEN (TABLE 17-7)

INSULIN INJECTION SITES

The site of insulin injection can affect absorption and bioavailability. For optimal absorption, pregnant women inject insulin into the abdomen, avoiding a 2-inch radius around the navel. Site rotation is important to prevent lipohypertrophy and lipoatrophy. The arms, thighs, and buttocks may be used if the patient has abdominal lipohypertrophy and lipoatrophy. Physical activity/exercise will accelerate absorption from extremity injection sites.

- **Insulin adjustment guidelines:**
  - Manipulation of caloric intake, meal plan, schedule for meals/snacks, or changes in injection site may obviate the need for altering the insulin dosage.
  - If more than two doses of insulin are changed at any one time, a follow-up telephone contact should take place within 1 to 3 days. In general, changes in each insulin dose should be individualized with 10% to 20% increments.
  - If a patient experiences nocturnal hypoglycemia (less than 60 mg/dL), the evening regimen of rapid-acting and intermediate-acting insulin may be split to give the former before dinner and latter before the important bedtime snack.
  - The goal is to first achieve normal AM fasting values and then focus on the rest of the glucose profile.

Table 17-4 Commonly Prescribed Insulins during Pregnancy

Type	Example	Category	Onset	Peak	Duration	Appearance
Rapid-acting (analogs)	Humalog (lispro)	B	<15 min	1–2 h	4–6 h	Clear
Bolus or for meals	NovoLog (aspart)	B	<15 min	1–2 h	4–6 h	Clear
Short-acting	Apidra (glulisine)	C	<15 min	1–2 h	4–6 h	Clear
Short-acting (regular)	Humulin	B	½–1 h	2–4 h	6–8 h	Clear
Usually for IV use	Novolin		½–1 h	2–4 h	6–8 h	Clear
Intermediate-acting (NPH)	Humulin N	B	1–2 h	4–6 h	12 h	Cloudy
Basal insulin	Novolin N		1–2 h	4–6 h	12 h	
Long-acting (analog)	Lantus (glargine)	C	1.5 h	Flat, maximum effect 5 h	24 h	Clear
Basal insulin						
Long-acting (analog)	Levemir (detemir)	B	1 h	Flat, maximum effect 5 h	12–24 h	Clear
Basal insulin						

Intermediate-acting and long-acting insulins are usually given before bedtime (HS).
Lantus is generally not recommended for use in pregnancy.
Rapid-acting insulin (Humalog/NovoLog) is used in the CSII pump.

Table 17-5	Calculating Split-Dose Weight-Based Insulin
Weeks of gestation	**TDD**
Week 1–18	0.7 unit/kg
Week 18–26	0.8 unit/kg
Week 26–36	0.9 unit/kg
Week 36–40	1 unit/kg
For obesity >150% of DBW	1.5–2 unit/kg
Week 0–6 postpartum	0.4 unit/kg
Calculate TDD as above (kg = maternal weight in pounds/2.2)	

- Fasting hyperglycemia may result from inadequate levels of insulin to cover the caloric intake from the previous night, the Somogyi effect, or the dawn phenomenon.
  - **Somogyi effect** is a hypoglycemic episode in the early morning (1:00 AM to 6:00 AM) that results in rebound hyperglycemia and an elevated prebreakfast glucose value. Assessment of 2:00 AM to 4:00 AM glucose values is necessary for diagnosis.
  - If nocturnal hypoglycemia is identified, patients should have the evening dose of intermediate- or long-acting insulin reduced. Delaying NPH administration until bedtime may help minimize nocturnal hypoglycemia. Otherwise, the caloric intake (especially protein) at the bedtime snack may be increased.
  - If nocturnal hypoglycemia is not identified, then increase the evening dose of intermediate- or long-acting insulin to lower the fasting glucose value.
  - The **dawn phenomenon** describes a period of insulin resistance that occurs as the day begins in the early morning (4:00 AM to 7:00 AM). This is characterized by prebreakfast fasting hyperglycemia and is probably caused by an exaggerated growth hormone or cortisol effect in conjunction with the morning waking process. Treatment involves cautious use of early morning (3:00 AM to 6:00 AM) rapid-acting insulin or, for patients using a CSII pump, a temporary increase in basal rate may blunt the rapid rise in glucose before breakfast. Late-evening NPH may also be helpful in these circumstances.
- If a postprandial glucose is elevated greater than 120 mg/dL despite a normal preprandial glucose level, the premeal rapid-acting insulin dose should be increased by 10% to 20%.
- The morning intermediate (NPH) or long-acting (Levemir) insulin will affect the pre- and postprandial lunch and predinner glucose values.
- The morning rapid-acting insulin will affect mostly the postbreakfast and to a lesser extent the pre- and postlunch glucose values.
- The predinner rapid-acting insulin will primarily affect the postdinner and bedtime glucose values.

Table 17-6	Split-Dose Pathway

Split-Dose Insulin Regimen
Total daily insulin dose (TDD)

2/3 TDD prebreakfast | 1/3 TDD evening

2/3 NPH mixed with 1/3 Rapid Acting analog Prebreakfast | 1/2 Rapid Acting analog Predinner | 1/2 NPH Prebedtime

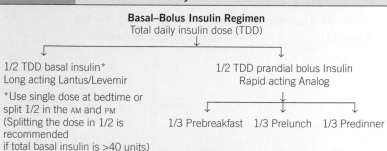

Table 17-7   Basal–Bolus Pathway

Basal–Bolus Insulin Regimen
Total daily insulin dose (TDD)

1/2 TDD basal insulin*
Long acting Lantus/Levemir

*Use single dose at bedtime or split 1/2 in the AM and PM (Splitting the dose in 1/2 is recommended if total basal insulin is >40 units)

1/2 TDD prandial bolus Insulin
Rapid acting Analog

1/3 Prebreakfast   1/3 Prelunch   1/3 Predinner

- Women with pregestational DM using CSII pumps will require more individualized management and adjustment of insulin basal rates and bolus doses with meals and snacks. Preprandial hyperglycemia can usually be corrected by increasing insulin basal rates (U/h) unless insufficient insulin was administered to normalize the postprandial glucose level with the previous meal. Postprandial hyperglycemia can be controlled by administering more insulin with the preprandial bolus by decreasing the insulin to CHO ratio (ICR), for example, changing from 1:15 to 1:10 (units/g).
- **Insulin corrections using supplemental rapid-acting insulin scale (SRAIS):**
  - For patients with pregestational DM (or GDM A$_2$ diagnosed during early pregnancy), use of an SRAIS will help optimize glycemic control more rapidly. Ideally, the amounts of insulin required to cover preprandial hyperglycemia ($\geq$100 mg/dL) should be incorporated into the split-dose or basal–bolus insulin regimens once there is a clear pattern of repetitive need for a supplemental correction dose.
  - Each time the fasting or preprandial glucose is measured, the patient should refer to the SRAIS and determine whether additional insulin is needed. This is done whether or not a scheduled insulin dose is needed (i.e., at lunchtime).
  - Before the bedtime snack or between 10:00 PM and 6:00 AM, only half of the indicated supplemental insulin dose should be given. In patients prone to nocturnal hypoglycemia, overnight dosing with rapid-acting insulin should probably be avoided.
  - Standardized sliding insulin scales have been used for many patients without taking into consideration the variable insulin sensitivity from one patient to the other (see Table 17-8). Instead, an individualized premeal adjustment scale should be developed for each patient based on the patient's TDD using the following formula:
    ○ One unit of insulin expected to lower a patient's blood glucose level by X mg/dL
    ○ For example, if a patient's calculated TDD insulin is 100 units (insulin resistant)
    ○ 1500/100 units = 15 mg/dL:
    ○ Add 1 unit of rapid-acting insulin for every 15 mg/dL above premeal target of 100 mg/dL
  - If a patient's calculated TDD insulin is 60 units (i.e., more insulin sensitive):
    ○ 1800/60 units = 30 mg/dL.
    ○ Add 1 extra unit of rapid-acting insulin for every 30 mg/dL above premeal target of 100 mg/dL.
  - When a consistent pattern for additional SRAIS is identified over a several days, the additional amount of insulin can then be added to the prescribed daily dose (e.g., 1 unit additional Humalog insulin at lunch is converted to 1 unit additional Humalog insulin with the morning dose; 1 unit additional Humalog insulin before dinner is

Table 17-8	Premeal Insulin Dose Adjustment Algorithm

For preprandial hyperglycemia correction using Humalog/NovoLog

BG (mg/dL)	Humalog/NovoLog (Units)
<100	0
100–140	2
141–160	3
161–180	4
181–200	5
201–250	6
251–300	8
>300	10

Use during the day only *BEFORE* breakfast, lunch, and dinner.
Use half the premeal insulin dose *BETWEEN* 10:00 PM to 6:00 AM.
DO NOT USE THIS ALGORITHM TO TREAT BLOOD GLUCOSES BETWEEN MEALS TO AVOID STACKING INSULIN

From de Veciana M, Evans AT. Chapter 17: Endocrine disorders: diabetes. In: Evans AT, ed. *Manual of obstetrics.* 7th ed. Philadelphia: Wolters Kluwer/Lippincott Williams and Wilkins, 2007.

converted to 1 unit additional of intermediate-acting (NPH) insulin or long-acting (Levemir) insulin with the morning dose or long-acting daily insulin).
- Postprandial hyperglycemia should not be covered in pregnancy unless values exceed 180 mg/dL to avoid "stacking insulin" increasing the risk for hypoglycemic reactions between meals.
- **Hospitalization for glycemic control optimization should be considered when:**
  - Organogenesis is taking place (prior to 7 to 8 weeks' gestation) if glycemic control is not optimal.
  - Patients fail outpatient dietary and insulin management despite education and reported compliance (e.g., fasting glucose values greater than 120 mg/dL; 1-hour postprandial values greater than 160 mg/dL). Continuous insulin infusion (CII) should be considered until good control is achieved for a period of 24 hours.
- **Continuous intravenous insulin infusion (CII) for inpatient antepartum glycemic control** should be considered for patients admitted with persistent hyperglycemia despite MDIs.
  - Calculate the antepartum ratio of total daily caloric intake to total daily insulin (e.g., 2000 calorie diet and 40 units insulin correspond to 1 unit of insulin per 50 calories).
  - Estimate the caloric intake for the time span of the infusion (nothing by mouth on 5% D/1/2 normal saline at 125 mL/h × 24 hour = 3 L = 150 g glucose).
  - Calculate the insulin dose required to cover the estimated caloric intake and then determine the rate of insulin infusion per hour.
  - Infusion rates are generally 0.25 to 3.0 units/h. Rates calculated at more than 5 units/h should be rechecked. Some advocate starting an infusion rate of 1.0 unit/h empirically and titrating up or down as needed.
  - A separate peripheral 5% dextrose solution is used with CII for hydration and caloric and potassium supplementation; the suggested solution is 5% dextrose in 1/2 normal saline at 125 mL/h.
  - Preparation of a CII solution: 100 units regular insulin is added to 1000 mL normal saline (1 unit regular insulin per 10 mL normal saline).
  - The plasma glucose should initially be monitored hourly, and the CII rate adjusted up or down as needed to achieve target glucose levels initially and euglycemia ultimately.

- If a patient is placed on an oral diet while on the CII, the hourly rate must be adjusted with the meal or snack to cover the insulin bolus for the CHOs. Calculate the number of CHO to be ingested and calculate the units of additional insulin needed to cover the meal intake. Then, divide this insulin bolus over 1 to 3 hours (based on complexity of calories) and add this dose to the basal insulin infusion rate starting with the meal. After the meal bolus, the CII rate is reduced back to a maintenance level based on glucose values.
- A computer-directed algorithm (e.g., the Glucommander) is available for CII infusion management. This computerized program takes into consideration the patient's response to the insulin infusion (i.e., insulin sensitivity) and calculates the appropriate adjustments to the insulin infusion rates. This computerized approach has been demonstrated to be a safe and effective method for glycemic control in pregnant and nonpregnant patients even in the setting of DKA (43).
- **Continuous Subcutaneous Insulin Infusion (CSII) Pump (programmable) (44)**
  - CSII pumps infuse rapid-acting analog insulin (lispro/Humalog or aspart/NovoLog) by means of a catheter placed into the subcutaneous tissue in the abdomen. The pumps are programmable on an hourly basis to infuse insulin as units per hour over a 24-hour period. Multiple basal rates are generally necessary during each 24-hour period to achieve optimal glucose management during pregnancy. The TDD of insulin consists of all basal insulin administered as units per /hour and all units of bolus insulin needed to cover meals and as correction doses for elevated glucose levels over a 24-hour period.
  - CSII pump therapy has become increasingly affordable and is covered by most insurance carriers.
  - There are limited data that CSII pump therapy is clearly superior to MDI therapy during pregnancy. However, extensive literature validates the benefits of CSII pump therapy particularly in patients with type 1 DM who are poorly controlled and prone to repetitive and persistent episodes of hypoglycemia.
  - Ideally, CSII pump therapy would be initiated prior to conception, but initiation during pregnancy with adequate supervision is acceptable and encouraged.
  - Good candidates for CSII pump therapy include highly motivated patients with a history of repetitive and persistent hypoglycemia or hypoglycemia unawareness, labile glycemic control despite compliance with medical therapy, gastropathy/hyperemesis with unpredictable glucose intake, extreme insulin sensitivity (TDD less than 25 units), and erratic work schedules (e.g., occasional night shifts).
  - For example: calculate the TDD (60 units); multiply 60 units × 0.5 = 30 units; divide 30 units by 24 hours for the third basal rate = 1.25 units/h; multiply the third basal rate (1.25 units/h) by 0.8 for the first basal rate = 1 unit/h; multiply the third basal rate (1.25 units/h) by 1.2 for the second basal rate = 1.5 units/h. Calculate the correction factor by dividing 1700 by TDD (60 units) = 28 units. Calculate the I:C ratio, divide 500 by the TDD (60 units) = 1 unit of insulin to 8 g CHO (1:8) (see Table 17-9).
  - **Continuous glucose monitoring (CGM) sensor devices** (which measure glucose levels from the interstitial tissues 288 times per day) can be used in conjunction with CSII pump therapy and have been integrated into some insulin pump systems. These devices enable the patient to constantly be aware of whether glucose levels are rising, steady, or falling. Pregnant women will be excellent candidates for the evolving CGM technology.
- **Illness.** When a pregnant woman with DM feels ill, experiences nausea and vomiting, or cannot tolerate the prescribed meal plan, she should be instructed as follows:
  - Discontinue the scheduled mixed-insulin or long-acting regimen until she can resume the CHO counting meal plan.

Table 17-9	CSII Pump Calculation for Pregnancy
1. Obtain TDD of multiple daily injections (MDIs) (all types of insulin)	Amount of MDIs of insulin over 24 h MDI TDD × 0.75 = _____TDD
2. Reduce MDI TDD by 25% when switching from MDIs to CSII	
3. To calculate TDD units/kg:	Wt calculated TDD =
a. Prepregnant: × 0.6 unit/kg	
b. Week 1–18: × 0.7 unit/kg	
c. Week 18–26: × 0.8 unit/kg	Current wt in kg × units/kg =
d. Week 26–36: × 0.9 unit/kg	Total units/24 h
e. Week 36–40: × 1 unit/kg	
f. Week 0–6 postpartum: × 0.4 unit/kg	
4. Choose the lower of the two TDD amounts for the rest of the calculations	Final TDD
5. Use 50% of TDD as total daily basal insulin	TDD × 0.5 = total daily basal insulin
6. To start the pump, the total daily basal insulin is divided into 3 basal rates with the third basal rate calculated as TDD divided by 24 h being the key value:	
a. The first basal rate is from 12 MN to 3:00 AM and equals third basal rate × 0.8.	
b. The second basal rate is from 3:00 AM to 8:00 AM and equals third basal rate × 1.2.	
c. The third basal rate is from 8:00 AM to 12 MN and equals TDD divided by 24 h.	
7. Correction factor (sensitivity factor)	1700 divided by the TDD = correction factor
8. Insulin-to-carbohydrate (I:C) ratio	
a. Grams of carbohydrate that 1 unit of insulin will cover	500 divided by the TDD = I:C ratio
b. Usually about 60% of the TDD during pregnancy	
After the first trimester, the ratio often changes to 60% bolus and 40% basal insulin due to the increasing insulin resistance associated with CHO intake.	

- Discontinue the meal plan until she feels well enough to resume. Increase fluid intake with water, clear broth, decaffeinated tea, or diet soda to prevent dehydration. If fluids are not tolerated, the woman should contact her physician or diabetes nurse specialist immediately.
- Continue to check glucose levels at the regularly scheduled times if fluids are tolerated. If PO fluids are not tolerated, monitor glucose levels more frequently (every 1 to 2 hours if necessary).
- Use the SRAIS to give rapid-acting insulin if glucose values exceed 100 mg/dL; the goal is to keep the levels close to 100 mg/dL.
- Ingest 4 oz of juice (15 g) or multiple Life Savers (10 cal each) if glucose values are less than 60 mg/dL. Glucagon should be used only if the patient becomes disoriented or unresponsive (see below).
- Be aware that recurrent hyperglycemia or hypoglycemia, as well as persistent significant ketonuria requires hospitalization. It takes an experienced patient with trained family members to handle an episode of significant illness at home.
- Watch for signs of DKA, as this requires hospitalization. Unlike in the nonpregnant patient, DKA may rarely occur in pregnancy with glucose levels as low as 200 mg/dL.

HYPOGLYCEMIA MANAGEMENT

Symptoms

- **Symptoms** of hypoglycemia include hunger, headache, sweating, weakness, tremulousness, nausea, numbness, blurred or tunnel vision, confusion, stupor, loss of consciousness, coma, and seizure. Pregnancy may exacerbate hypoglycemia unawareness. Episodes of hypoglycemia fall into one of these three categories based on severity:
  - Symptomatic but alert and oriented
  - Symptomatic with disturbed mental function (drowsy, lethargic, and disoriented)
  - Comatose, obtunded, or otherwise seriously disoriented

Guidelines
- **Guidelines for treating hypoglycemic episodes are as follows:**
  - Immediately, measure a fingerstick blood glucose (FSBG) level using a glucose meter.
  - Administration of glucose for treatment for hypoglycemia should occur when the patient is symptomatic and glucose value is less than 50 mg/dL. If greater than 50 mg/dL, the FSBG level should be rechecked in 10 to 15 minutes to confirm that the glucose level is rising.
  - If the patient is vomiting, minimally responsive, confused, or unconscious, glucagon (one vial intramuscular [IM] or intravenous [IV]) should be administered immediately. Onset of action is within 5 minutes. The unconscious patient should be turned on her side because she may experience emesis as consciousness returns. Glucagon is preferred over IV administration of D10 or D50 during pregnancy. This peptide hormone is more physiologic and has less propensity for subsequent rebound hyperglycemia. There may also be a less dramatic change in fetal glucose levels associated with glucagon use, theoretically making glucagon safer for the fetus.
  - If the patient is able to take glucose orally, fruit juice (4 ounces or a half cup) is preferred (grape, apple, or orange, in this order of preference). Glucola or glucose tablets may be substituted for fruit juice if the patient prefers. Foods such as milk, peanut butter crackers, cheese and crackers, or whole fruit have less readily available glucose (more complex carbohydrates and protein) and should not be used to treat an acute hypoglycemic reaction because of slower absorption and less rapid effect on the blood glucose. These foods will produce a more delayed and prolonged rise in the blood glucose and tend to overshoot the physiologically desired glucose range.
  - The glucose level should be rechecked within 10 to 15 minutes based on the patient's symptoms and response to the glucagon (or oral glucose).
  - Repeat small amounts of juice may be administered as necessary. The goal of treatment is to give just enough glucose to make the patient euglycemic (60 to 100 mg/dL) and not hyperglycemic.
  - An appropriately trained person should remain with the patient until she becomes fully conscious, stable, and euglycemic.
  - Large amounts of IV glucose should not be given except in the most unusual circumstances where the patient has been given such a large amount of insulin that the glucose level continues to drop despite the initial treatment.
  - Glucagon has the opposite effect of insulin. This hormone raises the blood glucose level by rapidly releasing glycogen stored in the liver and is used to counteract severe hypoglycemic reactions resulting from insulin when the women is unable to take calories orally. All women with insulin-requiring DM should have a glucagon kit at home/work, and family members/coworkers should be instructed on how to use the kit.

PREGNANCY MONITORING

- Maternal antepartum care should remain unchanged from the routine prenatal care for uncomplicated pregnancies with diet-controlled GDM. Outpatient visits should be scheduled every 1 to 3 weeks until 32 to 34 weeks and then weekly unless specific complications arise.

- Patients requiring oral agent(s) or insulin therapy for management of diabetes (GDM or pregestational DM) should have glycemic control assessed at least every 2 weeks until 32 to 34 weeks and weekly thereafter.

INTRAPARTUM MANAGEMENT

- In planning the timing and route of delivery for the pregnancy, the goal is to minimize maternal and neonatal morbidity while maximizing the likelihood for a vaginal delivery of a fully mature infant. Delivery earlier than 39 weeks proportionately increases the risk of neonatal respiratory distress and failed labor induction, while delivery closer to 40 weeks (the actual estimated date of delivery [EDD]) increases the risks of macrosomia, birth injury, and intrauterine fetal death. Note that after 37 weeks, the increase in fetal weight may be as much as 100 to 150 g/wk (2).

Timing of Delivery

- The optimal time for delivery for most patients with DM is between 39 and 40 weeks' gestation (2).
- Patients with GDM A_1 should be delivered at or proximal to the EDD unless there are extenuating circumstances for continuing the pregnancy (e.g., unfavorable cervix without fetal macrosomia and with reassuring antepartum fetal surveillance). Fetal surveillance should then be started as outlined above.
- Patients with well-controlled class A_2, B, C, and D diabetes should be allowed to progress to 39 weeks before delivery if possible. Selection of the exact gestational age for delivery depends on the certainty of pregnancy dating, glycemic control, cervical ripeness, and fetal status (well-being and size). Routine induction at 39 weeks does not appear to increase the risk of cesarean section and may reduce the risk of macrosomia.
- Patients with class F, R, H, T diabetes, poor glycemic control, or pregnancy complications (pregnancy-induced hypertension, intrauterine growth restriction, etc.) may be able to wait until 39 weeks for delivery, but this decision should be carefully individualized to their specific clinical situation with earlier delivery if indicated.
- Elective delivery at less than 39 weeks' gestation requires confirmation of fetal pulmonary maturity by amniocentesis. This does not apply to early delivery for specific obstetric or fetal indications (2). If pulmonary studies are not mature and the pregnancy is stable with optimal glycemic control, delivery may be delayed for another week and fetal lung status reevaluated. In well-controlled diabetic pregnancies, standard fetal lung maturity (FLM) indexes are considered valid. Otherwise, the presence of phosphatidylglycerol (greater than 3%) should be required.
- Use of regional anesthesia intrapartum is acceptable. A non–glucose-containing IV solution (normal saline or lactated Ringer solution) is preferable for the routine preanesthesia fluid bolus in order to avoid an inadvertent glucose load.

Route of Delivery

- **Vaginal delivery** is the preferred route if the fetus is vertex and not macrosomic by ultrasound evaluation immediately before the date of delivery. Induction of labor per standard protocols with cervical ripening and IV Pitocin is acceptable.
- **Cesarean section** is indicated for the usual obstetric indications.
  - The risk for shoulder dystocia in the general population is 0.3% to 0.5% of vaginal deliveries (2). Fetuses of diabetic pregnancies have a two to four times greater risk for "shoulder dystocia." This is due to the combination of normal head size with the increased chest and abdominal circumferences, with excessive fetal weight gain secondary to persistent hyperglycemia. This risk may be as high as 23% in deliveries of fetuses weighing ≥4000 to 4999 g. The shoulder dystocia risk increases substantially (up to 50%) if fetal weight is ≥4500 g.

- With suspected macrosomia in DM pregnancies, many advocate elective cesarean deliveries to avert the risk of shoulder dystocia. The decision regarding the appropriate route of delivery should be individualized for each patient.
- Sonographic EFW values have a variance of ±15%. In morbidly obese patients, the variance may be greater.
- The use of prophylactic peripartum antibiotics may be warranted particularly in the obese patient due to the increased risk of infection with DM.
- **Trial of labor after cesarean** (TOLAC) should be offered if the patient meets the usual criteria for TOLAC and macrosomia is not suspected.
- **External breech version** may be considered with stable DM. However, β-sympathomimetic tocolytics for uterine relaxation are relatively contraindicated because of the risk of hyperglycemia.

Insulin Management for Labor or Cesarean Section

- **Term spontaneous labor:**
  - After midnight on the day of delivery, all split-dose or basal–bolus insulin regimens should be discontinued. The patient should be NPO and monitor glucose values as if she were feeling ill, covering with rapid-acting insulin as needed.
  - Women using a CSII pump should be hospitalized for management at the onset of labor. The pump may be continued during labor, but infusion rates should be decreased by at least 50% and often to the lowest overnight basal rate. Placement of the pump infusion set on the upper part of the abdomen prevents the set from becoming dislodged during labor. Insulin requirements typically decrease dramatically after delivery of the placenta and postpartum.
    - ○ **Early labor.** Women should be instructed to drink fluids and sip fruit juices instead of the regular CHO counting meal plan. Hospital admission is indicated with the onset of labor for women with diabetes.
    - ○ **Latent-active labor.** Once hospitalized, the diabetic parturient should receive nothing by mouth (NPO) except for ice chips. IV fluid should be administered at 100 to 125 mL/h. The type of fluids should be chosen according to glycemic status. An optimal range for maternal FSBG values during labor should be 70 to 110 mg/dL (18).
- **Day before elective delivery.** The patient should follow the prescribed meal plan and insulin regimen the day before delivery. However, if injecting long-acting insulin (e.g., Levemir), this should be discontinued the day before delivery because of its prolonged action.
- **Day of induction of labor (IOL):**
  - ○ Overnight cervical ripening with a plan for serial IOL is acceptable. The patient should be NPO after midnight the night before the induction.
  - ○ The usual insulin regimen should be discontinued after midnight. Patients with a CSII pump may keep the device in place, but the infusion rate should be reduced and bolus settings adjusted as needed. Patients with a CGM device should be encouraged to place a new sensor the day prior to admission preferably in a location away from the lower abdomen (in case a cesarean section is necessary). The CGM device can obviate the need for frequent intrapartum fingerstick glucose values when readings are stable.
  - ○ A fingerstick glucose level should be measured at 6:00 AM and every 1 to 2 hours during IOL (or up to every 4 hours in stable diet-controlled GDM patients).
  - ○ If glucose values exceed 110 mg/dL, continuous IV insulin infusion (CII) (mixed in normal saline) should be initiated or basal rate adjustments should be made to the CSII pump if indicated.
  - ○ Urine ketones should be checked every 1 to 2 hours. If significant ketonuria (≥2+) is noted, IV fluids with glucose are started along with CII, and the capillary glucose level should be maintained at 70 to 110 mg/dL.

○ Routine IV fluids should be administered as normal saline or other non–glucose-containing solutions. Insulin should not be added to the routine IV fluids.

○ Labor should be induced using a standard oxytocin (Pitocin mixed in normal saline or lactated Ringer solution) induction protocol.

○ Inductions lasting more than 2 days should be avoided in patients with diabetes.

• **Day of elective cesarean section**

• NPO after midnight prior to surgery.

• The usual MDI insulin regimen should be discontinued after midnight. Patients using CSII pumps may drop the basal infusion rates 50% after midnight. Insulin pump bolus settings for Insulin to Carbohydrate ratio and Insulin sensitivity factor should also be adjusted at this time to account for the anticipated increased insulin sensitivity which will result intra- and postpartum.

• A fingerstick glucose level should be measured at 6:00 AM and every 1 to 2 hours until delivery.

• If glucose values exceed 110 mg/dL, CII should be initiated and adjusted each hour as needed until delivery occurs. CSII pump users may optimize intrapartum glycemic control by adjusting basal rates as needed.

• Surgeries should be scheduled early in the morning if possible to avoid prolonged periods without oral intake prior to hospital admission.

• Intrapartum CII should be considered (using the same protocol suggested for antepartum management) if glucose values are persistently greater than 110 mg/dL.

POSTPARTUM MANAGEMENT
Class A$_1$ GDM

• Monitor glucose levels after delivery with a fasting and 1-hour postprandial capillary glucose value when the patient has resumed a regular diet.

• Most patients will have normal glucose values in the immediate postpartum period.

• If glucose values are normal at discharge, a plasma fasting glucose level should be checked at 6 to 8 weeks postpartum.

  • **Fasting plasma glucose.** An FPG of less than 110 mg/dL (6.1 mmol/L) is normal in the nonpregnant state. A level of greater than 125 mg/dL (6.9 mmol/L) or a random plasma glucose of >200 mg/dL (11.1 mmol/L) on two occasions confirms the diagnosis of overt diabetes in the nonpregnant woman (3). A level of 110 to 125 mg/dL (6.1–6.9 mmol/L) suggests impaired fasting glucose, and a 2-hour 75-g OGTT is indicated for definitive classification.

  • **Two-hour 75-g OGTT.** A 2-hour glucose value less than 140 mg/dL (7.8 mmol/L) is normal. A patient with a 2-hour value >200 mg/dL (11.1 mmol/L) has DM and should be referred for further management. A 2-hour value of 140 to 199 mg/dL (7.8 to 11.0 mmol/L) represents impaired glucose tolerance (IGT) or "prediabetes" (80% will develop DM within 5 years).

Class A$_2$ GDM

• Management includes the same recommendations as class A$_1$, although glucose monitoring is different. Monitor glucose levels after delivery with a fasting and a postprandial glucose level when the patient resumes PO intake.

• The scheduled split-dose or basal–bolus insulin or oral agent(s) regimen should be discontinued in the immediate postpartum period.

• Administer rapid-acting insulin subcutaneously if preprandial glucose is greater than 180 to 200 mg/dL (4 to 6 units of rapid-acting insulin subcutaneously is usually adequate).

• If preprandial values are persistently greater than 180 to 200 mg/dL, a split-dose or basal–bolus insulin regimen should be resumed. See recommendations for classes B to T insulin-dependent DM regarding calculation of postpartum insulin dose.

- If the patient was taking oral agent(s) for glycemic control prior to delivery, the medication(s) may be resumed during the postpartum period with persistent hyperglycemia. There are limited data on breast-feeding with acarbose, glyburide, and Glucophage; however, this is not considered a contraindication for term infants (33).

Class B to T Diabetes Mellitus

- The goal in the first 3 to 5 days after delivery is to avoid hypoglycemia and to reduce the risk of DKA, severe hyperglycemia, and insulin reactions rather than achieving euglycemia. Glucose values of 80 to 160 mg/dL are acceptable. Patients with severe vascular complications may benefit from tighter control.
- CII is discontinued immediately after delivery unless the patient is experiencing persistent hyperglycemia (e.g., as occurs with infection or DKA).
- IV fluids may be administered as either non–glucose containing or 5% dextrose solutions. After a vaginal delivery, glucose infusion is generally not required because PO intake is resumed almost immediately. The postoperative patient will generally tolerate a 5% dextrose solution at 125 to 150 mL/h without insulin therapy because of the dramatic and rapid onset of postpartum insulin sensitivity. When oral intake resumes, the IV dextrose solution should be discontinued.
- Glucose control may be followed by measurement of either fasting and preprandial glucose values (better for class C and above) or fasting and 1-hour postprandial values.
- If repeated, rapid-acting insulin coverage is needed to treat persistent hyperglycemia (greater than 160 mg/dL); a regular schedule of split-dose or basal–bolus insulin should be resumed. The new TDD of insulin should be either approximately 50% of the prepregnancy dose (if the patient was in good control) or 25% to 33% of the end-pregnancy dose. The latter is generally chosen because this is usually more accurate and reflects tighter control. When the patient is ready to resume tighter glucose control, additional insulin can be sequentially added and the level of control gradually improved with a final goal of 80 to 110 mg/dL before meals. Once euglycemia is established, the SRAIS may be used to adjust the insulin dose as needed. Recommendations should be individualized.

Breast-feeding

- Lactation is an antidiabetogenic factor in which glucose is shunted preferentially for use as energy in milk production. This naturally lowers glucose levels in the mother without requiring increased insulin. Breast-feeding women with overt DM need to adjust insulin doses and meal plan to balance their bodies' requirements with those of milk production. Breast-fed babies have a much lower risk of developing DM than those exposed to cow's milk protein (34).
- **Insulin** requirements are usually reduced until lactation ceases and then return to normal levels. Breast-feeding may be contraindicated in the patient with severely complicated DM who cannot tolerate the added stress of lactation or if the patient must take a medication that is contraindicated with breast-feeding.
- **Calories.** To ensure adequate nutrition and avoid reactive hypoglycemia, the lactating mother (especially if insulin requiring) should test the blood glucose prior to breast-feeding. If the level is less than 100 mg/dL, the women should eat a snack (100 to 300 cal) with each nursing period, especially overnight. Meal plans should be individualized, as caloric requirements vary. Particular attention should be given to adequate calories at night to support feeding schedules (especially in pregestational DM patients). Ketonuria should be monitored as needed.
- **Fluids.** Adequate fluid intake of 2 to 3 quarts of liquid (primarily water) per day is needed (8 to 12 cups of liquid in a 24-hour period). The nursing mother should drink 6 to 8 ounces during each nursing period.

COMPLICATIONS

Diabetic Ketoacidosis (35)

- A medical emergency for both mother and fetus.
- Pregnant women with type 1 DM are at increased risk. DKA can on rare occasion also occur in patients with type 2 DM or GDM.
- Predisposing factors include decreased buffering capacity (respiratory alkalosis of pregnancy), pregnancy hyperemesis, "accelerated starvation" of pregnancy, increased insulin antagonists (HPL, prolactin cortisol), and stress.
- Precipitating factors include illness (gastrointestinal, pulmonary, urinary, or soft tissue infections), eating disorders, or poor compliance with insulin administration.
- Prompt recognition of DKA and treatment is imperative in order to protect the fetus and optimize perinatal outcome.
- Diagnosis of DKA is usually confirmed with presence of hyperglycemia (glucose greater than 200 mg/dL) and positive serum ketones. DKA in pregnancy, however, may occur with glucose values under 200 mg/dL
- The fetus is at high risk until maternal metabolic homeostasis is achieved; high plasma glucose levels and ketones are readily transported to the fetus, which may be unable to secrete sufficient amounts of insulin to prevent DKA in utero.
- Protocol for management of DKA:
  - Search for and treat the precipitating cause (e.g., infection, history of noncompliance).
  - Fluid resuscitation. Most pregnant women with DKA will have lost 7 to 10 L of free water at the time of diagnosis. Give physiologic fluid (0.9% NaCl) at 1000 mL/h for at least 2 hours. After the initial 2 L, change to hypotonic saline (0.45% NaCl) at 250 mL/h (more similar to electrolyte losses during osmotic diuresis) until serum glucose level is between 200 and 250 mg/dL. Once glucose levels are lower than 250 mg/dL, fluid should be changed to a glucose-containing solution (0.45% NaCl with 5% dextrose). Approximately 75% of fluid replacement should occur during the first 24 hours of treatment. A practical way to estimate the total fluid loss is 100 mL/kg actual body weight.
  - Potassium depletion with acute DKA can be substantial. With correction of metabolic acidosis, K^+ ions shift intracellularly leading to a rapid decline in potassium levels. If serum K^+ is low or normal, begin KCl (20 mEq/h) and reduce by 50% if patient is oliguric.
  - Insert a Foley catheter and monitor fluid balance (I&Os) carefully.
  - Insulin for correction of hyperglycemia.
    - Typically start with 10 to 15 units of regular insulin (0.1 unit/kg) as an IV bolus load.
    - Then initiate a CII at 5 to 10 units/h until glucose values are under 250 mg/dL. The goal is to normalize glucose values over a 4- to 8-hour period. Use of computer software–directed insulin infusion algorithms (e.g., Glucommander) when available can optimize glycemic control promptly.
    - When glucose level is less than 250 mg/dL, the CII rate should be decreased, usually to 2.0 to 4.0 units/h and subsequently down to the maintenance range of 0.5 to 2.0 units/h. Ideally, serum blood glucose levels should decline by 50 to 75 mg/dL/h until euglycemia is achieved.
    - CII should be continued until metabolic alterations have been corrected and the patient can resume a regular diet and transition to her usual subcutaneous insulin treatment regimen when acidosis has resolved.
    - Preparation of CII solution: 200 units of regular insulin added to 1000 mL normal saline (2 units regular insulin/10 mL normal saline).
  - Laboratory monitoring and additional tests:
    - Hourly with CII for DKA: serum glucose, urine ketones, and serum potassium.
    - At longer intervals: serum electrolytes, arterial blood gases, BUN, serum creatinine, blood acetone, CBC, serum osmolality.
    - Twelve-lead EKG should be checked if K^+ levels are significantly abnormal.

Chronic Hypertension

- Hypertension is a common comorbidity of diabetes, which may be found in 20% to 30% of women who have had diabetes for more than 10 years (2).
- Current evidence suggests that none of the antihypertensive medications commonly used in pregnancy (calcium channel blockers, β-blockers, methyldopa) are teratogenic, but they should only be prescribed or continued during pregnancy if required for optimization of blood pressure control.
- β-Blockers (e.g., labetalol) may blunt the sympathetic response that precedes hypoglycemia in women with pregestational diabetes, and their use is relatively contraindicated.
- Certain calcium channel blockers (e.g., diltiazem) may have renal protective benefits and may be an ideal choice for the pregnant patient with overt nephropathy and hypertension.
- Angiotensin-converting enzyme (ACE) inhibitors are commonly utilized in nonpregnant patients with nephropathy due to their renal protective benefits. It is not clear whether this class of drugs has teratogenic potential in the first trimester, but usage in the second trimester and beyond can significantly decreased fetal renal blood flow resulting in oligohydramnios and fetal compromise (36). Recent data suggest that in the first trimester, fetal risk from ACE inhibitors may result from hypertension itself rather than ACE exposure (37). Use of angiotensin receptor blockers (ARBs) and receptor antagonists probably carries a similar risk, but limited data are available.

Preterm Labor

- **Tocolytics:**
  - Magnesium sulfate is the preferred IV tocolytic agent for women with diabetes.
  - Indomethacin (oral or rectal in patients at less than 32 weeks of gestation) as well as nifedipine (until fetal lung maturity is established) have been used successfully with close follow-up.
  - The use of β-sympathomimetics should be approached with extreme caution because of the attendant risk of hyperglycemia and ketosis.
- **Steroids** to enhance fetal lung maturity also increase the risk of hyperglycemia and ketosis.
  - The benefits from use must be weighed against the possible adverse effects namely hyperglycemia (which may last several days).
  - When steroid use is felt to be necessary because of the high likelihood of an extremely premature delivery (less than 30 weeks of gestation), the patient should be hospitalized, glucose levels should be monitored closely, and a CII should be initiated if necessary to maintain glycemic control after steroid administration.
  - Use of steroids between 30 to 34 weeks of gestation should be carefully individualized.
  - Beyond 34 weeks, the use of steroids is not recommended, as benefits to the fetus do not outweigh risks to the mother.
- **Bed rest:**
  - If long-term bed rest is required, a 10% reduction in total calories may be necessary to prevent excess weight gain.
  - Insulin requirement may also increase due to the lack of physical activity.

PATIENT EDUCATION

Contraception

- Hormonal methods currently available include the combination oral contraceptive pill (OCP), combination contraceptive patch or NuvaRing, the progestin-only OCP, Implanon, and the long-acting progestins given intramuscularly.
- Virtually all combination hormonal contraceptives contain a low estrogen dosage of ethinyl estradiol (20 to 40 mg), but the formulations of progestins vary widely.
- Breast-feeding women with a history of GDM should be aware that using the progestin-only hormonal contraceptives has been associated with an almost threefold increased risk

for developing overt DM in their lifetime, compared to that seen with combination OCP use; the magnitude of this risk appears to correlate with the duration of uninterrupted use (38).

- ACOG recommends that oral contraceptive use in women with DM should be limited to otherwise healthy nonsmokers, less than 35 years old, with no evidence of hypertension, nephropathy, retinopathy, or other vascular disease (39).
- Metabolically neutral methods include barrier methods and the intrauterine device (IUD). The same contraindications apply as for patients without DM.

Recurrence of GDM and Risk of Overt DM

- Risk of recurrence of GDM in subsequent pregnancies has been quoted as 30% to 60%. Patients requiring medication therapy in addition to nutrition management for optimization of glycemic control are more likely to develop GDM in subsequent pregnancies.
- Up to 60% of women with a history of GDM will be diagnosed with overt diabetics during their lifetime. Therefore, DM screening every 1 to 3 years should be recommended if the postpartum 2-h 75-g OGTT screen is normal. Having a subsequent pregnancy or 10 lb increase from the postpartum weight may increase the risk of overt DM later in life. Conversely, a 10-lb reduction from the postpartum weight may reduce lifetime DM risk by as much as 50% (38).

Preconception Counseling for Pregestational Diabetes

Despite widespread underutilization, preconception care programs have consistently been associated with decreased morbidity and mortality (30). It is thus very important that women with overt DM postpone conception until glycemic control has been optimized. The following guidelines are recommended for preconception care (30):

- Glycemic control should be optimized to achieve euglycemia prior to conception (fasting blood glucose 70 to 99 mg/dL, preprandial values less than 100 mg/dL; 1-hour postprandial <140 mg/dL or 2-hour postprandial values ≤120 mg/dL) and a normal glycosylated hemoglobin value (the precise value varies with type of test and laboratory) before conception. Overall, the goal is to achieve an HbA_{1c} as close to normal as possible without causing significant hypoglycemia. Patients who are not prone to hypoglycemia may be able to achieve even tighter glycemic control ($HbA_{1c} < 6\%$) preconception.
- The patient should be advised to start taking a prenatal vitamin with 1 mg of folic acid preferably 3 months before attempting conception.
- The patient should be evaluated and treated if necessary for diabetic retinopathy, nephropathy, neuropathy, and cardiovascular disease/hypertension prior to conception. Laboratory evaluations/referrals should include
  - Twenty-four-hour urine collection for total protein and creatinine clearance.
  - Thyroid function should be evaluated and treated if abnormal.
  - Baseline retinal evaluation with photocoagulation performed if needed.
- A careful review of the patient's current medical management should screen for medications contraindicated for use during pregnancy such as ACE inhibitors, ARBs, statins, and most noninsulin therapies.
- Despite the absence of evidence of teratogenicity for most currently available oral medications, none are recommended in pregnancy. The standard of care, at present, is to transition these patients to insulin therapy preconceptionally (particularly with poor glycemic control) or as soon as pregnancy is confirmed. The possible exception to this is the use of Glucophage in nondiabetic, infertility patients with polycystic ovarian syndrome (PCOS) who are oligo-ovulatory. These women may benefit from higher fertility rates and lower miscarriage rates if Glucophage is continued throughout the first trimester (41). Some advocate continuation of Glucophage throughout pregnancy given their higher risk for developing overt glucose intolerance. However, this should be approached with caution as the safety of this practice has yet to be determined. The use of newer oral

hypoglycemic and oral antihyperglycemic agents appears promising in the latter half of pregnancy. However, data confirming safety for use in early pregnancy are not available.
• After the assessment, the patient and her family should be provided with prognostic information taking into consideration glycemic control, cardiovascular, renal, and ophthalmologic status to provide advice regarding potential risks with pregnancy (as outlined above). Potential contraindications to pregnancy should be candidly discussed.
• The patient should be counseled regarding the required time commitment, appropriate nutrition, exercise, and stress management strategies during pregnancy.

Genetics of Diabetes
• The health care provider should consider the possible benefit of genetic counseling for all women of childbearing age, especially if they have type 1 DM.
• The risk of fetal congenital anomalies, their correlation with poor glycemic control, and options for prenatal diagnosis should be discussed.
• The risk of a woman with type 1 DM having a child who subsequently will develop DM in childhood is approximately 1 in 40, compared with a risk of 1 in 20 if a child's father has type 1 DM (42). If both parents have type 1 DM, the risk of having an affected child may be as high as 15%. These patients should be informed regarding the rapid advances in genetic diabetes research so they may consider cord blood collection at delivery for stem cell storage.
• Having a parent with type 2 DM increases the chance of a child developing type 2 DM later in life by twofold to fourfold (43).

REFERENCES

1. American Diabetes Association. http://www.professional.diabetes.org/facts/. Accessed March 2013.
2. Moore TR, Catalano P. Diabetes and pregnancy. In: Creasy RK, Resnik R, eds. *Maternal–fetal medicine*. 6th ed. Philadelphia: WB Saunders, 2009; Chapter 46:953–993.
3. American Diabetes Association. Diagnosis and classification of diabetes mellitus. *Diabetes Care*. 2014;37(Suppl 1):S81–S90.
4. Buchanan TA. Metabolic changes during normal and diabetic pregnancies. In: Reece EA, Coustan DR, eds. *Diabetes mellitus in pregnancy*, 2nd ed. New York: Churchill Livingstone, 1995:59–77.
5. Coustan DR, Felig P. Diabetes mellitus. In: Burrows GN, Ferris TF, eds. *Medical complications during pregnancy*, 3rd ed. Philadelphia: WB Saunders, 1988:34–64.
6. Schaeffer LD, Wilder ML, Williams RH. Secretion and content of insulin and glucagon in human fetal pancreatic slices in vitro. *Proc Soc Exp Biol Med*. 1973;143:314–319.
7. Kitzmiller JL, Brown ER, Phillippe M, et al. Diabetic nephropathy and perinatal outcome. *Am J Obstet Gynecol*. 1981;141:741–751.
8. Miodovnik M, Rosenn BM, Khoury JC, et al. Does pregnancy increase the risk for development and progression of diabetic nephropathy? *Am J Obstet Gynecol*. 1996;174:1180–1189.
9. Reece EA, Lockwood CJ, Tuck S, et al. Retinal and pregnancy outcomes in the presence of diabetic proliferative retinopathy. *J Reprod Med*. 1994;39:799–804.
10. Chaturvedi N, Stephenson JM, Fuller JH. The relationship between pregnancy and long-term maternal complications in the Eurodiab IDDM complications study. *Diabetic Med*. 1995;12:494–499.
11. Sadler TW, Hunter ES III, Wynn RE, et al. Evidence for multifactorial origin of diabetes induced embryopathies. *Diabetes*. 1989;38:70–74.
12. Mills JL, Simpson JL, Driscoll SG, et al. Incidence of spontaneous abortion among normal and insulin-dependent diabetic women whose pregnancies were identified within 21 days of conception. *N Engl J Med*. 1988;319:1617–1623.
13. Rosenn B, Miodovnik M, Combs CA, et al. Glycemic thresholds for spontaneous abortion and congenital malformations in insulin-dependent diabetes mellitus. *Obstet Gynecol*. 1994;84:515–520.

14. Buchanan TA, Denno KM, Sipos GF, et al. Diabetic teratogenesis: In vitro evidence for a multifactorial etiology with little contribution from glucose per se. *Diabetes.* 1994;43: 656–660.

15. Becerra JE, Khoury MJ, Cordero JF, et al. Diabetes mellitus during pregnancy and the risks of specific birth defects: a population-based case-control study. *Pediatrics.* 1990;85:1–9.

16. Faranoff AA, Martin RJM, Miller MJ. Identification and management of problems in the high-risk neonate. In: Creasy RK, Resnik R, eds. *Maternal–fetal medicine.* 4th ed. Philadelphia: WB Saunders, 1999:1171–1172.

17. Silverman BL, Metzger BE, Cho NH, et al. Impaired glucose tolerance in adolescent offspring of diabetic mothers: Relationship to fetal hyperinsulinism. *Diabetes Care.* 1995;18:611.

18. International Association of Diabetes and Pregnancy Study Groups Consensus Panel. The International Association of Diabetes and Pregnancy Study Groups Recommendations on the Diagnosis and Classification of Diabetes during Pregnancy. *Diabetes Care.* 2010;33(3):676–682.

19. American College of Obstetricians and Gynecologists Committee on Practice Bulletins-Gynecology. ACOG Practice Bulletin. Gestational Diabetes, Number 137, August 2013.

20. Vandorsten JP, Dodson WC, Espeland MA. NIH Consensus Development Conference. Diagnosing Gestational Diabetes Mellitus. *NIH Consens State Sci Statements.* 2013;29(1):1–31.

21. American Diabetes Association. Clinical Practice Recommendations—Standards of Medical Care in Diabetes- 2014-Position Statement. Diabetes Care 2014;37(Suppl 1):S14–S80.

22. HAPO study Cooperative Research Group. Hyperglycemia an adverse pregnancy outcomes. *N Engl J Med.* 2008;358(19):1991–2002.

23. American College of Obstetricians and Gynecologists. Screening and Diagnosis of Gestational Diabetes Mellitus. Committee Opinion No. 504. *Obstet Gynecol.* 2011;118 Issue 3:751–753.

24. Carpenter MW, Coustan DR. Criteria for screening tests for gestational diabetes. *Am J Obstet Gynecol.* 1982;144:768–773.

25. Moreno-Castilla C, Hernandez M, Bergua M, Alvarez MC, Arce MA, et al. Low-carbohydrate diet for the treatment of gestational diabetes. *Diabetes Care.* 2013;36(8):2233–2238.

26. Jovanovic-Peterson L, Peterson CM, Reed GF, et al. Maternal postprandial glucose levels and infant birth weight: the Diabetes in Early Pregnancy Study. *Am J Obstet Gynecol.* 1991;164;103–111.

27. Jovanovic L. American Diabetes Association's Fourth International Workshop-Conference on Gestational Diabetes Mellitus: summary and discussion. Therapeutic interventions. *Diabetes Care.* 1998;21(Suppl 2):B131–B137.

28. de Veciana M, Major CA, Morgan MA, et al. Postprandial versus preprandial blood glucose monitoring in women with gestational diabetes mellitus requiring insulin therapy. *N Engl J Med.* 1995;333:1237–1241.

29. Kolterman OG. Glyburide in non-insulin dependent diabetes: an update. *Clin Ther.* 1992;14:196–219.

30. Kitzmiller J, Block J, Brown F, et al. Managing preexisting diabetes for pregnancy. *Diabetes Care.* 2008;31(5):1060–1079.

31. de Veciana M, Trail PA, Evans AT, et al. A comparison of oral acarbose and insulin in women with gestational diabetes. *Obstet Gynecol.* 2002;99(4 Suppl):S5.

32. Langer O, Conway DL, Berkus MD, et al. A comparison of glyburide and insulin in women with gestational diabetes. *N Engl J Med.* 2000; 343:1134–1138.

33. Briggs GG, et al. *Drugs in pregnancy and lactation,* 5th ed. Baltimore: Lippincott Williams & Wilkins, 1998:133,966.

34. Schrezenmier J, Jazla A. Milk and diabetes. *J Am Coll Nutr* 2000;19(Suppl):176S.

35. de Veciana M. Diabetes Ketoacidosis in Pregnancy. *Seminars in Perinatology* 2013;37: 267–273.

36. Buttar HS. An overview of the influence of ACE inhibitors on fetal-placental circulation and perinatal development. *Mol Cell Biochem.* 1997;176:61–71.

37. Li D-K, Yang C, Andrade S et al. Maternal exposure to angiotensin converting enzyme inhibitors in the first trimester and risk of malformations: a retrospective cohort study. *BMJ.* 2011;343:d5931.

38. Kjos SL, Peters RK, Xiang A, et al. Hormonal choices after gestational diabetes: subsequent pregnancy, contraception, and hormone replacement. *Diabetes Care.* 1998; 21:B50–B57.

39. American College of Obstetricians and Gynecologists Committee on Practice Bulletins-Gynecology. ACOG Practice Bulletin. The use of hormonal contraception in women with coexisting medical conditions. Number 18, July 2000.

40. Diabetes Control and Complications Trial Research Group. Pregnancy outcomes in the Diabetes Control and Complications Trial. *Am J Obstet Gynecol.* 1996;174:1343–1353.

41. Jakubowicz DJ, Iuorno MJ, Jakubowicz S, et al. Effects of metformin on early pregnancy loss in the polycystic ovary syndrome. *J Clin Endocrinol Metab.* 2002:87:524–529.

42. Tuomilehto J, et al. Evidence for importance of gender and birth cohort for risks of IDDM in offspring of IDDM parents. *Diabetologia.* 1995;38:975–982.

43. Pierce M, et al. Risk of diabetes in offspring of parents with non-insulin-dependent diabetes. *Diabetes Med.* 1994;11:481.

44. Davidson PC, Steed RD, Bode BW. Glucommander: a computer-directed intravenous insulin system shown to be safe, simple and effective in 120,618h of operation. *Diabetes Care* 2005;28(10):2418–2423.

45. Walsh J, Roberts R. *Pumping insulin: everything you need to succeed on an insulin pump.* 5th ed. San Diego: Torrey Pines Press, 2012.

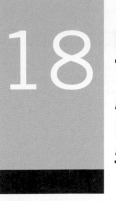

18

Endocrine Disorders: Thyroid, Parathyroid, Adrenal, and Pituitary Disease

Amy M. Valent and David D'Alessio

THYROID
Key Points
- Evaluation of thyroid function should be performed in patients with a history of thyroid disorder, medical conditions commonly associated with thyroid disease, strong family history, or suggestive symptoms.
- The recommended iodine intake in pregnancy is increased to 250 µg/d to compensate for increased renal iodine clearance and fetal and placental utilization (1,2).
- Thyroid hormone is critical for normal central nervous system development during embryogenesis. Women with normal thyroid function increase the production of thyroid hormone by 50% in the first trimester.
- Until method- and trimester-specific free T_4 levels are established, thyroid-stimulating hormone (TSH) is the most reliable means to assess thyroid function in pregnancy (1).

Background
Pregnancy Physiology
- TSH from the anterior pituitary stimulates thyroid production of thyroxine (T_4) and levothyronine (T_3), the important metabolic mediators and essential hormones for normal fetal and neonatal brain development. Iodine is required for T_4 and T_3 synthesis.
- Human chorionic gonadotropin (hCG) has direct thyroid-stimulating activity and transiently increases T_4 production in the first trimester.
  - TSH levels decrease in the first trimester via negative feedback as hCG peaks (3), and asymptomatic, mildly decreased TSH does not indicate hyperthyroidism. The median TSH during the first trimester is 0.8 mIU/mL (0.03 to 2.3 mIU/mL). TSH rises back to the normal range in the second and third trimesters.
- Levels of total thyroxine (TT_4) and triiodothyronine (TT_3) increase during pregnancy and remain 1.5 times above the normal nonpregnant reference range throughout pregnancy.
  - Thyroid-binding globulin (TBG) is the primary binding protein for T_4 and T_3 in plasma. Estrogen stimulation during pregnancy increases serum TBG production by 50%. *Free* T_4 (FT_4) and free T_3 (FT_3) are more accurate measures of thyroid status but must be interpreted carefully as trimester-specific normative ranges have not been established and results from common clinical assays vary (3).
- The transfer of maternal thyroid hormones across the placenta to the fetus varies, but thyroid autoantibodies, antithyroid medications, and iodine can passively cross the placenta and affect the fetus.
  - The placenta is relatively impermeable to TSH. A although uptake of T_4 and T_3 from the maternal circulation to the placenta is rapid, transfer to the fetus is regulated via placental deiodinases and thyroid hormone transporter proteins (4,5).

- Thyroid function in the newborn changes rapidly in the first 48 hours of life.
  - Fetal secretion of thyroid hormone is significant after the first trimester, and at the time of delivery, 20% to 30% of fetal thyroid hormones are of maternal origin.
  - Immediately after delivery, a significant fall in the newborn's temperature causes a rapid increase in TSH and thyroid hormone secretion. Following this burst of thyroid hormone, TSH declines exponentially within 48 hours due to negative feedback. In term infants, T_4 and T_3 remain elevated for approximately 6 weeks (6).
  - Delayed treatment of congenital hypothyroidism increases the risk for mental retardation and other neurologic sequelae. Newborn screening for hypothyroidism on days 2 to 4 of life is mandatory to prevent lifelong impairment (6).

HYPERTHYROIDISM
Key Points
- The prevalence of hyperthyroidism in pregnancy is 0.2%.
- Graves disease is the most common cause of hyperthyroidism in pregnancy.
- Standard treatment of Graves disease in pregnancy is with antithyroid drugs (ATD), using the lowest dose that reduces FT_4 to the upper end of the normal range.

Background
Definition
- Hyperthyroidism is defined by the suppression of serum TSH below the lower limits of the trimester-specific range and elevated serum FT_4 and/or FT_3 above the nonpregnant reference range.
- Subclinical hyperthyroidism is defined as a suppressed TSH concentration and serum FT_4 and/or FT_3 within the nonpregnant reference range.

Differential Diagnosis and Etiology
- Gestational transient thyrotoxicosis is characterized by elevated FT_4 and suppressed TSH levels in the first trimester, with the absence of a goiter, history of hyperthyroidism, or TSH receptor antibodies (TRAB). It is caused by the thyrotropic effects of hCG early in pregnancy and spontaneously improves with the decline of hCG in the second trimester. Gestational thyrotoxicosis is commonly associated with hyperemesis gravidarum, multiple pregnancies, and gestational trophoblastic diseases, but has not been correlated with poor pregnancy outcomes (7).
- Hyperemesis gravidarum is a clinical diagnosis of persistent vomiting, evidence of starvation (i.e., ketonuria) and 5% weight loss. It complicates 0.5% to 2% of pregnancies, and up to 60% to 70% of women will have suppressed TSH and elevated FT_4 levels.
- Trophoblastic hyperthyroidism is seen in up to 64% of women with placental tumors. The hyperthyroidism may be severe due to the thyrotropic activity of partially desialylated hCG. It is commonly treated by removal of the hydatidiform mole or chemotherapy-directed treatment for choriocarcinoma (7).
- Graves disease is an autoimmune disorder caused by the production of antibodies that bind to the TSH receptor and accounts for 85% to 95% of hyperthyroidism in pregnancy. TRAB can be measured in serum and have either thyroid-stimulating or thyroid-blocking effects. Measurement of thyroid-stimulating immunoglobulins (TSI) is a bioassay that distinguishes between these effects with stimulating activity being the early universal feature of Graves'. TSI cause general thyroid activation with increased growth, vascularity, and excess secretion of thyroid hormones independent of TSH. This is generally associated with signs and symptoms of thyrotoxicosis.
- The least common causes of thyrotoxicosis in pregnancy are toxic nodular goiter, functional adenomas, thyroiditis, or excessive intake of thyroid hormones.

Diagnosis and Evaluation

- The key features of Graves disease are abnormal thyroid function tests, a goiter, positive TRAB, and less commonly findings of Graves ophthalmopathy or dermopathy.
- Palpable thyroid masses or nodules should be evaluated with thyroid ultrasound and fine needle aspiration is recommended for nodules suspicious for malignancy (8). Radioactive iodine scans, used to visualize the functional anatomy of the thyroid in nonpregnant women, are contraindicated during pregnancy.

History and Physical Exam

- Thyroid hormones affect metabolism in virtually all tissues. Common clinical symptoms of hyperthyroidism include tachycardia, palpitations, weight loss, nervousness, muscle weakness, heat intolerance, hair loss, or excessive sweating. Findings specific for Graves disease are infiltrative dermopathy (pretibial myxedema) and exophthalmos, due to inflammation, edema, and hyaluronate accumulation in the extraocular muscles.

Diagnostic Testing

- Serum TSH measurement is the mainstay for the diagnosis of hyperthyroidism. If the TSH is low, FT_4 evaluation is recommended. Serum FT_3 assessment is advised if the FT_4 is within normal range.
- Circulating TRAB are present in greater than 90% of patients with active Graves disease. Antibodies fluctuate throughout gestation and decrease through the second and third trimesters (7). Commonly, values will increase in the postpartum period when patients may experience an exacerbation of Graves disease.

Pregnancy Complications

- Treatment is essential. Uncontrolled hyperthyroidism increases the risk for spontaneous abortion, preterm birth, preeclampsia, intrauterine growth restriction, low birth weight, and fetal demise (9,10).
- Thyroid storm is an accelerated, extreme presentation of hyperthyroidism that occurs in 1% of pregnancies and is a medical emergency. Patients present with usual signs and symptoms of hyperthyroidism in addition to fever, sinus tachycardia and/or atrial arrhythmia, heart failure, hyperbilirubinemia, and mental status changes (10).
- Fetal hyperthyroidism complicates 1% to 5% of pregnancies with Graves disease. Transfer of maternal antibodies to the newborn and the capacity for the neonatal thyroid to respond to TSI cause this condition. Findings suggesting fetal hyperthyroidism are a goiter on ultrasound, fetal heart rate greater than 160 bpm, evidence of heart failure, arrhythmias, advanced bone age, growth restriction, craniosynostosis, and hydrops (9).
- Fetal hypothyroidism is a risk of overtreatment with ATD or passive transfer of blocking thyroid antibodies. Cordocentesis, fetal blood sampling, should only be performed for cases in which definitive fetal thyroid function is uncertain from ultrasound assessment and the results would impact management (8,11).

Treatment

- Iodine-131 exposure is contraindicated in pregnancy for the risk of fetal thyroid ablation, and pregnancy should be avoided for at least 4 to 6 months after exposure (8,10).
- Women with Graves disease should have TRAB titers assessed at initial prenatal visit and between 22 and 26 weeks to assess the risk of neonatal hyperthyroidism. Measurement of TSI in the latter phase of the third trimester is predictive of neonatal hyperthyroidism.
- Medical management: Propylthiouracil (PTU) and methimazole (MMI) are antithyroid medications that inhibit thyroid hormone synthesis. PTU also decreases peripheral conversion of T_4 to T_3 and is the recommended thioamide drug in the first trimester. Embryopathy, primarily aplasia cutis, and choanal or esophageal atresia are rare complications of MMI and almost never seen with PTU. With the infrequent but potentially

fatal hepatotoxicity associated with PTU, therapy should be switched to MMI after the first trimester unless the patient is intolerant of MMI (2,8).

- Dosing: Initial treatment with PTU is 50 to 100 mg every 6 to 8 hours or MMI 10 to 20 mg every 12 hours (10). As symptoms improve and FT_4 decreases, the dosing of ATD is reduced. In stable patients, PTU is usually given two to three times daily and MMI once daily. The goal of therapy is to maintain FT_4 at or just above the upper limit of the nonpregnant reference range with the lowest ATD dose (8,10).
- FT_4 and TSH should be measured every 2 to 4 weeks after initiating ATD, and every 4 to 6 weeks after the FT_4 goal is reached to guide dose adjustments. Serum TSH may remain suppressed even after FT_4 responds and should not be used alone to guide treatment.
- Minor drug side effects include rash, urticaria, arthralgias, nausea, metallic taste, and pruritus, which often resolve spontaneously without significant sequelae.
- Agranulocytosis may occur in 0.5% of treated individuals, presenting with fever, sore throat, and neutropenia. Immediate discontinuation of thioamide drugs with the development of a sore throat and fever is recommended until a white blood cell count and differential has been performed (10).
- Although small amounts of PTU and MMI are found in breast milk, breast-feeding is considered safe in mothers taking these medications.
- Thyroidectomy is indicated if ATD are ineffective, adverse reactions occur, or with a symptomatic goiter. Surgery is optimally performed in the second trimester.

HYPOTHYROIDISM
Key Points
- Hypothyroidism has a prevalence of 0.3% to 1.5% in the United States and is 5 to 10 times more common in women than men (2).
- Iodine deficiency is the most common cause of hypothyroidism worldwide. In developed countries, autoimmunity is the most common etiology. Hashimoto disease (chronic lymphocytic thyroiditis) and atrophic thyroiditis are the two manifestations of autoimmune thyroid disease leading to hypothyroidism.
- Women are advised to reach an euthyroid state with serum TSH in the lower limit of normal prior to conception for optimal pregnancy outcomes (12,13).
- Pregnant women with preexisting hypothyroidism invariably require an increase in thyroxine dose by 30% in the first trimester.

Background
Definition
- Hypothyroidism is defined as a serum TSH elevated above the trimester-specific range and a FT_4 below the nonpregnant reference range.
- In subclinical hypothyroidism, there is elevated serum TSH with normal FT_4 levels.

Differential Diagnosis and Etiology
- Hypothyroid symptoms are nonspecific. Anemia, depression, and pregnancy can mimic many of the symptoms experienced.
- Hashimoto disease is the most common cause of primary hypothyroidism. It is characterized by a small firm goiter due to lymphocytic infiltration, painless inflammation, and destruction of thyroid cells.
- Prior ablative radioiodine therapy or thyroidectomy.
- Medications altering thyroid hormone (see Table 18-1).
- Endemic iodine deficiency.
- Secondary hypothyroidism from pituitary disease and TSH deficiency such as Sheehan syndrome, lymphocytic hypophysitis (LH), or history of hypophysectomy.
- Tertiary hypothyroidism due to hypothalamic disease is rare. Sarcoidosis and histiocytosis are the most common causes of tertiary hypothyroidism (10).

Table 18-1	Drugs that Affect Thyroid Function
Medications	**Mechanism**
Iodide, lithium, thioamides	Inhibit thyroid hormone synthesis
Glucocorticoids, ipodate sodium, propranolol, PTU, amiodarone	Inhibit T_4-to-T_3 conversion
Ferrous sulfate, sucralfate, cholestyramine, aluminum hydroxide	Inhibit absorption of thyroid hormone
Phenytoin, salicylates	Inhibit T_4 and T_3 protein binding
Iodide, lithium	Increase TSH
Glucocorticoids, dopamine agonists	Decrease TSH
Phenytoin, rifampin, phenobarbital, sertraline, carbamazepine	Increase thyroxine clearance

Diagnosis and Evaluation

History and Physical Exam

• Diagnosis in pregnancy is difficult because many of the symptoms associated with hypothyroidism are also common in pregnancy.

• Common clinical signs and symptoms of hypothyroidism may include the following: fatigue, lethargy, dry skin, weight gain, cold intolerance, impaired memory, edema, or depression. Goiter is common with iodine deficiency or Hashimoto thyroiditis.

Diagnostic Testing

• Measurement of serum TSH is the mainstay for the diagnosis of hypothyroidism. If the TSH is abnormal, antithyroid antibodies and FT_4 are recommended.

• Elevated anti-thyroid peroxidase antibodies (anti-TPO Ab) and antithyroglobulin antibodies (anti-Tg Ab) are consistent with thyroid autoimmunity and are associated with higher rates of miscarriage and preterm labor.

Pregnancy Complications

• Hypothyroidism is associated with an increased rate of spontaneous abortion, especially in women with positive antithyroid antibodies (8). Thyroid dysfunction increases the risks for pregnancy complications such as preeclampsia, placental abruption, prematurity, premature rupture of membranes, postpartum hemorrhage, intrauterine demise, and low birth weight (10,14).

• Maternal hypothyroidism is associated with impaired neuropsychological development in the child (15).

Treatment

Medications

• Synthetic levothyroxine (T_4) is the treatment of choice for hypothyroidism (16,17).

• If hypothyroidism is newly diagnosed in pregnancy, levothyroxine should be started at 1.5 to 2 μg/kg. Patients with malabsorption, complete thyroidectomy, or prior ablative radioiodine may require higher concentrations. Thyroxine is best taken on an empty stomach at bedtime or first thing in the morning. Calcium, antacids, sucralfate, and caffeine can interfere with absorption.

• Higher doses of levothyroxine are required in 85% to 90% of patients with prior hypothyroidism early in the first trimester (13,18). In these patients, increasing levothyroxine 30% (~2 additional tablets per week) once pregnancy is established decreases the risk of hypothyroidism in the first trimester. Patients should strive for an euthyroid state prior to conception and immediately seek care to have thyroid function studies performed when pregnancy is confirmed for optimal management (12,13,18).

- TSH should be measured 4 to 6 weeks after each dose adjustment and each trimester once the optimal serum TSH levels have been reached. During pregnancy, TSH goals are less than 2.5 mIU/L in the first trimester and 3.0 mIU/L in the second and third trimesters.
- TSH 4 to 10   Increase dose by 25 to 50 μg daily
- TSH 10 to 20   Increase dose by 50 to 75 μg daily
- TSH greater than 20   Increase dose by 75 to 100 μg daily
- Reduce levothyroxine to prepregnancy dose after delivery and recheck TSH 6 weeks later.

POSTPARTUM THYROID DYSFUNCTION

Key Points
- The prevalence of postpartum thyroid dysfunction (PPTD) is 5% to 10% (10,17,19).
- Women with autoimmune disorders such as type 1 diabetes mellitus, Addison disease, and systemic lupus erythematosus are at a higher risk for PPTD, a form of autoimmune thyroid disease (2,17,19,20).
- After one episode, patients have a 70% risk of recurrence in a subsequent pregnancy. The risk of permanent hypothyroidism is 20% to 64% and can occur as soon as the first year postpartum (17,19). Women with PPTD should have annual serum TSH screening.

Background
Definition
- PPTD is a transient autoimmune thyroiditis during the 1st year postpartum in women who were euthyroid prior to pregnancy.
  - The typical presentation is with a period of transient thyrotoxicosis, followed by transient hypothyroidism, and return to an euthyroid state by the end of the first year postpartum. Patients may present with transient isolated thyrotoxicosis or isolated hypothyroidism followed by an euthyroid recovery period.

Differential Diagnosis and Etiology
- Up to 50% of women with positive TPO-Ab during pregnancy develop PPTD. Thyroid gland inflammation due to lymphocytic thyroiditis is thought to result from the immunologic rebound following selective immunosuppression of normal pregnancy (19).
- Anemia and depression may cause symptoms similar to PPTD.

DIAGNOSIS AND EVALUATION

History and Physical
- Thirty percent of patients with PPTD are asymptomatic. In patients with underlying Hashimoto disease, a small firm goiter is palpable.
- Thyrotoxic symptoms are less pronounced than in Graves' disease, and elevations of FT_4 are lower. Frequent symptoms include fatigue, palpitations, nervousness, irritability, weight loss, and heat intolerance.
- Hypothyroid symptoms are often more significant and include fatigue, impaired memory and concentration, constipation, dry skin, cold intolerance, and myalgia/arthralgia.

Diagnostic Testing
- Typical laboratory parameters for hyper- and hypothyroidism are used for PPTD. Antithyroid antibodies are commonly associated with this disease.
- In contrast to Graves' disease, PPTD is distinguished by a substantially reduced uptake of radioactive iodine. Radioactive iodine is contraindicated in lactating mothers.

Treatment
- Antithyroid medications are not effective for treating hyperthyroidism of PPTD.
- Propranolol may be used to mitigate some of the symptoms of hyperthyroidism such as tremor, heat intolerance, and palpitations, providing relief during the hyperthyroid

phase. Patients should be educated to get adequate rest and hydration and avoid stimulants and symptom triggers.

- Hypothyroidism is treated with levothyroxine when the patient is symptomatic, planning or attempting pregnancy, currently pregnant, breast-feeding, or when serum TSH is abnormally elevated for greater than 6 months (17,19). The duration of levothyroxine therapy has not been firmly established, but patients may be weaned after 6 to 12 months of therapy to determine if the hypothyroid phase is permanent (2,10,17).

PARATHYROID DISORDERS
Key Points
- Primary hyperparathyroidism is a common endocrine disease with a prevalence of 2–3:1000 American women. However, hypoparathyroidism is less common in women of reproductive age, and the epidemiology in this group is not well defined (21,24).
- In pregnant women, hypercalcemia can be underestimated because of physiologic hypoalbuminemia, growing fetal calcium demands, and gestational hypercalciuria.

Background
Physiology in Pregnancy and Lactation
- Calcium regulation is critical for normal cell function and signaling. Pregnancy and lactation significantly alter calcium homeostasis. The parathyroid glands release parathyroid hormone (PTH), a peptide hormone that maintains calcium balance within a narrow range (21). PTH increases conversion of 25-OH vitamin D to the active 1, 25-OH vitamin D, increasing intestinal calcium absorption. PTH decreases renal clearance of calcium and increases osteoclast activity, causing calcium resorption from bone.
- During pregnancy, a total of 25 to 30 g of calcium is transferred to the fetus. The maternal intestinal calcium absorption doubles by the end of the first trimester, which is mediated by a twofold increase in 1, 25-dihydroxy vitamin D $(1,25(OH)_2D_3)$, the active form of vitamin D. Placental and maternal renal $1,25(OH)_2D_3$ synthesis is mediated by estrogen, human placental lactogen, prolactin, and parathyroid hormone–related peptide (PTHrP) as well as PTH (21).
- In pregnancy, total calcium concentrations in the blood decrease due to physiologic hypoalbuminemia (22). Maternal ionized calcium remains unchanged throughout pregnancy. PTH may be slightly suppressed or within the normal range. PTHrP is produced by the fetal parathyroid glands and the placenta, regulating active placental calcium transport to the fetus (21,22). These effects are mediated by the PTH receptor.
- Calcium lost through breast milk is 210 to 400 mg/d and as high as 1000 mg/d when breast-feeding twins. Mammary-derived PTHrP acts synergistically with low estradiol levels to drive bone resorption and renal calcium retention to adapt to the significant calcium demand (21,22).
- Following delivery, intestinal calcium uptake is reduced to nonpregnant levels, PTH is suppressed, and serum phosphorus increases. Calcitonin increases the first 6 weeks of the postpartum period, possibly playing a role in protecting the maternal skeleton from excessive resorption (21,22).

HYPERPARATHYROIDISM
Background
Definition
- Primary hyperparathyroidism: overproduction of PTH from adenomatous or hyperplastic parathyroid glands resulting in hypercalcemia
- Secondary hyperparathyroidism: a physiologic parathyroid response to low serum calcium concentration to maintain homeostasis

Differential Diagnosis and Etiology
- A single, benign parathyroid adenoma is the most common cause of primary hyperparathyroidism (80% to 90%). Parathyroid hyperplasia (10% to 20%) and carcinoma (less than 1%) are other primary causes.
  - Consider multiple endocrine neoplasia (MEN1 or MEN2A) in patients with multigland hyperplasia on surgical pathology.
- Hypercalcemia can be due to other causes such as chronic use of lithium, hematologic malignancies, vitamin D or A toxicity, excess 1,25 vitamin D production from granulomatous disease, hyperthyroidism, Addison disease, use of thiazide diuretics, and giant mammary hyperplasia and solid tumors that produce PTHrP.
  - Familial hypocalciuric hypercalcemia is an autosomal dominant condition caused by an inactivating mutation in the calcium-sensing receptor, resulting in hypercalcemia with normal PTH levels and low urinary calcium excretion. Patients are usually asymptomatic, and the key to diagnosis is the presence of family members with similar biochemistries. Homozygous mutations can cause severe neonatal hypercalcemia (22).
  - Ingestion of high amounts of calcium, especially in patients with transient renal insufficiency, can impact serum calcium (milk-alkali syndrome).

Diagnosis and Evaluation
History and Physical
- The vast majority of patients are asymptomatic with mildly elevated calcium levels.
- Signs and symptoms related to hypercalcemia are more evident with levels greater than 12 mg/dL. Presentation may include fatigue, shortened QT intervals, arrhythmias, abdominal pain, constipation, peptic ulcer disease, weakness, mental confusion, skeletal pain, nephrolithiasis, or renal impairment with high serum calcium and phosphate levels.

Diagnostic Testing
- Elevated ionized calcium and inappropriately normal or elevated intact PTH in the presence of increased urinary calcium levels are observed. The use of ionized calcium compensates for the dilutional effects of pregnancy on total calcium, and the measure of intact PTH is highly specific for the bioactive hormone.
- High-resolution ultrasound imaging of the parathyroid glands can assist in the diagnosis with 64% to 85% sensitivity reported. Imaging with isotopic scanning can be useful but should be avoided in pregnancy.

Pregnancy Complications
- Maternal complications occur in up to 67% of pregnancies complicated by primary hyperparathyroidism. Perinatal complications may result in a spontaneous abortion, fetal growth restriction, intrauterine or neonatal demise, low birth weight, prematurity, hypertensive crisis, preeclampsia, nephrolithiasis, hyperemesis, pancreatitis, and rarely life-threatening consequences of severe hypercalcemia (21,23).
- Neonatal complications have been shown to be as high as 80%. Chronically high levels of maternal calcium can suppress fetal PTH and cause hypocalcemia with or without tetany or seizures in over 50% of neonates. Permanent hypoparathyroidism from impaired fetal parathyroid development is rare.

Treatment
- Surgical intervention is the definitive management for primary hyperparathyroidism. However, inherent surgical risks must be taken into consideration with maternal and fetal risks and gestational age at diagnosis. With the known morbidity and mortality associated with hypercalcemia and high fetal loss rate in pregnancies with high serum calcium, surgical intervention is recommended for women with serum calcium levels greater than 11.0 mg/dL or worrisome symptoms. Surgery is optimal mid-second trimester of pregnancy.

- Conservative medical treatment of hyperparathyroidism requires adequate fluid hydration and correction of electrolyte abnormalities (21,24).
- Correct dehydration due to calciuresis with oral and intravenous (IV) fluid.
- Once hydration is assured, furosemide may increase urinary calcium loss.
- Calcitonin does not cross the placenta and can be used for acute lowering of serum calcium. The reduction in calcium is short lived due to tachyphylaxis.
- There are insufficient data to support the use of bisphosphonates and cinacalcet in pregnancy.

HYPOPARATHYROIDISM
Background
Definition
- Persistently low serum calcium and high serum phosphate measurement

Differential Diagnosis and Etiology
- The most common cause of hypoparathyroidism is prior removal or traumatic or autoimmune damage to the parathyroid glands.
- Hypomagnesemia can impair PTH release.
- Pseudohypoparathyroidism is an inherited syndrome of target tissue resistance to PTH. Albright syndrome type 1a is a variant presenting with short stature, obesity, round face, brachydactyly, and mental retardation (21).
- 22q11.2 deletion (DiGeorge syndrome) causes developmental delay, and greater than 60% of these patients have abnormal development of the parathyroids with hypocalcemia.
- Vitamin D deficiency, calcium chelators like citrate from blood transfusions, sepsis, and total parenteral nutrition may alter serum calcium levels.

Diagnosis and Evaluation
History and Physical
- Signs and symptoms of hypocalcemia may include the following: laryngeal stridor, dyspnea, numbness and tingling of digits and lips, positive Trousseau and/or Chvostek sign, carpal tunnel spasm, or changes in teeth, nails, and hair. Pseudohypoparathyroidism may be associated with a short fourth metacarpal.

Diagnostic Testing
- Low ionized calcium with concomitant high serum phosphorus levels and low intact PTH are consistent with hypoparathyroidism.
- Vitamin D deficiency, defined with a 25 hydroxy vitamin D (25(OH)D) level less than 10 ng/mL, may be associated with lower ionized calcium and high PTH levels (25).

Pregnancy Complication
- Maternal hypocalcemia increases the risk for preterm labor and fetal hyperparathyroidism, resulting in bone abnormalities. Adequate treatment can result in good outcomes (21).
- Severe vitamin D deficiency has been associated with an increased risk of preeclampsia, poor maternal weight gain, and calcium malabsorption. Neonatal risks of severe vitamin D deficiency include congenital rickets, small for gestational age, and neonatal hypocalcemia (25).

Treatment
- Vitamin D is the primary treatment. Low or absent PTH inhibits 25(OH)D conversion to $1,25(OH)_2D_3$, requiring active metabolite supplementation.
  - Calcitriol (0.5 to 3.0 μg daily) has a short half-life, relatively rapid onset of action, and low risks of toxicity in the short term. Doses are increased in the first trimester and adjusted throughout pregnancy. Supplement requirements are reduced or completely discontinued during lactation to avoid hypercalcemia during lactation (21,22).

- Ionized calcium or albumin-adjusted serum calcium in the low to mid-normal range is the optimal target in pregnancy (21). Levels may be monitored every 2 to 4 weeks to guide calcitriol adjustments throughout pregnancy and lactation (21,22). Daily calcium supplementation with at least 1 g/d is recommended.
- Acute and severe hypocalcemia can have grave consequences for both mother and fetus. Low calcium levels associated with neuromuscular symptoms should be treated with IV calcium (100 mg/h) until resolution. This should be followed by aggressive oral treatment with calcitriol and calcium.

ADRENAL DISORDERS
Key Points
- Primary adrenal insufficiency (AI) reduces fertility and thus is very uncommon in pregnancy.
- The incidence of pheochromocytoma is 1 in 50,000 pregnancies (26).
- Primary aldosteronism occurs in 0.5% to 5.0% of patients with hypertension.

Background
Pregnancy Physiology
- Pregnancy enhances the activity of the hypothalamic–pituitary–adrenal (HPA) axis and the renin–angiotensin–aldosterone system (RAAS). There is a progressive increase in maternal corticotropin-releasing hormone (CRH), adrenocorticotropic hormone (ACTH), total and free plasma cortisol, urinary free cortisol (UFC), androgens, aldosterone, and renin throughout pregnancy. This occurs without clinical evidence of glucocorticoid (Cushing syndrome [CS]) or mineralocorticoid (aldosteronism) excess (27).
- Increase in placental estrogen production stimulates synthesis of hepatic corticosteroid-binding globulin (CBG), increasing total plasma cortisol threefold compared to nonpregnant levels by the third trimester (28,29). The fetus is protected from excess cortisol by placental 11β-hydroxysteroid dehydrogenase, which converts bioactive cortisol to cortisone, a relatively inactive form (28).
- Ninety to ninety-five percent of fetal cortisol is maternally derived up to 33 weeks of gestation when the maternal contribution drops and the fetal adrenal glands take over (28).
- Aldosterone is the major mineralocorticoid hormone synthesized in the zona glomerulosa of the adrenal glands. Production increases 10- to 20-fold by the third trimester, increasing renal sodium retention and plasma volume expansion. Elevated renin production from the kidney, ovary, and maternal decidua is additive to estrogen in promoting hepatic angiotensinogen synthesis and angiotensin II secretion. Progesterone is a mineralocorticoid receptor antagonist in the distal renal tubule and attenuates the effects of increased aldosterone in pregnancy (28).
- The HPA axis gradually returns to a prepregnant state by 12 weeks postpartum. Lactating women have a blunted HPA response to stress with elevated prolactin and decreased estrogen levels compared to nonlactating women.

ADRENAL INSUFFICIENCY
Background
Definition
- Primary AI, Addison disease, due to destruction of the adrenal cortex results in deficiencies of cortisol, aldosterone, and adrenal androgens (androstenedione and dehydroepiandrosterone [DHEA]). In developed countries, the most common cause of AI is autoimmune and is three times more common in women.
- Secondary AI is due to reduced ACTH secretion, diminished stimulation of the adrenals, and atrophy of the cortical portion of the glands. This can be a result of pituitary or hypothalamic injury, but the most common cause is suppression of the HPA axis by

chronic use of exogenous glucocorticoids. The zona glomerulosa is not under primary control by ACTH, and aldosterone levels are normal in secondary AI.

Differential Diagnosis and Etiology

- The common presentation of primary AI is hyperpigmentation, fatigue, anorexia, and GI symptoms. Many of these are features of normal pregnancy. Anemia, hypothyroidism, and depression can also manifest similarly.
- Patients with Addison disease frequently have other autoimmune diseases such as hypothyroidism, type 1 diabetes mellitus, celiac disease, and hypoparathyroidism (30).
- Tuberculosis (TB) is the most common cause of primary AI in developing countries.
- Bilateral adrenal hemorrhage causing AI is the most common endocrine manifestation of the antiphospholipid syndrome (31). Coagulopathy and shock can also cause adrenal hemorrhage and AI.
- The adrenal glands have rich arterial supply and are common sites of tumor metastases and fungal infections that can cause AI.

Diagnosis and Evaluation

History and Physical Exam

- Signs and symptoms concerning for AI include (27,29,30) fatigue, malaise, lethargy, weight loss, postural hypotension, syncope, nausea, vomiting, anorexia, abdominal pain, and salt craving; hyperpigmentation in non–sun-exposed areas, old scars, and palmar creases is due to the actions of ACTH-related peptides on melanocortin-1 receptors. Bluish spots may be seen on mucosal surfaces such as the lips, gums, vagina, and rectum.
- Adrenal crisis: previously undiagnosed women may present with severe hypotension, hypovolemic shock, acute abdominal pain, vomiting, and fevers.

Diagnostic Testing

- Metabolic profile may show hypoglycemia, hyponatremia, and hyperkalemia but the absence of these abnormalities does NOT exclude AI.
- Paired plasma cortisol and ACTH should be measured. An ACTH greater than 100 pg/mL is consistent with primary AI (29).
- Serum and urinary cortisol levels are not reliable as they increase throughout gestation. However, basal morning (8 AM) plasma cortisol of less than 3 μg/dL is highly suspicious and should undergo further work up for AI.
- The synacthen/cosyntropin test is a measure of adrenal cortisol reserve. Injection of 250 μg ACTH is followed by measuring plasma cortisol at 30 and 60 minutes. Peak cortisol responses to ACTH stimulation are 60% to 80% above nonpregnant women, and trimester-specific cutoff points have been suggested (25 μg/dL, 29 μg/dL, and 32 μg/dL for the first, second, and third trimesters) (27,29).
- 21-Hydroxylase antibodies are positive in 90% of nonpregnant patients with autoimmune adrenal failure, and concurrent hypothyroidism is common. If antibodies are negative, consider imaging of the adrenals after delivery.
- For secondary AI, head MRI and assessment of other anterior pituitary hormones (luteinizing hormone [LH], follicle-stimulating hormone [FSH], prolactin, free T_4, TSH, growth hormone [GH]) are recommended.

Pregnancy Complications

- Before 1933, the mortality rate was 35% to 45% secondary to adrenal crises, but since the introduction and use of corticosteroids, maternal deaths have significantly declined. Mild cases may be undetected until the stress of labor, pregnancy complications, or immediately postpartum because of the protective transplacental passage of cortisol from the fetus to mother (28,30).
- Stressful conditions such as labor, delivery, infections, hyperemesis gravidarum, preeclampsia, or acute hemorrhage can precipitate an acute adrenal crisis.

- Risks for intrauterine growth restriction, low birth weight, and prematurity are increased in untreated or undiagnosed women with AI in pregnancy. Compliant, optimal glucocorticoid therapy prior to pregnancy reduces adverse pregnancy outcomes with high rates of success (27,32).

Treatment
Medications
- The goal of therapy is physiologic glucocorticoid replacement. Hydrocortisone is the preferred treatment. A daily dose of 12 to 15 mg/m^2 is divided to two-thirds in the morning upon awakening and one-third in the mid-afternoon to mimic normal diurnal variation (27). With the progressive increase in CBG during pregnancy, some women may require a 20% to 50% dose adjustment in the third trimester (27,29).
- 50 to 100 mg hydrocortisone IV every 6 to 8 hours is given throughout labor or a cesarean delivery and continued for 24 to 48 hours postdelivery. Hydrocortisone is quickly tapered to prepregnancy dose within 3 days of delivery and can be safely continued during lactation as less than 0.5% is excreted in breast milk.
- Continue prepregnant mineralocorticoid replacement with fludrocortisone 0.05 to 0.2 mg/d throughout pregnancy. Changes in blood pressure and electrolytes should be monitored throughout pregnancy to guide dose adjustments.
- Patients should increase oral hydrocortisone or take intramuscular glucocorticoid during "sick days" or stressful conditions. Medical identification bracelets are encouraged for women to be recognized during emergency situations (27).
- If an acute adrenal crisis is suspected, treatment should be given immediately. After obtaining a blood sample for cortisol, administer 100 to 200 mg IV hydrocortisone once and 50 to 100 mg every 6 hours with close monitoring of electrolytes, heart rate, and blood pressure. Saline resuscitation is useful to overcome the salt wasting and dehydration associated with mineralocorticoid deficiency. Hypoglycemia is treated with oral or IV glucose. Hydrocortisone exerts mineralocorticoid activity at high doses (29), and fludrocortisone is not needed if IV saline is provided.

CUSHING SYNDROME
Background
Definition
- CS is caused by chronic exposure to excessive glucocorticoids. The most common cause is the therapeutic use of exogenous steroids. Endogenous hypercortisolism is either ACTH dependent or ACTH independent. Cushing *disease* refers to overproduction of ACTH by a pituitary adenoma.

Differential Diagnosis and Etiology
- ACTH-independent adrenocortical adenomas (40% to 50%) account for a majority of cases during pregnancy compared to only 15% of cases in nonpregnant patients (30). Adrenal carcinomas have also been described (26).
- ACTH-dependent pituitary or other ectopic tumors result in excess ACTH secretion in approximately 33% of cases diagnosed during pregnancy.
- Carney complex is a rare (1%) primary nodular adrenocortical disease associated with abnormal skin pigmentation, myxomas, and schwannomas.
- ACTH-secreting pheochromocytoma, ACTH-independent adrenal hyperplasia, and aberrant expression of LH/hCG receptors are rare causes of CS (33).

Diagnosis and Evaluation
History and Physical
- Pregnancy is uncommon in women with CS because high levels of cortisol prevent normal follicular development and ovulation (13,30). Diagnosis during pregnancy is challenging, and mild cases may not be confirmed until the postpartum period.

- Signs and symptoms of this condition develop from chronic glucocorticoid exposure and may include the following (28): hypertension, hyperglycemia, peripheral edema, myopathy most apparent in large muscle groups, depression, mood lability, dermal atrophy leading to thin skin, easy bruising, violaceous striae, acne, hirsutism, or downy facial hair with temporal scalp hair regression. CS is commonly characterized with weight gain in a predominantly central distribution frequently with a prominent dorsocervical fat pad (buffalo hump), supraclavicular fat deposition, and perimalleolar edema (moon facies).

Diagnostic Testing
- UFC is recommended for the initial evaluation of pregnant women. Greater than three times the upper limit of nonpregnant normal range is considered abnormal.
- Women with CS lose the circadian rhythm of plasma free and total cortisol and have elevated midnight plasma or salivary cortisol levels (30).
- Because placental CRH can stimulate pituitary ACTH production, plasma levels must be interpreted carefully. If levels are very high, an ectopic source of ACTH should be considered. If ACTH levels are low, it should raise suspicion for an adrenal cause and imaging with CT or ultrasound is indicated.
- A high-dose dexamethasone suppression test (DST) can be diagnostically useful to separate patients with adrenal Cushing who do not suppress cortisol levels, and those with Cushing disease who are globally suppressed. However, DSTs have not been well standardized in pregnancy and can be confounded by the physiologically high plasma total cortisol levels leading to high rates of false-positive tests (28).
- Electrolyte abnormalities may be present from the mineralocorticoid action of cortisol.
- In the absence of a gold standard diagnostic algorithm, distinguishing CS in pregnancy relies on a composite of clinical history, signs on physical exam, and consideration of the usual diagnostic tests: 24-hour urine cortisol, midnight salivary cortisol, plasma ACTH, and DST in the context of gestational physiology.

Pregnancy Complications
- CS is associated with significant maternal morbidity reported to be as high as 70% in pregnancy.
- Pregnant women with CS have higher rates of hypertension (65% to 87%) and diabetes (25% to 61%) (30). CS has been associated with increased perinatal risks for postsurgical wound complications, preeclampsia, oligohydramnios, osteoporosis with fractures, and psychiatric disease. Untreated disease places the patient at risk for heart failure, renal insufficiency and pulmonary edema (28,34).
- Pregnancies complicated by CS have high fetal risks for prematurity (50% to 61%), spontaneous abortion, intrauterine demise, intrauterine growth restriction, and uncommonly fetal hypoadrenalism (28).

Treatment
- Untreated women have poor obstetric outcomes, and treatments are individualized based on gestational age and severity of disease.
- Definitive surgical therapy may be performed in pregnancy, optimally in the second trimester. Adrenalectomy for adrenal adenomas or carcinomas has resulted in a live birth rate of 87%. Transsphenoidal hypophysectomy for pituitary adenomas has been performed successfully with improved perinatal outcomes.
- Metyrapone inhibits 11β-hydroxylase, which is the final step in cortisol synthesis. It passes through the placenta, and nonteratogenicity, fetal virilization, or postpartum hypoadrenalism has been reported. Because of the increased mineralocorticoid effect, metyrapone may increase hypertension during therapy.
- Ketoconazole has not been well studied but has been successfully used in pregnancy. It is a steroidogenesis inhibitor and lowers circulating androgens. Women must be closely monitored for risks of hepatotoxicity and theoretic fetal risks for growth restriction and antiandrogenic effects.

PHEOCHROMOCYTOMA

Background

Definition

- A catecholamine-producing neuroendocrine tumor is arising from chromaffin cells in the adrenal medulla (30). Most cases are sporadic or unilateral and 10% are malignant, bilateral, or familial (28).

Differential Diagnosis and Etiology

- Pheochromocytoma is often overlooked in pregnancy as the clinical manifestations are similar to other pregnancy complications including preeclampsia, other hypertensive disorders of pregnancy, and peripartum cardiomyopathy. Panic attacks, hyperthyroidism, and intracranial tumors may all have features that overlap with pheochromocytoma.
- Because familial syndromes present in younger patients, pheochromocytomas in pregnancy are enriched for those related to MEN 2A & 2B, neurofibromatosis type 1, von Hippel-Lindau syndrome, and mutations in the succinate dehydrogenase B or D genes (28). The other components of MEN 2 are medullary thyroid carcinoma and hyperparathyroidism.

Diagnosis and Evaluation

History and Physical Exam

- Signs and symptoms most commonly featured with pheochromocytoma include (28,30) headache, diaphoresis, dizziness, and palpitations associated with sustained, labile, or paroxysmal hypertension. Patients may also experience anxiety, impending doom, fatigue, weight loss, tachycardia, arrhythmias, angina pectoris, pulmonary edema, heart failure, idiopathic dilated cardiomyopathy, cardiogenic shock, hypertensive retinopathy, papilledema, abdominal pain, diaphoresis, and hyperglycemia
- Women may become symptomatic in the supine position or in labor with the increase in intra-abdominal pressure, gravid uterine compression of the tumor, contractions, and increased sympathetic drive in labor

Diagnostic Testing

- Hyperuricemia, thrombocytopenia, edema, abnormal liver function, and proteinuria are less common in pheochromocytoma and would favor preeclampsia (26,35).
- Pregnancy does not alter catecholamine metabolism; nonpregnant parameters for pheochromocytoma can be used (36). Collection of a 24-hour urine for fractionated metanephrines and measures of catecholamines is both sensitive and specific; vanillylmandelic acid is another metabolite of catecholamine metabolism and can also be used. Plasma fractionated metanephrines is useful in patients with a high likelihood of disease (familial syndrome or known adrenal mass) but lacks specificity. Alpha- and beta-adrenergic blockers, calcium channel antagonists, and tricyclic antidepressants can cause physiologic elevations of circulating catecholamines and may contribute to false-positive results. However, these drugs typically do not elevate diagnostic studies to levels observed in pheochromocytoma (greater than two times the upper limit of normal).
- MRI is the preferred imaging modality to localize the tumor in pregnancy but is less reliable for extra-adrenal locations. A CT and metaiodobenzylguanidine scintigraphy (MIBG) also have diagnostic utility, but due to concerns for radiation exposure are commonly deferred to the nonpregnant state (35).

Pregnancy Complications

- Maternal and fetal mortality rates have recently been shown as high as 8% and 17% with the highest risks associated with women presenting with a hypertensive crisis (35). Antenatal diagnosis is associated with improved perinatal outcomes.

- Hypertension can lead to uteroplacental insufficiency and placental abruption with subsequent complications including but not limited to maternal seizures, stroke, coagulopathy, intrauterine fetal death, and intrauterine growth restriction.

Treatment
- Initiate and optimize medical pharmacotherapy as soon as pheochromocytoma is suspected. Phenoxybenzamine is the preferred alpha-blocker and titrated to achieve blood pressure control. Beta-blockers are added subsequently to oppose reflex tachycardia and catecholamine-induced arrhythmias. Initiation of alpha-blockade should precede beta-blocker administration to minimize the risk of unopposed alpha-adrenergic stimulation worsening a hypertensive crisis (26,35).
- Adrenalectomy is the definitive treatment for pheochromocytoma, and laparoscopy is the preferred approach. When diagnosed early in pregnancy, favorable outcomes have been reported with optimized blood pressure control prior to surgical intervention less than 24 weeks of gestation (26,30,35). When diagnosed after the second trimester, medical therapy, close maternal and fetal surveillance, and a scheduled cesarean delivery with concurrent tumor resection or delayed removal at 2 to 6 weeks postpartum are preferred management strategies (26,35).
- Careful patient monitoring to avoid hypotension and tachycardia is critical. Comanagement with anesthesia for appropriate pain management, preoperative sedation, and volume resuscitation can optimize maternal management.
- If pheochromocytoma is diagnosed and associated with a heritable syndrome, genetic testing should be discussed and offered.

PRIMARY HYPERALDOSTERONISM
Background
Definition
- Primary hyperaldosteronism is a common cause of secondary hypertension and hypokalemia resulting from mineralocorticoid excess.
- Like cortisol, aldosterone levels are higher in pregnant women likely driven by an increase in plasma renin.

Differential Diagnosis and Etiology
- Adrenocortical adenomas, first described by Conn, are the most common cause (60%) (37). Estrogen and ACTH may contribute to aldosterone secretion in these tumors. Worsening hypertension observed in pregnancy may occur due to supraphysiologic aldosterone levels that cannot be antagonized by progesterone.
- Idiopathic hyperaldosteronism is associated with bilateral micro- or macronodular adrenal hyperplasia and is found in 20% to 40% of cases (37).
- Glucocorticoid remediable aldosteronism (GRA) is an autosomal dominant condition and presents with early-onset hypertension, elevated aldosterone, and suppressed plasma renin activity (PRA). It accounts for less than 1% of primary hyperaldosteronism cases and has not been shown to increase the rate of preeclampsia.
- Aberrant LH/hCG and gonadotropin-releasing hormone (GnRH) receptor expression in the adrenal zona glomerulosa has been shown to modulate aldosterone secretion in pathologic tissue (30,38).

Diagnosis and Evaluation
History and Physical Exam
- Clinical presentations in pregnancy are similar to the nonpregnant state and manifest from potassium depletion and hypertension.
- Primary hyperaldosteronism must be distinguished from preeclampsia, eclampsia, secondary aldosteronism such as renovascular hypertension, malignant hypertension, and renal disease. Excessive consumption of licorice can cause pseudoaldosteronism.

- Signs and symptoms are mostly related to hypertension and hypokalemia (39,40): severe hypertension, heart failure, headache, generalized muscle weakness and cramping, polydipsia, polyuria, and nocturia.

Diagnostic Testing

- Hypokalemia, increased potassium excretion, metabolic alkalosis with mild hypernatremia, hypomagnesemia, and proteinuria are commonly observed (39,40).
- Diagnosing primary hyperaldosteronism is difficult as aldosterone increases 5- to 20-fold and PRA increases three- to sevenfold throughout the pregnancy. Despite these quantitative differences, renin should still be suppressed by autonomous aldosterone production. Thus, the ratio of PRA to aldosterone and an elevated plasma aldosterone to PRA ratio (≥50) drawn at 8:00 AM may be used to screen in pregnancy. Patients should not be on spironolactone or eplerenone for 6 weeks before these labs are drawn.
- A high plasma aldosterone (greater than 10 ng/dL) after a 2 L IV infusion of normal saline over 4 hours between 8:00 AM and 12:00 PM is a test to confirm the diagnosis if screening is positive.
- In secondary aldosteronism, there are elevations in aldosterone and PRA.
- GRA is identified with the presence of tetrahydroaldosterone, 18-hydroxycortisol, and 18-oxycortisol in the urine. DST over 3 days will suppress ACTH production and through negative feedback regulation will suppress aldosterone production. The gold standard test for diagnosis is long-amplification PCR for the chimeric gene (37).
- Once primary hyperaldosteronism is established, adrenal imaging by MRI is useful in distinguishing aldosterone-producing adenomas from bilateral hyperplasia.

Pregnancy Complications

- Elevated circulating aldosterone and untreated primary aldosteronism places women at risk for cardiovascular events including arrhythmias, myocardial infarction, and stroke (37). Pregnant women are at higher risk for preeclampsia, HELLP syndrome, placental abruption, gestational diabetes, cesarean delivery, and uncontrollable hypertension (28,30,39).
- Fetal risks for prematurity, intrauterine growth restriction, and intrauterine fetal demise are increased, particularly with uncontrolled hypertension.
- One-third of women will remain hypertensive after definitive surgical management in pregnancy due to the long-term effects of hypertension on the maternal vasculature and renal function (37).
- Some patients with hyperaldosteronism have normal blood pressure values throughout gestation followed by sustained, severe pressures postpartum when progesterone levels decline, but aldosterone levels continue to be elevated (40). Women should be worked up 6 to 8 weeks postpartum with persistent hypertension.

Treatment

- The primary goal of treatment is blood pressure control.
- Spironolactone, a mineralocorticoid antagonist, crosses the placenta and is commonly used for medical management of primary hyperaldosteronism. It is contraindicated in pregnancy due to the potent antiandrogenic effects, causing genital ambiguity in male fetuses (30). Eplerenone is a more selective aldosterone receptor antagonist than spironolactone and has shown to successfully improve blood pressure and potassium in pregnancy without the feminization of male genitals but has not been well studied.
- Laparoscopic adrenalectomy can be performed successfully in the second trimester with improvement of blood pressure and potassium levels.
- Antihypertensive medications including labetalol, amiloride, and calcium channel antagonists are used for blood pressure management (39). Nifedipine is an effective treatment

in pregnancy because it resembles mineralocorticoid antagonists, competes with aldosterone binding at the mineralocorticoid receptor, and blocks aldosterone-induced recruitment to the receptor (39).

PITUITARY DISORDERS
Key Points
- Prolactinomas are the most common cause of persistent hyperprolactinemia and account for approximately 50% pituitary tumors.
- The diagnostic features of Sheehan syndrome is failure of postpartum lactation and restoration of normal menstruation.
- Gestational diabetes insipidus (DI) is a rare endocrinopathy in pregnancy with an incidence of 4 in 100,000 pregnancies.

Pregnancy Physiology
- The anterior pituitary (adenohypophysis) has five different cell types that produce and release peptide hormones: pro-opiomelanocortin (POMC) and associated derivatives (e.g., ACTH and β-lipotropin), prolactin, GH, LH, FSH, and TSH.
- The posterior pituitary lobe (neurohypophysis) releases oxytocin and vasopressin.
- Placental estrogen stimulates hyperplasia and hypertrophy of lactotrophs increasing the anterior pituitary volume by twofold. Elevated lactotroph activity promotes prolactin synthesis, which peaks at 150 to 250 ng/mL before delivery to prepare breast tissue for lactation. Circulating prolactin is also influenced by sleep, physical activity, food consumption, breast stimulation, and thyroid function.
- In postpartum women who do not breast-feed, serum prolactin decreases to prepregnancy levels within 3 months. In lactating women, basal circulating prolactin levels remain elevated but with periodic spikes due to nursing. Pituitary glandular enlargement returns to normal shape, size, and volume within 6 months after delivery.
- Plasma GH begins to increase at approximately 10 weeks of gestation and plateaus at 28 weeks of gestation. Pituitary GH release in the first half of the pregnancy is of pituitary origin, but a GH variant made by placental syncytiotrophoblasts increases later in gestation.
- FSH and LH decrease by 6 to 7 weeks of gestation due to negative feedback by estradiol, progesterone, and inhibin.
- Vasopressinase is made in the placenta and rapidly inactivates ADH, increasing the metabolic clearance rate of ADH three- to fourfold during pregnancy. Vasopressinase activity remains elevated until delivery, decreasing thereafter at an exponential rate of 25% per day.

DIABETES INSIPIDUS
Background
Definition
- Central DI is an idiopathic or acquired disorder characterized by failure of arginine vasopressin (AVP) secretion. The most common causes are surgery in the sella, trauma, or diseases that infiltrate the pituitary such as tumors, metastases to the hypothalamus, Langerhans cell histiocytosis, or sarcoidosis. Syndromes of inherited DI are rare.
- Nephrogenic DI is due to impairment of AVP signaling at the distal tubule and the inability to concentrate urine despite normal or elevated plasma concentrations of AVP. Common causes include hypokalemia and hypercalcemia, acute and chronic kidney diseases, and chronic lithium chloride treatment.
- Gestational DI is a condition resulting from abnormal AVP secretion, degradation, or response. It can be due to excessive vasopressinase activity or transient reduction of vasopressinase degradation because of abnormal liver function (41).

Differential Diagnosis and Etiology
- Psychogenic or primary polydipsia and certain medications (lithium, diuretics, anticholinergics) can share similar symptoms of DI.
- Diabetes mellitus, chronic renal disease, and other metabolic disorders can present with polydipsia and polyuria.
- Gestational DI can present in the following distinct clinical settings (41):
  - Women with hereditary DI, asymptomatic carriers, or those with previous neurosurgery/trauma are at higher risk for diagnosis during pregnancy when the metabolic AVP clearance is increased.
  - Transient AVP-resistant but dDAVP-(desmopressin-2 amino acid substitute of AVP) responsive DI, occurring during gestation or the early puerperium period, is the most common type seen during pregnancy. It is commonly associated with multiple pregnancies or with pregnancies complicated by liver abnormalities (preeclampsia, acute fatty liver of pregnancy, HELLP syndrome).
  - Postpartum DI may be observed secondary to Sheehan syndrome with significant obstetrical hemorrhage.

Diagnosis and Evaluation
History and Physical Exam
- DI is diagnosed by clinical history, hypernatremia without other major electrolyte abnormalities, increased serum osmolality with inappropriately low urine osmolality, and high urine output. Common signs and symptoms patients may present with include the following (42): weakness, fatigue, postural dizziness, polydipsia, abdominal pain, nausea, vomiting, or polyuria (greater than 3 L/d).

Diagnostic Tests
- In a hypernatremic patient, early morning low urine osmolality (less than 200 mOsm/L) with elevated serum osmolality (greater than 285 mOsm/L) is suggestive of DI.
- Diagnosis is confirmed by the water deprivation test, but these are not commonly performed in pregnancy as it can lead to severe dehydration.
- Nephrogenic DI is diagnosed by the failure to increase urine osmolarity and decrease serum sodium following administration of exogenous AVP.
- Metabolic panel, liver function testing, 24-hour urine total protein, and complete blood count should be obtained to rule out pregnancy disorders such as preeclampsia, diabetes, acute fatty liver, and HELLP that may be associated with DI.
- MRI is helpful to identify pathologic lesions (loss of the bright signal typical of the posterior pituitary).

Pregnancy Complications
- Clinical presentation is typically acute, and DI can be associated with significant pregnancy complications. Polyhydramnios, neonatal polyuria, and intrauterine fetal demise have been reported.

Treatment
- Desmopressin or dDAVP is a synthetic, modified form of vasopressin and the treatment of choice for gestational DI. It is not degraded by placental vasopressinase and can be used to manage central DI or pregnancy-induced DI (43). It is available in IV (1 to 2 µg), intranasal (5 to 10 µg/d), and oral tablet forms (100 to 300 µg/d). No risk of fetal malformations has been reported from drug exposure.
- Nephrogenic DI is treated with thiazide diuretics (hydrochlorothiazide 50 to 100 mg daily) and salt restriction to induce mild sodium depletion, enhancing proximal tubular resorption and decreases urine output.

PROLACTINOMA
Background
Definition
- Prolactinoma is an anterior pituitary tumor derived from prolactin-secreting lactotroph cells.
  - Microadenomas: less than 10 mm; more than 90% of prolactinomas
  - Macroadenomas: greater than 10 mm.

Differential Diagnosis and Etiology
- Women with prolactinomas are generally infertile or anovulatory because hyperprolactinemia impairs the hypothalamic–pituitary–ovarian axis, decreasing pulsatile GnRH secretion.
- Hyperprolactinemia without a tumor visualized on imaging and no identifiable secondary causes are considered idiopathic.
- Secondary causes of hyperprolactinemia include but are not limited to hypothyroidism, renal insufficiency, hypothalamic and pituitary diseases, and neurogenic etiology such as spinal cord lesions, breast stimulation, and chest wall lesions. Lactotrophs are under tonic inhibition by dopamine. Sellar lesions that compress the pituitary stalk interfere with this regulation causing hyperprolactinemia.
- Pituitary glandular enlargement can be caused by apoplexy or hemorrhagic necrosis of an adenoma, Sheehan syndrome, or lymphohypophysitis.
- Medications and substances inhibiting dopamine secretion can increase prolactin levels, including phenothiazines, various antidepressants, metoclopramide, methyldopa, cocaine, opiates, verapamil, and high-dose estrogens.

Diagnosis and Evaluation
History and Physical Exam
- Amenorrhea or oligomenorrhea and galactorrhea are the most common symptoms in women of reproductive age. Many women present with infertility and are diagnosed prior to pregnancy.

Diagnostic Testing
- Hyperprolactinemia is the cardinal feature in nonpregnant women and usually correlates with tumor size. In nonpregnant women, microadenomas generally have prolactin levels greater than 100 ng/mL and tumors greater than 1 cm have greater than 200 ng/mL.
- In women with a known prolactinoma prior to pregnancy:
  - Prolactin should not be routinely monitored in pregnancy.
  - Patients should be evaluated with prolactin levels 2 months after delivery. Prolactin levels have been reported to normalize or decrease by 50% to 60% in microadenomas and 64% to 72% macroadenomas compared to pregestational levels.
- MRI of the pituitary is the best imaging study to detect pituitary adenomas for both pregnant and nonpregnant individuals. Prepregnancy baseline imaging should be obtained and does not have to be repeated in pregnancy unless there are clinical features that raise concern for glandular enlargement.
- Baseline automated visual fields (i.e., Humphrey visual fields) should be obtained for all women with a prolactinoma. Patients with a microadenoma do not require routine testing unless optic chiasm compression is suspected. Macroadenomas should be tested each trimester (44).
- If marked elevations or changes in serum prolactin occur, measure serum drug screen, TSH, FT_4, metabolic panel, and insulin-like growth factor-1 to rule out secondary causes of hyperprolactinemia.

Pregnancy Complications

- Symptomatic enlargement is seen in 1.4% to 2.2% of microadenomas and 15.5% to 37% of macroadenomas that were not radiated or surgically treated prior to pregnancy (44). Macroadenomas have a greater propensity of symptomatic growth and need to be followed closely through the pregnancy. Symptoms primarily include headaches and visual disturbances.
- Macroadenoma enlargement rarely results in pituitary apoplexy or neurosurgical complications, but the highest risk is seen in the third trimester.
- Microsurgical resection of prolactinoma is associated with a long-term restoration of normal prolactin levels of approximately 60% to 80% microadenomas and 15% to 30% macroadenomas. Surgery has risks of death (0.3% cases) and cerebrospinal fluid (CSF) leak (0.4%).

Treatment

- Medical therapy and successful transsphenoidal surgery for prolactinomas usually result in restoration of normal gonadal function and pregnancies.
- Goals of treatment are to prevent optic chiasm compression, suppress prolactin production, induce ovulation, preserve pituitary function, and prevent tumor recurrence.
- Dopamine agonists are first-line therapy, decreasing tumor size and prolactin secretion. Bromocriptine is the drug of choice in women with prolactinomas in pregnancy (44). It has been well studied and can be used to restore fertility without increased fetal or maternal risks. Cabergoline, a long-acting dopaminergic agonist, is a safe alternative to bromocriptine with fewer gastrointestinal side effects but not as well studied in pregnancy.
  - Safety of continuous treatment during pregnancy has not been established, and therapy should be discontinued once pregnancy is confirmed (44).
  - Continuous dopamine agonist therapy in pregnancy is considered with tumor margins outside the intrasellar boundaries.
  - Most common side effects are nausea, vomiting, and postural hypotension and can be minimized by starting with a low dose (0.625 to 1.25 mg/d) and increasing slowly over a 2- to 3-week period.
- Clinical evaluation for headaches and visual changes should be assessed every 3 months with microadenomas and every 1 to 2 months with macroadenomas. Imaging and automated visual field assessments should be performed with suspicion for tumor enlargement (44). Confirmation of symptomatic tumor enlargement should prompt reinstituting bromocriptine therapy immediately.
- Transsphenoidal surgery or delivery, if gestational age appropriate, should be considered when the response to medical therapy is suboptimal or with worsening visual compromise. Glucocorticoids are not effective to reduce tumor size.
- If the adenoma is very large or elevates the optic chiasm, the patient is at high risk for significant tumor enlargement in pregnancy. Pregnancy should be discouraged until the adenoma has been treated by transsphenoidal surgery, postoperative radiation, or prolonged dopamine agonist therapy to decrease tumor size.
- Breast-feeding has not been shown to enhance tumor growth, and postpartum tumor regression has been reported on radiological evaluation in lactating women (44).
- Oral contraceptives are safe for women with prolactinomas and have not been shown to cause tumor growth.

SHEEHAN SYNDROME AND LYMPHOCYTIC HYPOPHYSITIS

Background

Definition

- Sheehan syndrome (SS) is a hypopituitarism caused by ischemic infarction or pituitary necrosis from severe hypotension or shock due to significant postpartum hemorrhage and hypovolemia.

- LH is an autoimmune disorder with both humoral and cellular-mediated lymphocytic infiltration and enlargement and destruction of the pituitary gland. Pituitary dysfunction ranges from partial to full anterior hypophysitis, infundibuloneurohypophysitis, and panhypophysitis. It is highly associated with pregnancy and postpartum.

Differential Diagnosis and Etiology
- Pregnancy is associated with physiologic enlargement of the pituitary gland, and ischemia may occur with mild compression of the superior hypophyseal artery that is the major blood supply of the adenohypophysis. When challenged with a substantial hemorrhage and hypotension, changes in arterial pressure places the pituitary at risk for vascular insufficiency, ischemic damage, and necrosis. An arrest of blood flow to the pituitary can also result from vasospasm, thrombosis, or vascular compression, and the severity of disease is related to the degree of distribution and duration of insult. Women with a small sella size are at a higher risk.
- Pituitary apoplexy is an acute hemorrhagic infarction of a pituitary adenoma that occurs spontaneously or in response to hypotension. Patients present with headache, visual changes, and/or symptoms of acute AI. Accurate diagnosis is required as apoplexy is unresponsive to conservative therapy and often requires transsphenoidal decompression, which is contraindicated with Sheehan syndrome.
- Empty sella syndrome is an anatomic abnormality often noted incidentally on pituitary imaging in persons with no history of pituitary-related disease. Abnormalities in pituitary endocrine function occur in approximately 20% of cases and can mimic the deficiency aspects of Sheehan's. Women with chronic hypertension, obesity, or previous intracranial injury, radiation, or surgery have risk factors for pituitary dysfunction.

Diagnosis and Evaluation
History and Physical Exam
- Criteria for the diagnosis of SS:
  - History of severe postpartum hemorrhage, shock, or hypotension requiring significant resuscitation or blood transfusion
  - Failure of postpartum lactation
  - Failure to resume normal menstrual cycles after delivery
  - Evidence of varying degrees of anterior pituitary dysfunction/failure
  - MRI showing empty sella turcica
- Diagnosis is usually made based on history, clinical presentation of hypopituitarism, and empty sella on brain MRI or CT.
  - Panhypopituitarism with deficiencies of ACTH, LH, FSH, TSH, and GH is present in 55% to 86% of individuals and from time of inciting even to diagnosis of Sheehan syndrome may be a few months to several years but women may present with select deficiencies.
  - Posterior pituitary hormone deficiency causing DI is uncommon although atrophy of the neurohypophysis and supraventricular and paraventricular nuclei have been identified in greater than 90% of women with SS.
- Definitive diagnosis for LH requires histopathologic confirmation on pituitary biopsy.
- Clinical signs and symptoms vary with the severity of pituitary injury, and diagnosis is often delayed. Acute clinical presentation of Sheehan syndrome is rare and may present with headache, tachycardia, hypotension, postpartum seizure, poor wound healing, or coma. Chronic SS or LH may present with bradycardia, hypotension, varying degrees of hypopituitarism, infertility, anemia, or skin or hair changes.

Diagnostic Testing
- Basal hormone levels of prolactin, FT_4, TSH, cortisol, ACTH, FSH, LH estradiol, and insulin-like growth factor 1 (IGF-1) may be useful in diagnosis.
- Dynamic pituitary function testing is usually required for a more detailed workup.

- GnRH stimulation test is used to evaluate pituitary gonadotropin secretion. Low FSH and LH with low estradiol are commonly seen.
- Insulin tolerance test is the preferred choice to assess GH and ACTH reserve, resulting in low GH, ACTH, and cortisol secretion.
- Hyponatremia due to hypothyroidism and ACTH deficiency is the most common electrolyte disorder. GH-deficient hyperlipidemia may be significant.
- Pituitary antibodies are inconsistently observed with LH and not routinely ordered.
- MRI is the most sensitive imaging modality for hypothalamic–pituitary assessment. Early, acute forms of Sheehan's will show nonhemorrhagic enlargement of the gland followed by involution and atrophy when empty sella develops. LH will demonstrate homogenous, enhancing pituitary mass with suprasellar extension.

Treatment
- Goal of treatment is replacement of deficient hormones.
- Replacement of thyroid, adrenal, and gonadal hormones are life saving, improve health outcomes, and correct anemia and pancytopenia commonly observed.
- GH replacement is useful in some cases to improve overall well-being, lipid profile, cardiovascular health, and body composition. However, the ultimate benefit of this treatment is still under debate, and the drug is very expensive.
- Pregnancy has been shown to improve hypopituitarism, stimulating pituitary remnants.
- Transsphenoidal surgery for decompression and debulking of the inflammatory mass with LH should be reserved for progressive visual impairment, persistent neurologic dysfunction, unresponsive to medical therapy, or radiologic evidence of symptomatic enlargement.
- Pituitary mass reduction in LH can be achieved with pituitary surgery, dopamine agonists (bromocriptine), glucocorticoids, immunosuppressive drugs (azathioprine), or pituitary radiotherapy but long-term efficacy and success is unclear (45).

REFERENCES

1. World Health Organization. *Reaching optimal iodine nutrition in pregnant and lactating women and young children: a joint statement.* Geneva, Switzerland: 2007.
2. Stagnaro-Green A, Abalovich M, Alexander E, et al. Guidelines of the American Thyroid Association for the diagnosis and management of thyroid disease during pregnancy and postpartum. *Thyroid.* 2011;21(10):1081–1125.
3. Fereidoun A, Ladan M, Atieh A, et al. Establishment of the trimester-specific reference range for free thyroxine index. *Thyroid.* 2013;23(3):354–359.
4. Burrow G, Fisher D, Larson P. Maternal and fetal thyroid function. *N Engl J Med.* 1994;331:1072–1075.
5. Loubière LS, Vasilopoulou E, Glazier JD, et al. Expression and function of thyroid hormone transporters in the microvillous plasma membrane of human term placental syncytiotrophoblast. *Endocrinology.* 2012;153(12):6126–6135.
6. Schmaltz C. Thyroid hormones in the neonate: an overview of physiology and clinical correlation. *Adv Neonatal Care.* 2012;12(4):217–222.
7. Mestman JH. Hyperthyroidism in pregnancy. *Curr Opin Endocrinol Diabetes Obes.* 2012;19(5):394–401.
8. Krajewski DA, Burman KD. Thyroid disorders in pregnancy. *Endocrinol Metab Clin North Am.* 2011;40(4):739–763.
9. Azizi F, Amouzegar A. Management of hyperthyroidism during pregnancy and lactation. *Eur J Endocrinol.* 2011;164(6):871–876.
10. Casey BM, Leveno KJ. Thyroid disease in pregnancy. *Obstet Gynecol.* 2006;108(5):1283–1292.
11. Bliddal S, Rasmussen AK, Sundberg K, et al. Antithyroid drug-induced fetal goitrous hypothyroidism. *Nat Rev Endocrinol.* 2011;7(7):396–406.
12. Kothari A, Girling J. Hypothyroidism in pregnancy: pre-pregnancy thyroid status influences gestational thyroxine requirements. *BJOG.* 2008;115(13):1704–1708.

13. Yassa L, Marqusee E, Fawcett R, et al. Thyroid hormone early adjustment in pregnancy (the THERAPY) trial. *J Clin Endocrinol Metab.* 2010;95(7):3234–3241.

14. Cleary-Goldman J, Malone FD, Lambert-Messerlian G, et al. Maternal thyroid hypofunction and pregnancy outcome. *Obstet Gynecol.* 2008;112(1):85–92.

15. Haddow JE, Palomaki GE, Allan WC, et al. Maternal thyroid deficiency during pregnancy and subsequent neuropsychological development of the child. *N Engl J Med.* 1999;341(8):549–555.

16. Reid SM, Middleton P, Cossich MC, et al. Interventions for clinical and subclinical hypothyroidism in pregnancy. *Cochrane Database Syst Rev.* 2010;(7):CD007752.

17. De Groot L, Abalovich M, Alexander EK, et al. Management of thyroid dysfunction during pregnancy and postpartum: an Endocrine Society clinical practice guideline. *J Clin Endocrinol Metab.* 2012;97(8):2543–2565.

18. Alexander E, Marqusee E, Lawrence J, et al. Timing and magnitude of increases in levothyroxine requirements during pregnancy in women with hypothyroidism. *N Engl J Med.* 2004;351:241–249.

19. Stagnaro-Green A. Approach to the patient with postpartum thyroiditis. *J Clin Endocrinol Metab.* 2012;97(2):334–342.

20. Stagnaro-Green A, Akhter E, Yim C, et al. Thyroid disease in pregnant women with systemic lupus erythematosus: increased preterm delivery. *Lupus.* 2011;20(7):690–699.

21. Kovacs CS. Calcium and bone metabolism disorders during pregnancy and lactation. *Endocrinol Metab Clin North Am.* 2011;40(4):795–826.

22. Cooper MS. Disorders of calcium metabolism and parathyroid disease. *Best Pract Res Clin Endocrinol Metab.* 2011;25(6):975–983.

23. Hong MK, Lin YC, Wei YC, et al. Parathyroid adenoma with hypertensive crisis and intracerebral hemorrhage mimicking hemolysis, elevated liver enzymes, low platelets syndrome. *Obstet Gynecol.* 2011;117(2 Pt 2):498–500.

24. Som M, Stroup JS. Primary hyperparathyroidism and pregnancy. *Proc (Bayl Univ Med Cent).* 2011;24(3):220–223.

25. Mulligan ML, Felton SK, Riek AE, et al. Implications of vitamin D deficiency in pregnancy and lactation. *Am J Obstet Gynecol.* 2010;202(5):429.e1–e9.

26. Lansdown A, Rees DA. Endocrine oncology in pregnancy. *Best Pract Res Clin Endocrinol Metab.* 2011;25(6):911–926.

27. Yuen KC, Chong LE, Koch CA. Adrenal insufficiency in pregnancy: challenging issues in diagnosis and management. *Endocrine.* 2013;44(2):283–292.

28. Abdelmannan D, Aron DC. Adrenal disorders in pregnancy. *Endocrinol Metab Clin North Am.* 2011;40(4):779–794.

29. Lebbe M, Arlt W. What is the best diagnostic and therapeutic management strategy for an Addison patient during pregnancy? *Clin Endocrinol (Oxf)* 2013;78(4):497–502.

30. Monticone S, Auchus RJ, Rainey WE. Adrenal disorders in pregnancy. *Nat Rev Endocrinol.* 2012;8(11):668–678.

31. Mehdi AA, Salti I, Uthman I. Antiphospholipid syndrome: endocrinologic manifestations and organ involvement. *Semin Thromb Hemost.* 2011;37(1):49–57.

32. Björnsdottir S, Cnattingius S, Brandt L, et al. Addison's disease in women is a risk factor for an adverse pregnancy outcome. *J Clin Endocrinol Metab.* 2010;95(12):5249–5257.

33. Achong N, D'Emden M, Fagermo N, et al. Pregnancy-induced Cushing's syndrome in recurrent pregnancies: case report and literature review. *Aust N Z J Obstet Gynaecol.* 2012;52(1):96–100.

34. Choi WJ, Jung TS, Paik WY. Cushing's syndrome in pregnancy with a severe maternal complication: a case report. *J Obstet Gynaecol Res.* 2011;37(2):163–167.

35. Biggar MA, Lennard TW. Systematic review of phaeochromocytoma in pregnancy. *Br J Surg.* 2013;100(2):182–190.

36. Kamoun M, Mnif MF, Charfi N, et al. Adrenal diseases during pregnancy: pathophysiology, diagnosis and management strategies. *Am J Med Sci.* 2014;347:64–73.

37. Escher G. Hyperaldosteronism in pregnancy. *Ther Adv Cardiovasc Dis.* 2009;3(2):123–132.

38. Albiger NM, Sartorato P, Mariniello B, et al. A case of primary aldosteronism in pregnancy: do LH and GNRH receptors have a potential role in regulating aldosterone secretion? *Eur J Endocrinol.* 2011;164(3):405–412.
39. Krysiak R, Samborek M, Stojko R. Primary aldosteronism in pregnancy. *Acta Clin Belg.* 2012;67(2):130–134.
40. Ronconi V, Turchi F, Zennaro MC, et al. Progesterone increase counteracts aldosterone action in a pregnant woman with primary aldosteronism. *Clin Endocrinol (Oxf)* 2011;74(2):278–279.
41. Karaca Z, Kelestimur F. Pregnancy and other pituitary disorders (including GH deficiency). *Best Pract Res Clin Endocrinol Metab.* 2011;25(6):897–910.
42. Kalelioglu I, Kubat Uzum A, Yildirim A, et al. Transient gestational diabetes insipidus diagnosed in successive pregnancies: review of pathophysiology, diagnosis, treatment, and management of delivery. *Pituitary.* 2007;10(1):87–93.
43. Schrier RW. Systemic arterial vasodilation, vasopressin, and vasopressinase in pregnancy. *J Am Soc Nephrol.* 2010;21(4):570–572.
44. Bronstein MD, Paraiba DB, Jallad RS. Management of pituitary tumors in pregnancy. *Nat Rev Endocrinol.* 2011;7(5):301–310.
45. Foyouzi N. Lymphocytic adenohypophysitis. *Obstet Gynecol Surv.* 2011;66(2):109–113.

19 Hematologic Complications

Tondra Newman and David F. Colombo

KEY POINTS

- Anemia is the most common medical complication of pregnancy.
- "Physiologic anemia" of pregnancy is a consequence of disproportionate expansion in red cell mass and blood volume.
- Pregnancy is a state of hypercoagulability. Alteration in hormonal milieu, increase in coagulation factors, and a decrease in anticoagulants and fibrinolysis activity actuate this process.
- Hematologic cancers in pregnancy are rare. Pregnancy does not usually affect the course of the disease, and treatment is generally not withheld during pregnancy.

NORMAL PHYSIOLOGY

Background

- Pregnancy-associated changes (1):
  - Increased plasma volume
  - Increased formed elements: erythrocyte mass, platelets, and leukocytes
  - Adjusted coagulation factors
- Upper and lower limits of these changes in the hematologic elements are somewhat variably defined, but general ranges can be appreciated (Table 19-1) (2).

RED BLOOD CELLS

Background

- Increases in both the number of red blood cells (RBCs) and plasma volume occur until near term and then gradually return to prepregnancy levels by 6 weeks postpartum.
- Plasma volume increases to three times that of red cell volume. Expansion begins at 6 weeks and increases significantly until 34 weeks gestation (50% over baseline).
- RBC volume expansion is more gradual than plasma volume from around 10 weeks until term (20% to 30% over baseline).
- A greater increase in plasma volume than red cell volume leads to a decrease in the hemoglobin–hematocrit, resulting in the "physiologic anemia" of pregnancy.
- Multiple-gestation pregnancy is associated with an even larger increase in blood volume.
- An increase in red cell and plasma volume provides for the increased perfusion needs of the fetal–placental unit, accommodates maternal oxygen demands, and gives a margin of safety associated with blood loss during delivery (2).

ANEMIA

Background

- Anemia is the most common medical complication of pregnancy.
- Globally, as many as 41.8% of pregnant women are anemic. The prevalence in the United States has not been well studied; however, WHO approximates 18% in industrialized countries (3,4).

Table 19-1	Normal Pregnancy Values of the Different Blood Elements
Blood element	**Pregnancy values**
Red blood cells (hematocrit)	
Second trimester	31.2%–35.5%
Third trimester	31.9%–36.5%
White blood cells	$9–15 \times 10^9$ cells/L
Platelets	$140–400 \times 10^9$ cells/L
Coagulation factors	
Fibrinogen	Increased up to 200%
Prothrombin	No change
V	No change
VII	Increased up to 200%
VIII	Increased up to 300%
IX	Slight increase
X	Increased up to 200%
XI	Slight decrease
XIII	Slight decrease

Adapted from Kilpatrick SJ. Anemia and pregnancy. In: Creasy RK, Resnik R, Iams JD, eds. *Maternal-fetal medicine principles and practice.* 6th ed. Philadelphia: W.B. Saunders, 2009:869–884.

- Rate is influenced by smoking status, high altitudes, race, and chronic medical conditions.
- The most common causes of anemia are nutritional-related iron deficiency and acute blood loss.
- Hgb levels less than 6 g/dL and greater than 14 g/dL are associated with adverse maternal and fetal outcomes (5).
- Recent studies have re-examined the association between maternal anemia and adverse perinatal outcomes. In the setting of moderate to severe anemia, there is an increased risk of prematurity, low birth weight, and fetal death (6–8).
- The inability to expand blood volume or chronic hypoxia may explain the underlying pathophysiology influencing fetal outcomes (6).
- In addition to increased maternal–fetal risk associated with anemia, long-term metabolic and developmental outcomes in children are still being investigated (7).
- Delayed cord clamping following birth has been shown to demonstrate a higher hematocrit in neonates. There is no evidence of maternal or neonatal compromise as once speculated (9).

Definition
- The acceptable lower limit for hemoglobin is 10 g/dL (normal of 14.0 ± 2.0 g/dL).
- Given the normal physiologic hemodilution of pregnancy, the Centers for Disease Control and Prevention defines anemia in pregnancy as follows (10):
  - Hgb less than 11.0 g/dL in the first and third trimesters
  - Hgb less than 10.5 g/dL in the second trimester

Evaluation
History and Physical
- Signs and symptoms range from subclinical with mild anemia to nonspecific in those with moderate to severe anemia. Symptoms may include:
  - Fatigue
  - Weakness
  - Anorexia

- Headache
- Dyspnea on exertion
- The first prenatal visit should include universal screening for anemia, including questions relating to a history of anemia, personal and family history of bleeding diathesis, and other blood disorders.

Laboratory Tests
- Routine prenatal laboratory studies should include a CBC.
- The hemoglobin/hematocrit should be repeated during the third trimester (about 28 to 32 weeks) and more frequently if indicated.
- Hemoglobin less than 10 g/dL is abnormal in pregnancy and should trigger an evaluation for etiology of anemia (11).
- In the presence of low hemoglobin levels, RBC indices are helpful in deciding the pathophysiology of the anemia.
- Further evaluation may include
  - Urinalysis
  - Iron studies
  - Reticulocyte count
  - Peripheral blood smear
  - Stool for ova and parasites
  - Stool for occult blood (guaiac test)
  - Bone marrow studies rarely indicated in pregnancy
- Certain ethnicities should have screening tests for specific conditions.
  - African American patients should have a hemoglobin electrophoresis to evaluate for sickle cell trait and thalassemia.
  - Patients from the Mediterranean, the Middle East, India, and Southeast Asia are at risk for thalassemia, which also can be identified on hemoglobin electrophoresis.

SPECIFIC ANEMIAS
- Acquired causes of anemia
  - Iron deficiency anemia
  - Folate deficiency anemia
  - B_{12} deficiency
  - Anemia of chronic disease
  - Acquired hemolytic anemia
  - Aplastic anemia
  - Hemorrhagic anemia

Iron Deficiency Anemia
Background
- Most common cause of anemia in pregnancy.
- Antepartum iron deficiency is associated with low iron levels in the infant at 1 year of life but has not been demonstrated to be associated with fetal anemia (10).

Etiology
- Most reproductive-age women have inadequate prenatal iron stores entering pregnancy.
- Factors contributing to iron deficiency include the following:
  - Dietary insufficiency, malabsorption, or iron supplement intolerance
  - Bleeding prior to or during pregnancy
  - Multiple gestation, which increases iron requirements and may be responsible for a greater blood loss at delivery
  - Concurrent antacid use may prevent iron absorption
  - Poor dietary habits or pica (an appetite for inedible substances, such as clay or dirt)
  - Short interpregnancy interval

- Pregnancy exhausts maternal iron stores because of increased maternal blood production and fetal growth needs.
  - An approximate iron deficit of 580 mg occurs in pregnancy.
- Conventional diets, even with a focus on iron-rich food, contain about 15 mg of daily iron and do not meet the additional iron requirement of pregnancy.
- Dietary iron intake of 27 mg/day is recommended during pregnancy.
- In total, pregnancy requires approximately 1 g of elemental iron
  - 450 mg for RBC expansion
  - 270 mg for fetal iron
  - 170 mg for basal loss
  - 150 mg for delivery loss
- Eighty percent of available functional iron is found in the Hgb of RBCs.

Evaluation
Laboratory Studies
- Iron deficiency anemia (IDA) manifests abnormal lab findings after maternal iron stores are significantly depleted.
  - Characterized by a microcytic, hypochromic anemia.
  - Decreased mean corpuscular volume (MCV) approximately to a borderline level of 70 to 80 fL (normal = 90 ± 10 fL).
  - Serum iron falls below 40 µg/dL.
  - Since iron is transported bound to transferrin, the unsaturated total iron-binding capacity (TIBC) rises above 400 µg/dL.
  - Serum ferritin (abnormal less than 12 µg/dL) correlates well with bone marrow stores, making a bone marrow examination rarely necessary (12).
    - Ferritin is an acute-phase reactant and may be elevated in the presence of inflammation (normal ferritin with normal C-reactive protein is not consistent with IDA) (13).
    - An alternative to ferritin measurement is soluble transferrin receptor (sTfR), which identifies decreased rate of erythropoiesis, levels greater than 4.4 mg/L suggest iron deficiency in tissues (14).

Diagnosis
Differential Diagnosis
- Includes anemia of chronic disease and heterozygous thalassemia
- Thalassemia minor produces a mild anemia with a borderline low MCV but should not exclude the diagnosis of IDA.
- Serum ferritin level, which is highly sensitive and specific for IDA, should help differentiate.

Treatment
Prophylaxis
- In the absence of a laboratory diagnosis of iron deficiency, clinical studies have failed to show a consistent benefit for routine iron supplementation in terms of outcome such as low birth weight or preterm delivery (15–18).

Medications
- Most common oral iron replacement formulations contain inorganic nonheme supplements.
  - Limited information is available on organic heme iron supplements but appear to demonstrate better improvement in iron stores postpartum in comparison to placebo or nonheme iron (19).
- Ferrous sulfate 325-mg tablets contain 65 mg of elemental iron.
- Intestinal absorption, approximately 10% of dietary intake, permits absorption only up to 15 mg of iron without signs of iron intolerance.

- Given the limits of daily absorption and the well-recognized gastrointestinal intolerance to iron, TID oral dosing is unnecessary.
- Alternative treatments to oral therapy are parental iron, subcutaneous erythropoietin, and darbepoetin.
  - Parental iron formulations are iron dextran (IM/IV), iron sucrose (IV), and sodium ferric gluconate (IV). Iron sucrose and sodium ferric gluconate are better tolerated.
  - Parental iron should be considered in setting of oral iron noncompliance or intolerance, malabsorption syndrome, and significant anemia less than 8.5 g/dL.
  - No benefit of parental (IV) iron therapy over oral iron therapy when Hgb evaluated 30 days after initiation of therapy (20).
- Reticulocytosis should be observed after 7 to 10 days, and an increase of 1 g/dL should be seen within 14 days after initiation of iron therapy.
- If severe anemia (less than 6 g/dL) is present in the antepartum period, blood transfusion should be considered for fetal and maternal indications.
- Iron supplementation should continue for 6 months after anemia resolves to replace iron stores.

Side Effects
- The dose of elemental iron correlates with the symptoms listed below and dosing should be reduced for intolerance (10):
  - Nausea, vomiting
  - Abdominal cramps
  - Diarrhea
  - Constipation
- Childhood poisoning. Note: Maternal iron preparations are the second most common cause of childhood poisoning in the United States (after aspirin).

Folate Deficiency Anemia
Background
- Folic acid deficiency is the most common cause of megaloblastic anemia in the United States.
  - It complicates 1% to 4% of pregnancies in the United States and approximately 30% worldwide (2,10).
  - Folate requirement increases from 50 µg/day in the nonpregnant state to 400 µg/day during pregnancy.
- Folate is a component of tetrahydrofolate (THF), which plays an important role in nucleic acid synthesis and maturation.
- Folate is solely obtained from the diet and absorbed in the proximal jejunum. Prime dietary sources are leafy vegetables, legumes, and animal protein.
- Similar predisposing factors to IDA in pregnancy, along with other specific considerations:
  - Ongoing hemolysis (e.g., hemoglobinopathies)
  - Seizure disorders treated with anticonvulsants, which interfere with metabolism
  - Chronic disease promoting malabsorption, e.g., gluten-induced enteropathy and tropical sprue
- Likely confounded with socioeconomic or nutrition status, folic acid deficiency has been associated with such pregnancy complications as birth defects, low birth weight, abruptio placentae, and prematurity (21).

Etiology
- Folate stores are limited and easily depleted within 3 to 4 months in times of increased demand (e.g., pregnancy and lactation) (2).
- Low levels of folic acid result in disruption of nucleic acid synthesis, cellular division impairment, and accumulation of homocysteine.

Evaluation
History and Physical
- Deficiencies in either folic acid or B_{12} can present with hyperpigmentation, low-grade fever, glossitis, skin changes, and other nonspecific symptoms of anemia.
- However, the concomitant presence of neurologic symptoms is diagnostic of B_{12} deficiency and is almost never seen with folic acid deficiency.

Laboratory Tests
- Macrocytic anemia and megaloblasts present in the bone marrow; MCV is usually greater than 110 fL.
- The macrocytosis can be masked by concomitant iron deficiency or thalassemia (2% to 5%).
- Peripheral smear may demonstrate neutropenia, thrombocytopenia, and hypersegmented granulocytes.
- Serum folate levels are decreased to less than 2.0 µg/L (normal 2.0 to 15 µg/L).
- Red cell folate concentration (an indicator of severity of deficiency) is usually less than 160 µg/L (normal 160 to 640 µg/L).
- Plasma homocysteine and methylmalonic acid levels will differentiate between folate deficiency and vitamin B_{12} deficiency. Methylmalonic acid is normal in folate deficiency.

Treatment
Medications
- The recommended daily dose of folic acid is 1 mg for uncomplicated pregnancies.
- With treatment, an increased reticulocyte count should be seen within 3 to 4 days.
- If neurologic symptoms are present, a B_{12} level should be measured. Folic acid will correct the anemia, but not the neurological symptoms.
- Oral folic acid is sufficient for treatment. If folic acid antagonists are being used, parenteral folic acid is indicated.

Patient Education
- Prevention or reduction of neural tube defects
  - Folic acid can be used preconceptionally for the prevention (or reduction) of both first-time and recurrent neural tube defects (see Chapter 30, Teratogens and Birth Defects).

B_{12} Deficiency Anemia
Background
Etiology
- Vitamin B_{12} is readily available in conventional diets, and deficiency is rarely due to inadequate ingestion, except in strict vegetarians.
- Intrinsic factor is important to absorption and is produced by the fundic parietal cells.
  - The same cells are responsible for hydrochloric acid secretion, which frees cobalamin (B_{12}) from the ingested animal protein.
- Freed cobalamin is bound to intrinsic factor and absorbed in the ileum.
- Inadequate synthesis and production of intrinsic factor or malabsorption syndromes are the most common causes, as a result of these conditions listed below (1):
  - Autoimmune inhibition of intrinsic factor production a.k.a. pernicious anemia (rare in this age group) and Zollinger-Ellison syndrome
  - Previous gastric or intestinal surgery (i.e., gastric bypass and ileal resection)
  - Intestinal parasites, HIV
  - Atrophic gastritis, severe pancreatitis, or inflammatory bowel disease (Crohn disease)
  - Medications (i.e., antihistamines and proton pump inhibitors)
- Neurological symptoms are related to damage to the posterior column of the spinal cord.

Evaluation
Laboratory Tests
- A radioimmunoassay is used to measure B_{12} serum levels.

- Vitamin B$_{12}$ levels may fall to 80 to 120 pg/mL during pregnancy; levels below 50 pg/mL are indicative of B$_{12}$ deficiency.
- Low levels of vitamin B$_{12}$, but normal levels of folate are expected
- The Schilling test is used to measure B$_{12}$ absorption but is contraindicated in pregnancy secondary to use of radioactive cobalt.
  - However, if vitamin B$_{12}$ deficiency is present, a Schilling test must be done at a safe time after delivery to rule out pernicious anemia.
- Elevated serum bilirubin and lactic dehydrogenase levels may also be demonstrated (2).

Treatment
Medications
- Treatment is vitamin B$_{12}$ 1 mg intramuscular daily for 1 week, then every week for 4 to 8 weeks, and continues at monthly intervals indefinitely.
- Serum B$_{12}$ levels should respond within 6 weeks. Reticulocytes should increase within 3 to 5 days.

Anemia of Chronic Illness
Background
- Intestinal disease (e.g., peptic ulcer disease)
- Parasitic disease (e.g., malaria, helminthes)
- Chronic or subclinical infection (e.g., chronic renal or liver disease)
- Chronic inflammatory process (e.g., rheumatoid arthritis)
- Neoplasia
- Human immunodeficiency virus

Evaluation
Laboratory Tests
- Normochromic, normocytic (or microcytic) anemia usually unresponsive to iron therapy.
- The diagnosis of an underlying condition requires a high index of suspicion followed by careful history and physical examination.
- Treatment is guided by the specific cause.

APLASTIC ANEMIA
Background
- Aplastic anemia in pregnancy has widely varying reported outcomes.
  - Pregnancy may be a causative factor in pre-existing aplastic anemia. Potential pathologic mechanisms suggested are hormonal inhibition of erythropoiesis or the bone marrow's inability to respond to normal stressors of pregnancy.
  - Conflicting evidence is termination of pregnancy only promoted recovery in one-third of the cases (22).
- The two most common causes of death in patients with aplastic anemia are infection and hemorrhage (23).

Etiology
- Aplastic anemia is defined as pancytopenia with a hypocellular bone marrow and no increase in reticulocytosis, in the absence of malignancy or myeloproliferative disease.
- Seventy percent to eighty percent of cases are idiopathic. The remaining have been associated with a multitude of causes, including medications, solvents (e.g., benzene), agricultural pesticides/fertilizers, and recreational drugs (e.g., MDMA, ecstasy) (22).

Evaluation
- History should be detailed and evaluate for recent medication use, potential occupational exposure, and family history for inherited causes. Fanconi anemia is most commonly associated; however, patients with history of paroxysmal nocturnal hemoglobinuria (PNH) and myelodysplastic syndrome may also share genetic properties with aplastic anemia (2).

- Clinical presentations include (23):
  - Profound pallor
  - Petechiae
  - Bleeding
  - Epistaxis
  - Infection

Laboratory Test
- Pancytopenia is found on the CBC. Severe cases demonstrate ANC less than 500, platelets less than 20,000, and anemia with a retic count less than 1%.
- Bone marrow aspirate and biopsy are necessary to make the diagnosis (cellularity less than 25%) and to exclude other causes for pancytopenia (24).

Treatment
- Bone marrow transplant (BMT) with an HLA-matched donor is first-line treatment.
  - High dose immunosuppressive therapy used in conjunction with the transplant makes BMT relatively contraindicated in pregnancy (22).
- Alternative immunosuppressive agents include androgen therapy, antithymocyte globulin (ATG), steroids such as prednisone, or monoclonal antibody therapy directed against helper T cells.
  - Androgen therapy is contraindicated especially with female fetuses.
  - ATG therapy is not widely used in pregnancy.
  - Monoclonal antibody therapy, that is, cyclosporine, in adjunction with a granulocyte–macrophage colony stimulator has demonstrated no fetal toxicity and favorable pregnancy outcomes.
- Supportive care remains the mainstay of treatment in pregnancy and includes serial blood and platelet transfusions, treatment of infection, and stimulation of hematopoiesis with steroids (22,25).
- Recommendation for pregnancy termination remains uncertain unless maternal condition worsens.
- Maternal and fetal mortality rates depend on severity of disease and resource availability.

PAROXYSMAL NOCTURNAL HEMOGLOBINURIA
Background
Etiology
- Disorder results from an acquired somatic mutation of the PIG-A gene, which encodes for glycosyltransferase enzyme, on chromosome X.
  - This key enzyme makes glycophosphatidylinositol (GPI), which is essential for transmembrane formation in anchoring CD55 and CD59, two integral regulatory proteins in complement activation.

Epidemiology
- A rare disorder with one to two cases per million individuals
  - Twenty-five percent of cases discovered during pregnancy, although limited information available (1,2).

Diagnosis
Clinical Manifestations
- Clinical manifestations due to susceptibility of intravascular hemolysis:
  - Hemolysis
  - Hematuria (night hemolysis lead to morning tea-colored urine)
  - Thrombosis
  - Bone marrow failure
- Pregnant women experience severe anemia, preterm delivery, thrombocytopenia, low birth weight, and neonatal and maternal death.

- Twenty percent maternal mortality depending on severity of the enzyme deficiency (2)
- Thrombosis is the leading cause of death in PNH.
  - Anticoagulation with low molecular weight heparin (LMWH) until 6 weeks postpartum is advised.
- Lab findings include severe anemia with low reticulocyte count.
  - Fifty percent present with pancytopenia consistent with aplastic anemia (22)

Treatment
- Eculizumab, a monoclonal antibody therapy against complement 5, has demonstrated improvement in hemolysis, hemoglobin levels, and transfusion requirements (1).
- Early detection of infection is paramount.
- Transfusion support as needed.

Inherited causes of anemia
- Hemoglobinopathies
- Inherited hemolytic anemia

HEMOGLOBINOPATHIES
Background
- Normal hemoglobin is a tetramer with two sets of paired alpha (α), beta (β), delta (δ), or gamma (γ) chains.
  - α-Globin gene pair is located on chromosome 16, along with the embryonic zeta (ζ) globin gene.
  - β-globin gene is located on chromosome 11, along with the embryonic epsilon (ε) globin, two fetal γ-globins, and a δ-globin gene.
- The principle hemoglobin in adults, namely hemoglobin A$_1$, is composed of two α chains and two β-chains and constitutes 97% of adult hemoglobin (2).
- Hemoglobin A$_2$, which is normally less than 2% or 3% of the total adult hemoglobin, is composed of two α-chains and two δ-chains.
- Fetal hemoglobin F, two α-chains and two γ-chains, produced after 6 weeks postconception, predominates between 12 and 24 weeks' gestation and is slowly replaced by A$_2$ by a few weeks following delivery.
  - In normal adults, hemoglobin F accounts for less than 1% of total hemoglobin.
- Embryonic hemoglobin, Hgb Gower consists of two ε and two ζ chains. It is not found in the fetus after the first trimester or in adults.
- Hemoglobinopathies are inherited single-gene disorders and affect the globin chains of the hemoglobin tetramer. Comprised of two main classes:
  - Quantitative disorders: Thalassemia syndrome, which is characterized by inadequate production of structural normal hemoglobin, is named according to the hemoglobin affected.
  - Structural disorders: Sickle cell disease characterized by a change in the amino acid configuration of the hemoglobin leading to its dysfunction (26).

Alpha-thalassemia
Background
- Commonly found in Southeast Asian, African, and Mediterranean populations
Etiology
- Manifestation of gene deletions in the α-globin chain genes.
  - May inherit in conjunction with β-globin disorders and portends less severity in Hb SS or Hb SA.
- The clinical severity is based on number of alleles deleted.
  - The genotype of normal individuals is aa/aa.

- The carrier state is represented by –a/aa and is clinically silent.
- α-Thalassemia minor: deletion in two of four copies of α-globin. Trans deletion (–a/–a) is more common in African descent and cis deletion (—/aa) is common in Asians.
- Hemoglobin H disease is seen with a deletion of three α-chains (—/–a).
- Hb Bart is the absence of all four α-chains (––/––) and is incompatible with life.
- Less common, a mutation results in a normal α-globin gene
  - Hb Constant Spring: long unstable α-chain due to stop codon mutation
  - Hb Quong Sze: substitution impairing αβ dimer
  - α^{TSaudi}: point substitution likely affecting stability or translation of mRNA

Evaluation
- History and physical and laboratory findings all determined by severity (27)
  - α-Thalassemia minor is usually clinically asymptomatic, except during great stress. It is usually an incidental finding in pregnancy.
    - A mild microcytic, hypochromic anemia with poikilocytosis and anisocytosis is sometimes seen.
    - Evidence of iron deficiency may develop in pregnancy.
  - Hemoglobin H disease
    - Occurs mostly in Southeast Asians
    - Chronic moderate hemolytic anemia is present with reticulocytosis, microcytosis, hypochromasia, and poikilocytosis.
    - Splenomegaly and occasionally hepatomegaly is found along with hemochromatosis.
    - Hb H (a tetramer of β-chains) and Hb Bart are both evident.
      - Newborns carry 2% to 10% of Bart's hemoglobin (an abnormal tetramer of γ-chains).
  - Hemoglobin Bart
    - The fetus will generally experience second-trimester hydrops and result in intrauterine death.
    - Bart's hemoglobin predominates
    - These pregnancies are notable for a high incidence of preeclampsia (2).
    - Unusual in those of African descent
- Couples at risk should be identified early and offered genetic screening.
  - Carrier state may only be identified by molecular genetic testing.
  - In those found to be carriers, genetic counseling should be encouraged for inheritance risk determination (28).
  - Prenatal diagnosis with CVS, amniocentesis, and cordocentesis are all options, if mutation or deletion is previously identified in the parents.
  - Free fetal DNA will become more widely available to evaluate for hemoglobinopathies, at this time approximately 65% are detected (29).
  - Prior to pregnancy, preimplantation genetic diagnosis is also available.

Treatment
Medications
- In α-thalassemia minor, folate may need to be supplemented.
- α-Thalassemia carriers and minors usually do not behave different from normal gestations.
- In hemoglobin H disease, transfusions may be needed for severe anemia; otherwise, limited evidence is available regarding pregnancy outcome.

Beta-thalassemia
Background
- Similar ethnic, Mediterranean and African, predisposition as α-thalassemia.
- Mutation in β-globin chain gene leads to variable or no production of Hb A; this promotes red cell weakness and manifests as a chronic hemolytic anemia.
- Ineffective erythropoiesis encourages hemolysis, and extramedullary hematopoiesis leads to hemochromatosis.

Etiology
- β-Thalassemia minor is the heterozygous state.
- β-Thalassemia major is the homozygous state.
  - Cooley's anemia (severe form)
  - β-Thalassemia intermedia
- Pregnancy rarely occurs because of delayed pubertal growth and anovulation.

Evaluation
- Laboratory findings of moderate to severe microcytic, hypochromic anemia (low MCV) with a relatively high red cell count and target cell morphology
  - Hemoglobin A_2 is elevated above 3.5% (usually 3.5% to 7%) and Hb F slightly elevated.
  - Serum iron and ferritin concentrations are elevated.
- The clinical manifestations are variable in β-thalassemia minor.
- Thrombotic events complicate more pregnancies in those affected by β-thalassemia major and intermedia.
- Genetic testing performed is DNA analysis with PCR.
- Iron overload may be present from prior transfusions.

Treatment
- Folic acid supplementation may be necessary.
- Transfusions therapy in severe anemia is usually performed with aggressive iron chelation therapy (i.e., deferoxamine) to prevent iron accumulation.
  - Deferoxamine has a teratogenic potential but has been safely used in the second and third trimester without fetal compromise.

Complications
- Infants who survive with this anemia have a course that is marked by profound, transfusion-dependent anemia, growth delay, delayed sexual development, and heart failure by puberty.
- Pregnant women with evidence of cardiac impairment from iron overload have less favorable outcomes and high maternal morbidity/mortality.
- Pregnancies also experience higher rates of preterm delivery, third-trimester intrauterine death, and growth restriction.

Sickle Cell Anemia
Background
- Autosomal recessive disorder originating from a point mutation, which results in a β-chain substitution and production of defective hemoglobin.
- Severity of disorder influenced by zygosity of inheritance.
- Best perinatal outcomes in prenatal care coordinated by multidisciplinary team to include the obstetrician, hematologist, and anesthesiologist.
- Since 1 in 500 births in the African American population is affected by Hb SS, sickle cell disease is now part of the universal newborn screening in the United States (2).

Etiology
- A single nucleotide change (alanine → thymine) in the coding sequence creates a substitution of glutamic acid to valine. Subsequent production of HbS has the following manifestations:
  - In a setting of low oxygen tension, RBCs become sickle shaped with decreased elasticity and increased fragility.
    - Microvascular obstruction with rigid RBCs leads to vasoocclusive crises in long bones, chest, back, and abdomen.
    - Increase in adhesion and coagulation factors also encourages RBC adhesion and platelet aggregation worsening the vasoocclusive cycle.
    - Normal physiologic changes of pregnancy promote more sickling especially in the later gestation. Sickling in placental vessels and intervillous space may be associated with adverse perinatal events.

- Shortened life span of RBCs (protective in malaria endemic countries)
  - Skeletal adaptations occur secondary to marrow cavity expansion.
- Inability to concentrate urine (hyposthenuria) may occur as a result of renal papillary necrosis and loss of deep medullary nephrons.
- By adolescence, functional asplenia has occurred as a result of repetitive microinfarctions. Therefore, increased risk of infections with encapsulated organisms (i.e., *Streptococcus. pneumonia*, *Haemophilus. flu*, meningococcus).
- Other single amino acid substitutions can cause defective hemoglobin that lead to rigid RBCs with reduced solubility and a changed oxygen affinity.
  - Hb C, a point mutation of alanine > guanine, substitutes adenine for glutamic acid.
  - Hb Sb thalassemia (discussed in previous section).

Diagnosis
- The course of Hgb S disease prior to pregnancy frequently predicts how the woman will do in pregnancy. Avoid hypovolemia and hypoxemia in any trimester (2)
- Genetic counseling and prenatal diagnosis should be offered (28,29)
- Hemoglobin electrophoresis is the diagnostic test.
  - Moderate anemia with irreversibly sickled RBCs on peripheral smear. Normal, target, fragmented, and nucleated cells may also be seen.
  - Hemoglobin electrophoresis shows greater than 80% hemoglobin S and elevated Hgb F.
  - Solubility test (e.g., Sickledex) is inadequate for distinguishing between genotypes.

Clinical Manifestations
- β-Chain synthesis does not reach sufficient levels to cause symptoms until about 6 months of age.
- Children with Hgb SS are at increased risk for certain infections:
  - Sepsis
  - Meningitis
  - Pneumonia
  - Osteomyelitis
  - Urinary tract infections
- Respiratory manifestations are secondary to vasoocclusion or infection.
  - Acute chest syndrome: pulmonary infiltrate, fever, pleuritic chest pain, and tachypnea. Treat if infectious, otherwise supportive care with hydration, pain relief, adequate oxygen.
  - Leading cause of death is from acute chest syndrome or pulmonary embolism.
- Cardiovascular manifestations are secondary to the condition's hyperdynamic state.
  - Cardiomegaly (50% with left ventricular hypertrophy)
  - Prolonged PR interval
  - Increased risk for gestational or worsening pulmonary hypertension, preeclampsia, and intrauterine growth restriction (IUGR)
- Frequent complications in pregnancy: (30)
  - Antepartum admission
  - Thrombotic events
  - Placental abruption
  - Vasoocclusive episodes
  - Postpartum infections
- Vasoocclusive target areas:
  - Extremities
  - Lungs
  - Spleen, splanchnic bed
  - Kidneys
  - Brain (CVA, moyamoya)
  - Eyes (retinopathy)

- Perinatal complications include small-for-gestational age (SGA) neonate, preterm labor, and premature rupture of membranes (30) In efforts to decrease the likelihood of developing pre-eclampsia, a daily lose-dose (81 mg) aspirin may be considered after 12 weeks gestation.

Treatment
- Folic acid supplementation of 5 mg/day is recommended.
- Iron supplementation is not helpful in treating anemia. Most patients have iron overload due to transfusion history (26).
- Sickle cell crises must be treated with generous fluid support, oxygen supplementation, pain management, and blood transfusions as indicated.
- Hydroxyurea is an antineoplastic agent that encourages production of hemoglobin, and decreases the severity of sickling and frequency of pain crises. Concerns for fetal toxicity, so controversial in pregnancy.
- Blood transfusion to treat vasoocclusive crises and anemia:
  - Partial exchange transfusion targets a concentration of hemoglobin A greater than 40% to 50% and a hematocrit between 25% and 30%.
  - Evidence has shown a decrease in number of vasoocclusive crises, but no difference in perinatal outcome (31).
  - Prophylactic transfusions are not recommended but may be performed in setting of severe anemia (Hgb less than 6), acute chest syndrome, preoperative, sepsis, acute renal failure, or protracted pain crisis.
  - Transfusion therapy risks include 25% rate of alloimmunization, 20% rate of delayed transfusion reaction, iron overload, and 1:2,000,000 risk of HIV (2,31).

Procedures
- Careful monitoring for asymptomatic bacteriuria and urinary tract infections is necessary.
- Fetal surveillance should be started in the late second to early third trimester with non-stress tests and sonographic evaluation for growth and amniotic fluid index (AFI).
- Labor and delivery are managed on the basis of obstetric principles.
  - Cesarean section should be performed only for obstetric indications. Regional anesthesia is preferred to general anesthesia.
  - Venous thromboembolism (VTE) prophylaxis postpartum is recommended.
- Influenza vaccine should be within a year and penicillin prophylaxis continued. Administer pneumococcal vaccine every 5 years.

Patient Education
- Limited evidence of good quality to advise one contraception method over another; however, depot medroxyprogesterone acetate has been suggested to decrease the incidence and severity of vasoocclusive crises. No studies evaluate the risk of thromboembolism with combined hormonal contraception (32).
- Permanent sterilization should be considered when the patient has completed childbearing.
- Termination of the pregnancy because of maternal sickle cell anemia is largely unwarranted and should be considered on an individual basis.

Sickle Cell Trait (Hb SA)
Evaluation
- Carriers will be heterozygous for the condition and have one abnormal and one normal β-chain (1:12 African Americans) on Hgb electrophoresis.
- Family history is important (28)

Clinical Manifestations
- Sickle cell trait is associated with increased rates of pyelonephritis in pregnancy (26).
  - In one study, carriers had a higher incidence of pyelonephritis despite similar rates of asymptomatic bacteria or acute cystitis compared to normal pregnant women.
  - Urinalysis should be performed at each visit with urine cultures every trimester.

- Patients at increased risk of early spontaneous abortion and multiple gestations but appears to have low risk of preterm delivery at less than 32 weeks (30).
- In settings of significant hypoxemia, sickle cell trait may be associated with:
  - Vasoocclusive disease
  - Sudden death at high altitudes (e.g., when exercising a mile above sea level or when in a suddenly depressurized aircraft)
  - Severe concurrent illness (26)

Hemoglobin SC Disease
- Double heterozygous for hemoglobin S and hemoglobin C
  - Carrier rates for Hgb C trait in African Americans are 1:30.
  - Normal life span but subject to rapid and severe anemic crisis from splenic sequestration. Also, increased tendency in those affected to experience bone marrow necrosis with fat-forming emboli.
  - During pregnancy, Hb SC can behave like SS with an increase in IUGR, PP infection, and antepartum admission. However, patients usually have better perinatal outcomes (1).
- Similar in presentation to hemoglobin S/β-thalassemia

OTHER ABNORMALITIES IN HEMOGLOBIN RESULTING IN HEMOLYTIC ANEMIA

HEREDITARY SPHEROCYTOSIS
Background
- Autosomal dominant disorder arises from a mutation in erythrocytes' structural proteins, spectrin and ankyrin. It is the most common cause of inherited hemolytic anemia.
- The incidence of the disease is estimated at 1 per 5000 among those of European descent.
- The expression of the disorder is due to increased erythrocyte osmotic fragility. Mild cases frequently go undetected until pregnancy (2).

Evaluation
- Hyperproliferative anemia on CBC and microspherocytes are found on peripheral smear.
- Increased erythrocyte fragility in hypotonic saline is noted on osmotic fragility testing.
- Hemolytic crisis may be incited by infection, trauma, and pregnancy.

Treatment
- Most affected patients have undergone splenectomy, and pregnancy outcomes are favorable.
- If splenectomy has not been previously done, the treatment of the anemia should be supportive with transfusion as necessary (31).
- Folic acid supplementation is given.
- Patients are also at risk for cholelithiasis from pigmentary gallstones produced by chronic hemolysis.
- The pneumococcal vaccine can be safely given in pregnancy.

GLUCOSE 6-PHOSPHATE DEHYDROGENASE DEFICIENCY
Background
Etiology
- This X-linked disorder promotes a defect in the erythrocyte enzyme G6PD, an essential mediator in the G6PD/NADPH pathway. The pathway is also known as the pentose phosphate pathway and functions to protect the erythrocyte from oxidation.
- Makes RBC susceptible to a variety of oxidizing agents:
  - Analgesics
  - Sulfa drugs
  - Antimalarials
  - Quinines

Epidemiology
- A common enzyme deficiency and can be identified in 10% of African American men but in only 3% of African American women.
- Greeks, Sardinians, and Sephardic Jews have more severe hemolysis when exposed to oxidizing agents and fava beans (1).
  - Closely related to favism, fava bean consumption produces a hemolytic reaction.

Evaluation
- Female heterozygous activity varies (Lyon hypothesis) but usually is intermediate in severity (2).
- Pregnant women may be predisposed to miscarriage, IUGR, and hemolytic episodes in the third trimester.
  - Urinary tract infections may be more common, and it may be prudent to screen patients at risk for the disorder before treatment.
  - Heterozygotes may experience symptoms if a male fetus is affected by disease.
- The affected fetus is at risk for neonatal jaundice from chronic hemolytic anemia.
  - Hydrops may result
  - Breast-fed infants may be at risk if exposed to oxidants or fava beans ingestion by the mother (1).

Treatment
Hemolytic episodes during pregnancy require a prompt discontinuation of the causative medication.
- Transfusion support as warranted.

Patient Education
- Screening by PCR for the defect should be considered before treating a patient at-risk.
- Screen the newborn infants at-risk in setting of hyperbilirubinemia.
- Genetic counseling should be offered (28)

AUTOIMMUNE HEMOLYTIC ANEMIA
Background
- Warm-reactive antibody (IgG) are directed against Rh factors on the erythrocyte's surface.
- Cold-reactive antibody (IgM), usually anti-I or anti-i, also targets the RBC surface but differs from IgG pathophysiology:
  - A combination of intra- and extravascular hemolysis. More commonly extravascular hemolysis from complement activation (2)
  - Demonstrates little affinity at the physiologic temperature of 37°C

Etiology
- Most causes in women are idiopathic; however, pregnancy is an associated factor.
- Warm antibodies may be seen with malignancy (chronic lymphocytic leukemia [CLL], lymphoma) SLE, viral infection, and drug ingestion (i.e., penicillin, α-methyldopa).
- Cold antibodies may be seen with mycoplasma infections, infectious mononucleosis (Epstein-Barr virus [EBV]), and lymphoreticular neoplasms.

Diagnosis
- Mild to moderate macrocytic anemia with leukocytosis, and reticulocytosis; peripheral smear demonstrates microcytes, poikilocytosis
- Positive direct and/or indirect Coombs test
- May be seen in conjunction with thrombocytopenia (Evans syndrome) (2)

Treatment
- Glucocorticoids, intravenous immunoglobulin (IVIG) for severe cases, and supportive transfusion as needed.

- Splenectomy is an alternative treatment for warm agglutinins. If refractory to splenectomy and steroid therapy, immunosuppression is the next line of therapy.
- Hydration and maintaining body temperature are important with cold-reactive antibodies.
  - Plasmapheresis or immunosuppression may be required in severe cases.

THROMBOCYTOPENIA
Background
- Platelet counts are decreased in pregnancy. The etiologic mechanism is unclear; possibly related to the physiologic autoimmune state of pregnancy. Severely, low levels should be evaluated for other etiologies.

Etiology
- Due to the natural decline in pregnancy, gestational thrombocytopenia is very common in pregnancy. It accounts for approximately two-thirds of thrombocytopenia cases (33).
  - Patients are usually asymptomatic and platelet counts rarely drop below 70,000 cells/µL. These patients are not at risk for any further sequelae.
  - Platelet count normalizes within 1 week after delivery, 3 months at the most.
  - Regional anesthesia usually given at counts greater than 70,000.
- Pathogenic thrombocytopenia generally results from inadequate production, increased consumption, or increased destruction of platelets.
  - Inadequate production from nutritional deficiency, congenital thrombocytopenia, aplastic anemia, and infiltrative bone marrow malignancies are examples.
  - Increased consumption occurs in disseminated intravascular coagulation (DIC).
  - Increased destruction as a result of acquired, autoimmune, or viral causes:
    ○ Antibodies directed against the platelets (idiopathic thrombocytopenia purpura [ITP])
    ○ Thrombotic thrombocytopenia purpura (TTP)/hemolytic uremic syndrome (HUS)
    ○ Certain drugs (heparin, quinidine)
    ○ HIV
    ○ Autoimmune conditions (SLE)
    ○ Antiphospholipid syndrome (APS)

ACQUIRED CAUSES OF THROMBOCYTOPENIA
Idiopathic Thrombocytopenia Purpura
Etiology
- Most common cause of thrombocytopenia during the early trimesters and most common autoimmune disorder in pregnancy (34).
- Thrombocytopenia a result of destruction mediated by antibody binding; destruction outperforms new platelet production.

Evaluation
Clinical Manifestations
- Based on personal history of bleeding or excessive bruising
- Since IgG is selectively transported across the placenta, fetal thrombocytopenia may be present.
  - Corticosteroid and IVIG are not effective in reducing rate of occurrence.
    ○ Maternal platelet count is *not* directly proportional to fetal counts; however, procedures to evaluate fetal platelet counts complications outweigh any theoretical benefit of information. These procedures have not been shown to demonstrate reduction of neonatal bleeding episodes.
  - Fetal complications from ITP are usually mild and transient.
  - DDX: NAIT (neonatal alloimmune thrombocytopenia), a condition resulting in maternal autoimmunization against fetal platelet antigen.

○ Most common cause of NAIT is sensitization against HPL 1a (PLAT or Zwa). The clinical manifestations are profound; severe thrombocytopenia, ecchymosis, petechiae, and intracranial hemorrhage in 10% to 20% of cases (34).

○ Cordocentesis is indicated in this condition to determine fetal platelet count. IVIG has been shown to be effective and mode of delivery should be by cesarean.

Laboratory Tests
- Platelet count less than 100,000 cells/µL, peripheral smear with enlarged platelets
- Antiplatelet antibody assays are not specific enough to be diagnostic and is not recommended for routine monitoring

Treatment
- Current management focuses on glucocorticoid administration (1 mg/kg/day), IVIG, platelet transfusion prior to surgery or for acute bleeding, and splenectomy in refractory cases (34).
  - Platelet counts greater than 50,000 cells do not require treatment is experts' consensus; however, what is unclear is the platelet level for prophylactic replacement in pregnancy.
  - Counseling prior to steroid treatment should include disclosure about weight gain, bone loss with prolonged usage, worsening hypertension, and onset of hyperglycemia. Steroid effects are usually seen in 3 to 7 days and last for 2 to 3 weeks but are still a short-term therapy.
  - IVIG reduces antiplatelet antibody production and binding; however, it is associated with high cost, headache, nausea, elevated liver transaminases, transient neutropenia, and a severe anaphylactic reaction in IgA-deficient persons.
  - If splenectomy is indicated, the procedure is usually performed after the second trimester.
- Rituximab, a monoclonal antibody treatment, has been suggested as an alternative first line of therapy for chronic and refractory ITP adult patients.
  - FDA class C, although some case series demonstrates a safe use of rituximab in pregnancy.
    ○ Further prospective studies are needed to evaluate efficiency and maternal and neonatal safety. Some cancer studies have demonstrated an initial suppression of B-lymphocyte development but a return to normal by 6 months of age.

Thrombotic Thrombocytopenia Purpura/Hemolytic Uremic Syndrome
Etiology
- Microangiopathic condition usually developing in the second or third trimester. It initiates a cascade of thrombocytopenia, hemolytic anemia, and end-organ failure.
  - End-organ damage is secondary to ischemia from numerous consolidations of intravascular platelet plugs.
- TTP associated with autoimmune disorders, female sex, recent viral illness, and pregnancy. HUS has also been associated with recent *Escherichia coli* O157:H7 infection, chemotherapy, and bone marrow transplants.
- The condition has a high recurrence rate of 50% in subsequent pregnancies (35).

Evaluation
Clinical Manifestations
- TTP manifests as a triad with severe thrombocytopenia, CNS disturbances (i.e., headaches, altered consciousness, sensory motor defects, seizures), and hemolytic anemia. It can easily be confused for HELLP especially in someone with chronic hypertension.
  - Lactate dehydrogenase (LDH)-to-aspartate aminotransferase (AST) ratios may be helpful, as concurrent preeclampsia will exhibit two to four times higher AST values and have lower total LDH-to-AST ratios.
  - Up to 80% will have renal dysfunction confusing the diagnosis further (35).

- HUS manifests as a pentad with severe thrombocytopenia, CNS disturbances, renal dysfunction, fever, and hemolytic anemia.
  - High maternal and neonatal morbidity. Most occur in the postpartum period as acute renal failure. Chronic kidney insufficiency in 25% of patients and neonatal morbidity is related to maternal status and prematurity.

Laboratory Tests
- CBC will demonstrate low hemoglobin and low platelets with a peripheral smear confirming hemolysis with schistocytes, helmet cells.
- ADAMTS13, a von Willebrand factor (vWF) protease, that clears abnormal large-sized vWF and prevents intravascular platelet agglutinin, has been shown to have decreased activity in TTP. No role for ADAMTS13 has been found in HUS (36).

Treatment
- Plasmapheresis is the gold standard of care to remove precipitating factors from serum.
  - Corticosteroids may also be given to encourage response to the plasmapheresis.
- Platelet transfusion is not recommended, as it will perpetuate the condition. If active bleeding present, factor/platelet-deficient fresh frozen plasma (FFP) may be given (33).

Disseminated Intravascular Coagulation (DIC)
Etiology
- There are many diverse causes of DIC (37).
  - In abruption placenta, the bleeding diathesis results from consumption of fibrinogen and platelets in the retroplacental clot as well as activation of the fibrinolysis system.
  - In septic abortion or a retained IUFD, decomposition of the fetus and placenta causes passage of thromboplastic material into the maternal circulation initiating a consumptive coagulopathy.
  - In a severe intrauterine infection due to gram-negative or anaerobic bacteria, endotoxin activation of the coagulation system perpetuates DIC events. The release of microthrombi can cause end organ ischemia.
- DIC implies a general intravascular activation of the coagulation, platelet, and fibrinolysis systems (34).

Evaluation
Clinical Manifestations
- The range of presentations is highly variable and depends on the etiology.

Laboratory Tests
- Depending on the severity, any of the following can be seen:
  - Decreased hemoglobin–hematocrit
  - Decreased platelet count
  - Prolonged partial thromboplastin time (PTT)
  - Prolonged bleeding time
  - Decreased fibrinogen
  - Elevated fibrin degradation products (FDPs)
- Fibrinogen levels will fall precipitously prior to the appearance of significant thrombocytopenia.
- The degree of laboratory abnormalities does not always correlate with the clinical picture.

Treatment
- Definitive management requires evacuation of the uterus to stop release of tissue thromboplastin and coagulopathy cycle.
- In some situations, supportive therapy may be necessary with ventilator support, circulatory support with vasopressors, and replacement of products as needed.
- Hypofibrinogenemia is managed by transfusions of FFP or cryoprecipitate.

- In situations of severe thrombocytopenia (platelet count below 50,000 per mL), platelet transfusions are indicated.

Preeclampsia
Etiology
- Thrombocytopenia may be present in up to 50% of pregnancies complicated by preeclampsia (33).
  - May develop during the postpartum period
  - A severe variant of preeclampsia, HELLP syndrome:
    - Hemolysis (peripheral blood smears with schistocytes and increased LDH)
    - Elevated liver enzyme test (greater than 2 SD or 70 units/L)
    - Low platelets (less than 100,000 cells/μL)
    - Similar findings in TTP-HUS (35)
- Endothelial wall damage causes fibrin deposits (especially in the glomerular capillaries of the kidneys) and arteriolar spasm from platelet release of serotonin and ADP:
  - Platelet adhesion and consumption
  - Hemolytic anemia
- Generally, consumption of coagulation factors has not been demonstrated. In fact, evidence of hypercoagulability exists with increased fibrinogen levels and elevated fibrin degradation products (35).

Treatment
Procedures
- Delivery with removal of the placenta is the definitive treatment for preeclampsia–eclampsia.
- Thrombocytopenia will spontaneously resolve in the following days after delivery and platelet transfusions are rarely indicated.
- Steroid administration's efficacy to boost platelet recovery is uncertain, but it does appear to temporarily improve laboratory abnormalities.

Acute Fatty Liver
Etiology
- A very rare cause of thrombocytopenia in pregnancy (1/16,000). Usually presents in the third trimester and is more common in multiple gestations (38).
- Fatty infiltrates in the liver and kidney microvascular impair function and create a cascade of disseminated problems.
- More than half of cases also have concurrent preeclampsia (35).

Evaluation
Clinical Manifestations
- Clinical manifestations of nausea/vomiting, epigastric pain, anorexia, and jaundice progress to renal dysfunction (diabetes insipidus), elevated liver enzymes, hypoglycemia, and bleeding. Renal failure, coagulopathy, ascites, and encephalopathy are late findings (35,39).
  - Active bleeding results from deficiency of coagulation factors secondary to impaired hepatic function and acquired antithrombin deficiency.

Laboratory Tests
- CBC with mild leukocytosis (greater than 15,000), low platelets, and moderately elevated LFTs (greater than 300 international units/dL) are evident; significant elevation in alkaline phosphatase and conjugated bilirubinemia, profound hypoglycemia, and metabolic acidosis on blood gas are also demonstrated (35).
- Liver biopsy is not required for definitive diagnosis, but histologic finding in AFLP is diffuse low-grade centrilobular microvesicular fatty infiltrates.
- Computer tomography (CT) is more sensitive than ultrasound or magnetic resonance imaging (MRI) in detecting fatty infiltration, but all imaging methods lack good predictive value to be used as a definitive modality.

Treatment

Procedures

- Expedient delivery necessary for maternal recovery.
- Supportive care is the mainstay for treatment in AFLP. The focus is on strict fluid balance, correction of coagulopathy, hypoglycemia surveillance and treatment, and prophylactic broad spectrum antibiotic coverage including antifungal (38).
- Plasma exchange is effective short-term therapy to sustain liver function and enable hepatocellular regeneration. Results are transient but allow time until liver transplant (40).
- Liver transplant is not necessary in most cases as hepatic function usually recovers spontaneously (38).

MECHANISMS OF NORMAL HEMOSTASIS

Background

- Hemostasis is a complex process involving three interacting systems:
  - Platelet function
  - Coagulation factors
  - Fibrinolysis
- Coagulation factors widely vary during pregnancy:
  - Factor VIII, fibrinogen, VII, and X are all increased.
  - No consistent changes in V or prothrombin.
  - Protein S is decreased.
- Regulation of the process involves both promotion and inhibition to ensure optimal conditions. Abnormalities in either can lead to a bleeding diathesis or thrombus formation (41).
- The relative stasis of circulation leading to "hypercoagulability" and anatomic changes of pregnancy increase the risk of venous thrombosis.

PLATELETS

Physiology

- Vascular damage leads to exposure of thromboplastic elements, vWF, GpV1, or GpIa-IIa ($\alpha_2\beta_1$ integrin), and cause platelets to adhere to exposed collagen.
  - vWF and platelets interact via the glycoprotein Ib/IX/V complex receptor.
  - Platelets may also directly adhere to subendothelial tissue by GpIa–IIa or GpV1.
- Once adherent to the damaged vasculature, the platelets are activated, assemble together, and prompt the coagulation cascade.
  - GpV1, TXA_2 and ADP all play a role in activation.
  - Thrombin also plays a role, after binding to protease-activated receptor 1 and 4 (PAR-1, PAR-4).
  - GIIb/IIIa binding with fibrinogen is most important in platelet aggregation.
  - Factors contained in α-granules promote further aggregation or clotting.
- Formation of the platelet plug is the first step in obtaining hemostasis.

COAGULATION FACTORS

Physiology

- Soluble plasma proteins interact to provide fibrin deposits where the platelet plug has formed.
- Coagulation enzymes, initially present in proenzyme forms, are activated; this catalyze and amplify activation of other cofactors.
- The resulting cascade ultimately leads to formation of thrombin (Fig. 19-1).
  - Thrombin converts fibrinogen to fibrin, in addition to activating factors V, VIII, VII, XI, and XIII in the cascade.
  - The soluble fibrin monomers are stabilized by cross-linking into fibrin polymers (mediated by factor XIIIa) and bind to the platelet plugs.

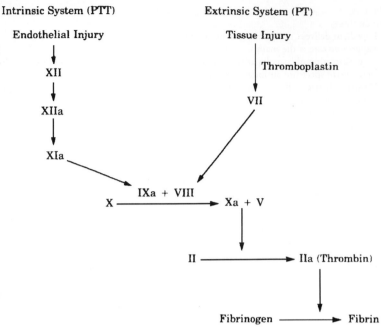

Intrinsic System (PTT) Extrinsic System (PT)

Figure 19-1. The classic coagulation cascade. The intrinsic system is activated by endothelial damage and is reflected by measurement of the partial thromboplastin time (PTT). The extrinsic system is activated by tissue damage and is reflected by measurement of the prothrombin time (PT). Proenzymes are generally cleaved to make the activated form (e.g., II → IIa), and these often catalyze the conversion of other proenzymes.

- The coagulation cascade can be initiated by an intrinsic or extrinsic pathway. The actual process is less separate than implied, and the final product is an interaction between both.
  - The intrinsic pathway is so named because all necessary elements exist in the plasma.
    - The intrinsic pathway contains factors XII, XI, IX, and VIII.
  - The extrinsic system is activated by factors available from adjacent activated platelets activated on the cell membrane and "extrinsic" to the circulating blood.
    - Primary instigator is the exposure of tissue factor (TF) after injury so that it is available to bind circulating factor VII.
    - The extrinsic pathway contains tissue thromboplastin and factor VII.
  - Merging of the intrinsic and extrinsic pathways forms the common pathway, which contains factors X, V, prothrombin time (PT), and fibrinogen and leads to the generation of fibrin.
- Main screening tests of the coagulation cascade reflect these pathways:
  - The PTT reflects the intrinsic system.
  - The PT reflects the extrinsic system.
- Regulation of the system involves a delicate balance of activation and inhibition.
  - Extrinsic pathway activation is time sensitive. Tissue factor pathway inhibitor (TFPI) binds factor Xa, and the complex inhibits the TF–factor VII complex. The intrinsic pathway is then charged with further coagulation by formation of IXa.
  - Antithrombin III is the best known inhibitory protein, because of its potentiating interaction with heparin in inhibiting Xa and thrombin.

Σ-dependent protein inhibitor–protein Z inhibits Xa as well.
- Protein S and protein C inactivate factors Va and VIIIa, mediated by thrombin.
- Similar thrombin-mediated mechanism of inhibition by α_2-microglobulin and heparin cofactor II.
- In normal pregnancy, factors VII, VIII, X, fibrinogen, and vWF are all elevated, resulting in a procoagulant state (42).

FIBRINOLYSIS
Background
Etiology
- Fibrinolysis limits the size of the fibrin clot formed.
- The release of tissue plasminogen activator (tPa), in the presence of fibrin, converts plasminogen to plasmin.
- Plasmin lyses the fibrin clot into degradation products and along with urokinase-type plasminogen activator (UPA) restores fluidity to the blood.
  - Inhibitory factors, PAI-1, PAI-2, and TAF1 all play a role to counterbalance.
- Defects in this system can lead to thrombotic complications or premature clot dissolution causing delayed bleeding.

DISORDERS OF HEMOSTASIS
- The ability to maintain hemostasis when challenged by vaginal delivery or cesarean section is the physiologic goal during pregnancy.
- Patients with congenital disorders predisposing them to hemorrhagic or thromboembolic events may or may not be diagnosed prior to pregnancy (42).

Evaluation
History and Physical
- An assessment of the patient's experience with hemostatic challenges, that is, surgery or trauma, should be obtained during the initial prenatal evaluation.
  - The pattern of bleeding should guide the appropriate investigation.
  - Abnormal bleeding after a dental extraction, especially if delayed or a blood transfusion required, may indicate a bleeding disorder.
- Platelet deficiency, either in number or in function, will frequently manifest by mucosal bleeding either spontaneously or with minor challenges (41):
  - Epistaxis
  - Gingival bleeding
  - Gastrointestinal bleeding
  - Menorrhagia, especially at menarche
- Hemarthrosis or deep muscle hematomas are characteristic of coagulation factor deficiencies.
- Bleeding problems may be immediate or delayed even if adequate hemostasis was obtained at the time of surgery.
- Disorders of fibrinolysis are suggested in the following situations:
  - Delayed bleeding
  - Poor wound healing
  - Unexplained thromboembolic events
- Patients may have an exaggerated response to aspirin or other nonsteroidal anti-inflammatory drugs.

Laboratory Tests
- Laboratory evaluation should be triggered by an abnormal bleeding history and focused on those hemostatic elements most likely to be abnormal.
- Routine lab studies beyond PT and PTT and platelet count have a very low yield in the absence of an abnormal history and are not necessary before routine procedures.

ACQUIRED DISORDERS OF HEMOSTASIS

Etiology

- There are multiple sources of disordered hemostasis:
  - Hepatic dysfunction
  - Vitamin K deficiency
  - Anticoagulant medications
  - Antibodies to coagulation factors
  - Hematologic malignancies
  - Platelet disorders
  - Disseminated intravascular coagulation

CONGENITAL DISORDERS OF HEMOSTASIS

von Willebrand Disease

Background

- The most common congenital bleeding disorder affecting 1% of the population.
- Primarily an autosomal dominant condition.
- vWF is responsible for platelet adhesion to the damaged endothelial surface.
  - Deficiency or activity dysfunction leads to platelet dysfunction and resulting bleeding diathesis.
  - Complexes with factor VIII procoagulant
  - Factor VIII is also carried by vWF; a deficiency in the vWF will lead to a deficiency in factor VIII (similar to hemophilia).
- The etiology of the condition varies.
  - Type I, a quantitative deficiency of normal factor, is the most common type, accounting for about 80% of cases.
  - Type II results from a qualitative deficiency and consists of four subtypes (34).
    - ○ Type IIA form large and intermediate vWF multimers with a decreased affinity for platelets.
    - ○ Type IIB is characterized by increased affinity for GpIB thus platelets and promotes rapid clearance from plasma.
      - − DDAVP is contraindicated and leads to thrombocytopenia.
    - ○ Type IIM has a reduced interaction for GpIb on platelets.
    - ○ Type IIN is characterized by impaired binding to factor VIII.
  - Type III is a rare autosomal recessive disease characterized by absent vWF.

Evaluation

Clinical Manifestations

- Uncertain clinical spectrum ranges from subclinical to severe.
- The condition may not become apparent until the patient undergoes surgery or becomes pregnant.
- Classically, the signs that lead to the diagnosis of von Willebrand disease are:
  - Positive family history
  - Positive personal history of excessive bruising or bleeding, especially at menarche
- Peripartum complications may include postpartum hemorrhage, perineal hematomas, surgical site bleeding, and anesthesia complications.

Laboratory Tests

- As previously noted, the coagulation factors, vWF and factor VIII, are frequently elevated in pregnancy. Patients with von Willebrand disease will often experience amelioration in their condition because of an elevation in these factors.
  - If the disease is mild, the elevation may be sufficient to raise both ristocetin cofactor and factor VIII to normal levels.
  - As the disease becomes more severe, this elevation in the factors may not be sufficient to provide normal hemostasis.

- Characteristic of vWD is a prolonged bleeding time and PTT.
  - Only if the factor VIII level is less than 25% to 30% will the PTT be prolonged.
  - Similarly, the vWF must be less than 30% to cause a prolonged bleeding time (43).
- If both are normal and suspicion continues, then one can check a specific vWF panel, which usually consists of
  - Plasma vWF antigen
  - Ristocetin cofactor activity
  - Factor VIII coagulant activity
  - Multimeric analysis
- Be aware that these factor levels can vary greatly from day to day.
- Repeat testing in the third trimester may be required to demonstrate an abnormality.
- Patients with von Willebrand disease may also be monitored with serial bleeding times.
  - If the bleeding time is normal at term and factor VIII coagulant activity is at least 30% to 40%, no special treatment is required (43).
  - If the bleeding time is elevated to greater than 20 minutes, then therapy should be initiated in the expectation of delivery.
- The most important assay for the functional activity of vWF is based on the antibiotic ristocetin to initiate platelet agglutination.
  - The ristocetin test best approximates the level and function of vWF to cause platelet adhesion in vivo to the damaged endothelial surface.
  - It also correlates well with clinical bleeding and a prolonged bleeding time.
- Electrophoresis may also demonstrate abnormalities in the vWF protein.

Treatment
Medications
- Desmopressin (DDAVP), a synthetic vasopressin, causes release of stored vWF from the endothelial cells.
  - No adequate and controlled studies are available regarding DDAVP use in pregnancy, although it has been used without deleterious effects (43).
  - The max dose of DDAVP is 0.3 µg/kg by slow IV infusion in active bleeding.
  - Variable response so should test during an in emergent situation. Consider for prophylaxis prior to any procedure if factor VIII or vWF is less than 50 international units/dL.
  - Daily administration may result in water intoxication, hyponatremia, hypertension, and tachyphylaxis.
- vWF concentrate (Humate-P in the United States).
  - Fifty to sixty units per kilogram is administered over 10 minutes and can be repeated every 12 hours.
  - The risk of virus transmission is greatly reduced by a pasteurization process.
  - Indicated for types IIb and III as those are unresponsive to DDAVP.
- If neither of these is appropriate or available, then cryoprecipitate 0.24 bags per kg at the onset of labor, followed by 0.12 bags per kg every 12 hours for up to 7 days, may be used in an emergency (Table 19-2).

Risk Management
- Patients with von Willebrand disease are candidates for the hepatitis B vaccine because they are at risk for numerous transfusions of blood products.
- Newborns born to mothers with severe types are at risk for intracranial hemorrhage (ICH). Delivery mode has not demonstrated an improvement in prevention of this condition, but operative deliveries should be avoided. Male infants' von Willebrand status should be confirmed prior to circumcision.
- If regional anesthesia is performed, DDAVP prophylaxis should be given and the epidural catheter should be discontinued as soon as possible given the risk for postpartum bleeding.

Table 19-2			
Plasma product	**Components**	**Use**	**Indications**
Fresh frozen plasma (1 unit = 250 mL)	Plasma, fibrinogen, antithrombin III, all coagulation factors (high concentration of factors V and VIII)	Use immediately after thawing or store at 1°C–6°C for up to 24 h	Massive transfusion, bleeding in setting of coagulopathy, heparin reversal, alternatives in specific factor deficiencies
Cryoprecipitate (concentrate of factors as result a slow controlled thaw of FFP)	Fibrinogen, vWF, factor VIII, factor XIII, and fibronectin An assumption of 80 international units of factor VIII and 150 mg of fibrinogen per unit will help determine the number of units needed for transfusion	Use within 6 h postthawing	Active hemorrhage or preprocedure prophylaxis in patients with significant hypofibrinogenemia (<100 mg/dL). Also alternative for factor XIII deficiency or bleeding in vWF unresponsive to DDAVP
Cryoreduced plasma	Plasma and all factors except contain decreased levels of fibrinogen, factor VIII, factor XIII, and vWF	Stable for up to 5 y (at or below −20°C)	Plasma exchange in TTP or HUS

Adapted from Circular of Information for the Use of Human Blood and Blood Components. AABB; 2009.

HEMOPHILIA A

Background

- Hemophilia A is due to a deficiency of factor VIII.
- It is a sex-linked recessive disorder that usually affects males.
- An acquired form is even rarer but may result from autoimmune conditions, such as pregnancy, malignancy, SLE, rheumatoid arthritis, and pemphigoid, which generate autoantibodies against factor VIII.
- Prenatal diagnosis is important because the mothers are obligate carriers, and the male fetus has a 50% risk of inheritance.
  - Fetal blood can be tested for factor VIII procoagulant activity and compared with the amount of the multimeric form (the complex of vWF and factor VIII procoagulant).
  - Prenatal diagnosis can be made by direct assays for the abnormal gene on the X chromosome by restriction endonuclease analysis (34).

Evaluation

- Diagnosis usually based on family history.
- Carriers of the gene rarely have clinical manifestations (44).
  - Factor VIII levels are approximately 50%, which is sufficient to provide normal hemostasis.
  - Lower levels are rare but can occur by X inactivation (Lyon hypothesis)
- Factor VIII levels less than 25% of normal are clinically apparent as a bleeding disorder.
  - In pregnancy, factor VIII levels increase, but treatment is necessary if the level remains below 50% of normal.
  - Very low or absent amounts of factor VIII coagulant activity are consistent with severe hemophilia.

Treatment
- Cryoprecipitate or factor VIII transfusions are used to replenish the levels to at least 60% of normal.
  - Cryoprecipitate was previously preferred to factor VIII transfusions to decrease the risks of hepatitis and HIV.
- Recombinant human factor VIII is now available without the risk of HIV or hepatitis (34).
- Mild conditions may be treated with DDAVP.
- Acquired forms are treated by immune suppression with steroids and/or cyclophosphamide, depending on if childbearing is complete.
- Delivery mode not contributory to neonatal bleeding risk; however, operative vaginal deliveries, invasive monitoring, and neonatal circumcision should be avoided in hemophilic patients.

HEMOPHILIA B
Background
- Hemophilia B, an uncommon sex-linked recessive disorder, is due to a deficiency of factor IX.
- Prenatal diagnosis is as important as in hemophilia A.

Evaluation
- Presentation is indistinguishable from hemophilia A.
- The diagnosis is made by an assay specifically for factor IX (45).
  - Unlike VIII, factor IX does not increase in pregnancy and levels maybe decreased in carriers.

Treatment
Medications
- Similar to hemophilia A, mild conditions may not require treatment.
- If the levels fall below 50 international units/dL, treatment is warranted with factor IX. Cryoprecipitate does not contain sufficient amounts to correct the deficiency (45).

OTHER CONGENITAL DISORDERS OF HEMOSTASIS
Background
- These other conditions can involve problems with fibrinolysis or platelet function, and most are rare.

Etiology
- Factor XIII deficiency may present with delayed bleeding problems.
  - Factor XIII is responsible for establishing cross-links between fibrin monomers, thus stabilizing the fibrin clot. Deficiency of this factor leads to a bleeding diathesis and poor wound healing (34).
  - Affected newborns characteristically will have bleeding from the umbilical cord stump.
- Factor XII deficiency manifest as bleeding problems, thrombosis, and recurrent miscarriages.
- The following autosomal recessive bleeding problems are related to platelet dysfunction (34):
  - Gray platelet syndrome is characterized by α-granule deficiency.
  - Bernard-Soulier, an abnormality of GpIb-IX-V complex, requires platelet transfusions.
    - Regional anesthesia is contraindicated.
    - Risk of postpartum hemorrhage increased so prophylactic platelet transfusion may be indicated.
    - Absent response to ristocetin or donor plasma
    - Immune suppression to promote delay platelet destruction, DDAVP, recombinant activated factor VII, and HLA compatible platelet transfusions are alternative options.
    - Prenatal diagnosis is available when family mutation is known.

- Glanzmann thrombasthenia is characterized by an abnormality of GpIIb-IIIa and has similar manifestations as Bernard-Soulier described above.
- Wiskott-Aldrich, Chédiak-Higashi, and Hermansky-Pudlak syndrome are all storage pool disorders.
  - ○ Wiskott-Aldrich syndrome is X linked and is associated with a shorter life expectancy.
  - ○ Hermansky-Pudlak syndrome is an autosomal recessive condition also associated with oculocutaneous albinism and yellow granule accumulation in reticuloendothelial cells. More common in Puerto Rican population (34).

CONGENITAL DISORDERS PREDISPOSING TO THROMBOSIS
Background
Etiology
- There are a number of inherited disorders that have an increased risk for thrombosis:
- Factor V Leiden (FVL) mutation
- Protein S deficiency
- Protein C deficiency
- Antithrombin III deficiency
- Elevated levels of factor VII and fibrinogen (46,47)
- Persons with a personal history of venous thromboemolism (VTE), a first-degree relative (parent or sibling) with history of an inherited high-risk thrombophilia (antithrombin deficiency, FVL homozygous, prothrombin homozygous, or compound heterozygous for FVL and prothrombin), or first-degree relative with VTE before age 50 in the absence of other risk factors should be tested for an inherited thrombophilia (41).
  - Screening for *inherited* thrombophilias is otherwise not recommended for recurrent fetal loss, placental abruption, IUGR, or preeclampsia.
- Chronic conditions associated with liver and kidney dysfunction may predispose individuals to acquire these hypercoagulable disorders.
- Diagnostic testing should be performed ≥6 weeks from thrombotic event, while patient is not pregnant or taking anticoagulation.
  - Testing for protein C, protein S, and AT deficiencies are not reliable while on anticoagulation or with an acute thrombosis.
  - From the inherited etiologies listed, testing for protein S deficiency is unreliable in pregnancy due to a physiologic decrease in activity (cutoff values of less than 30% and less than 24% in the second and third trimester should be used instead of nonpregnancy values) (48).
  - FVL is reliable on anticoagulation if DNA analysis performed; otherwise, testing is unreliable when protein C resistance assays are performed.

FACTOR V LEIDEN
- This mutation is the most common, carried by approximately 5% to 8% of the general population, and is transmitted in autosomal dominant fashion (47).
- A point mutation in the gene coding for factor V.
  - The defective factor V molecule is resistant to the normal proteolytic effects of activated protein C, thus causing an increased tendency toward recurrent thrombosis.
- Its prevalence among patients with recurrent thromboembolic events is considerably higher.
  - FVL appears to account for a much larger proportion of otherwise unexplained thromboembolic events than the other known hereditary deficiencies. This is likely due to the frequency of the mutation in the overall population.
- In pregnant women with FVL, activated protein C resistance appears to be at particularly increased risk for thrombotic complications.

- In one small study of patients with arterial or venous thromboembolic events during pregnancy or the puerperium, the incidence of activated protein C resistance was 78% (49).
- Another study in a low-risk obstetric population noted a 30% incidence of thrombotic complications among the 3% of women with the FVL mutation (50).
- This mutation may also be associated with recurrent pregnancy loss (51).

ANTITHROMBIN III DEFICIENCY

- Antithrombin is an important inactivator of thrombin and factor Xa, thus a vital inhibitor of coagulation.
- Inherited defects of antithrombin are uncommon with a prevalence estimated to be approximately 2 per 1000 in the population (52).
- Stratified into two types:
  - Type I is a quantitative deficiency and is the least thrombogenic.
  - Type II is a defect in the heparin-binding region in the AT gene and results in a qualitative defect that is highly thrombogenic.
- Diagnosis should be considered after all other acquired forms of thrombophilia have been ruled out and is performed by a functional AT activity assay.
- AT deficiency is associated with an increased risk of VTE and pregnancy loss.
- Given the high risk of thromboembolism during pregnancy and the puerperium, women with AT deficiency should be placed on VTE history–dependant dosing of thromboprophylaxis with LMWH or unfractionated heparin (41).

ANTIPHOSPHOLIPID SYNDROME

Background
Etiology
- Characterized by the presence of a group of antiphospholipid (aPL) antibodies along with defined clinical events related to thrombosis.
  - APS should not be diagnosed if less than 12 weeks or more than 5 years separate the positive aPL test and the clinical manifestation.
  - Diagnostic criteria for APS are specific as detailed in Table 19-3 (53).
  - Indications for aPL antibody testing are outlined in Table 19-4.
- APS is *associated* with (54):
  - Recurrent pregnancy losses (typically after 10 to 12 weeks' gestation)
  - Arterial and venous thromboses
  - Autoimmune thrombocytopenia
  - Placental insufficiency and infarction
  - Intrauterine growth restriction
  - Severe preeclampsia
- The groups of aPL antibodies defined in APS and measured as part of the workup are
  - Lupus anticoagulant (LAC)
  - Anticardiolipin antibodies (ACA) IgG and IgM
  - Anti-β_2 glycoprotein-I IgG and IgM
- Multiple aPL positivity is associated with a more severe course of the disease, increasing significantly the rate of thrombosis.
- The APS can occur secondary to an autoimmune process such as systemic lupus erythematosus, but it is frequently seen in the absence of autoimmune disease.

Treatment
Medications
- Preventive treatment with subcutaneous heparin and low-dose aspirin is now widely used during pregnancy in women with prior pregnancy losses or thrombotic events secondary to the aPL antibody syndrome (54).

Table 19-3	International Consensus Statement on Revised Criteria for the Classification of the Antiphospholipid Syndrome[a]

Clinical criteria

1. Vascular thrombosis

One or more clinical episodes of arterial, venous, or small vessel thrombosis occurring within any tissue or organ and confirmed by objective unequivocal findings on appropriate imaging studies or histopathology. For histopathology confirmation, thrombosis should be present without significant evidence of inflammation in the vessel wall

2. Complications of pregnancy

(a) One or more unexplained deaths of morphologically normal fetuses at or after the 10th wk of gestation

(b) One or more premature births of morphologically normal newborns at or before the 34th wk of gestation secondary to placental insufficiency, eclampsia, or severe preeclampsia by standard definitions

(c) Three or more unexplained consecutive SAB before the 10th wk of gestation with maternal anatomic or hormonal abnormalities and paternal and maternal chromosomal causes excluded

Laboratory criteria

Anticardiolipin antibodies

Anticardiolipin IgG or IgM antibodies present at moderate or high levels in serum or blood on two or more occasions at least 12 wk apart

Lupus anticoagulant antibodies

Lupus anticoagulant antibodies detected in plasma on two or more occasions at least 12 wk apart, according to the guidelines of the International Society on Thrombosis and Hemostasis

[a]A diagnosis of definite APS requires the presence of at least one of the clinical criteria and at least one of the laboratory criteria. No limits are placed on the interval between the clinical event and the positive laboratory findings

Anti-β_2 glycoprotein-I antibody of IgG and/or IgM isotype in serum or plasma (in titer > the 99th percentile), present on two or more occasions, at least 12 wk apart

---

[a]Antiphospholipid antibody syndrome (APS) is present if at least one of the clinical criteria and one of the laboratory criteria that follow are met.

Adapted from Miyakis S, Lockshin MD, et al. International consensus statement on an update of the classification criteria for definite antiphospholipid syndrome (APS). *J Thromb Haemost*. 2006;4:295–306.

ANTICOAGULANT MEDICATIONS

Background

Etiology

• Indications in pregnancy for anticoagulation include a preexisting condition, such as a prosthetic heart valve, previously diagnosed inherited thrombophilia, or an acute antepartum thromboembolic event in the current pregnancy (41).

• Anticoagulant medications have the potential for significant complications in pregnancy, and their use must be carefully regulated. Clinical practice guidelines during pregnancy are guided by prior history of VTE, presence of an inherited thrombophilia, or additional high-risk factors (55).

• Warfarin is an oral vitamin K antagonist. It suppresses the intrinsic coagulation pathway and is largely contraindicated in pregnancy due to teratogenicity and fetal hemorrhagic complications.

| Table 19-4 | Indications for Antiphospholipid Antibody Testing |

Recurrent spontaneous abortion[a]
Unexplained second- or third-trimester fetal death
Severe preeclampsia prior to 34 wks' gestation
Unexplained venous thrombosis[b]
Unexplained arterial thrombosis
Unexplained stroke
Unexplained transient ischemic attack or amaurosis fugax
Systemic lupus erythematous or other connective tissue disease
Autoimmune thrombocytopenia
Autoimmune hemolytic anemia
Livedo reticularis
Chorea gravidarum
False-positive serologic test for syphilis
Unexplained prolongation in clotting assay
Unexplained severe IUGR

[a]Three or more SAB with no more than one live birth.
[b]Superficial venous thrombosis is not included in the clinical criteria.

- Warfarin crosses the placenta. Congenital anomalies may occur with exposure anytime during pregnancy but is most common with in utero exposure between 6- and 13-week gestation. Substitution of heparin prior to 6 weeks eliminates the risk of embryopathy.
  ○ Warfarin embryopathy is associated with nasal hypoplasia and/or stippled epiphyses in the first trimester exposure and dorsal/ventral midline dysplasia leading to optic atrophy, mental retardation, spasticity, and hypotonia with exposure in any trimester. In one-third of embryopathy cases, limb hypoplasia is present (56).
- Warfarin has been found not to pass into breast milk in nursing mothers, so breast-feeding is safe postpartum.
- Use should be restricted to those situations in which long-term therapy with heparin is not possible or has significant deleterious consequences, that is, the presence of mechanical heart valves.
- Heparin does not cross the placenta and is the preferred anticoagulation therapy in pregnancy (57).
  - Unfractionated heparin has the advantage of being reversible. Four hours after discontinuation, the anticoagulation effect is nearly absent. A more rapid reversal can be obtained by use of protamine sulfate.
  - Recent studies, some of them conducted on pregnant women, suggest that LMWHs are comparable if not superior in safety and efficacy to traditional unfractionated heparin in the treatment and prevention of VTE (56).
  - Long-term therapy with higher doses of heparin can cause osteoporosis as well as increase the risk of maternal hemorrhage.

HEMATOLOGIC MALIGNANCIES

- Nonspecific symptoms of the malignancy may delay diagnosis during pregnancy as they are often mistaken for normal physiologic occurrences of pregnancy.
- Diagnostic procedures are safe during pregnancy; however, some staging modalities, that is, positron emission tomography (PET) scans, should not be utilized.
- Management decisions are difficult and must consider the risk to mother for delay of treatment and fetal risk with treatment.
  - Expectant management is reasonable in chronic or indolent malignancy.

- In aggressive types or in setting of progressing disease, therapy delay until the second trimester may not be feasible.
- Considerations of management (58):
  - All systemic therapies cross the placenta.
  - Although increased metabolism is suspected with normal physiologic changes of pregnancy, no current evidence supports adjusted dose in pregnancy.
  - In the first trimester, the risk of fetal malformation and spontaneous abortions (SAB) are increased. Counseling should involve consideration of pregnancy termination, especially if antimetabolite or alkylating agent is indicated.
  - In the second and third trimester, treatment appears to be safe in pregnancy. IUGR, prematurity, and neonatal complications of bone marrow suppression and sepsis may occur.
  - Radiation should be limited to deliver a total fetal dose of less than 0.1 Gy (10 rad).
  - No long-term adverse effects on childhood malignancies or childhood development are reported.
  - Specific cytotoxic drugs may be excreted into breast milk and to the fetus, so breastfeeding may be contraindicated.
  - During the initial year after treatment, conception for subsequent pregnancies may be delayed.
  - Most treatment protocols are based on experts' opinion due to the limited pregnancy safety data from randomized trials in this setting.
  - Prophylaxis for thromboembolism indicated given the extreme increase in hypercoagulability as a result of the pregnancy and compounded by malignancy.
  - Nutritional support, including total parenteral nutrition, is usually reserved for compromised patients.
  - Granulocyte colony–stimulating factors (G-CSF) and recombinant erythropoietin may be used for prolonged or severe myelosuppression in pregnancy.
- Reproductive counseling should advise to avoid pregnancy in the immediate 2 to 3 years after diagnosis and treatment, as relapse is more common during this time. Progesterone-only agents are the safest for contraception.

LYMPHOMAS
- Lymphomas are subdivided into Hodgkin (HL) and non-Hodgkin lymphoma (NHL).

Hodgkin Lymphoma (HL)
Background
- Forth most common malignancy in pregnancy (1:1000 to 6000)
- Concurrent pregnancy frequency is likely a consequence of high prevalence during the reproductive ages, especially the nodular-sclerosing subtype.
- Two types of HL: classical HL and nodular lymphocyte–predominant HL.
  - Classical HL is the most common and consists of four subtypes: nodular sclerosing, mixed cellularity, lymphocyte depleted, and lymphocyte rich.
  - Nodular lymphocyte–predominant HL is rare and only comprises 5% of patients diagnosed with HL.
- Clinical presentation is variable but usually related to spread of the increasing lymphadenopathy of the neck, mediastinum, and axilla. It ultimately progresses below the diaphragm and may spread to extralymphatic tissues.
- Prognosis and treatment are largely based on the stage at the time of presentation and are similar to nonpregnant women. Potentially curable in most cases even at advanced stages.

Etiology
- Still relatively unknown, proposed to be associate with a viral etiology. Genetic, environmental, and autoimmune-related factors have also been discussed.
  - Those with a prior EBV-related mononucleosis have a two- to threefold risk of developing HL; however, only 20% to 40% of HL tumors contain EBV genome.

Diagnosis
- Giant cells derived mainly from B cells infiltrate the affected tissue. These giant cells are called Reed-Sternberg cells.
  - Reed-Sternberg cells are only present in up to 1% of affected tissue; therefore, fine needle aspiration may miss abnormal cells. Bone marrow or lymph node biopsy is recommended for diagnostic purposes.
  - B-cell component relates to the symptoms of fever, night sweats, and greater than 10% weight loss that may develop.
- Staging of HL with the Ann Arbor staging system is a description of number and position of lymph nodes involved.
- Staging evaluation to determine the extent of disease is primarily radiologic, as laparotomy with splenectomy is now rarely done.
  - Conventional staging in nonpregnant women is bone marrow biopsy, CT of the chest/abdomen/pelvis, and PET scan.
  - Staging in pregnancy is performed by CT of the chest only with abdominal shielding along with MRI for postdiaphragmatic disease. PET scan is withheld until after delivery and likely posttreatment to evaluate treatment response.
- Even in setting of disseminated disease, precise staging in pregnancy is unwarranted because multiagent chemotherapy is the first-line therapy at all stages.

Treatment
- First-line treatment: ABVD (doxorubicin, bleomycin, vinblastine, dacarbazine)
- Large case series demonstrate increase in fetal malformations if chemotherapy is administered during the first trimester but no significant adverse outcomes when administered in the second or third trimester (58).
- If delaying treatment until the second trimester compromises maternal outcome, termination of pregnancy should be considered and treatment started immediately.
- Once favored for early-localized disease above the diaphragm, radiation therapy with abdominal shielding is no longer recommended because of risk of fetal teratogenicity and potential under treatment.

Non-Hodgkin Lymphoma (NHL)
Background
- Less common malignancy that occurs on a spectrum from indolent to aggressive lymphomas and includes all other lymphoid malignancies of B-cell, T-cell, NK-cell, or plasma cell origin.
  - Rising prevalence due to increasing maternal ages, general increase in NHL disease, and growing incidence of HIV-associated NHL.
- Approximate classifications:
  - High-grade aggressive disease: Burkitt's, primary mediastinal B cell, mantle cell lymphoma, and large B cell
  - Intermediate-grade aggressive disease: T-cell lymphoma, diffuse B-cell lymphoma
    o Diffuse B cell is the most common (30% to 40%) of NHLs and occurs at all ages.
  - Indolent diseases, that is, follicular or marginal zone lymphoma and multiple myelomas, are seen in older age groups. Diagnosis in pregnancy is associated with a poor prognosis.
- In this heterogeneous group of lymphomas, therapy and prognosis are dependent on histology. Cure rates decrease as stage of disease advances.
- Some NHL types express hormone-related receptors in reproductive organs, which contribute to disease progression and tumor growth at a higher rate than age-matched nonpregnant women.
  - Burkitt's lymphoma is mostly known for this phenomenon and is the second most common NHL. Characterized by rapid tumor growth, increased CNS and bone marrow involvement, and increased risk for tumor lyses and relapse.

- ○ Burkitt's lymphoma is responsible for almost half childhood lymphomas. Although a lower incidence in adults is noted, the median age in adults (30 years) makes occurrence in pregnancy possible.
- The overall 5-year relative survival rate in NHL is 69.3% (59).

Etiology
- Multifactorial as environmental, genetics, and chronic immune stimulation may all play a role in development (60).

Diagnosis
- Lymphoma does not affect the course of pregnancy, and the pregnancy does not impact the course of the lymphoma.
- Presentation varies based on subtype, and involvement of extranodal sites is more common than HL (61).
  - Diffuse lymphoma presents with B symptoms, lymphadenopathy, mediastinal mass, and extranodal site involvement.
  - Burkitt's presents with signs and symptoms of intra-abdominal masses consequential of extranodal site involvement.
  - Large B-cell lymphoma commonly manifests as superior vena cava syndrome or progressive dyspnea, from a large mediastinal mass with dense fibrosis.
- Diagnosis is performed by bone marrow or lymph node biopsy.
- Staging is similar to Hodgkin's: Ann Arbor system with same staging modalities.

Treatment
- NHL's first-line treatment is usually chemotherapy.
  - CHOP (cyclophosphamide, adriamycin, vincristine, prednisone) therapy is most widely used in conjunction with radiotherapy or monoclonal antibodies.
  - Rituximab is an anti-CD20 monoclonal antibody that has been shown to improve outcomes in indolent or aggressive malignancies with weekly administration.
    - ○ Retrospective case series described 153 pregnancies exposed to rituximab mainly in the second or third trimester of pregnancies; serious complications were related to maternal and neonatal immunosuppression with subsequent infection. Not associated with increase in congenital malformations (62).
    - ○ Recommendations to delay pregnancy during and up to 12 months following treatment is related to the potential depletion of maternal and fetal B cells up to 6 months.
  - Therapeutic component of radiation may be delayed until after delivery.
- More aggressive forms of chemotherapy used in Burkitt's (CODOX-M/IVAC) contain agents that are not usually recommended in pregnancy. These regimens should be considered as less potent agents are not as affective in promoting remission. Treatment with relapse is usually ineffective (58).
  - Profound and prolonged myelosuppression may result and stem cell transplantation maybe indicated.
- Expectant management early in pregnancy is reasonable in indolent cases, but is usually treated with chemotherapy in later trimesters.
- Palliative steroids to alleviate B symptoms are appropriate in women who desire treatment delay until later gestational age.

LEUKEMIA
Background
- Leukemia is divided into chronic and acute and then subdivided into histologic categories.
  - Two-thirds are myeloid and one-third are lymphoid in origin.
  - Use of cell surface markers, histochemical staining, and careful examination of the leukemic cells in peripheral blood and bone marrow allow for a precise determination of category.

- Increased rates of abortion, fetal growth restriction, preterm delivery, and perinatal mortality (usually related to preterm delivery) have been demonstrated in leukemia-affected pregnancies; A function of disease-related effects of coagulopathy, maternal anemia, and decreased placental perfusion.
  - Maternal response to therapy is the most influential factor on pregnancy outcomes and perinatal mortality.
  - Metastasis of maternal leukemia to the placenta or fetus is very rare (63).
- The fertility of patients with acute disease is diminished; however, for those in remission after childhood treatment, the fertility rates are good especially if treated prior to puberty.
- Oral contraception is the method of choice because ovulation is suppressed and menstrual flow is diminished, thus preventing menorrhagia in patients both with acute disease and in remission.

Epidemiology
- The incidence is estimated to be less than 0.9 to 1.2 cases per 100,000 women per year (64).

Acute Leukemia
Background
- Three common types in pregnancy: acute lymphocytic leukemia (ALL), acute promyelocytic leukemia (APML), and acute myeloid leukemia (AML)
  - ALL is more common in childhood.
    - Diagnosis in adults has a grave prognosis. ALL in pregnancy are usually survivors with a previous diagnosis.
    - Most likely to present with lymphadenopathy.
  - AML comprises the majority of acute leukemia in pregnancy.
  - APML is a variant of AML associated with translocation between chromosomes 15:17.
    - May present with life-threatening hemorrhage and increase likelihood of developing DIC.
- All are rapid progressing (63).

Diagnosis
- Diagnosis is usually by peripheral blood smear evaluation, bone marrow biopsy with flow cytometry, and cytogenetic analysis. An increased total leukocyte count with neutropenia, anemia, and thrombocytopenia are common findings.

Treatment
- Given the dismal prognosis of leukemia in the absence of therapy and lack of documented side effects of chemotherapy in utero, chemotherapy should not be withheld or significantly delayed regardless of gestational age at diagnosis (58).
  - In the first trimester, the patient should be offered termination with subsequent induction of chemotherapy.
    - Reports of limb deformities and cardiac dysfunction are available following first-trimester therapy.
  - If abortion is refused or diagnosis is made after the start of second trimester, chemotherapy should be started immediately.
  - Delivery planning is imperative to allow greater than 3 weeks between last treatment and delivery for bone marrow recovery and fetal drug excretion. After 32 weeks, consider delivery and then therapy induction.
- Management is based on the type of leukemia (61).
  - AML usually treated with cytarabine and an anthracycline.
    - Anthracyclines, daunorubicin and idarubicin, are associated with higher incidence of pregnancy complications including IUGR, neonatal pancytopenia, prematurity, and IUFD.
    - Doxorubicin, an anthracycline used in breast cancer, has a better pregnancy profile and maybe considered as the choice for gestation.

- APL receives ATRA: retinoic acid, an anthracycline, and cytarabine.
  - Cardiac and neurologic malformations increase with use of ATRA in the first trimester.
  - Delay in starting an anthracycline along with ARTA increases risks of relapse and ATRA resistance.
- ALL treatment is usually modified to avoid the use of methotrexate, so various regimens have been employed.
- Methotrexate is associated with aminopterin syndrome, cranial dysostosis, micrognathia, and ear anomalies (61).

Chronic Leukemia
Background
- The diagnosis is usually chronic myelogenous leukemia (CML) if encountered in pregnancy, as CLL tends to target individuals over 50 years (61).
- CML makes up 10% of all types of leukemia (63).
  - Characterized by the presence of the oncogene, BCR/ABL, which promotes and maintains the leukemic clone
    - Ninety-five percent of patients have the balanced translocation of t (9:22), which produces the BCR-ABL oncogene.
  - Slow progressing malignancy, whose course is unaffected by pregnancy

Diagnosis
Clinical Manifestation
- CML undergoes three clinical phases: chronic phase, accelerated phase, and a blast phase (blast crisis).
  - Ninety percent of CML are diagnosed in chronic phase with increased neutrophils, normal platelets, and low blast ratio in bone marrow biopsy (63).
- In early CML, 50% are asymptomatic. Others may experience indiscriminate symptoms or symptoms associated with leukocytosis (WBC greater than 100,000 cells/μL) (63).
  - May induce leukostasis, tumor lysis syndrome, and disseminated intravascular coagulopathy
  - Leukostasis, a condition of hyperviscosity, manifests as headaches, tinnitus, or dyspnea.
- Diagnosis made with peripheral blood smear (neutrophilia with marked immature myeloid cells), followed by bone marrow biopsy and cytogenetic analysis to evaluate for gene mutation (61).

Treatment
- Imatibinib, a tyrosine kinase inhibitor, targets BCR/ABL oncogene in CML and is now first-line treatment (58).
  - Animal studies have demonstrated a teratogenic effect. Retrospective case series support that the frequency of congenital malformations was higher in women exposed to imatibinib at various gestational ages (65,66).
  - Remission is dependent on continuation of therapy and may be achieved in 18 months.
  - Risk of relapse is higher with discontinuation.
  - Alternative therapies, interferon and hydroxyurea, cytogenetic response is inferior to imatibinib. Hydroxyurea has consistently been found to be teratogenic and should not be used. Interferon does not cross the placenta and is a viable option for those wanting to discontinue imatibinib during pregnancy (58).
- If the patient suffers a blast crisis, chemotherapy is necessary, and management of the pregnancy should be similar to that of acute leukemia.
  - Leukophoresis is an alternative for a rapid, short-term cytoreduction in symptomatic leukocytosis. This should be followed by induction of imatibinib (66).

MYELOPROLIFERATIVE NEOPLASMS

- Comprised of essential thrombocythemia (ET), polycythemia vera (PV), and primary myelofibrosis (PMF) and is also known as the Philadelphia-negative myeloproliferative neoplasms (MPN)
- Peak incidence is 50 to 70 years of age. However, ET has a second peak in reproductive age, and 15% of PV occurs less than 40 years of age, so a concurrent pregnancy is possible (67).
- The condition is a result of a mutation in hemopoietic stem cells inducing RBC overproduction. It follows a chronic course and may transform to acute leukemia.
  - JAK2V617F mutation is found in a majority of PV cases and approximately half of ET and PMF. It is unclear if isolated complications result from the mutation being present in pregnancy (68).
- Pregnancy compounds the prothrombotic nature of MPN, so most major complications are thrombosis-related.
  - ET and PV have similar perinatal complications: fetal loss especially in the first trimester, placental abruption, IUGR, postpartum thrombotic events, or hemorrhage. PMF seems to share only the increase in fetal loss, as there are no reports of maternal or adverse pregnancy complications (67).
- Contraceptive counseling is imperative in women with MPN. In the event of an unplanned pregnancy, the significant fetal and maternal risk should be clearly outlined.

Management

- Aspirin has demonstrated decreased thrombosis formation in this condition.
  - Aspirin should be continued in pregnancy in the absence of a contraindication.
  - LMWH should be considered in the setting of additional risk factors and dosed according to indication.
- Venesection or cytoreductive therapy with interferon-α therapy as needed to maintain platelet counts less than 400,000 and packed cell volume (PCV) less than 0.42 to 0.45 (67).
  - May experience drastic increase during postpartum period in platelets and RBCs
- Monitor blood counts closely in pregnancy with monthly CBCs and fetal surveillance for growth.

REFERENCES

1. Lee A, Okam M. Anemia in pregnancy. *Hematol Oncol Clin North Am.* 2011;25(2):241–259.
2. Kilpatrick SJ. Anemia and pregnancy. In: Creasy RK, Resnik R, Iams JD, eds. *Maternal-fetal medicine principles and practice.* 6th ed. Philadelphia: W.B. Saunders, 2009:869–884.
3. McLean E, Cogswell M, Egli I, et al. Worldwide prevalence of anaemia, WHO Vitamin and Mineral Nutrition Information System, 1993–2005. *Public Health Nutr.* 2009;12(4):444–454.
4. Adebisi OY, Strayhorn G. Anemia in pregnancy and race in the United States: Blacks at risk. *Fam Med.* 2005;37:655–662.
5. Kozuki N, Lee A, Katz J. Moderate to severe, but not mild, maternal anemia is associated with increased risk of small-for-gestational-age outcomes. *J Nutr.* 2012;142(2):358–362.
6. Tzur T, Weintraub A, Sergienko R, Sheiner E. Can anemia in the first trimester predict obstetrical complications later in pregnancy? *J Matern Fetal Neonatal Med.* 2012;25(11):2454–2457.
7. Murray-Kolb LE, Beard JL. Iron deficiency and child and maternal health. *Am J Clin Nutr.* 2009;89:946S–950S.
8. U.S. Preventive Services Task Force. Routine iron supplementation during pregnancy. [Review.] *JAMA.* 1993;270:2848–2854.
9. Andersson O, Hellstrom-Westas L, Andersson D, et al. Effect of delayed versus early umbilical cord clamping on neonatal outcomes and iron status at 4 months: a randomized controlled trial. *BMJ.* 2011;343:d7157.

10. American College of Obstetricians and Gynecologists. ACOG Practice Bulletin Number 95: Anemia in pregnancy. *Obstet Gynecol.* 2008;112:201–207.

11. Mei Z, Cogswell ME, Looker AC, et al. Assessment of iron status in US pregnant Women from the National Health and Nutrition Examination Survey (NHANES), 1999–2006. *Am J Clin Nutr.* 2011;93:1312–1320.

12. Walsh T, O'Broin S, Geary M, et al. Laboratory assessment of iron status in pregnancy. *Clin Chem Lab Med.* 2011;49(7):1225–1230.

13. Breymann C, Honegger C, Holzgreve W, et al. Diagnosis and treatment of iron-deficiency anaemia during pregnancy and postpartum. *Arch Gynecol Obstet.* 2010;282:577–580.

14. Akesson A, Bjellerup P, Bremme K, et al. Soluble transferrin receptor: longitudinal assessment from pregnancy to postlactation. *Obstet Gynecol.* 2002;99:260–266.

15. Pena-Rosas JP, Viteri FE. Effects and safety of preventive oral iron or iron plus folic acid supplementation for women during pregnancy. *Cochrane Database Syst Rev.* 2009;(4):CD004736.

16. Reveiz L, Gyte GM, Cuervo LG, et al. Treatments for iron-deficiency anaemia in pregnancy. *Cochrane Database Syst Rev.* 2007;2:CD003094.

17. Cogswell ME, Parvanta I, Ickes L, et al. Iron supplementation during pregnancy, anemia, and birth weight: a randomized controlled trial. *Am J Clin Nutr.* 2003;78:773–781.

18. Siega-Riz AM, Hartzema AG, Turnbull C, et al. The effects of prophylactic iron given in prenatal supplements on iron status and birth outcomes: a randomized controlled trial. *Am J Obstet Gynecol.* 2006;194:512–519.

19. Cao C, O'Brien K. Pregnancy and iron homeostasis: an update. *Nutr Rev.* 2013;71(1):35–51.

20. Krafft A, Breymann C. Iron sucrose with and without recombinant erythropoietin for the treatment of severe postpartum anemia: a prospective, randomized, open-label study. *J Obstet Gynaecol Res.* 2011;37(2):119–124.

21. Lassi Z, Salam R, Haider B, et al. Folic acid supplementation during pregnancy for maternal health and pregnancy outcomes. *Cochrane Database Syst Rev.* 2013;(3):CD006896.

22. Shetty A, Anwar S, Acharya S. Aplastic anaemia in pregnancy. *J Obstet Gynaecol.* 2011;31(1):77–78.

23. Choudry VP, Gupta S, Gupta M, et al. Pregnancy associated aplastic anemia: a series of 10 cases with review of literature. *Hematology.* 2002;7:233–238.

24. Marsh J, Ball S, Yin J, et al. Guidelines for the diagnosis and management of aplastic anaemia. *Br J Haematol.* 2009;147(1):43–70.

25. Kwon J, Lee Y, Shin J, et al. Supportive management of pregnancy-associated aplastic anemia. *Int J Gynaecol Obstet.* 2006;95(2):115–120.

26. American College of Obstetricians and Gynecologists. Practice Bulletin No. 78: Hemoglobinopathies in pregnancy. *Obstet Gynecol.* 2007;109(1):229–237.

27. Leung T, Lao T. Thalassemia in pregnancy. *Best Pract Res Clin Obstet Gynaecol.* 2012;26(1):37–51.

28. American College of Obstetricians and Gynecologists. ACOG Committee Opinion Genetic screening for hemoglobinopathies No. 238. *Int J Gynaecol.* 2001;74(3):309–310.

29. Barrett A, McDonnell T, Chan K, et al. Digital PCR analysis of maternal plasma for noninvasive detection of sickle cell anemia. *Clin Chem.* 2012;58(6):1026–1032.

30. Yu C, Stasiowska E, Stephens A, et al. Outcome of pregnancy in sickle cell disease patients attending a combined obstetric and haematology clinic. *J Obstet Gynaecol.* 2009;29(6):512–516.

31. Rogers D, Molokie R. Sickle cell disease in pregnancy. *Obstet Gynecol Clin North Am.* 2010;37(2):223–237.

32. Haddad L, Curtis K, Legardy-Williams J, et al. Contraception for individuals with sickle cell disease: a systematic review of the literature. *Contraception.* 2012;85(6):527–537.

33. Bockenstedt P. Thrombocytopenia in pregnancy. *Hematol Oncol Clin North Am.* 2011;25(2):293–310.

34. Lockwood CJ, Silver R. Coagulation disorders in pregnancy. In: Creasy RK, Resnik R, Iams JD, eds. *Maternal-fetal medicine principles and practice.* 6th ed. Philadelphia: W.B. Saunders, 2003:825–854.

35. Sibai B. Imitators of severe preeclampsia. *Obstet Gynecol.* 2007;109(4):956–966.

36. George J. ADAMTS13, thrombotic thrombocytopenic purpura, and hemolytic uremic syndrome. *Curr Hematol Rep*. 2005;4(3):167–169.

37. Letsky EA. Disseminated intravascular coagulation. *Best Pract Res Clin Obstet Gynaecol*. 2001;15:623–644.

38. Dey M, Reema K. Acute fatty liver of pregnancy. *North Am J Med Sci*. 2012;4(11):611–612.

39. Fesenmeier M, Coppage K, Lambers D, et al. Acute fatty liver of pregnancy in 3 tertiary care centers. *Am J Obstet Gynecol*. 2005;192(5):1416–1419.

40. Seyyed Majidi M, Vafaeimanesh J. Plasmapheresis in acute fatty liver of pregnancy: an effective treatment. *Case Re Obstet Gynecol*. 2013;2013:615975.

41. American College of Obstetricians and Gynecologists. Inherited thrombophilias in pregnancy. Practice Bulletin No. 113. *Obstet Gynecol*. 2010;116:212–222.

42. Brenner B. Haemostatic changes in pregnancy. *Thromb Res*. 2004;114:409–414.

43. Mannucci PM. Treatment of von Willebrand's disease. *N Engl J Med*. 2004;351:683–694.

44. Giangrande PLF. Management of pregnancy in carriers of haemophilia. *Haemophilia*. 1998;4:779–784.

45. Yang MY, Ragni MV. Clinical manifestations and management of labor and delivery in women with factor IX deficiency. *Haemophilia*. 2004;10:483–490.

46. Nachman RL, Silverstein R. Hypercoagulable states. *Ann Intern Med*. 1993;199:819–827.

47. Kujovich JL. Thrombophilia and pregnancy complications. *Am J Obstet Gynecol*. 2004;191:412–424.

48. Lockwood CJ. Thromboembolic Disease in pregnancy. In: Creasy RK, Resnik R, Iams JD, eds. *Maternal-fetal medicine principles and practice*. 6th ed. Philadelphia: W.B. Saunders, 2003:855–867.

49. Hallak M, Senderowicz J, Cassel A, et al. Activated protein C resistance (factor V Leiden) associated with thrombosis in pregnancy. *Am J Obstet Gynecol*. 1997;176:889–893.

50. Dizon-Townson DS, Nelson LM, Jang H, et al. The incidence of the factor V Leiden mutation in an obstetric population and its relationship to deep venous thrombosis. *Am J Obstet Gynecol*. 1997;176:883–886.

51. Ridker PM, Miletich JP, Buring JE, et al. Factor V Leiden mutation as a risk factor for recurrent pregnancy loss. *Ann Intern Med*. 1998;128:1000–1003.

52. Wells PS, Blajchman MA, Henderson P, et al. Prevalence of antithrombin deficiency in healthy blood donors: a cross-sectional study. *Am J Hematol*. 1994;45:321–324.

53. Miyakis S, Lockshin MD, Atsumi T, et al. International consensus statement on an update of the classification criteria for definite antiphospholipid syndrome (APS). *J Thromb Haemost*. 2006;4:295–306.

54. Carp HJA. Antiphospholipid syndrome in pregnancy. *Curr Opin Obstet Gynecol*. 2004;16:129–135.

55. Bates S, Greer I, Pabinger I, et al. Venous thromboembolism, thrombophilia, antithrombotic therapy, and pregnancy: American College of Chest Physicians Evidence-Based Clinical Practice Guidelines (8th Edition). *Chest*. 2008;133(6 suppl):844S–886S.

56. Ageno W, Crotti S, Turpie AGG. The safety of antithrombotic therapy during pregnancy. *Expert Opin Drug Saf*. 2004;3:113–118.

57. Pabinger I, Grafenhofer H. Anticoagulation during pregnancy. *Semin Thromb Hemos*. 2003;29:633–638.

58. Rizack T, Mega A, Legare R, et al. Management of hematological malignancies during pregnancy. *Am J Hematol*. 2009;84(12):830–841.

59. Howlader N, Ries L, Mariotto A, et al. Improved estimates of cancer-specific survival rates from population-based data. *J Natl Cancer Inst*. 2010;102(20):1584–1598.

60. Mills GB. Immunology of cancer in pregnancy. In: Allen HH, Nisker JA, eds. *Cancer in pregnancy*. Mt. NY: Futura, 1986.

61. Cohen J, Blum K. Evaluation and management of lymphoma and leukemia in pregnancy. *Clin Obstet Gynecol*. 2011;54(4):556–566.

62. Decker M, Rothermundt C, Holländer G, et al. Rituximab plus CHOP for treatment of diffuse large B-cell lymphoma during second trimester of pregnancy. *Lancet Oncol*. 2006;7(8):693–694.

63. Pejovic T, Schwartz PE. Leukemias. *Clin Obstet Gynecol.* 2002;45:866–878.
64. Catanzarite VA, Ferguson JE II. Acute leukemia and pregnancy: a review of management and outcome, 1972–1982. *Obstet Gynecol Surv.* 1984;39:663.
65. Pye S, Cortes J, Apperley J, et al. The effects of imatinib on pregnancy outcome. *Blood.* 2008;111(12):5505–5508.
66. Apperley J. Issues of imatinib and pregnancy outcome. *J Natl Compr Canc Netw.* 2009;7(10):1050–1058.
67. Barbui T, Finazzi G. Myeloproliferative disease in pregnancy and other management issues. *Hematol Am Soc Hematol Educ Prog.* 2006;246–252.
68. Harrison C, Robinson S. Myeloproliferative disorders in pregnancy. *Hematol Oncol Clin North Am.* 2011;25(2):261–265.

20 | Immunologic Complications

Jill G. Mauldin and Donna D. Johnson

KEY POINTS

- Immunologic diseases are common in pregnancy.
- The complications encountered during pregnancy are related to the type of autoimmune disease.
- Most patients can have a successful pregnancy outcome with a multidisciplinary team approach to their care and careful monitoring.

SYSTEMIC LUPUS ERYTHEMATOSUS (SLE)

Background

- A disease of fluctuating immune dysfunction.
- Disease manifestations vary within a patient as well as across populations of patients.
- Pregnancy complicated by systemic lupus erythematosus (SLE) is not uncommon as SLE has a predilection for females of childbearing years.
- Ten times more common in women than men.
- More common in African Americans than Caucasians.

Evaluation

- If a patient with SLE is contemplating pregnancy or is pregnant, assessment of her disease is important. Ideally, preconceptional assessment and counseling should be performed because of the potential for adverse impact on pregnancy outcome.
- Renal insufficiency is an important risk factor for maternal and fetal complications.
  - Renal function is more important than precise renal histology.
  - Urinalysis, creatinine clearance, and 24-hour urine are important for counseling and pregnancy prognosis.
- Presence or absence of hypertension should be documented.
- Autoimmune antibodies associated with SLE flares and adverse outcomes should be assessed preconceptionally and in the first trimester.
  - ANA
  - Anti-dsDNA
  - Lupus anticoagulant
  - Anticardiolipin antibodies
  - Anti-SS-A
  - Anti-SS-B
- Baseline complement levels (C3, C4, and CH50) should be drawn.
- Important to evaluate the complete blood count and platelets in the first trimester (1).

Diagnosis

- Rarely diagnosed for the first time during pregnancy.
- Diagnosis requires a thorough history, physical exam, and laboratory tests.
- Clinical manifestations: malar rash, discoid rash, photosensitivity, oral ulcers, polyarthritis, serositis, renal disorder, neurologic disorder (seizures, psychosis, organic brain

syndrome, and stroke), and hematologic disorders (hemolytic anemia, leukopenia, lymphopenia, and thrombocytopenia).
- Immunologic tests associated with SLE: antinuclear antibodies, anti-SSA (Rho), anti-SSB (La), anti-RNP, anti-Sm, anti-dsDNA, and antiphospholipid antibodies.
- Four or more of the above clinical or laboratory features must be present to establish the diagnosis of SLE (2).
- The natural history of the disease is for flares to occur.
- Diagnosis of a flare in pregnancy may be difficult (3).
  - Fatigue, joint aches, or changes in the skin may mark a flare or may be symptoms of normal pregnancy.
  - Some laboratory findings used to assess disease activity, such as sedimentation rate, platelet counts, and hemoglobin, are altered by pregnancy.
  - May be confused with preeclampsia.

Treatment
- Is the same in pregnancy as in the nonpregnant state with a few caveats.
- Caution should always be exercised when using drugs in pregnancy because limited data are available for many drugs.
- The benefit of treatment should clearly outweigh any potential risk to the fetus.
- Immunosuppressive agents
  - Glucocorticoids/corticosteroids, such as prednisone and hydrocortisone:
    ○ Are inactivated by the placenta.
    ○ Are associated with cleft lip in animals but never documented in humans
    ○ Place patients at higher risk for gestational diabetes and hypertension (3)
  - Glucocorticoids/corticosteroids, such as dexamethasone and betamethasone:
    ○ Cross the placenta and should be used only if there is the intent to treat the fetus
    ○ Should be avoided because of the concern of fetal growth
  - Azathioprine:
    ○ Is generally considered safe to use
    ○ Has been associated with fetal cytopenias and intrauterine growth restriction in some reports (3)
  - Antimalarial agents, such as hydroxychloroquine:
    ○ In the past, these drugs have been discontinued during the pregnancy due to concerns of ophthalmologic damage.
    ○ More recent reports have not revealed any congenital, ophthalmologic, or auditory abnormalities.
    ○ Discontinuation in pregnancy may precipitate a flare (4).
  - Cyclophosphamide
    ○ An alkylating agent.
    ○ First trimester use should be avoided if possible as it may be teratogenic.
    ○ Second and third trimester usage appears safer but may be associated with intrauterine growth restriction (1).
  - Methotrexate
    ○ An abortifacient
    ○ Associated with specific malformations such as craniosynostosis, cleft palate, and ear and eye abnormalities (3)
- Nonsteroidal anti-inflammatory agents (NSAIDs):
  - Do not appear to be teratogenic
  - May be used in very limited amounts and for a short duration but should particularly be avoided in the third trimester
  - Associated with premature closure of the ductus arteriosus and may lead to primary pulmonary hypertension
  - Associated with fetal oliguria and subsequent oligohydramnios (1)

- Antihypertensive agents
  - Important to have good blood pressure control during pregnancy, especially if the patient has preexisting renal disease.
  - Antihypertensive therapy is discussed in detail in Chapter 12.
  - Angiotensin-converting enzyme (ACE) inhibitors should be stopped once pregnancy is diagnosed.
  - Use of ACE inhibitors in the second and third trimesters is associated with severe and irreversible fetal renal abnormalities (1).

Complications

Maternal
- Pregnancy may be inadvisable in situations such as uncontrollable hypertension, rapid deterioration of renal function, or severe neurologic or cardiopulmonary involvement due to the increased risk of maternal morbidity and mortality.
- Whether or not flares are more common in pregnancy is still debatable (1,3,5).
- Features of SLE that appear to be protective of flares and subsequent progression of disease in pregnancy are quiescent disease for 6 to 12 months preconceptionally, normal renal function, nephritis in complete remission, and normal blood pressure before conception.
- A serum creatinine of greater than 1.6 mg/dL is associated with an increased risk of hypertension, proteinuria, and further renal impairment (6).
- Multidisciplinary management is often necessary to ensure the best maternal and fetal outcome.

Pregnancy
- Preterm delivery
  - Rate is 24% to 59% compared to 5% to 15% in the general population.
  - Most common causes are preeclampsia, nonreassuring fetal status, and possibly a higher incidence of premature rupture of the membranes.
  - Major cause of perinatal morbidity and mortality.
  - Increases the risk of cesarean section (5).
- Preeclampsia
  - Two-thirds of patients with preexisting renal disease will develop preeclampsia compared to only 14% of patients with SLE without renal involvement.
  - It may be impossible to distinguish a lupus flare from preeclampsia.
  - Clinical signs of active SLE, such as inflammatory arthritis, rash, adenopathy, and rising anti-dsDNA titers, favor the diagnosis of lupus nephritis (1).

Fetal
- Increased fetal loss rate
  - Includes both first spontaneous abortions and intrauterine fetal demise.
  - Median loss rate is 29% in SLE patients compared to 15% in the general population.
  - Creatinine greater than 1.6 mg/dL is associated with a fetal loss rate of 45%.
  - Antiphospholipid antibodies are also associated with increased fetal wastage (6).
  - Late second- and third-trimester losses may be reduced with antenatal fetal testing (see Chapter 32).
  - Educate patients regarding fetal kick counts at 28 weeks (1).
- Intrauterine growth restriction
  - May be detected by the use of serial growth ultrasounds.
- Congenital heart block
  - Most strongly associated with anti-SS-A (Ro) (1).
  - Affects less than 2% of the offspring of antibody-positive patients (5).
  - Can be detected by auscultation with Doppler or ultrasound.
  - Characterized by persistent fetal bradycardia leading to congestive heart failure and hydrops fetalis (7).

- Mortality is at least 20%.
- Surviving infants will require a pacemaker.
- Considered the only nonreversible component of neonatal lupus erythematosus.

Neonatal
- Neonatal lupus erythematosus
  - Clinical manifestations include photosensitive rash, thrombocytopenia, and liver function abnormalities.
  - Anti-SS-A (Ro) and to a lesser extent anti-SS-B (La) antibodies are associated with neonatal lupus erythematosus.
  - In patients with these antibodies, approximately 25% of their offspring will develop this neonatal condition (5).
  - Neonatal lupus erythematosus is transient and disappears by 6 months of life (7).

ANTIPHOSPHOLIPID SYNDROME (APS)
Diagnosis
- The diagnosis of antiphospholipid syndrome (APS) must include one clinical criterion and one laboratory test (5,8).
- Nonobstetrical clinical criteria include
  - One or more episodes of arterial, venous, or small vessel thrombosis in any tissue or organ.
    - Thrombosis must be confirmed by imaging, Doppler studies, or histopathology.
    - For histopathologic confirmation, thrombosis should be present without significant evidence of inflammation in the vessel wall.
- Obstetrical clinical criteria include
  - One or more unexplained deaths of a morphologically normal fetus at or beyond the 10th week of gestation.
  - One or more premature births of morphologically normal neonates at or before 34 weeks due to severe preeclampsia or placental insufficiency.
  - Three or more unexplained consecutive spontaneous abortions before 10 weeks of gestation.
- Laboratory criteria
  - Anticardiolipin antibodies
    - Medium or high titer of immunoglobulin IgG or IgM isotype in the blood on two occasions, at least 12 weeks apart.
  - Anti-β_2 glycoprotein 1–dependent antibodies:
    - Should be measured by standard enzyme-linked immunosorbent assay
    - May be IgG or IgM isotype in the blood on two occasions, at least 12 weeks apart
  - Lupus anticoagulant antibodies
    - The name of the antibody is misleading as many patients do not have SLE and have difficulty with thrombosis, not bleeding.
    - Should be present in the blood on two occasions, at least 12 weeks apart.
    - Should be detected in accordance with the guidelines of the International Society of Thrombosis and Hemostasis in the following steps:
      - Prolonged phospholipid-dependent coagulation demonstrated on a screening test, such as activated partial thromboplastin time, kaolin clotting time, or dilute Russell viper venom time
      - Failure to correct the prolonged coagulation time on the screening test by mixing with normal, platelet-poor plasma
      - Shortening or correction of the prolonged coagulation time on the screening test by the addition of excess phospholipids
      - Exclusion of other coagulopathies, such as factor VIII inhibitor, or heparin

- Anticardiolipin, lupus anticoagulant, and anti-β_2 glycoprotein 1–dependent antibodies can be found in healthy patients, so testing should be limited to patients with clinical features of APS.
- Primary APS usually occurs in patients without clinical evidence of other autoimmune disorders.
- Secondary APS occurs in patients with autoimmune or other diseases (5).

Treatment

- The goal of therapy is to improve maternal and fetal outcome by prevention of pregnancy losses, preeclampsia, and intrauterine growth restriction and to prevent arterial or venous thrombosis.
- Although large, controlled, randomized trials are lacking, low-dose aspirin and heparin remain the mainstays of therapy in patients with prior obstetrical complications (9).
- The patient may be given aspirin prior to conception.
- Patients with obstetrical complications or prior thrombosis may be treated with prophylactic regimens of anticoagulation (10).
  - Standard heparin
    - 5000 units every 12 hours in the first trimester and 10,000 units in the last two trimesters
  - Low molecular weight heparin
    - Enoxaparin 40 mg or dalteparin 5000 units once a day
- Treatment with heparin and low-dose aspirin reduces the risk of pregnancy loss.
- In pregnancy, antenatal fetal testing and serial growth ultrasounds are indicated.
- Iatrogenic preterm delivery is often indicated (9).
- Postpartum management depends on whether or not a patient has had a thrombotic event.
  - If a patient has had a prior thrombosis, prophylactic anticoagulation is recommended and warfarin is acceptable.
  - If a patient has only a poor obstetrical history, management is more controversial.
    - Prophylactic anticoagulation therapy is suggested for 6 weeks after delivery by some experts.

Complications

- Thrombotic
  - Arterial and venous thromboses are the most common complications of APS.
  - Overall prevalence of thrombosis in individuals with APS is 30%.
  - The annual rate of the first event is 1%.
  - The annual rate of recurrence in all APS patients not receiving anticoagulation is 10% to 29% (11).
- Obstetrical
  - Recurrent pregnancy loss
    - Preembryonic and embryonic loss
      - These losses occur between conception and the 4th week (preembryonic period) and the 5th through the 9th week (embryonic period).
      - As many as 10% to 20% of these patients will test positive for lupus anticoagulant or anticardiolipin antibodies (12).
      - Recurrent pregnancy loss is defined as three or more consecutive losses in this time period (5).
    - Fetal period
      - Ranges from 10th week of gestation until term.
      - Fetal death criteria apply only to morphologically normal fetuses.
      - Approximately 80% of patients with APS have had one fetal death compared to fewer than 25% of patients without APS.
    - In patients with prior fetal deaths, antepartum fetal testing is indicated.

- Preeclampsia
  - The median rate of gestational hypertension and preeclampsia is 32% to 50% (8).
  - A common indication for delivery in patients with APS.
  - The rate of preeclampsia is not reduced by treatment with heparin, aspirin, or steroids.
- Placental insufficiency
  - Characterized by poor fetal growth or fetal distress.
  - Occurs in approximately 30% of patients with APS.
  - One of the primary indications for preterm delivery.
  - Serial growth ultrasounds can detect early growth aberrations (8).

IMMUNE THROMBOCYTOPENIA PURPURA (ITP)
Background
- This is a common autoimmune disorder encountered during pregnancy.
- The most common reason for significant thrombocytopenia in the first trimester (13).
- Female to male prevalence is 3:1.
- Seventy percent of women diagnosed with this are less than 40 years of age.

Diagnosis
- Common signs and symptoms include petechiae, ecchymoses, easy bruising, menorrhagia, epistaxis, and gingival bleeding.
- There are no definitive symptoms, signs, or diagnostic tests for immune thrombocytopenia purpura (ITP). The diagnosis is one of exclusion.
- Immune thrombocytopenia purpura is suspected if the first-trimester platelet count is less than 100,000 mm³ and declines during pregnancy.
- The differential diagnosis for thrombocytopenia in pregnancy is extensive.
  - Gestational thrombocytopenia is the most common cause.
    - Accounts for 74% of pregnant women with thrombocytopenia.
    - Diagnosis of exclusion.
    - The typical woman has platelet counts between 100,000 and 150,000 mm³.
    - Women with platelet counts less than 70,000 mm³ are less likely to have gestational thrombocytopenia.
    - Usually occurs in the late second or third trimester.
    - The patient has no prior history suggestive of thrombocytopenia such as ecchymoses.
  - Preeclampsia can be associated with low platelet count.
    - Usually accompanying hypertension and proteinuria
  - Infection, such as human immunodeficiency virus or malaria, can cause thrombocytopenia.
  - Some drugs are associated with thrombocytopenia:
    - Heparin, sulfonamides, penicillin, rifampin, and quinine
  - Thrombocytopenia can be caused by diseases such as SLE, APS, and thrombotic thrombocytopenic purpura (13).

Treatment
- Treatment is recommended in patients with platelet counts less than 30,000 mm³ or with active bleeding.
- As a pregnant patient approaches term, the platelet count should be 50,000 mm³ to ensure adequate hemostasis at delivery (13).

Medications
- Corticosteroids may be used.
  - Efficacious and inexpensive.
  - 1 to 2 mg/kg/d is usually started.

- o Once the platelet count reaches 75,000 to 100,000 mm³, the dose is reduced to maintain the platelet count in this range.
  - o Side effects include hypertension and glucose intolerance (13).
- High-dose intravenous immunoglobulin (IVIg)
  - The typical dose is 1 to 2 g/kg infused over 6 to 8 hours (13).
  - IVIg is effective in two-thirds of patients.
  - The effect persists for 4 weeks.
  - IVIg is more expensive than corticosteroids but has fewer side effects that are usually mild including headache, chills, and nausea.

Procedures
- Splenectomy
  - Considered when refractory to corticosteroids and IVIg (13)
  - Ideally performed in the second trimester
- Platelet transfusion
  - Recommended when a patient is actively bleeding or when the platelet count is less than 20,000 mm³

Complications
- Maternal hemorrhage from vaginal lacerations or cesarean section
  - Can be minimized if the platelet count is greater than 50,000 mm³
- Neonatal thrombocytopenia
  - Occurs in 3% to 4% of newborns.
  - Bleeding complications are uncommon in newborns with mildly depressed platelet counts.
  - Intracranial hemorrhage, a very serious complication, occurs in less than 1% of infants.
  - Maternal platelet count correlates poorly with neonatal platelet counts.
  - The best method of obstetrical management to prevent fetal intracranial hemorrhage is controversial.
    - o Determination of the fetal platelet count prior to delivery is not recommended.
      - – Current methods of assessing fetal platelet counts can be unreliable and are associated with mortality risks of 1% to 2% (which is at least as high as the risk of neonatal thrombocytopenia).
      - – Fetal scalp sampling.
        - * This technique is difficult in early labor because the presenting part is usually at a high station.
        - * Sampling can lead to a falsely low platelet count as clumping of the platelets can be problematic.
        - * The fetus has already been subjected to the potential ill effects of labor before the platelet count is determined.
      - – Percutaneous umbilical blood sampling has been utilized to determine fetal platelet counts.
        - * It provides an accurate platelet count.
        - * It is expensive and requires personnel and equipment that are not available at most hospitals.
        - * Has largely been abandoned because the complication rate may be as high as 4.6% (fetal hemorrhage) (14).
    - o Most authors advocate performing a cesarean section only for obstetrical indications since the incidence of intracranial hemorrhage is so low.
      - – At the root of the controversy is that cesarean section has not been proven to reduce the incidence of intracranial hemorrhage.
      - – A cesarean section does contribute to increased cost and maternal morbidity (14).
      - – Intracranial hemorrhage may actually precede intrapartum events (15).

RHEUMATOID ARTHRITIS (RA)
Background
- Systemic, chronic inflammatory disorder characterized by symmetrical polyarthritis.
- Relatively common occurring in 1% to 2% of the population.
- Three times more common in females than males.
- The incidence of the disease increases with age.

Diagnosis
- Classic symptoms are pain and swelling in more than one joint.
- Upper extremities are usually affected first.
- Rheumatoid factor autoantibody is present in 80% to 90% of patients.

Treatment
- Anti-inflammatory agents are used and are discussed above under SLE.
- Amelioration of symptoms occurs in three-fourths of pregnancies.
  - If a patient's symptoms improve, the initial relief occurs in the first trimester and is sustained.

Complications
- Three recent population-based studies found women with rheumatoid arthritis to have a significantly higher risk of preeclampsia and cesarean delivery (5).

SCLERODERMA
Background
- Scleroderma is an uncommon autoimmune disorder that usually affects women in the fourth decade of life.
- Scleroderma may be divided into two forms:
  - CREST (Calcinosis, Raynaud phenomenon, esophageal hypomotility, sclerodactyly, and telangiectases) is the localized form.
  - Systemic or generalized form:
    - Involves the skin, joints, gastrointestinal tract, lungs, heart, and kidneys

Evaluation
- Systemic scleroderma can cause damage to multiple organs.
  - Pulmonary: fibrosis
    - Vital capacity should be assessed with pulmonary function tests as these patients are at risk for restrictive lung disease.
  - Cardiac: cardiomyopathy
    - Use echocardiogram to estimate the ejection fraction.
  - Gastrointestinal: malabsorption and reflux
    - Weight and nutritional parameters can be determined.
  - Kidneys: renal insufficiency
    - Renal function should be measured before conception.
  - Hypertension: renal, cardiac, vascular, and CNS effects

Complications
- Gastrointestinal reflux
- May be treated with histamine blockers or proton pump inhibitors
- Renal crisis
- Antihypertensive therapy may be used to ameliorate.
- The most effective antihypertensive therapy is an ACE inhibitor.
  - Because of the high associated maternal and fetal mortality, the profound benefit of using an ACE inhibitor may outweigh the fetal risk (16).

SJÖGREN SYNDROME

Background

- Sjögren syndrome is a rare autoimmune disorder.
- Characterized by dry eyes and mouth.

Complications

- Sjögren syndrome is associated with intense and varied autoantibodies.
- These patients can have anti-SS-A (Ro) and anti-SS-B (La), either of which may lead to a congenital heart block in the offspring (17).

Patient Education

- Patients with immunologic disorders should receive education about the effect of their specific disease on pregnancy and the effect of pregnancy on their disease.
- Ideally, patients with underlying immunologic disorders will seek preconception counseling.

REFERENCES

1. Baer AN, Witter FR, Petri M. Lupus and pregnancy. *Obstet Gynecol Surv.* 2011;66:639–653.
2. Petri M. Treatment of systemic lupus erythematosus: an update. *Am Fam Physician.* 1998;57:2754–2760.
3. Lockshin MD, Sammaritano LR. Lupus pregnancy. *Autoimmunity* 2003;36:33–40.
4. Costedoat-Chalumeau N, Amoura Z, Huong, DLT, et al. Safety of hydroxychloroquine in pregnant patients with connective tissue diseases. Review of the literature. *Autoimmun Rev.* 2005;4:111–115.
5. Borchers AT, Naguwa SM, Keen CL, et al. The implications of autoimmunity and pregnancy. *J Autoimmun.* 2010;34:J287–J299.
6. Mascola MA, Repke JT. Pregnancy and rheumatic disease: obstetric management of the high-risk lupus pregnancy. *Rheum Dis Clin North Am.* 1997;23:119–132.
7. Shillingford AJ, Weiner S. Maternal issues affecting the fetus. *Clin Perinatol.* 2001;28:31–70.
8. Branch DW, Holmgren C, Goldberg JD. Antiphospholipid syndrome: ACOG Practice Bulletin, #132. *Obset Gynecol.* 2012;120:1514–1521.
9. Empson M, Lassere M, Craig JC, et al. Recurrent pregnancy loss with antiphospholipid antibody: a systematic review of therapeutic trials. *Obstet Gynecol.* 2002;99:135–144.
10. Bates SM, Greer IA, Middeldorp S, et al. VTE, Thrombophilia, antithrombotic therapy, and pregnancy: antithrombotic therapy and prevention of thrombosis, 9th ed: American College of Chest Physicians Evidence-Based Clinical Practice Guidelines. *Chest.* 2012;141 (2 suppl):e691S–e736S.
11. Galli M, Barbui T. Antiphospholipid syndrome: definition and treatment. *Semin Thromb Hemost.* 2003;29:195–203.
12. Geis W, Branch DW. Obstetric implications of antiphospholipid antibodies: pregnancy loss and other complications. *Clin Obstet Gynecol.* 2001;44:2–10.
13. Provan D, Stasi R, Newland AC, et al. International consensus report on the investigation and management of primary immune thrombocytopenia. *Blood.* 2010;115:168–186.
14. Stavrou E, McCrae KR. Immune thrombocytopenia in pregnancy. *Hematol Oncol Clin N Am.* 2009;23:1299–1316.
15. Silver RM. Management of idiopathic thrombocytopenic purpura in pregnancy. *Clin Obstet Gynecol.* 1998;41:436–448.
16. Lidar M, Langevitz P. Pregnancy issues in scleroderma. *Autoimmun Rev.* 2012;11(6–7): A515–A519.
17. Mecacci F, Pieralli A, Bianchi B, et al. The impact of autoimmune disorders and adverse pregnancy outcome. *Semin Perinat.* 2007;31:223–226.

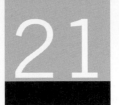

Vascular Complications
Wendy F. Hansen and Samantha Mast

VASCULAR COMPLICATIONS
Key Points
- The most common times for presentation of rupture or dissection of aneurysms during pregnancy are the third trimester, labor, or the puerperium.
- Intracranial hemorrhage (ICH) complicates approximately 3.7 to 9.0 per 100,000 pregnancies, and maternal mortality approaches 40%.
- The reported mortality for cerebral infarction is nearly 10%.
- Pregnant women with mechanical prosthetic heart valves are at high risk for thrombosis and thromboembolism and require close monitoring and therapeutic levels of anticoagulation.
- The optimal regimen for anticoagulation that minimizes both maternal and fetal risks is yet to be determined.

ANEURYSMS OF THE AORTA AND ITS BRANCHES
Background
Definition
- An aneurysm is the presence of a focal dilatation of all three layers of a vessel wall, in direct communication with the lumen, due to congenital or acquired weakness in the vessel wall.
- Dissection is present when an intimal tear occurs in a major vessel, allowing formation of an aneurysm.
- The three most common sites for intra-abdominal aneurysms: (a) aorta, (b) iliac arteries, and (c) spleen.

Pathophysiology
- All of the following factors have been reported to play a role in the risk of aortic dissection and rupture of arterial aneurysms during pregnancy:
  - Congenital disorders including Marfan syndrome, Ehlers-Danlos syndrome, Turner syndrome, Loeys-Dietz syndrome, aortic coarctation, and the mucopolysaccharidoses (1).
  - Takayasu arteritis, a chronic progressive granulomatous vaso-occlusive disorder of unknown etiology that primarily affects women of childbearing age (2).
  - Trauma, infection, or cocaine abuse (1)
  - Increased wall pressure in the proximal aorta, especially in late pregnancy, which may occur due to cardiovascular changes associated with pregnancy such as increased cardiac output, stroke volume, and blood volume (3)
  - Changes in progesterone concentrations may alter vessel wall integrity.

Epidemiology
- In the absence of Marfan syndrome or Ehlers-Danlos syndrome, arterial aneurysms are uncommon in people less than 40 years of age.
- The most common times for presentation of dissection or rupture during pregnancy are the third trimester, labor, or the puerperium.
- Splenic artery aneurysms are four times more common in females than males, and 80% are discovered incidentally (4).

Evaluation

History and Physical

- Common symptoms of aortic aneurysm rupture or dissection include
  - Sudden onset of chest or abdominal pain, often described as severe or "tearing." Pain may radiate to midscapular area or be migratory.
  - Nausea, vomiting, light-headedness, and other vasovagal symptoms.
  - Pain or tingling in extremities.
  - Neurologic symptoms such as syncope.
- The rupture of a splenic artery aneurysm will be associated with severe left upper quadrant pain or epigastric pain, left shoulder or flank pain, and hemodynamic instability (4).
- Physical findings with dissection or ruptured aneurysm may include
  - Tachycardia, hypotension, or hypertension
  - Anxiety
  - Decreased pulses and blood pressure differences between extremities

Diagnosis

- Symptoms of aneurysmal rupture may mimic more common conditions, so a high index of suspicion is necessary. As this condition threatens maternal and fetal well-being, rapid diagnosis is imperative.
- Various imaging modalities are used to diagnose dissection and aneurysm rupture. Modalities that utilize ionizing radiation are not contraindicated (5).
  - Magnetic resonance image (MRI) without contrast is the recommended first-line imaging study during pregnancy.
  - Computed tomography (CT) of the chest (with shielding of the uterus) results in little fetal radiation exposure and has sensitivity equivalent to MRI.
  - Chest radiography may show mediastinal widening, but a normal radiograph does not exclude the diagnosis.
  - Echocardiography will demonstrate abnormalities of the thoracic aorta and is useful if the patient is clinically unstable.
  - Abdominal ultrasound does not require radiation, but in late pregnancy, the gravid uterus may impede imaging of the abdominal aorta and its branches.

Treatment

- Immediate management should be aimed at maternal stabilization, including aggressive treatment of hypertension, if present, with an intravenous beta-blocker; administration of oxygen by face mask to optimize placental gas exchange; obtaining blood products for possible transfusion; and close maternal and fetal observation.
- Ascending aortic dissections (type A) require emergent surgical repair. Mortality rate may be as high as 1% to 3% per hour over the first several hours and up to 25% in the first 24 hours (1).
- Descending aortic dissections (type B) may initially be treated medically. When aortic dissection is diagnosed before the third trimester, surgical repair should be performed, but if the diagnosis is made in the third trimester and the dissection is stable, expectant management is preferred. Repair should be undertaken after cesarean delivery, either at or near term, or if maternal condition worsens (1).
- Splenectomy is the treatment of choice for a ruptured splenic artery aneurysm. Asymptomatic splenic aneurysms detected before or during pregnancy should be treated before term (6).

Complications

- Aortic rupture is frequently catastrophic, and mortality is high. As many as 50% of aortic dissections in women younger than 40 occur during pregnancy and the postpartum period, although pregnancy itself is unlikely to represent an independent risk factor (7).

- Splenic artery aneurysms are associated with 75% maternal mortality and 95% fetal mortality; combined maternal and fetal survival is rare (6).
- Renal artery aneurysms are rare. Rupture leads to retroperitoneal hemorrhage and is associated with a high mortality rate. This entity should be considered among the causes of retroperitoneal hemorrhage in pregnancy (8).

PREGNANCY-RELATED STROKE

- Rare but potentially devastating event estimated to occur in 34 per 100,000 deliveries with an estimated mortality rate of 1.4 per 100,000 deliveries (9,10).
- Risk factors for pregnancy-related stroke include age greater than 35 (OR 2.0), African American race (OR 1.5), migraines (OR 16.9), thrombophilia (OR 16.0), lupus (OR 15.2), heart disease (OR 13.2), hypertension (OR 2.61 to 10.39), thrombocytopenia (OR 6.0), sickle cell disease (OR 9.1), diabetes (OR 2.5), substance abuse (OR 2.3), smoking (OR 1.9), anemia (OR 1.9), and postpartum hemorrhage (OR 1.9) (9).
- Pregnancy-related stroke can be pregnancy induced or pregnancy incidental and categorized into two broad types: intracranial hemorrhage and ischemic (11).
- Treatment decisions are based on the type of stroke. History and physical are insufficient to answer the question, and imaging with CT or MRI should be done as quickly as possible after symptom onset.
- Other rare causes of pregnancy-related stroke include cardioembolism, paradoxical embolism, choriocarcinoma, amniotic fluid embolism, air embolism, and moyamoya disease.

INTRACRANIAL HEMORRHAGE

Background

ICH occurs in 3.7 to 9.0 out of 100,000 pregnancies (12). Approximately half are due to rupture of a saccular aneurysm or of an arteriovenous malformation (AVM), with the other half a consequence of hypertension or trauma. The highest risk for ICH occurs in the postpartum period (13).

Definition

- A saccular (berry) aneurysm is an aneurysm commonly found at the bifurcation of major vessels of the circle of Willis, with 85% occurring along divisions of the internal carotid artery. Multiple aneurysms are found in 20% of patients.
- An AVM results from congenital anomalies such as arteriovenous fistulae, resulting in direct arteriovenous shunting. They are seen most commonly in the frontoparietal and temporal regions but can occur anywhere in the brain.
- Other risk factors for AVM formation include family history of aneurysm, female gender, current cigarette use, or cocaine abuse (13).

Pathophysiology

- Controversy exists as to whether the risk of hemorrhage from AVMs is increased during pregnancy, with recent large retrospective cohort studies refuting a theory of increased risk. Any relationship is likely to be coincidental as the most common time for rupture is age 20 to 40 years, the prime childbearing years (13–15).
- The risk of rupture of a known AVM in pregnancy is estimated at 3.5%. Reasons given for an increased risk of bleeding include increased cardiac output and increased blood volume.
- The risk of rupture of a saccular aneurysm increases as pregnancy advances, possibly due to the increased blood volume of late pregnancy or due to hormonal fluctuations (14).
    - Maternal hypertension or preeclampsia increases the risk of rupture.

Epidemiology
- AVMs occur in approximately 0.01% of the population (16) and are twice as common in men as in women.
- The prevalence of saccular aneurysms in the general population is estimated to be 3.6% to 6% (11).
- The risk of ICH due to a ruptured berry aneurysm is estimated as 1:10,000 pregnancies (11).
- Risk factors associated with ICH in pregnancy include hypertensive disease (including preeclampsia), coagulopathy, maternal age greater than 35, African American race, tobacco abuse, and increasing parity (13,17).

Evaluation
History and Physical
- Symptoms and signs of ICH include a severe headache of sudden onset, meningismus, seizures, altered level of consciousness, vomiting, and focal neurologic deficits.

Genetics
- Saccular aneurysms are more common in women with coarctation of the aorta or adult polycystic kidney disease.

Diagnosis
- Pregnant women in whom ICH is suspected should undergo cranial CT or MRI scanning. Unenhanced CT scanning may reveal blood in the subarachnoid space or within the ventricles; if negative, a contrast-enhanced CT scan should be obtained.
- If performed accurately, this imaging method will identify 95% of ICHs, but the detection rate falls to 30% by 96 hours after the event.
- If CT indentifies a subarachnoid hemorrhage, angiography for diagnosis and localization of aneurysms is imperative (14).
- A lumbar puncture to assess for blood stained or xanthochromic fluid should follow a negative CT scan. If such fluid is found, cerebral angiography should be performed to identify the site of bleeding. Occasionally, vascular spasm occurs at the site of hemorrhage, and a repeat angiogram may be required.
- Abdominal shielding should be employed during all radiographic studies.

Treatment
Procedures
- Women known to have a saccular aneurysm or AVM should have definitive management before becoming pregnant. If the patient becomes pregnant before treatment, intervention would be recommended only if expansion or hemorrhage were to occur. Radiosurgery (Gamma Knife) has not been evaluated in pregnancy due to the use of high-dose ionizing radiation (15,16).
- It is clear that some women with a stable intracranial AVM will have uneventful pregnancies, and expectant management with neurosurgical consultation is advisable.
- If hemorrhage occurs, immediate evaluation is necessary and therapy should be guided by neurosurgical principles. An increased risk of death without treatment and a high incidence of rebleeding argue for the liberal use of surgical intervention.
  - Surgery is recommended in the presence of coma, space-occupying hematoma, hydrocephalus, or increased intracranial pressure.
  - Treatment using interventional radiology techniques may be possible in some cases.
- Saccular aneurysms less than 4 mm in diameter are usually stable, while those that are more than 5 to 7 mm in diameter are more likely to bleed.
- The treatment of saccular aneurysms, whether ruptured or unruptured, should be individualized, with the decision for surgical or medical management based primarily on neurosurgical principles.

- If the gestational age is less than 26 weeks, surgical treatment is almost always indicated.
- If the gestational age is more than 26 weeks, the fetal condition should be considered in surgical decision making, and either delivery followed by surgical repair or expectant management may be appropriate.
- Surgical management of aneurysmal ICH is associated with lower maternal and fetal mortality (18).
- Decision making regarding route of delivery in women with intracranial aneurysms is impaired by limited data. The risk of aneurysm rupture during pregnancy, delivery, and the puerperium is not increased and has been estimated to be 0.05%, similar to the average risk in the general population (15,19).
- Cesarean delivery is often recommended because of concerns for increased intracerebral vascular pressure during labor or with Valsalva. There is no evidence that cesarean improves outcomes for mother or fetus and should be reserved for obstetric indications (11,14).
  - Cesarean delivery is recommended for hemorrhage occurring in the third trimester.
  - Vaginal delivery is acceptable for women with aneurysms that rupture before the third trimester or those that are treated surgically. A passive second stage of labor and operative vaginal delivery are recommended to avoid the increased intracranial pressure associated with expulsive efforts.

Referrals/Counseling
- Some women with ICH during pregnancy will have long-term reduction in decision-making capacity or may even be left in a persistent vegetative state. An ethics consultation service may be helpful in guiding decision making in such cases (20).

Complications
- ICH accounts for 5% to 12% of all maternal deaths (9,11–14).
- The maternal mortality from ICH is 20% (13).

EMBOLIC STROKE AND CEREBRAL VENOUS THROMBOSIS
Background
Definitions
- Transient ischemic attack (TIA) is the sudden but short-lived onset of a focal neurologic deficit, caused by brain ischemia.
- Stroke, which may be caused either by hemorrhage or by cerebral embolism, is also sudden in onset and focal, but without the rapid resolution seen in TIA.
- Cerebral venous thrombosis (CVT) most often involves the superior sagittal sinus but may occur anywhere in the cerebral venous circulation. It occurs more commonly in preeclampsia, sepsis, and when abnormalities of the clotting system are present.

Epidemiology
- The overall incidence of cerebral infarction (arterial and venous combined) is approximately 0.9 to 24 per 100,000 deliveries (10,12).
  - The incidence of embolic stroke is estimated as 4 to 11 per 100,000 deliveries. The occurrence is distributed fairly evenly throughout pregnancy (10,12).
  - CVT occurs in 0.7 to 24 per 100,000 deliveries and occurs much more commonly in the postpartum period (12). If CVT occurs early in pregnancy, it is likely to recur later in the pregnancy or in the puerperium.

Evaluation
Any pregnant woman who experiences new-onset or increased frequency of cerebral ischemic symptoms should be hospitalized for diagnostic evaluation and treatment.

History and Physical
- The symptoms of CVT include headache, vomiting, seizures, lethargy, and drowsiness.
- Progressive, atypical headache resistant to analgesia develops in more than 90% of patients and may develop over the course of several days, leading to an average time between symptom onset and diagnosis of 7 days (21).
- Physical findings include papilledema, hemiplegia, and altered speech, sensation or vision, including visual field deficits or blindness.

Laboratory Tests
- Blood tests include complete blood count, erythrocyte sedimentation rate, serum glucose, coagulation studies, evaluation for thrombophilia, and tests for anticardiolipin antibodies.
- The incidence of prothrombotic mutations in patients with CVT may be as high as 40% with many women having multiple mutations (22).

Diagnosis
- Electrocardiography, echocardiography, and cranial MRI/MRV scanning are indicated, and cerebral angiography should be considered (11).

Differential Diagnosis
- The differential diagnosis of cerebral ischemic symptoms includes cerebral embolism, CVT, ICH, mass lesions, seizure disorder, migraine, and eclampsia.

Treatment
- Labor is not contraindicated, but a passive second stage and operative vaginal delivery are often recommended to avoid increases in intracranial pressure.
- Cesarean delivery may be advisable when CVT occurs near term.

Medications
- Aspirin in low doses (81 mg/d) is recommended for all women with TIAs, embolic stroke, and current or previous CVT.
- Heparin is the anticoagulant of choice in pregnancy due to its inability to cross the placenta. Low molecular weight heparin (LMWH) may provide better safety and efficacy than unfractionated heparin (UFH) in the initial treatment of CVT (23).
  - Heparin is indicated in women with recurrent TIAs to prevent recurrences.
  - Intravenous heparin is used in patients with acute embolic stroke or CVT once ICH has been excluded.
  - Long-term heparin therapy is often advised for women with embolization from a left atrial mural thrombus in the setting of atrial fibrillation.
  - Heparin is utilized for 6 to 8 weeks postpartum in all women who have had stroke or CVT, as the postpartum period presents a high risk for thrombotic and embolic events.
- Although available data are insufficient to develop guidelines, thrombolytic therapy with recombinant tissue plasminogen activator (rt-PA) or streptokinase may be employed in pregnant patients who otherwise meet the criteria for use of such agents, including early presentation to the hospital after onset of symptoms, absence of cerebral hemorrhage, and presence of a significant neurologic deficit (24).
- In patients with CVT and increased intracranial pressure, the use of dexamethasone or mannitol should be considered to reduce cerebral edema.

Referrals/Counseling
- The diagnostic evaluation and treatment planning should be performed in conjunction with a neurologist.
- Physical and occupational therapy are helpful in facilitating recovery.

Complications
- The reported mortality of cerebral infarction in pregnancy varies widely, ranging from 0% to 15% (9).
- The mortality of CVT temporally related to pregnancy is 0% to 9%, significantly lower than that in nonpregnant patients (25,26).

Patient Education
- Once a patient has been diagnosed with cerebral infarction, patient education should include smoking cessation, control of hypertension, lipid-lowering therapy, and possibly long-term anticoagulation.
- Estrogen-containing oral contraceptives are contraindicated.
- Although the risk is low, any of these entities may recur in a future pregnancy, and patient education should include discussion of these risks. Women should be treated with LMWH during future pregnancies (26).

MECHANICAL PROSTHETIC HEART VALVES
Another serious vascular complication is thrombosis of an artificial heart valve. While cardiovascular complications of pregnancy are covered in Chapter 4, the topic of artificial heart valves is emphasized here due to the high propensity to thromboembolism and the competing needs for maternal and fetal health.

Background
- Pregnant women with mechanical prosthetic heart valves are at significant risk for thromboembolism (~2.6%) and death (3.3%) (27). Continuous therapeutic anticoagulation with frequent monitoring is required.
- Data on the efficacy of anticoagulation in pregnancy are limited to several small case series. The optimal regimen for anticoagulation has yet to be determined. Choice of anticoagulation regimen should be made after a fully informed discussion of risks with the pregnant woman.

Treatment
Medications
- Warfarin
  - Although evidence suggests that warfarin is the most effective anticoagulant in the presence of a mechanical heart valve, there is strong evidence that warfarin is most teratogenic during the 6th to 12th week of gestation, whereas use of warfarin late in pregnancy predisposes to fetal ICH or intrauterine fetal demise (28).
  - The risk for pregnancy complications in patients treated with sodium warfarin is higher when the mean daily dose exceeds 5 mg daily (29).
- LMWH
  - Should be used with caution for anticoagulation in patients with mechanical prosthetic heart valves, as reports of thrombosis and stroke in both pregnant and nonpregnant women have been published. Careful monitoring of peak and trough levels is required (30).
  - The use of LMWH during pregnancy is associated with an increased risk of prosthetic valve thromboses (29,30).
- While data do not exist from clinical trials to determine the optimal regimen to minimize both maternal and fetal risks, some form of anticoagulation is preferable to no anticoagulation, and one of the following regimens could be considered (29,30):
  - Adjusted-dose twice-daily LMWH throughout pregnancy with frequently monitored anti-Xa levels 4 hours after subcutaneous injection to maintain the anti-Xa level between 0.7 and 1.2 units/mL.
  - Adjusted dose UFH every 12 hours to prolong the 6-hour postinjection aPTT at 2.0 to 2.5 times baseline.

- UFH or LMWH (as above) until the 13th week with conversion to warfarin for weeks 13 through 35 (target INR 2.5 to 3.5) when UFH or LMWH is resumed.
- In those women deemed to be at highest risk of thromboembolism, may consider warfarin throughout pregnancy until conversion to LMWH or UFH near delivery.
- The addition of low-dose aspirin should be considered in high-risk women with prosthetic heart valves (29,30).

Patient Education
- Patients with known vascular complications require careful preconceptional assessment and counseling.
- The safety of pregnancy for these patients should not be presumed until a full assessment has been completed and discussed with the patient.
- The occurrence of vascular complications during pregnancy requires extensive patient counseling and education regarding risks and management options.

REFERENCES
1. Braverman AC. Acute aortic dissection: clinician update. *Circulation.* 2010;122:184–188.
2. Hauenstein E, Frank H, Bauer JS, et al. Takayasu's arteritis in pregnancy: review of the literature and discussion. *J Perinat Med.* 2010;38(1):55–62.
3. Robinson R. Aortic aneurysm in pregnancy. *Dimens Crit Care Nurs.* 2005;24:21–24.
4. Al-Habbal Y, Christophi C, Muralidharan V. Aneurysms of the splenic artery—a review. *Surgeon.* 2010;8(4):223–231.
5. Sahni G. Chest pain syndromes in pregnancy. *Cardiol Clin.* 2012;30(3):343–337.
6. Ha JF, Phillips M, Faulkner K. Splenic artery aneurysm rupture in pregnancy. *Eur J Obstet Gynecol Reprod Biol.* 2009;146(2):133–137.
7. Thalmann M, Sodeck GH, Domanovits H. Acute type A aortic dissection and pregnancy: a population based study. *Eur J Cardiothorac Surg.* 2011;39(6):e159–e163.
8. Soliman KB, Shawky Y, Abbas MM, et al. Ruptured renal artery aneurysm during pregnancy, a clinical dilemma. *BMC Urol.* 2006;6:22.
9. James AH, Bushnell CD, Jamison MG, et al. Incidence and risk factors for stroke in pregnancy and the puerperium. *Obstet Gynecol.* 2005;106:509–516.
10. Scott CA, Bewley S, Rudd A, et al. Incidence, risk factors, management, and outcomes of stroke in pregnancy. *Obstet Gynecol.* 2012;120(2 Pt 1):318–324.
11. Davie CA, O'Brien P. Stroke and pregnancy. *J Neurol Neurosurg Psychiatry.* 2008;79:240–145.
12. Edlow JA, Caplan LR, O'Brien K, et al. Diagnosis of acute neurological emergencies in pregnant and postpartum women. *Lancet Neurol.* 2013;12:175–185.
13. Bateman BT, Schumacher HC, Bushnell CD, et al. Intracerebral hemorrhage in pregnancy: frequency, risk factors, and outcome. *Neurology.* 2006;67:424–429.
14. Khan M, Wasay M. Haemorrhagic strokes in pregnancy and puerperium. *Int J Stroke.* 2012. [Epub ahead of print]
15. Kim YW, Neal D, Hoh BL. Cerebral aneurysms in pregnancy and delivery: pregnancy and delivery do not increase the risk of aneurysm rupture. *Neurosurgery.* 2013;72:143–150.
16. Friedlander RM. Arteriovenous malformations of the brain. *N Engl J Med.* 2007;356:2704–2712.
17. Jung SY, Bae HJ, Park BJ, et al. Parity and risk of hemorrhagic strokes. *Neurology.* 2010;74(18):1424–1429.
18. Dias MS, Sekhar LN. Intracranial hemorrhage from aneurysms and arteriovenous malformations during pregnancy and the puerperium. *Neurosurgery.* 1990;27:855–866.
19. Groenestege AT, Rinkel GJE, van der Bom JG. The risk of aneurismal subarachnoid hemorrhage during pregnancy, delivery, and the puerperium in the Utrecht population: case-crossover study and standardized incidence ratio estimation. *Stroke.* 2009;40:1148–1151.
20. Finnerty JJ, Chisholm CA, Chapple H, et al. Cerebral arteriovenous malformation in pregnancy: presentation and neurologic, obstetric, and ethical significance. *Am J Obstet Gynecol.* 1999;181:296–303.

21. Ferro JM, Cahnao P, Stam J, et al. Prognosis of cerebral vein and dural sinus thrombosis: results of the international study on cerebral vein and dural sinus thrombosis (ISCVT). *Stroke*. 2004;35:664–670.
22. Klai S, Fekih-Mrissa N, Mrissa R, et al. Maternal cerebral venous thrombosis, uncommon but serious disorder, pathologic predictors and contribution of prothrombotic abnormalities. *Fibrinolysis*. 2013;24:269–272.
23. Coutinho JM, Ferro JM, Canhao P, et al. Unfractionated or low-molecular weight heparin for the treatment of cerebral venous thrombosis. *Stroke*. 2010;41:2575–2580.
24. Leonhardt G, Gaul C, Nietsch HH. Thrombolytic therapy in pregnancy. *J Thromb Thrombolysis*. 2006;21:271–276.
25. Nasr DM, Brinjikji W, Cloft HJ, et al. Mortality in cerebral venous thrombosis: results from the national inpatient sample database. *Cerebrovasc Dis*. 2013;35:40–44.
26. Saposnik G, Barinagarrementeria F, Brown RD, et al. Diagnosis and management of cerebral venous thrombosis: a statement for healthcare professionals from the American Heart Association/American Stroke Association. *Stroke*. 2011;42:1158–1192.
27. Sillesen M, Hjortdal V, Vejlstrup N, et al. Pregnancy with prosthetic heart valves—30 years' nationwide experience in Denmark. *Eur J Cardiothorac Surg*. 2011;40(2):448–454.
28. Reimold SC, Rutherford JD. Valvular heart disease in pregnancy. *N Engl J Med*. 2003;349:52–59.
29. Bonow RO, Carabellow BA, Chatterjee K, et al. 2008 focused update incorporated into the ACC/AHA 2006 guidelines for the management of patients with valvular heart disease: a report of the American College of Cardiology/American Heart Association Task Force on Practice Guidelines. *J Am Coll Cardiol*. 2008;52(13):e1–e142.
30. Bates SM, Greer IA, Pabinger I, et al. Venous thromboembolism, thrombophilia, antithrombotic therapy, and pregnancy. American College of Chest Physicians evidence based clinical practice guidelines (8th Edition). *Chest*. 2008;133(6 suppl):844S–866S.

22 Thromboembolic Disorders

Christian A. Chisholm, Andra H. James and
James E. Ferguson II

KEY POINTS

- The risk of venous thromboembolism during pregnancy and the puerperium is 0.5 to 2.0 per 1000 women, a four-to fivefold increase over the nonpregnant state.
- Women with genetic and acquired thrombophilias incur a higher risk of thrombosis during pregnancy.
- The risk for venous thromboembolism is approximately similar in all trimesters and postpartum; however, the risk of pulmonary embolism is highest postpartum and, in particular, following cesarean delivery.
- The treatment of venous thromboembolism during pregnancy is heparin based; with rare exceptions, warfarin derivatives are contraindicated in pregnancy but not during the puerperium or lactation.

VENOUS THROMBOEMBOLISM

Background

Definition

- Thromboses in the deep venous system or deep vein thrombosis (DVT) and pulmonary embolism (PE) are collectively known as venous thromboembolism (VTE). VTE occurs more frequently in pregnant women, with an incidence of 0.5 to 2.0 per 1000 pregnancies, roughly four to five times higher than in the nonpregnant population. The risk for VTE is further elevated in the postpartum period (1,2).
- Pulmonary emboli, which occur in less than 1 in 1000 pregnancies, cause about 10% of maternal deaths in the United States (3). Most PE in pregnancy originates from DVT. Other causes include fat, amniotic fluid, and air emboli.

Pathophysiology

- A combination of normal physiologic changes of pregnancy and external influences contributes to the increased risk of VTE by altering all three components of the Virchow triad.
  - Hormone-related increases in the hepatic synthesis of components of the clotting cascade: fibrinogen, prothrombin, and factors VII, VIII, IX, and X. In the postpartum period, concentrations of factors V, VII, and IX are further elevated.
  - Relative stasis of flow in the venous circulation, particularly in late pregnancy due to compression of the inferior vena cava by the expanding uterus.
  - Endothelial injury, most often occurring at delivery and particularly after operative delivery. Medical complications of pregnancy associated with endothelial dysfunction (e.g., preeclampsia) may also increase the risk of VTE.

Epidemiology

- Risk factors for VTE in pregnancy (2,4)
  - Patient characteristics: age greater than 35 years, parity ≥3, African American race, positive family history (first-degree relatives)
  - Medical conditions: heart disease, blood disorders including sickle cell disease, autoimmune disorders including lupus and antiphospholipid syndrome, hypertension, diabetes, inflammatory bowel disease

- Obesity
- History of superficial thrombophlebitis (STP), varicose veins
- Smoking
- Surgery in pregnancy
- Complications of pregnancy:
  - Assisted reproduction, multiple gestation, hyperemesis, urinary tract infection, diabetes, antepartum hemorrhage, anemia
- Peripartum complications:
  - Preeclampsia, stillbirth
- Complications of delivery and the puerperium:
  - Cesarean delivery (especially emergency cesarean delivery), postpartum infection, postpartum hemorrhage, transfusion

Evaluation

History and Physical
- STP may present with inflammation, local edema, and pain, commonly at intravenous (IV) catheter sites.
- DVT is associated with pain, erythema, and edema, and most commonly occurs in a lower extremity.
  - The physical findings include tenderness to palpation of the involved extremity and asymmetric edema resulting in unequal calf circumferences (discrepancy of greater than 2 cm). DVT is more common in the left lower extremity, presumably due to relative compression of the left common iliac vein by the right common iliac artery.
  - Homans sign (calf tenderness on dorsiflexion of the foot) is neither sensitive nor specific for DVT in pregnancy, as most DVT in pregnancy occurs in the iliofemoral system.
- PE may present with dyspnea, substernal or pleuritic chest pain, tachypnea, apprehension, and cough.
  - Significant emboli may present with cardiovascular collapse, shock, and/or death.
  - Signs include tachycardia, jugular venous distension, parasternal heave, rales, hemoptysis, fever, diaphoresis, a pleural rub, and an S_3 murmur.

Laboratory Tests
- In pregnant women suspected of having a PE, the laboratory testing may include
  - Arterial blood gases:
    - Usually reveal arterial hypoxemia (P_aO_2 less than 70 mm Hg) without hypercarbia (normal P_aCO_2 in pregnancy = 28 to 32 mm Hg) or an increased alveolar–arterial oxygen gradient (greater than 15).
    - PE is unlikely if the P_aO_2 is greater than 85 mm Hg.
  - D-dimer is a degradation product formed during the lysis of fibrin by plasmin.
    - D-dimer concentrations (measured by ELISA) of less than 500 μg/mL in nonpregnant individuals essentially exclude PE (posttest probability less than 5%) (5).
    - D-dimer concentrations are normally increased in pregnancy. Cases of DVT and PE have been reported with negative D-dimer levels; consequently, D-dimers should not be used to exclude DVT and PE in pregnancy (6).

Genetics
- Hereditary thrombophilia (one or more) will be identified in at least 20% to 50% of women who experience VTE during pregnancy (2).
- Testing for hereditary thrombophilia is appropriate in women with a history of VTE, as results of testing may affect the thromboprophylactic regimen (1).
- General population screening for thrombophilia is not recommended, as the prevalence of some of these conditions is high, but the absolute risk of thromboembolism is low (7).
- Thrombophilias are discussed elsewhere in this chapter.

Diagnosis

Clinical Manifestations

- STP is diagnosed by physical examination, which will demonstrate inflammation and tenderness, and often a palpable thrombus.
- The clinical suspicion of DVT generally requires confirmation by imaging.

Imaging Techniques

- The diagnosis of DVT may be confirmed by a variety of imaging modalities (1,6).
  - Venous ultrasonography has a 95% sensitivity and 96% specificity for the diagnosis of symptomatic proximal DVT in the general population. However, it is less accurate for calf and iliac vein thrombosis (8). Due to the high proportion of DVT occurring above the inguinal ligament, accuracy of ultrasound is likely reduced during pregnancy. Two components of venous ultrasound are utilized in this imaging modality:
    - Compression ultrasound: The presence of a thrombus prevents coaptation of the vein walls.
    - Duplex Doppler ultrasound: The absence of venous flow in the femoral system as measured by Doppler techniques indicates a proximal occlusion. This is valuable for assessing for the presence of iliac thrombosis. Color Doppler imaging may further enhance the value of this modality.
  - Occasionally, additional imaging may be required such as magnetic resonance venography or magnetic resonance direct thrombus imaging (Fig. 22-1) (1).
- A number of imaging tests used in the evaluation of the patient with suspected of PE involve radiation exposure for the fetus. The total fetal radiation exposure in a woman requiring chest radiography, ventilation/perfusion ($\dot{V}/\dot{Q}$) imaging, and pulmonary angiography is estimated as 0.5 rad (5 mGy), substantially lower than the 1.0-rad exposure (10 mGy) threshold thought to increase slightly the risk of childhood malignancies (9). These tests should never be withheld in a pregnant woman suspected to have pulmonary thromboembolism, given the mortality of this condition.
  - Chest radiography will demonstrate vascular congestion, elevation of the hemidiaphragm, atelectasis, and pulmonary edema in up to 70% of patients with PE and will exclude pneumonia as an alternate diagnosis. Chest radiography results in less than 0.001 rad fetal radiation per exposure (less than 0.01 mGy) (9).
  - Electrocardiography may show tachycardia. The classic findings of acute cor pulmonale (right axis deviation with $S_1Q_3T_3$ and nonspecific T-wave inversion) usually are seen only in massive PE.
  - Ventilation/perfusion ($\dot{V}/\dot{Q}$) scan results in a fetal radiation exposure of 0.1 to 0.37 mGy (9).
    - A $\dot{V}/\dot{Q}$ scan or perfusion scan alone should be performed next if the chest radiograph is normal (6) (a normal perfusion scan essentially excludes PE, and the additional imaging time and radiation exposure of the ventilation phase can be avoided.)
    - The presence of a $\dot{V}/\dot{Q}$ mismatch is very reliable for diagnosing PE in pregnancy (6).
    - Matching $\dot{V}/\dot{Q}$ defects may be seen in women with underlying pulmonary disease, and angiography may be necessary to diagnose or exclude PE.
    - The primary reason to choose $\dot{V}/\dot{Q}$ scan over computed tomographic pulmonary angiography (CTPA) is the increased radiation exposure to maternal breast tissue with CTPA (approximately a four- to eightfold increase) (6).
  - CTPA is the diagnostic test of choice if the chest radiograph is abnormal or unavailable (6) (and has become the first-line imaging test for PE in many institutions). Fetal radiation exposure is estimated at 0.006 to 0.096 rad per procedure (0.06 to 0.96 mGy) (9).
    - CTPA may be considered diagnostic (posttest probability greater than 85%) when positive and exclusionary (posttest probability less than 1%; negative predictive value ~99%) when negative.
    - If venous ultrasonography or additional imaging studies are abnormal, treatment for DVT should be initiated (Fig. 22-2).

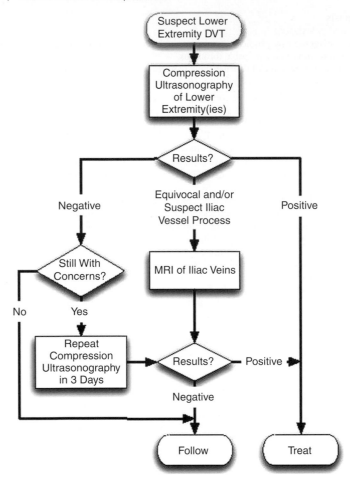

Figure 22-1. Recommended algorithm for evaluation of the pregnant patient with suspected deep venous thrombosis.

Differential Diagnosis
- For a pregnant patient presenting with cardiovascular collapse, the differential diagnosis includes amniotic fluid embolism, hemorrhage, narcotic overdose, myocardial infarction, pulmonary thromboembolism, and tension pneumothorax. Stabilization is usually necessary before undertaking a full diagnostic evaluation.
- When the clinical suspicion for pulmonary thromboembolism is high, anticoagulation with intravenous heparin should be initiated even before the diagnosis is confirmed.

Treatment
- Superficial thrombophlebitis (STP):
  - STP is treated with warm compresses, analgesia (acetaminophen), elevation, and oral antibiotics (if signs of infection are present).

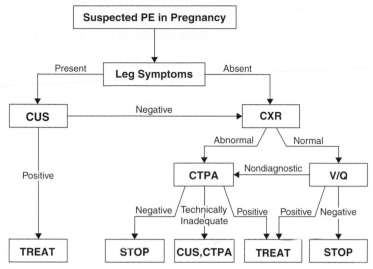

Figure 22-2. ATS/STR diagnostic algorithm for suspected PE in pregnancy. (Reprinted with permission of the American Thoracic Society. Copyright © 2013 American Thoracic Society. From Leung AN, Bull TM, Jaeschke R, et al. An official American Thoracic Society/Society of Thoracic Radiology clinical practice guideline: evaluation of suspected pulmonary embolism in pregnancy. *Am J Respir Crit Care Med.* 2011;184(10):1200–1208. Official Journal of the American Thoracic Society.)

- As embolism does not occur from the superficial veins, anticoagulation is not necessary. However, it may be useful to manage symptoms.
- Risk for DVT is not increased.
- DVT in pregnancy is managed with therapeutic-level heparin therapy, most commonly low molecular weight heparin (LMWH). Elevation of the involved extremity and early ambulation after resolution of pain and inflammation are important components of treatment for DVT.
- With suspected PE in pregnancy, the initial treatment and monitoring should include (1,10):
  - Administration of oxygen by face mask
  - Evaluation for the need for thrombolysis (presence of hypotension or cardiogenic shock)
  - Intensive monitoring of cardiovascular and respiratory status
  - Opioid analgesia as needed for pain relief and mild pulmonary vasodilatation
  - IV unfractionated heparin (UFH) given acutely in doses to prolong the activated partial thromboplastin time (aPTT) to 1.5 to 2.5 times normal, followed by outpatient treatment with adjusted-dose UFH or LMWH (see below)

Medications

Pharmacologic interventions to prevent and treat thrombosis in pregnancy rely primarily on the use of UFH or LMWH.

- Nomenclature for anticoagulation regimens used during pregnancy (1):
  - Low-dose prophylaxis: a fixed dose of anticoagulant given subcutaneously one to two times per day without use of routine monitoring to verify a therapeutic prolongation of the aPTT or therapeutic increase in anti-Xa levels, for example:

- ○ Low-dose UFH
- ○ Low-dose LMWH
- Adjusted-dose prophylaxis: anticoagulation administered to achieve traditional therapeutic effects.
  - ○ Adjusted-dose UFH is given two to three times per day subcutaneously or by continuous IV infusion. Typical midinterval aPTT prolongation is 1.5 to 2.5 times normal (2).
  - ○ Adjusted-dose LMWH is given subcutaneously (only), and a therapeutic increase in anti-Xa level (0.6 to 1.0 units/mL) (10) 3 to 4 hours after injection is desired.
- Unfractionated heparin (UFH)
  - Traditional method of heparin administration during pregnancy. Consequently, there is extensive experience with this method.
  - Molecular weight (MW): 3000 to 30,000 (mean 15,000) Da, with a negative charge.
  - Unreliable pharmacokinetics when administered subcutaneously with only 20% to 30% bioavailability.
  - Does not cross the placenta.
  - Binds to and increases the activity of antithrombin, a potent inhibitor of thrombin.
  - Short half-life of 1.5 hours. With IV administration, there is no detectable level 6 hours after discontinuation.
  - Therapeutic effect is measured by the aPTT or by anti-Xa levels.
  - Protamine sulfate is used when emergent reversal of anticoagulation is necessary.

Complications
- Osteoporosis—2% risk of vertebral fracture.
- Heparin-induced thrombocytopenia (HIT) is rare in pregnancy and likely occurs with less frequency than the 3% rate encountered in nonpregnant patients (10).

Administration
- Low-dose UFH: A commonly advocated approach is
  - 5000 units SQ q12h in the first trimester
  - 7500 units SQ q12h in the second trimester
  - 10,000 units SQ q12h in the third trimester
    - ○ In general, aPTT does not need to be performed unless the daily dose exceeds 15,000 units/d. The main reason to perform aPTT is to prevent excessive anticoagulation.
- Adjusted-dose UFH (SQ): Most often used in long-term treatment after 4 to 5 days of IV UFH. Initial dose of 10,000 units every 8 hours or 140 units/kg every 8 hours with an aPTT performed 4 hours after injection. Large doses (in excess of 30,000 units/d) are common during pregnancy.
- Adjusted-dose UFH (IV): Most often used in the acute treatment of a DVT or PE during pregnancy and postpartum. An institutional heparin nomogram should be followed, whether that be standard care (a bolus of 5000 units given over 5 minutes, followed by 1000 to 2000 units/h) or weight based (loading dose of 80 units/kg, followed by 18 units/kg/h) (11). Therapeutic target is aPTT 1.5 to 2.5 times control. An aPTT should be performed 6 hours after the loading dose.
- LMWH is increasingly used during pregnancy and is the most commonly used anticoagulant during gestation. There is a relative lack of controlled trials in pregnant women, with resultant unanswered questions about proper dosing and monitoring of anticoagulant levels. However, the potential advantages of LMWH (fewer bleeding complications, less frequent HIT) have made its use common.
  - Mean MW 3600 to 6500 Da.
  - Does not cross the placenta.
  - Anti-Xa levels are generally recognized as the most sensitive method for measuring anticoagulant effect.
  - Bioavailability is 85% to 90%.
  - Enoxaparin is available in 40-, 60-, 80-, 100-, 120-, and 150-mg syringes.

Complications
- HIT is very rare.
- Risk of osteoporosis is reduced compared to UFH.
- Difficult to reverse with protamine sulfate (10).

Administration
- In nonpregnant patients, once-daily administration of LMWH may be recommended for acute treatment of thromboembolism; however, alterations in the hemostatic system associated with pregnancy change the pharmacokinetics of LMWH and commonly require twice-daily dosing. LMWH is *not* given intravenously. Current recommendations include
  - Low-dose LMWH: There is little consensus concerning the proper dosing regimen. Two regimens commonly reported in the literature are
    - Once-daily regimen, for example, enoxaparin 40 mg qd.
    - Twice-daily regimen, for example, enoxaparin 30 to 40 mg per q12h.
    - The authors recommend the twice-daily approach for LMWH.
  - Adjusted-dose LMWH:
    - A twice-daily regimen: Enoxaparin 1 mg/kg q12h or dalteparin 100 units/kg q12h. Based on the pharmacokinetics of enoxaparin, anticoagulant effect should be measured 3 to 4 hours after injection (12), by peak anti-Xa levels targeting 0.6 to 1.0 units/mL (1). It is not known how often levels should be measured. Recommendations from monthly to each trimester have been made (10).

Special Considerations
- LMWH therapy is often changed to UFH at 35 to 37 weeks' gestation.
- Administration of epidural/regional anesthesia within 24 hours of LMWH injection may increase the risk of epidural hematoma, a serious complication.
- LMWH should not be given for at least 2 hours after removal of an epidural/spinal catheter (13).
- Coumarin: Coumarins such as warfarin (Coumadin) are restricted during pregnancy to very special circumstances such as artificial heart valves because of fetal hazards. Coumarins can be used postpartum. Consequently, pregnancy is one of the few situations where heparin is used for a prolonged period of time.
  - Warfarin derivatives cross the placenta, are teratogenic between 6 and 12 weeks of gestation, can cause fetal bleeding at any stage of pregnancy, and are associated with a high fetal loss rate. Their use is restricted to the second and early third trimester in certain cases of thrombogenic artificial heart valves as detailed in Chapter 21. Warfarin can be used safely in the postpartum period and during breast-feeding.
  - Warfarin is an antagonist of vitamin K, thereby decreasing the production of vitamin K–dependent clotting factors II, VII, IX, and X along with protein C (PC) and protein S (PS).
  - Warfarin is metabolized in the liver and kidneys. The half-life is 20 to 60 hours with a duration of effect of 2 to 5 days.
  - The anticoagulation effect of warfarin depends on the clearance of the functional clotting factors from the systemic circulation.
  - The earliest changes in the international normalized ratio (INR) occur 24 to 36 hours after the first dose. The early changes in the INR do not reflect the body's ability to prevent clot expansion or prevent new thromboses. Rather, the antithrombotic effect—the ability to prevent both clot expansion and new clot formation—depends on the inhibition of factor II (prothrombin), which does not occur until around day 5 of treatment.
  - Loading doses of warfarin (10 mg/d or more) *should not be used*, as they do not inhibit thrombosis any more rapidly and may potentiate a hypercoagulable state via early depletion of PC and PS, which have a much shorter half-life than prothrombin: 8 versus 50 hours.

- The paradoxical hypercoagulable state from depletion of PC and PS necessitates the concomitant use of a heparin or other anticoagulant for the first 4 to 5 days of warfarin treatment.
- Initial dosing should approximate the chronic maintenance dose, which is 4 to 6 mg/d. Typical target INR is 2.0 to 3.0.
- Monitoring: INR monitoring should be performed daily until a therapeutic range is maintained for at least 2 consecutive days. INR monitoring should then be performed two to three times per week until stable. Under very stable circumstances, monitoring can be reduced to once every 4 weeks.
- Complications: Maternal bleeding. The risks to the fetus are dose dependent and include intracranial hemorrhage and fetal death.

Prophylaxis
Guidelines for prophylaxis of selected patients at high risk of VTE can be found in Table 22-1.

Guidelines for cesarean for the peripartum interval include the following:
- Any patient receiving thromboprophylaxis during pregnancy should receive thromboprophylaxis postpartum.
- Women undergoing cesarean delivery should receive thromboprophylaxis with pneumatic compression devices (1).
- Patients with multiple risk factors for DVT or PE should receive thromboprophylaxis with pneumatic compression devices and LMWH (1,10).

Complications
- Long-term complications of DVT include
  - Postthrombotic syndrome (pain, edema, and hyperpigmentation)
  - Deep venous insufficiency
  - Venous stasis ulcers

Patient Education
- Women with a confirmed VTE during pregnancy or the puerperium should be advised to avoid estrogen-containing oral contraceptives.

GENETIC AND ACQUIRED THROMBOPHILIAS
Background
Definition
Thrombophilia is "the tendency to the occurrence of thrombosis" and may be genetic or acquired. The most common acquired thrombophilia is the antiphospholipid syndrome and is discussed in Chapter 10. Guidelines for prophylaxis to prevent VTE in patients with genetic thrombophilias are presented in Table 22-1. The most frequently encountered genetic thrombophilias are discussed below:

Factor V Leiden (G1691A) Mutation
Pathophysiology
- Mutation in nucleotide 1691 (G → A) of the factor V gene's 10th exon results in a substitution of glutamine for arginine at position 506 in the factor V polypeptide (factor V Q506).
- The resultant amino acid substitution impairs the activated PC and PS complexes' proteolytic inactivation of factor Va leading to an augmented generation of thrombin.
- Pregnancy-associated reductions in PS act to enhance factor V Leiden prothrombotic effects.

Epidemiology
- Present in 5% to 9% of white European populations; it is much more rare in Asian and African populations. Overall prevalence in the general population of 1% to 15% (7).

Table 22-1	Guidelines for Prophylaxis of Selected Pregnant Patients at High Risk of VTE	

Patient details	Antenatal recommendation	Postpartum recommendation
Low-risk thrombophilia[a] without previous VTE	Surveillance only or prophylactic LMWH or UFH	Surveillance only or postpartum low-dose LMWH or UFH[d] if the patient has additional risk factors[e]
Low-risk thrombophilia[a] with a single previous episode of VTE—not receiving long-term anticoagulation therapy	Low-dose LMWH/UFH or surveillance only	Low-dose LMWH or UFH for 4–6 wk postpartum
High-risk thrombophilia[b] without previous VTE	Low-dose LMWH or UFH	Low-dose LMWH or UFH for 4–6 wk postpartum
High-risk thrombophilia[b] with a single previous episode of VTE—not receiving long-term anticoagulation therapy	Low-dose or adjusted-dose LMWH/UFH regimen	Low-dose or adjusted-dose LMWH/UFH for 6 weeks (therapy level should be at least as high as antepartum treatment)
No thrombophilia with previous single episode of VTE associated with transient risk factor that is no longer present—excludes pregnancy- or estrogen-related risk factor	Surveillance only	Low-dose LMWH or UFH[c]
No thrombophilia with previous single episode of VTE associated with transient risk factor that was pregnancy- or estrogen-related	Low-dose LMWH or UFH[c]	Low-dose LMWH or UFH for 4–6 wk postpartum
No thrombophilia with previous single episode of VTE without an associated risk factor (idiopathic)—not receiving long-term anticoagulation therapy	Low-dose LMWH or UFH[c]	Low-dose LMWH or UFH for 4–6 wk postpartum
Thrombophilia or no thrombophilia with two or more episodes of VTE (provoked or not)—not receiving long-term anticoagulation therapy	Low-dose or adjusted-dose LMWH or UFH	Adjusted-dose LMWH or UFH for 6 wk

Table 22-1	Guidelines for Prophylaxis of Selected Pregnant Patients at High Risk of VTE (*Continued*)	
Patient details	**Antenatal recommendation**	**Postpartum recommendation**
Thrombophilia or no thrombophilia with (a) two or more episodes of VTE—receiving long-term anti-coagulation therapy— and (b) long-term anticoagulation any indication	Adjusted-dose LMWH or UFH	Resumption of long-term anticoagulation therapy

[a]Low-risk thrombophilia: factor V Leiden heterozygous; prothrombin G20210A heterozygous; protein C or protein S deficiency.

[b]High-risk thrombophilia: antithrombin deficiency; double heterozygous for prothrombin G20210A mutation and factor V Leiden; factor V Leiden homozygous or prothrombin G20210A mutation homozygous.

[c]Surveillance without anticoagulation is supported as an alternative approach by some experts.

[d]Postpartum anticoagulation with low-dose LMWH 40 mg daily or 30–40 mg every 12 hours, using higher doses when additional risk factors are present. LMWH is preferred to UFH except when rapid reversal may be needed.

[e]First-degree relative with a history of thrombotic episode before age 50 y or other major thrombotic risk factors (e.g., obesity, prolonged immobility).

LMWH, low molecular weight heparin; UFH, unfractionated heparin; VTE, venous thromboembolism.

Adapted from James A. Practice Bulletin No. 123: Thromboembolism in pregnancy. *Obstet Gynecol.* 2011;118(3):718–729; Bates SM, et al. VTE, thrombophilia, antithrombotic therapy, and pregnancy: Antithrombotic Therapy and Prevention of Thrombosis, 9th ed.: American College of Chest Physicians Evidence-Based Clinical Practice Guidelines. *Chest.* 2012;141(2 suppl):e691S–e736S.

Evaluation
Laboratory Tests
• Tests are DNA based and reliable during pregnancy.

Genetics
• Autosomal dominant

Diagnosis
Clinical Manifestations
• Heterozygosity for factor V Leiden mutation is present in approximately 40% of pregnant patients with thromboembolic disease (7).
• Heterozygosity is associated with an absolute thrombosis risk of less than 1.2% during pregnancy and the puerperium in women with no family history of VTE and 3.1% for those with such a history (10).
• Homozygosity for the mutation is rare (less than 1%) and confers a 4.8% absolute risk of thromboembolism during pregnancy and the puerperium among women with no family history of VTE and 14.0% with such a history (10).
• Compound heterozygosity for factor V Leiden and the prothrombin G20210A mutation is rare (0.01%) and is associated with an absolute risk of thromboembolism during pregnancy of 4.7%.

- This risk is increased to greater than 20.0% for women with factor V Leiden mutations and a prior personal history of VTE (7).

Factor II (Prothrombin G20210A) Mutation

Pathophysiology
- Mutation in the promoter located in the 3'-untranslated region of the prothrombin gene (G20210A) leads to increased (150% to 200%) circulating levels of prothrombin and an increased risk of thromboembolism.

Epidemiology
- Present in 2% to 5% of the general population (7)

Evaluation
Laboratory Tests
- Tests are PCR based and reliable during pregnancy.

Genetics
- Autosomal dominant

Diagnosis
Clinical Manifestations
- Among pregnant patients with a VTE, the mutation is found in approximately 17% (7).
- Heterozygosity is associated with an absolute risk of VTE during pregnancy and postpartum of 1.0% among women with no family history of VTE and 2.6% with such a history (10).
- Homozygosity is rare (less than 1%) and is associated with a 3.7% risk of VTE in pregnancy and postpartum among women with no family history of VTE (7,10).
- This risk is increased to greater than 17% for women with factor II mutations and a prior personal history of VTE (7).

Antithrombin Deficiency

Pathophysiology
- Numerous point mutations, deletions, and insertions result in circulating concentrations of antithrombin insufficient to oppose the action of thrombin (factor IIa) and other activated clotting factors, including IXa, Xa, XIa, and XIIa (7).

Epidemiology
- Present in 0.02% of the general population (7)

Evaluation
Laboratory Tests
- Concentrations unchanged during normal pregnancy.
- Concentrations reduced in patients with nephrotic syndrome.
- Heparin therapy interferes with measurement of antithrombin concentrations.
- Two classes of AT deficiency:
  - Type I (quantitative deficiency)
    - Most common
    - Concomitant reduction in both antigenic protein levels and activity
  - Type II (qualitative deficiency)
    - Normal antigenic levels but decreased activity

Genetics
- Usually autosomal dominant

Diagnosis
Clinical Manifestations
- Significant lifetime risk of thromboembolism
- Present in 1% of pregnant patients with thromboembolism (7)

- Antithrombin concentrations:
  - Mild deficiency: antithrombin activity 70% to 85%.
  - Severe deficiency: antithrombin activity less than 60%—VTE risk 0.7% during pregnancy and puerperium in those without a positive family history versus 3.0% with such history. The risk increases to 40% if there is a personal history of prior VTE.
  - Consider AT concentrates for women with AT deficiency who are pregnant or postpartum and have a personal history of VTE or new-onset or recurrent VTEs, AT levels less than 60% with a compelling family history and those with very low levels of AT (less than 40%) (14).

Protein C Deficiency
Pathophysiology
- PC is a vitamin K–dependent anticoagulant that works in conjunction with PS to inhibit factors Va and VIIIa.
- Deficiencies in PC result from numerous mutations.
- Two primary types are recognized (7).
  - Type I—both immunoreactive and functionally active PC levels are decreased.
  - Type II—immunoreactive levels are normal but functionally active levels are decreased.

Epidemiology
- Present in 0.2% to 0.4% in the general population (7)

Evaluation
Laboratory Tests
- Levels remain unchanged or may increase up to 135% during pregnancy.
- Liver disease may reduce levels.
Genetics
- Autosomal dominant

Diagnosis
Clinical Manifestations
- In patients without a family history, the risk of thromboembolism during pregnancy is 0.7% and 1.7% for those with a positive family history (10).
- In heterozygous individuals with a personal history of VTE, the risk of thromboembolism approximates 4% to 17% if PC levels are less than 60 (7).
- Homozygous individuals present with neonatal purpura fulminans at birth and extensive necrosis—pregnant women are unlikely to be encountered.

Protein S Deficiency
Pathophysiology
- PS is a vitamin K–dependent hepatic glycoprotein that acts as a cofactor for PC by promoting the binding of PC with the platelet surface membrane.
- Three phenotypes:
  - Type I—reduced total and free immunoreactive forms
  - Type II—normal free immunoreactive levels but reduced APC cofactor activity
  - Type III—normal total immunoreactive but reduced free immunoreactive levels

Epidemiology
- Present in 0.03% to 0.13% of the general population (7)

Evaluation
Laboratory Tests
- Free PS levels fall significantly during pregnancy.
- Liver disease may reduce levels.

Genetics
• Autosomal dominant

Diagnosis
Clinical Manifestations
• In patients without a family history, the risk of thromboembolism during pregnancy is 0.5% versus 6.6% for those with a positive family history (10).
• In heterozygous individuals with a personal history of VTE, the risk of thromboembolism approximates 0% to 22% if PS free antigen levels are less than 55% (7).
• Homozygous individuals present with neonatal purpura fulminans at birth and extensive necrosis—pregnant women are unlikely to be encountered.

Other Thrombophilias
• Hyperhomocysteinemia has been associated with an increased incidence of VTE in non-pregnant women; however, it does not appear that homozygosity for MTHFR C667T alone leads to an increased risk of VTE during pregnancy (10).
• Other thrombophilias exist that appear to exert little independent risk of VTE, and there is insufficient evidence to recommend screening for these thrombophilias (7). This group includes alternative mutations in the factor V gene, a *PAI-1* mutation, protein Z deficiency, and activity-enhancing mutations in various clotting factor genes.

Patient Education
• Reproductive-age patients with VTE outside of pregnancy require detailed evaluation and counseling prior to undertaking pregnancy.
• A number of the etiologies for VTE have a genetic basis that requires counseling regarding maternal and fetal risks including the risk of transmission to the fetus.
• Women on anticoagulation therapy require education regarding the risks of anticoagulant medications with pregnancy and treatment options prior to and during pregnancy.

REFERENCES

1. James A. Practice Bulletin No. 123: Thromboembolism in pregnancy. *Obstet Gynecol.* 2011;118(3):718–729.
2. James AH. Prevention and treatment of venous thromboembolism in pregnancy. *Clin Obstet Gynecol.* 2012;55(3):774–787.
3. Berg CJ, et al. Pregnancy-related mortality in the United States, 1998 to 2005. *Obstet Gynecol.* 2010;116(6):1302–1309.
4. Abdul Sultan A, et al. Risk factors for first venous thromboembolism around pregnancy: a population based cohort study from England. BMJ 2013;347:f6099.
5. Cutts BA, Dasgupta D, Hunt BJ. New directions in the diagnosis and treatment of pulmonary embolism in pregnancy. *Am J Obstet Gynecol.* 2013;208(2):102–108.
6. Leung AN, Bull TM, Jaeschke R, et al. An official American Thoracic Society/Society of Thoracic Radiology clinical practice guideline: evaluation of suspected pulmonary embolism in pregnancy. *Am J Respir Crit Care Med.* 2011;184(10):1200–1208.
7. Lockwood C, Wendel G. Practice Bulletin No. 124: Inherited thrombophilias in pregnancy. *Obstet Gynecol.* 2011;118(3):730–740.
8. Kearon C, Ginsberg JS, Hirsh J. The role of venous ultrasonography in the diagnosis of suspected deep venous thrombosis and pulmonary embolism. *Ann Intern Med.* 1998;129(12):1044–1049.
9. Groen RS, Bae JY, Lim KJ. Fear of the unknown: ionizing radiation exposure during pregnancy. *Am J Obstet Gynecol.* 2012;206(6):456–462.
10. Bates SM, et al. VTE, thrombophilia, antithrombotic therapy, and pregnancy: Antithrombotic Therapy and Prevention of Thrombosis, 9th ed.: American College of Chest Physicians Evidence-Based Clinical Practice Guidelines. *Chest.* 2012;141(2 suppl):e691S–e736S.

11. Raschke RA, et al. The weight-based heparin dosing nomogram compared with a "standard care" nomogram. A randomized controlled trial. *Ann Intern Med.* 1993;119(9):874–881.

12. Casele HL, et al. Changes in the pharmacokinetics of the low-molecular-weight heparin enoxaparin sodium during pregnancy. *Am J Obstet Gynecol* 1999;181(5 Pt 1):1113–1117.

13. Horlocker TT, et al. Executive summary: regional anesthesia in the patient receiving antithrombotic or thrombolytic therapy: American Society of Regional Anesthesia and Pain Medicine Evidence-Based Guidelines (Third Edition). *Reg Anesth Pain Med.* 2010;35(1):102–105.

14. James AH, Konkle BA, Bauer KA. Prevention and treatment of venous thromboembolism in pregnancy in patients with hereditary antithrombin deficiency. *Int J Womens Health.* 2013;2013(5):233–241.

Infectious Complications

Bonnie J. Dattel

KEY POINTS

- Bacterial and viral infections are common in pregnancy with the potential for severe consequences due to the physiologic changes of pregnancy.
- Treatment regimens for pregnant women must take into account the physiologic changes of pregnancy, the risks to the fetus, and optimal maternal health.
- Women should be screened for common infections during pregnancy and receive appropriate preventive treatment based on the specific organisms identified.

URINARY TRACT INFECTIONS

Urinary tract infections are frequently encountered medical complications of pregnancy.
- The three types of urinary tract infection in pregnancy are
  - Asymptomatic bacteriuria (ASB)
  - Cystitis
  - Pyelonephritis
- The uropathogens most commonly isolated in ASB are similar to those in cystitis and pyelonephritis. *Escherichia coli* is the primary pathogen in 65% to 80% of cases. Other pathogens include *Klebsiella pneumoniae, Proteus mirabilis, Enterobacter* species, *Staphylococcus saprophyticus,* and group B β-hemolytic *Streptococcus.*

Asymptomatic Bacteriuria

Background
Definition
Asymptomatic bacteriuria is defined as persistent bacterial colonization of the urinary tract without urinary symptomatology.

Epidemiology
- ASB occurs in 2% to 7% of pregnant women.
- The prevalence of ASB in pregnant and nonpregnant women is similar; therefore, pregnancy is not believed to predispose to ASB.
- However, ASB is more likely to become symptomatic and progress to pyelonephritis secondary to the physiologic changes of pregnancy (1). If untreated, 20% to 30% of pregnant women with ASB will develop acute pyelonephritis.

Treatment
Treatment should be considered when two clean catch specimens are positive for the same bacteria 10^5 colony-forming units, or a single catheterized specimen is positive for 10^2 bacteria of the same species (see Table 23-1).

Follow-up
- A negative repeat culture obtained approximately 10 days after completion of therapy is necessary to document successful treatment.

Table 23-1	ACOG Recommended Oral Therapy for ASB or Acute Cystitis
Agent	**Dosage**
Trimethoprim–sulfamethoxazole	160–180 mg q12h for 3 d
Nitrofurantoin macrocrystals	50–100 mg q6h for 3 d
Nitrofurantoin monohydrate/macrocrystals	100 mg q12h for 3 d
Cephalexin	250–500 mg q6h for 3 d
If antibiotic sensitivities are available:	
Ampicillin	250–500 mg q6h for 3 d
Amoxicillin	250–500 mg q8h for 3 d
Trimethoprim	200 mg q12h for 3 d
Sulfisoxazole	2-g loading dose, then 1 g q6h for 3 d

Maternal and Fetal Complications
- Acute pyelonephritis increases maternal risk for sepsis, respiratory insufficiency, anemia, and transient renal dysfunction.
- ASB increases the risks of preterm labor, preterm birth, and low birth weight.
- Therefore, all pregnant women should be screened for ASB early in pregnancy.

Pyelonephritis
- Acute pyelonephritis is most commonly treated with hospitalization and intravenous antibiotics.
- Intravenous therapy is usually continued until the patient is afebrile for 24 to 48 hours and symptomatically improved. The patient can then be changed over to outpatient oral antibiotics to complete a total of 10 days of therapy.
- Recommended antimicrobial regimens include
  - Trimethoprim–sulfamethoxazole, 160/800 mg q12h
  - Ampicillin, 1 to 2 g q6h, plus gentamicin, 1.5 mg/kg q8h
  - Ceftriaxone, 1 to 2 mg q24h
  - A third-generation cephalosporin first-line agent
- Suppressive therapy. Women treated for pyelonephritis are placed on antibiotic suppression for the remainder of the pregnancy and periodically screened for recurrence. Choices for suppression are
  - Nitrofurantoin, 50 to 100 mg hs or
  - Cephalexin, 250 to 500 mg hs
- All other women treated for urinary tract infections should have periodic rescreening for infection with cultures or urine dipstick for nitrates or leukocyte esterase. If infection recurs, patients are treated and then placed on chronic suppression.

PNEUMONIA
Background
Etiology
- Pneumonia is an infection with inflammation involving the parenchyma, distal bronchioles, and alveoli (2).
- Approximately two-thirds of cases of pneumonia are bacterial in origin, with two-thirds of those caused by *Streptococcus pneumoniae*. This is followed by *Haemophilus influenzae* and atypical pathogens such as *Mycoplasma* and *Legionella*.
- Two common viral agents are influenza A and varicella, which can be particularly menacing during pregnancy (2).
- Opportunistic infections with fungi and protozoans are especially noted in immunocompromised patients.

Table 23-2	Microbiologic Isolates from Pregnant Patients (Decreasing Frequency of Occurrence)

No organism isolated
Streptococcus pneumoniae or *Haemophilus influenzae*

Atypical bacterial agents
Mycoplasma or *Legionella*

Viral agents
Influenza A or varicella-zoster virus

Fungal/protozoal agents

Enteric bacterial
Escherichia coli or *Klebsiella pneumoniae*

Epidemiology

Pneumonia occurs in the pregnant population with a frequency equal to that of the general population.

Diagnosis

- Laboratory tests to aid diagnosis of pneumonia include anteroposterior and lateral shielded chest x-ray, sputum Gram stain and culture, blood cultures, and complete blood count with differential.
- In bacterial pneumonia, lobar consolidation is usually observed, with pleural effusion present in about 25% of cases. Leukocytosis may be present. Blood cultures are positive in about one-third of cases.
- In viral pneumonia, the respiratory symptoms may not be impressive initially, but the pregnant patient can rapidly develop respiratory failure. Chest x-ray findings include a unilateral patchy infiltrate (2).

Treatment

- Broad-spectrum antibiotic coverage is recommended. If the patient's condition worsens, anaerobic and gram-negative coverage can be supplemented.
- Once intravenous therapy is discontinued, oral therapy is continued for a total of 10 to 14 days (Tables 23-2 and 23-3).

Table 23-3	Therapy for Pneumonia

Antibiotic therapy for pneumonia
- Ampicillin, 2 g IV q6h
- Ceftriaxone, 1–2 g IV q24h
- Cefotaxime, 1 g IV q6–8 h
- Erythromycin, 500 mg to 1 g IV q6h
- Azithromycin, 250 mg PO q12h
- Gentamicin, 1.5 mg/kg IV initially, then 3 mg/kg/d
- Clindamycin, 900 mg IV q8h

Antiviral therapy (if needed)
- Amantadine (for influenza)
- Ribavirin (for influenza)
- Acyclovir (for varicella)

TUBERCULOSIS
Background
- Tuberculosis (TB) is the leading infectious disease in the world. The majority of patients presenting with TB have pulmonary disease.
- Progression of TB is not affected by pregnancy.
- There is no evidence to suggest an increased incidence of preterm labor or other adverse pregnancy outcomes in cases of treated TB (3).

Treatment
- The currently recommended initial treatment of drug-susceptible TB disease in pregnancy is
  - Isoniazid (INH) and rifampin daily, with the addition of ethambutol initially.
  - Pyridoxine (50 mg qd) should always be given with INH in pregnancy because of the increased requirements for this vitamin in pregnant women.
- If drug susceptibility testing of the isolate of *M. tuberculosis* reveals it to be susceptible to both INH and rifampin, then ethambutol can be discontinued.
- If pyrazinamide is not used in the initial regimen, INH and rifampin must be given for 9 months instead of 6 months.
- The treatment of any form of drug-resistant TB during pregnancy is extraordinarily difficult and should be handled by an expert with experience with the disease (2).
- The treatment of asymptomatic TB (positive PPD) should be delayed until after delivery unless there is evidence of recent infection.
- Because the risk of INH hepatitis is increased in the postpartum period, patients must be monitored closely for hepatotoxicity.

Complications for the Fetus
- Congenital infection of the infant also can occur via aspiration or ingestion of infected amniotic fluid. If a caseous lesion in the placenta ruptures directly into the amniotic cavity, the fetus can ingest or inhale the bacilli. Inhalation or ingestion of infected amniotic fluid is the most likely cause of congenital TB if the infant has multiple primary foci in the lung, gut, or middle ear.
- The mortality rate of congenital TB has been close to 50%, primarily because of failure to suspect the correct diagnosis.

CHORIOAMNIONITIS AND ENDOMYOMETRITIS
- In an uncomplicated pregnancy, there is no change in vaginal flora except for a progressive increase in colonization by *Lactobacillus*.
- A pregnancy complicated by bacterial vaginosis, preterm labor, or premature rupture of membranes predisposes the woman to chorioamnionitis.
- Postpartum, there are dramatic changes in the makeup of vaginal flora. There is a marked increase in the number of anaerobic species by the third postpartum day. Predisposing factors to anaerobic colonization include trauma, lochia, suture material, and multiple intrapartum vaginal examinations (4,5).

Chorioamnionitis
Background
Chorioamnionitis is an infection that involves the amniotic cavity and the chorioamniotic membranes. Microscopically, bacteria and leukocytes are noted between the amnion and the chorion.

Pathogens
Chorioamnionitis is most commonly the result of ascending contamination of the uterine cavity and its contents by the lower genital tract flora, although systemic infections can infect the uterus via blood (Table 23-4).

Table 23-4	Chorioamnionitis Organisms	
Aerobes		**Anaerobes**
Gram negative		**Gram negative**
E. coli		Fusobacterium sp.
Other gram-negative bacilli		Gardnerella vaginalis
		Bacteroides fragilis
		Bacteroides sp.
Gram positive		**Gram positive**
Streptococcus agalactiae		Peptostreptococcus sp.
Enterococcus faecalis		Peptococcus sp.
Staphylococcus aureus		Clostridium sp.
Streptococcus sp.		**Facultative**
		Mycoplasma hominis
		Ureaplasma urealyticum

Risk Factors

Risk facts for intra-amniotic infection include ruptured membranes before labor, labor duration, preterm labor, internal fetal monitoring, cervical examinations during labor, nulliparity, young age, meconium-stained amniotic fluid, cervical colonization (e.g., with gonorrhea or group B *Streptococcus* [GBS]), and bacterial vaginosis.

Diagnosis
- The diagnosis is made by clinical examination, based on maternal and fetal manifestations of intrauterine infection.
  - Maternal manifestations include fever, tachycardia, uterine tenderness, foul-smelling amniotic fluid, and maternal leukocytosis (unreliable).
  - Fetal manifestations include tachycardia and possibly a non–reassuring fetal heart rate pattern.

Treatment
- Intravenous antibiotics should be initiated immediately on diagnosis.
- Prompt intrapartum administration of broad-spectrum antibiotic therapy (Table 23-5) results in better maternal and fetal outcomes than when therapy is delayed until after delivery.

Table 23-5	Chorioamnionitis: ACOG Recommendations Intravenous Therapy

Intrapartum:
- Ampicillin, 2 g q4–6 h
- Penicillin, 5 million units q4–6 h plus gentamicin (aminoglycoside), 1.5 mg/kg q8h

If cesarean section is performed, then at cord clamp add:
- Clindamycin, 900 mg q8h
- Metronidazole, 500 mg q12h

Alternatively, possible extended-spectrum, single-agent therapy may include (less information regarding efficacy)
- Cefotetan, 2 g q12h
- Ampicillin/sulbactam, 1.5–3 g q6h, or
- Ceftizoxime, 1 g q8h, or
- Ticarcillin/clavulanic acid, 3.1 g q4–6 h, or
- Piperacillin, 3–4 g q4–6 h

Complications for the Mother and Fetus
- The average interval between diagnosis of chorioamnionitis and delivery is from 3 to 7 hours.
- There has never been a defined "critical time interval" after which maternal and neonatal complications increase. Recent studies have indicated that longer diagnosis-to-delivery times do not correlate with worsening prognosis of either mother or newborn.
- Because there is little evidence that cesarean delivery offers an advantage over vaginal delivery, route-of-delivery decisions should be based on standard obstetric indications (5).

GROUP B *STREPTOCOCCUS*
Background
- GBS is a leading cause of neonatal bacterial sepsis in the United States (6). Incidence has been decreasing after the release of revised disease prevention guidelines in 2002.
- *Streptococcus agalactiae* is a gram-positive coccus that colonizes the lower gastrointestinal tract of approximately 10% to 30% of all pregnant women in the United States. Secondary spread to the genitourinary tract commonly ensues.
- Colonization of the genitourinary tract creates the risk for vertical transmission during labor or delivery, which may result in invasive infection in the newborn during the first week of life. This is known as early-onset GBS infection and constitutes approximately 80% of GBS disease in newborns.
- Invasive GBS disease in the newborn is characterized primarily by sepsis, pneumonia, or meningitis (7). The incidence of invasive GBS decreased from 0.47/1000 LB in 1999 to 2001 to 0.34/1000 LB in 2003 to 2005 ($p < 0.001$) (6).

Evaluation
Recommendations for Prophylaxis
The Centers for Disease Control and Prevention (CDC) recommends following a screening-based approach for the prevention of neonatal GBS disease.

Screening-Based Approach
- All pregnant women should be screened by culture at 35 to 37 weeks of gestation for anogenital GBS colonization.
- Patients should be informed of the screening results and of potential benefits and risks of intrapartum antimicrobial prophylaxis for GBS carriers.
- Culture techniques that maximize the likelihood of GBS recovery should be used. Because lower vaginal and rectal cultures are recommended, cultures should not be collected by speculum examination. The optimal method for GBS screening is collection of a single standard culture swab or two separate swabs of the distal vagina rectum. Swabs may be placed in a transport medium if the microbiology laboratory is off-site. The sample should be identified as being specifically for GBS culture.
- Laboratories should report the results to the delivery site and to the physician who ordered the test. GBS prenatal culture results must be available at the time and place of delivery.

Treatment
- Intrapartum chemoprophylaxis should be offered to all pregnant women identified as GBS carriers by culture at 35 to 37 weeks of gestation.
- If the results of GBS culture are not known at the time of labor, intrapartum antimicrobial prophylaxis should be administered if one of the following risk factors is present:
  - Less than 37 weeks of gestation
  - Duration of membrane rupture of 18 hours or more
  - Temperature of 100.4°F (38.0°C) or more
- Women with GBS bacteriuria in any concentration in the current pregnancy or who previously gave birth to an infant with an early onset of the disease should receive intrapartum antimicrobial prophylaxis.
- Women with negative vaginal and rectal cultures within 5 weeks of delivery do not require intrapartum antibiotics regardless of gestational age.

- Oral antimicrobial agents should not be used to treat women who are found to be colonized with GBS during prenatal screening. Such treatment is not effective in eliminating carriage or preventing neonatal disease (8).
- Routine intrapartum antibiotic prophylaxis for GBS-colonized women undergoing cesarean section deliveries without labor or membrane rupture is not recommended.

Medications

Intrapartum chemoprophylaxis

- For intrapartum chemoprophylaxis, intravenous penicillin G (5 million units initially and then 2.5 million units every 4 hours) should be administered until delivery.
- Intravenous ampicillin (2 g initially and then 1 g every 4 hours until delivery) is an acceptable alternative to penicillin G, but penicillin G is preferred because it has a narrow spectrum and thus is less likely to select for antibiotic-resistant organisms.
- For penicillin-allergic women, clindamycin (900 mg IV q8h until delivery) or erythromycin (500 mg IV q6h until delivery) may be used, although GBS resistance to clindamycin is increasing. (Penicillin G does not need to be administered to women who have a clinical diagnosis of amnionitis and who are receiving other treatment regimens that include agents active against streptococci.) (8)

HUMAN IMMUNODEFICIENCY VIRUS

Background

Etiology

Perinatal transmission of HIV accounts for virtually all new HIV infections in children.

Epidemiology

Women presented approximately 20% of the cases of AIDS reported to the CDC through 2003 (9). In the year 2000, an estimated 6000 to 7000 HIV-infected women gave birth, and an estimated 280 to 370 infants were infected in the United States. Of these HIV infected women, one in eight did not receive prenatal care and one in nine did not have HIV testing before giving birth. The CDC estimates that the number of infants born with HIV each year dropped from 1650 (1991) to fewer than 200 (2004).

Treatment

Procedures

In 1994, following clinical trials that demonstrated a two-thirds reduction in perinatal HIV transmission with zidovudine (ZDV) therapy for infected pregnant women and their infants, the Public Health Service (PHS) issued guidelines for the use of ZDV during pregnancy. This was followed by recommendations for universal HIV counseling and voluntary testing of pregnant women in July 1995 (10) (Table 23-6).

Table 23-6	Zidovudine Therapy for the Prevention of Perinatal Transmission of HIV
Time period	**Therapy**
Antepartum	100 mg ZDV five times per day PO after 14 wk of gestation
Intrapartum	2 mg/kg body weight ZDV infused IV over 1 h, then 1 mg/kg body weight by continuous infusion until delivery
Neonatal	Oral ZDV syrup, 2 mg/kg body weight every 6 h for 6 wk; first dose at 8–12 h of age if possible (may be given IV in newborns unable to take oral feeds)

From Dattel BJ. Antiretroviral therapy during pregnancy: beyond AZT (ZDV). *Obstet Gynecol Clin North Am.* 1997;24:645–657.

Risk Factors for Transmission
- Transmission of HIV infection from the mother to child is influenced by many factors.
- Known correlates of HIV-1 transmission include high maternal plasma viremia, advanced clinical HIV disease, reduced maternal immunocompetence, prolonged duration of time after rupture of the amniotic membranes before delivery, vaginal delivery, direct exposure of the fetus to maternal blood during the delivery process, and prematurity or low birth weight of the newborn (11).
- There is no single factor that, by itself, seems to accurately predict whether an individual woman will transmit HIV to her child.

Antiretroviral Therapy
- ZDV monotherapy remains the standard for the prevention of vertical transmission of HIV, but it is not adequate for the treatment of pregnant women infected with HIV.
- Optimal therapy is two nucleoside analog revised transcriptase inhibitors and a protease inhibitor. This regimen has significant beneficial effects on CD4 counts, viral load, and survival in comparison with ZDV monotherapy (12,13).
- These treatment recommendations are based on the following risk for perinatal transmission:
  - Twenty percent among 396 women who do not receive antiretroviral drugs
  - Ten percent of 710 women taking ZDV alone
  - Four percent of 186 women receiving oral antiretroviral drugs
  - One percent of these taking three drug combinations
- ZDV alone is no longer a preferred agent for the treatment of HIV in the nonpregnant patient but is considered a first-line agent during pregnancy.
- Nevirapine should not routinely be initiated in treatment-naïve women with CD4 cell carry greater than 250 cells/mm^3 because of potential hepatotoxicity and fatal risk.
- Recommended regimens include
  - ZDV + lamivudine + lopinavir/ritonavir or atazanavir/ritonavir
- Alternatives include
  - Zid + lamivudine + nelfinavir.
  - ZDV + lamivudine + nevirapine if CD4 less than 250.
  - ZDV + lamivudine + ritonavir-boosted saquinavir on darunavir.
  - Alternatively, nucleoside reverse transcriptase inhibitors (NRTI)/nonnucleoside reverse transcriptase inhibitors (NNRTIs) with good placental passage (tenofovir, emtricitabine, or abacavir) can be used if ZDV toxicity, such as severe anemia, develops.
- Low CD4 counts of less than 200 cells/mm^3 suggest more advanced disease. Women with low counts should receive ZDV and a multiple drug regimen (HAART therapy) (12).
- Data suggest that patients with low viral loads (i.e., less than 2500 copies of HIV RNA per mL) are at lower risk of disease progression than those with high (2500 to 20,000 copies of HIV RNA per mL) or very high (greater than 20,000 copies of HIV RNA per mL) viral loads, indicating a relationship between increasing viral load and vertical transmission from the mother to fetus/infant.

Development of a Treatment Plan
- To develop an appropriate treatment plan, the physician must know the status of the HIV-1–infected pregnant patient's CD4 count and viral load.
- Intrapartum ZDV therapy is not required if viral load is less than 400.

OTHER VIRAL DISEASES

Influenza
Background
Influenza is an acute, communicable infection that occurs primarily in winter months. Because of its high infectivity and frequency of genetic mutation, novel strains of orthomyxovirus influenza, the etiologic agent, often cause major epidemics.

Diagnosis
- Generalized symptoms of headache, fever, myalgia, malaise, cough, and substernal chest pain appear abruptly within 1 to 2 days after infection.
- Physical examination may reveal basilar rales.
- The chest x-ray may show bilateral interstitial infiltrates.
- Gram stains of sputum show insignificant numbers of bacteria and mononuclear cells.
- Identification of the virus within exfoliated epithelial cells after reaction with fluorescent conjugates of an influenza antiserum is the only rapid method of definitive diagnosis.
- The virus can be cultured from nasopharyngeal washings, nasal swabs, and throat swabs.
- Serum antibody is detectable 2 to 3 weeks after infection by hemagglutination inhibition, neutralization, or complement fixation antibody testing. Paired specimens are necessary for the diagnosis.

Prognosis
Influenza generally is a self-limited disease, but serious morbidity and mortality do occur.

Mother
- Pregnant women are a high-risk group during influenza epidemics.
- Increased mortality is caused by viral pneumonia itself and by superimposed staphylococcal and gram-negative enteric pneumonias.
- Rates of spontaneous abortion are as high as 25% to 50%.

Fetus
- Influenza virus can be transmitted transplacentally to the fetus.
- Many studies of large numbers of patients have failed to link influenza and congenital malformations. However, serious maternal illness with hypoxia can cause premature labor and abortion.

Treatment
- Hospitalization of pregnant women is required if febrile or with pulmonary symptoms due to high rates of pneumonia especially in the third trimester.
- Antiviral prophylaxis should be initiated as soon as possible in pregnant women. Studies from 2009 to 2010 influenza season demonstrated less severe disease and fewer deaths.
- Oseltamivir is generally preferred: 75 mg two times per day for 5 days.
- Pregnant women who are seriously ill should be hospitalized.
- Bacterial superinfection should be treated empirically on the basis of presumed pathogens. Nafcillin and either a third-generation cephalosporin or gentamicin would be adequate initial therapy, which can be modified later on the basis of culture results.
- The CDC recommends that all pregnant women receive flu vaccine regardless of gestational age.

Measles
Background
Measles (rubella) is a highly contagious, exanthematous, common childhood disease with peak incidence in the spring. Widespread vaccination had reduced the number of cases in the United States. However, worldwide measles remain a significant cause of morbidity and mortality making it the fifth most common cause of death in children under 5 years of age (14).

Diagnosis
- Small, irregular, bright red spots (Koplik spots) that are diagnostic of measles appear on buccal and sometimes other mucosal membranes at the end of the 10- to 14-day incubation period.
- Catarrhal symptoms of coryza, cough, keratoconjunctivitis, and fever are prominent early in the illness.
- The maculopapular rash begins on the face and spreads downward to the extremities.
- The rash, which often becomes confluent, fades in the same sequence.
- Patients who are partially immune have milder catarrh, fewer Koplik spots, and a more discreet and fainter rash.

- Measles virus can be identified by immunofluorescent testing in smears from nasal secretions, sputum, and oropharyngeal surfaces and by culture of these specimens.
- Fourfold or greater increases in hemagglutination inhibition, neutralizing, or complement-fixing antibodies can be demonstrated in convalescent serum drawn 2 to 3 weeks after infection.

Prognosis
Mother
- Morbidity from the respiratory symptoms and rash and mortality from the infrequent complications of encephalitis and myocarditis are the same for pregnant and nonpregnant women.
- Spontaneous abortions and premature deliveries are common.

Fetus
- Measles virus penetrates the placenta, and newborns have or develop typical exanthematous lesions.
- Most reports, but not all, indicate no increase in congenital malformations in infants born to infected mothers (15,16).

Treatment
Management
- Supportive measures of bed rest, fluids, antipyretics, expectorants, and steam inhalation reduce morbidity.
- Immune serum γ-globulin (0.5 mL/kg) given within 6 days after exposure minimizes or prevents measles symptomatology.
- Secondary bacterial complications, particularly pneumonia, are treated with appropriate antibiotics.

Prevention
- Pregnant women who are exposed to measles and who are susceptible (i.e., do not have antibody) should receive γ-globulin. Infants born to women with active measles should receive γ-globulin (0.25 mL/kg).
- Women who have not had measles or documented measles immunity should receive two doses of the live virus vaccine, 1 month apart, at least 30 days before becoming pregnant. Vaccine is contraindicated during pregnancy (see Table 23-7).
- Women without documented immunity by history or serology or those patients vaccinated before 1980 should be revaccinated with two doses of the live virus vaccine before becoming pregnant because of waning immunity.

Rubella
Background
- Rubella (German measles) is a highly contagious exanthematous disease of childhood and early adulthood.
- Despite the availability of effective vaccines, up to 20% of women of childbearing age do not possess rubella antibody (17).

Diagnosis
- Fever, cough, conjunctivitis, headache, arthralgias, and myalgias occur after a 14- to 21-day incubation period and a 1- to 5-day prodromal period.
- Postauricular, occipital, and cervical lymphadenopathies are prominent early findings. Arthritis is a frequent occurrence in adult women.
- The maculopapular rash begins on the face, spreads downward, and subsequently fades in the same top-to-bottom order.
- The illness lasts from a few days to 2 weeks.
- Rubella virus can be isolated from pharyngeal secretions, blood, urine, and stools.

Table 23-7	Immunization for Viral Infections During Pregnancy					
Variable	**Influenza**	**Measles**	**Rubella**	**Mumps**	**Poliomyelitis**	**Hepatitis B**
Risk of disease to pregnant women	Increase in morbidity and mortality, particularly during epidemics	Significant morbidity; low mortality; not altered by pregnancy	Low morbidity and mortality; not altered by pregnancy	Low morbidity and mortality; not altered by pregnancy	Increased incidence and severity in pregnancy	Possible increase in severity in pregnant women from nutritionally deprived backgrounds
Risk of disease to fetus or newborn	Increased rate of abortion; no increase in malformations	Significant increase in abortion rate; no malformations reported	High rate of abortion and congenital rubella syndrome in first trimester	Slightly increased fetal mortality in serious infections; no confirmed congenital abnormalities	Anoxic fetal damage reported; 25% mortality in neonatal disease; paralysis but no increase in congenital abnormalities	Hepatitis B is transmitted transplacentally, sometimes causing neonatal hepatitis; no increase in congenital defects or abortions
Vaccine	Inactivated type A and type B virus vaccines	Live attenuated virus vaccine	Live attenuated virus vaccine	Live attenuated virus vaccine	Live attenuated virus vaccine (Sabin) or killed virus vaccine (Salk)	Recombinant subunit vaccine (HBsAg)
Risk of vaccine to fetus	None confirmed	None confirmed	None confirmed; teratogenicity is suspected	None confirmed	None confirmed	Unknown
Indications for vaccination during pregnancy	Recommended for patients with serious underlying disease	Contraindicated	Contraindicated	Contraindicated	Not recommended for adults except in epidemics or close contact with a suspected case	Recommended for pregnant women at high risk
Comments	Amantadine may be of value in influenza A infections, but because of possible teratogenicity, its use should be avoided	0.25 mL/kg immune serum globulin to exposed susceptible women within 6 d of exposure	Serologic testing of women in childbearing age should determine need for vaccination	Passive immunization with mumps is not indicated	Salk vaccine indicated for nonimmunized women traveling in endemic areas (see text for details)	Immune serum globulin has failed to prevent hepatitis B in newborns; hepatitis B immune globulin and vaccine should be given to newborns (see text for details)

HbsAg, hepatitis B surface antigen; d, day.
Adapted from Leontic EA, Respiratory disease in pregnancy. *Med Clin North Am.* 1977;61:111.

- Increases in hemagglutination inhibition, neutralizing, and complement-fixing antibodies are demonstrable 2 to 4 weeks after infection. Most laboratories presently use enzyme-linked immunosorbent assay (ELISA) or latex agglutination testing of paired sera to detect recent infection.

Prognosis
Mother
- Morbidity from the rash, respiratory illness, arthritis, and infrequent encephalitis are the same for pregnant and nonpregnant women. Fatality is rare.
- Spontaneous abortion and stillbirth are two to four times more frequent in pregnancies complicated by rubella.

Fetus
- Direct infection of the fetus occurs.
- If the disease is acquired during the first trimester of pregnancy, the risk of fetal malformation or death ranges from 10% to 34%.
- Acquisition of infection later in pregnancy results in fewer and usually less deleterious fetal abnormalities.
- Manifestations of congenital rubella include cataracts, blindness, cardiac anomalies (patent ductus arteriosus, ventricular septal defect, pulmonary valve stenosis), deafness, mental retardation, cerebral palsy, violaceous birthmarks, hepatosplenomegaly, thrombocytopenic purpura, hemolytic anemia, lymphadenopathy, encephalitis, and cleft palate (18).

Treatment
Management
- Supportive measures of bed rest, fluids, and acetaminophen for treatment of headache and arthritis usually suffice for this mild, self-limited illness.
- Therapeutic abortion should be considered except in instances in which infection is known to occur in the third trimester of pregnancy. During 2001–2004, the median number reported was 13. Since 2001, only five infants with congenital rubella have been reported.
- Epidemiologic evidence suggests rubella is no longer endemic in the United States.

Prevention
- Prepubertal and nonpregnant postpubertal women without documented antirubella antibodies should be immunized with live attenuated rubella vaccine.
- Women who are vaccinated should not become pregnant for 3 months after vaccination.
- Neither accidental immunization of a pregnant woman nor exposure to virus shed by recently immunized children has resulted in fetal infection (see Table 23-7).
- Rubella vaccine exposure in pregnancy is not an indication for termination.

Mumps
Background
Mumps is a contagious disease of children and young adults (18).

Diagnosis
- Fever, myalgia, malaise, and headache of variable severity occur after a 2- to 3-week incubation period.
- Parotitis is the most prominent feature, and this finding establishes the diagnosis.
- Mastitis and oophoritis can occur in postpubertal women.
- The demonstration of immunoglobulin M (IgM) antibody by immunofluorescent techniques or a fourfold or greater increase in serum complement-fixing antibody confirms the diagnosis.

Prognosis
Mother
- The morbidity from parotitis and the complications of mastitis, oophoritis, and encephalitis are the same for pregnant and nonpregnant women.
- Spontaneous abortions are more frequent in women who are infected during the first trimester of pregnancy.

Fetus. There has been a growing controversy concerning the development of congenital endocardial fibroelastosis (19).

Treatment
Management
- Administer symptomatic treatment to relieve the discomfort of fever and parotitis.
- Passive immunization with hyperimmune mumps immunoglobulin is no longer recommended because the drug is not of value.

Prevention
Vaccination with live attenuated mumps virus is suggested for nonpregnant postpubertal women who have not had mumps parotitis (see Table 23-7).

Poliomyelitis
Background
Poliomyelitis, currently a rare illness in pregnancy, was, in the prevaccine era, more common and more severe in pregnant than in nonpregnant women of similar age (20). This increase in incidence was attributed to hormonal changes in pregnancy and to greater exposure to young children.

Diagnosis
- Fever, headache, coryza, nausea, vomiting, and sore throat precede the characteristic paralytic phase, which is marked by hyperesthesia, muscle pain, and flaccid paralysis.
- Poliovirus can be isolated from feces, serum, and cerebrospinal fluid (CSF).
- Increases in neutralizing and complement-fixing antibodies are demonstrable in serum obtained at 2 and 4 weeks after infection.

Prognosis
Mother
- In the prevaccine era, morbidity and mortality were higher in the pregnant than in the nonpregnant state.
- The incidence of abortion is increased.

Fetus
- There is no increase in the incidence of congenital abnormalities with intrauterine infection.
- Paralysis and growth retardation occur in infants infected in utero. Neonatal poliomyelitis has a mortality of approximately 25%.

Treatment
Management
- Isolation procedures are required for infected mothers and newborns to prevent spread of the infection through excretory products.
- Supportive care to prevent deformities and, if necessary, to maintain adequate maternal ventilation is indicated during the acute illness.

Prevention
- If immediate protection against poliomyelitis is needed because of travel to an endemic area, a single dose of oral vaccine is given unless time permits the schedule required for the inactivated vaccine (see Table 23-7).
- The inactivated vaccine is recommended for booster injections because the live attenuated oral vaccine has, on rare occasions, caused poliomyelitis in adults.

COXSACKIE VIRUSES
Background
Coxsackie virus serotypes A and B cause a wide spectrum of brief, self-limited illnesses involving one or more organ systems (20).

Diagnosis
- Herpangina, lymphonodular pharyngitis, and rhinopharyngitis indistinguishable from rhinovirus-induced common colds occur in pregnant women infected with coxsackievirus A. Aseptic meningitis is caused by both serotypes. Pleurodynia is caused by infections with coxsackievirus B.
- Coxsackievirus can be isolated from pharyngeal secretions and feces, but for practical purposes, culture is rarely performed.
- Because of the large numbers of serotypes, serologic proof of infection—demonstration of fourfold or greater increases in neutralizing or complement-fixing antibody—is impractical except in epidemics.

Prognosis
Mother
- The coxsackievirus-induced illnesses are self-limited and are not associated with significant maternal mortality.
- The incidence of abortion is not increased.

Fetus
- Coxsackievirus A infections are of no consequence to the fetus.
- Coxsackievirus B infections cause serious illness (myocarditis and encephalitis) and fetal mortality in the perinatal period. The most common defect associated with coxsackievirus B infection is tetralogy of Fallot, but definitive evidence linking this or other congenital abnormality to coxsackievirus B infections is lacking.

Treatment
Management
- Symptomatic treatment is indicated for the mother, and supportive treatment is indicated for the fetus with myocarditis or encephalitis.
- Newborns who survive infection usually do not have residual defects.

Prevention
No vaccine is available.

Varicella (Chickenpox)-Zoster
Background
- Varicella is a common childhood illness caused by the varicella-zoster herpes virus that is characterized by cutaneous vesicles that crust and scab. It is transmitted by droplets or by direct contact with an infected person and is highly contagious to susceptible persons after household exposure.
- Most cases occur in children so that 95% of adults show serologic evidence of immunity (21).
- The mean incubation period of varicella is 15 days, with a range of 10 to 21 days.
- Infectivity occurs from 2 days before the onset of skin lesions until 5 days after the lesions have crusted.
- Childhood varicella usually is uncomplicated, and although varicella is uncommon in adults, adulthood varicella carries increased risks of death from pneumonia.

Diagnosis
- Before the onset of rash, a 1- to 2-day prodromal period of fever, headache, malaise, and anorexia may occur. Prodromal symptoms increase with age.
- Characteristic skin lesions appear on the trunk, scalp, face, and extremities. In a normal host, rash progresses in stages over a 1-week period: maculae, papule, vesicle, pustule, and crusted lesion.

- If present, fever lasts 1 to 3 days. All organ systems may be involved.
- Pneumonia and hepatitis are the primary serious complications.

Treatment
Healthy Woman Presenting for Preconceptional Counseling or First Prenatal Visit
- If a woman has a positive history of chickenpox, she is considered immune; therefore, a question about a history of chickenpox should be included during preconceptional counseling and at the initial prenatal visit.
- Women with a negative or equivocal history should have a serum varicella titer drawn to determine their immune status (varicella IgG).
- Also, because the vaccine may not be as immunogenic as past natural infection, patients who have been vaccinated should have serologic testing for varicella titers.
- Because the vaccine consists of a modified live virus, nonimmune women who are *not* pregnant can receive the vaccine but should avoid pregnancy for 1 month thereafter.
- Nonimmune pregnant women should receive the vaccine postpartum; the vaccine is not contraindicated with breast-feeding (22)
- There is no risk for pregnant women of acquiring varicella from children with recent varicella vaccination.

A Nonimmune Pregnant Woman Exposed to Chickenpox
- A person with chickenpox is infectious from 2 days before the appearance of typical lesions until 5 days after the vesicles crust over.
- It is important to note that 85% of adults who do not recall having had chickenpox nevertheless have protective antibody levels.
- In a potentially exposed patient, determining her varicella titer first is preferable to administering varicella-zoster immunoglobulin (VZIG), because VZIG is relatively expensive (~$400 for the usual adult dose) and because it is not stocked in local pharmacies. The patient's serum must be collected within 10 days of the earliest exposure because only by then can it be determined if the antibody detected is an indication of protection from prior exposure versus antibody response to the current exposure.
- VZIG must be administered within 96 hours of exposure, and it provides no benefit when administered after the onset of symptoms. VZIG reduces the rates of clinical varicella in exposed persons, but it has not been shown to prevent adverse fetal effects; therefore, VZIG's only purpose is to prevent or reduce the severity of illness in the mother (22).

A Pregnant Woman with Chickenpox
- All patients with suspected varicella infection should be isolated and evaluated with only varicella-immune medical staff in attendance.
- The diagnosis is usually clinical. Fever, malaise, and the characteristic rash appear 10 to 21 days after exposure.
- The care is isolated palliation.
- The most dangerous maternal complication is varicella pneumonia. When varicella pneumonia develops in pregnant women, the morbidity and mortality are comparatively high. Supportive oxygen and ventilator therapy should be used as indicated. There is general agreement that intravenous antiviral therapy should be given to pregnant women with any respiratory embarrassment associated with chickenpox.
- Antiviral therapy consists of inhibitors of herpes DNA polymerase (acyclovir, famciclovir, and valacyclovir). There are insufficient data regarding the risk/benefit ratio of giving these antivirals to pregnant varicella patients without pulmonary symptoms (22).

Chickenpox in the Immediate Peripartum Period
- When maternal chickenpox breaks out close to the time of delivery, the mother may infect the baby before there has been adequate time for her to produce and transfer protective antibodies across the placenta. These newborns suffer high morbidity and mortality rates.

- If mothers contract chickenpox between 5 days before and 2 days after delivery, their newborns should receive VZIG. Because VZIG does not always prevent neonatal chickenpox in this scenario, acyclovir may be a useful supplement in their management. Pediatric consultation is advised (22).

Maternal Complications
- Varicella infection may range from a trivial illness with a few skin lesions to a major life-threatening episode. The infection can result in complications such as pneumonia, encephalitis, visceral dissemination, or hemorrhagic varicella.
- Varicella acquired later in pregnancy, particularly in the third trimester, appears to be associated with increased morbidity, with a greater severity of pneumonia, a higher incidence of hospitalization, and an increased requirement for mechanical ventilation, compared to that acquired earlier in pregnancy (23).

Fetal Complications
- Fetal involvement has been traditionally divided into three forms:
  - "Varicella embryopathy" stemming from maternal disease occurring before 20 weeks of gestation
  - Congenital varicella resulting from maternal infection from 20 weeks of gestation until term, but more commonly close to term
  - Neonatal disease occurring when the pregnant patient has active lesions around the time of delivery (24)
- There is a wide range of fetal anomalies attributed to varicella-zoster. The risk of fetal anomalies correlates with the trimester in which infection occurred
  - First-trimester infection = 0.5% to 6.5%
  - Second- and third-trimester infection = 0% to 1.1% (25)

Fetal varicella infection is associated with maternal infection within the first 20 weeks of gestation. It can include low birth weight as well as dermatologic, neurologic, ophthalmologic, skeletal, gastrointestinal, and genitourinary abnormalities.

Herpes Zoster
Endogenous reactivation of latent varicella zoster not associated with significant risk of congenital varicella syndrome. Passage to fetus is rare. Treatment is similar to nonpregnant adults.

CYTOMEGALOVIRUS
Background
Definition
Cytomegalovirus (CMV) is a member of the herpesvirus family of double-stranded DNA viruses.
- It is the most common congenital viral infection with birth prevalence of 0.5% (26).
- It inserts itself into host cells creating characteristically large cells with prominent intranuclear inclusion bodies.
- The replicative cycle of CMV is divided into three periods: immediate-early, early, and late. Monoclonal antibodies against proteins from these three periods have been used to detect the presence of the virus, using rapid viral diagnostic techniques such as the shell vial culture–enhancement system (26).

Epidemiology
- On the basis of antibody testing, CMV infects 50% to 60% of women of childbearing age (27). Pregnant women usually acquire CMV infection initially by exposure to body excretions (saliva, urine) of young children or by intimate sexual contact (28).
- The virus is present in the urine of approximately 5% of pregnant women. Increased cervical excretion of CMV is seen in the third trimester.
- Virus shedding is much more common in women younger than 30 years. Interestingly, the majority of congenital CMV infections occur in infants of women younger than 30 years of age (27).

- CMV is the most common viral cause of intrauterine infection, and it is the major infectious factor known to be associated with congenital mental retardation and deafness (29). It has been estimated that the overall burden of congenital CMV infection to the health care delivery system is in excess of $1 billion (30).
- The period of greatest risk for fetal disease and subsequent neurologic impairment is the first 22 weeks of gestation.
- Fetal infection may follow either primary or recurrent maternal infection. Primary maternal CMV infection is associated with a more serious and a much higher incidence of congenital infection than recurrent maternal CMV infection (31).
- Primary maternal CMV infection affects approximately 1% of all pregnancies, and the infection carries a 50% risk of intrauterine transmission, with a 10% risk of symptomatic congenital sequelae at birth or in early infancy (32).
- Although the rate of recurrent maternal CMV infection is about 10 times greater than that of primary maternal CMV infection, the risk of intrauterine infection from recurrent maternal CMV infection is only about 1% (26,33).

Diagnosis
- Adult infections usually are asymptomatic. Symptomatic infections resemble infectious mononucleosis and present with low-grade fever, malaise, lymphadenopathy, and hepatosplenomegaly.
- Laboratory studies show leukocytosis with atypical lymphocytes, abnormalities in hepatocellular function, and a negative heterophile antibody test for mononucleosis.
- CMV can be cultured from blood, saliva, urine, and cervical mucus. Because many patients excrete CMV, the demonstration of increases in antibody titers in convalescent serum is the most accurate means of documenting a newly acquired infection.
- Identification of the virus can be accomplished with anti-CMV antibodies. Polymerase chain reaction (PCR) can be used to identify the presence of CMV DNA in amniotic fluid, urine, blood, and saliva (27).

Prognosis
Mother
- CMV infection is self-limited and without any increased morbidity or mortality in pregnancy.
- The infection also is not known to increase the incidence of abortion or premature delivery.

Fetus
- Infection of the fetus occurs either in utero by transplacental passage of the virus or at birth when the fetus traverses an infected birth canal.
- It has been estimated that the prevalence of intrauterine CMV infections is between 0.2% and 2.5% of births.
- Abnormalities of variable severity affect approximately 10% of infected infants and include microcephaly, diminished mentation, chorioretinitis, hearing loss, intracranial calcifications, and hepatosplenomegaly. Intrauterine infection can also result in stillbirth.
- Additionally, 5% to 20% of asymptomatic congenitally infected infants will experience late manifestations that include neuromuscular disturbances, auditory damage, and visual impairment (27).
- Hyperimmunoglobulin therapy of pregnant women with primary CMV is a promising but investigational approach.

Treatment
Management
Administer symptomatic treatment to relieve discomfort. Ganciclovir, an antiviral agent, is efficacious in the treatment of CMV retinitis and GI disease. Its value in pregnancy is unknown.

Prevention

No vaccine is currently available. Prenatal diagnosis of congenital CMV can be accomplished with serologic testing of amniotic fluid.

VIRAL HEPATITIS

Background

Viral hepatitis (hepatitis A, B, or C) is one of the most serious diseases in the United States and is the most common cause of jaundice during pregnancy (34).

- Hepatitis A has an incubation period of 25 to 40 days. Infection is transmitted by the fecal–oral route. Maternal transmission to the fetus does not occur.
- Hepatitis B has a 50- to 180-day incubation period and is transmitted by contaminated blood, saliva, breast milk, and semen. Pregnant women who are infected transmit the virus transplacentally to the fetus and at birth. Neonatal hepatitis seldom occurs if the mother is a chronic carrier or acquires hepatitis early in pregnancy; the risk is high when infection occurs late in pregnancy.
- Hepatitis C, which occurs in the same settings as hepatitis B, has an incubation period of approximately 9 weeks. Infection with hepatitis C virus (HCV), a small RNA virus, is characterized by persistent viremia. Two studies demonstrate that the risk of vertical transmission is low, with rates of approximately 6% (35). The risk of transmission correlates with the HCV viral titer in the mother (35).

Diagnosis

Clinical Symptoms

- Except for fever being more common in hepatitis A and prodromal arthralgias occurring in 20% of patients with hepatitis B, the clinical presentations of both viruses are similar, being marked by anorexia, nausea, and malaise.
- Jaundice with hepatic tenderness and enlargement occurs in the first weeks following the onset of symptoms. Pruritus may also be present.
- In hepatitis A, the onset of jaundice is associated with rapid improvement in symptoms. Hepatitis B infection causes more prolonged symptomatology and jaundice.
- Aspartate aminotransferase (AST), alanine aminotransferase (ALT), and lactate dehydrogenase (LDH) are markedly elevated, signifying hepatocellular damage. The serum bilirubin also is increased significantly, whereas the serum alkaline phosphatase is minimally elevated.

Antibody Studies

- Hepatitis A infection is diagnosed by demonstrating hepatitis A IgM antibody or by culturing the virus from stool.
- Hepatitis B infection is diagnosed by demonstrating hepatitis B surface antigen (HBsAg) in serum and increases in hepatitis B core antibody (HBcAb) and hepatitis B surface antibody (HBsAb). Hepatitis B e antigen (HBeAg) is present in HBsAg-positive sera, and its persistence is associated with chronic hepatitis and increased infectiousness.
- Hepatitis C is diagnosed by detection of antibodies using a second-generation enzyme immunoassay. Confirmation is accomplished using a radioactive immunoblot assay (RIBA).

Prognosis

Mother

- An increased severity of illness has been reported in pregnant women from nutritionally deprived backgrounds. Whether this association applies in developed countries is uncertain.
- Viral hepatitis is associated with an increased risk of premature labor.

Fetus

- The risk of fetal infection depends on the timing of the maternal infection.
- Hepatitis B virus is transferred from mother to infant in 75% of cases when infection occurs in the last trimester of pregnancy and in only 10% of cases when infection occurs earlier.

- Neonatal hepatitis is more common in infants whose mothers are infected in the last trimester.
- Congenital defects are not increased in infants born to infected mothers.
- Because infection with HCV is chronic, no difference can be determined regarding infection rate of the fetus and the timing of the primary infection.

Treatment
Management
- Bed rest and diet should accord with the patient's desires and tolerance.
- Hepatitis B immune globulin is recommended for newborns born to HBsAg-positive women, particularly if infections occurring in the second half of pregnancy. HBV vaccine should be given concomitantly with immune globulin with additional doses at 1 and 6 months.
- Two indications for use of antiviral therapy during pregnancy:
  - Treatment of chronic disease in mother
  - Decrease risk of transmission
- Lamivudine and telbivudine are preferred.

Prevention
- Human immune serum globulin, 0.02 mL/kg to a total of 2.0 mL, is given as prophylaxis for hepatitis A.
- Human immune serum globulin, 0.04 mL/kg to a total of 4.0 mL, is given as prophylaxis for hepatitis B. Alternatively, hepatitis B immune globulin, 0.05 to 0.07 mL/kg, can be given twice, once within 7 days of exposure and again 25 to 30 days after the first injection.
- Hepatitis B vaccine is available for individuals at high risk of infection, and pregnancy is not considered a contraindication.
- No prophylaxis or treatment is available for pregnant women with HCV infection or their infants.
- All newborns now receive their first hepatitis B immunization before discharge from the nursery.

RABIES
Background
Definition
Rabies is an almost invariably fatal infection that is transmitted by exposure to salivary secretions containing the neurotropic virus (36).

Etiology
Most human cases result from bites or licks of an infected animal, usually a dog. On occasion, respiratory infection occurs when persons enter caves inhabited by rabid bats.

Treatment
- Because prevention is paramount in this disease, which has an incubation period of 10 days to 1 year, the critical decisions relate to prophylaxis.
- The following are guidelines for determining prophylaxis:
  - Dogs and cats that are considered healthy should be observed for signs of rabies. If disease does not develop in 10 days, prophylaxis is unnecessary. If the animal dies, the brain should be examined for the presence of virus. Rabies is proved by identifying viral antigen, by virus isolation, or by finding Negri bodies. If rabies is found, the patient is treated with a single dose of rabies immune globulin, 20 international units/kg, and a course of human diploid cell vaccine, five 1-mL doses IM, to be given on days 0, 3, 7, 14, and 28. Serum for rabies antibody testing should be collected 2 to 3 weeks after the last dose. If no antibody response occurs, a booster dose should be given.
  - If the animal escapes or is suspected of being rabid, or if the bite is from a wild animal (e.g., skunks, raccoons, or foxes), treatment with rabies immune globulin and human diploid cell vaccine is instituted.

PARVOVIRUS B19

Background

Definition

Parvovirus B19 is a common cause of human infection worldwide.

Etiology

- The virus is transmitted by the respiratory route.
- Parvovirus B19 is present in blood, and although viremia is rare, infection can also be transmitted by blood and blood products (37).

Epidemiology

- Women of childbearing age show an average annual seroconversion rate of 1.5%.
- There is no evidence of reinfection in immunocompetent individuals.

Pathogenesis

Parvovirus B19 has a special predilection for the erythroid system.

- It attacks the final stage of the red blood cell line in the bone marrow, causing both hemolysis and red blood cell aplasia, resulting in anemia without reticulocytosis.
- Occasionally, the virus may strike all cell lines, resulting in pancytopenia.
- The fetus can be severely affected because the half-life of red blood cells in the fetus is 50 to 75 days, and production has to be increased in order to maintain a normal blood volume.

Diagnosis

- Parvovirus B19 cannot be cultured directly on traditional culture media.
- Maternal serum evaluation for parvovirus B19–specific IgG and IgM is most commonly used for diagnosis of acute infection.
- The diagnosis of congenital infection includes neonatal evaluation of IgG-, IgM-, and IgM-specific parvovirus B19 serologies as well as PCR amplification of viral DNA.
- Ultrasound Doppler velocimetry to evaluate for fetal anemia (see Chapter 31).

Treatment

- Whenever clinical evidence of nonimmune hydrops fetalis is noted on sonogram, or if exposure to the virus is suspected in a pregnant woman, serologic testing should be offered.
- Termination of pregnancy should not be recommended to an affected woman because the virus is not related to an increased risk of congenital malformations.
- Once the acute maternal infection is proved serologically, serial sonograms are recommended to search for signs of hydrops fetalis as a complication of severe fetal anemia. Follow-up should be continued for 12 weeks after the diagnosis of maternal infection. If signs of fetal hydrops appear after 20 weeks of gestation, a decision should be made whether to manage the case conservatively or to perform diagnostic cordocentesis and intrauterine transfusion as indicated. The parameters to be tested in fetal blood include karyotype, hemoglobin, white blood count, platelet count, as well as specific IgM, IgG, and viral DNA. Should the fetus suffer from severe anemia (hemoglobin less than 8 g/dL), intrauterine transfusion should be considered, preferably during the same procedure.

Maternal Complications

- The most common clinical presentation of parvovirus B19 infection is erythema infectiosum or fifth disease. This is a relatively mild influenza-like disease, accompanied by low-grade fever and a characteristic "slapped cheek" rash.
- In adults, the most common symptom is arthralgia, which may last for several weeks; occasionally, arthritis appears as polyarthritis or oligoarthritis.
- In about 20% of the population, the infection has no clinical manifestations despite positive serologies.

Fetal/Neonatal Complications
- Nonimmune fetal hydrops resulting from intrauterine fetal parvovirus B19 infection is a well-known, though rare, phenomenon. Both aplastic anemia and myocarditis may contribute to the development of fetal hydrops (38).
- There is no evidence of increased risk of birth defects in infants with maternal B19 infection.

The risk of fetal death from parvovirus B19 infection is calculated at 9% of B19-infected pregnancies.

GENITAL INFECTIONS
Herpes Simplex
Background
- Herpetic infections usually are caused by type 2 virus, but type 1 is responsible for 15% of genital herpes infections.
- Both viruses are transmitted by person-to-person contact; approximately 5% of pregnant women have histories of symptomatic disease, and 13% will have clinical reactivation of infection at the time of delivery (39).
- Serologic surveys suggest that at least 20% of people have had prior infections with herpes simplex virus (HSV) type 2 (36).

Diagnosis
- Herpetic vesicles, 1 to 22 mm in diameter, develop on the genitalia and skin surfaces. These pruritic lesions rupture in 2 to 3 days, forming painful, shallow ulcers.
- Accompanying signs and symptoms include low-grade fever, malaise, and regional adenopathy. Jaundice and encephalitis are infrequent complications.
- The illness lasts from 7 to 10 days; recurrences are common.
- Pregnant women infected for the first time shed virus for 8 to 100 days; patients with recurrences shed virus for 6 to 40 days. Asymptomatic shedding in women with a history of genital herpes occurs on approximately 1% of days; the duration of shedding is 1 to 2 days.
- The appearance and distribution of the lesions permit a presumptive clinical diagnosis. Definitive proof of herpes infection requires identification of virus in infected specimens by direct immunofluorescent testing or by culturing virus in tissue cultures.
- Specific serologic tests for the HSV-specific glycoprotein G2 have sensitivities of 80% to 98%, but false negatives may occur early in the course of infection. Other serologic evaluations are of limited clinical use because of the lack of IgG-specific tests.

Prognosis
Mother
- The morbidity from these self-limited infections and the rarity of death, usually from encephalitis, are unaffected by pregnancy.
- An increased incidence of abortion and premature delivery is associated with primary genital herpes but not with recurrent infection.

Fetus
- Local (skin), central nervous system (CNS), or disseminated herpetic infections develop in 30% to 50% of newborns delivered to mothers with primary herpes and 5% to those with recurrent disease develop infections.
- Disseminated infections are associated with high mortality and serious neurologic sequelae in survivors.
- Infections in newborns with intrauterine herpes simplex infections are characterized by a rash at birth, congenital malformations, and a less fulminant course. The congenital malformations include microcephaly, encephalitis, chorioretinitis, and cerebral atrophy.

Treatment
Management
Acyclovir, valacyclovir, and famciclovir decrease the duration of a primary genital herpes infection and the frequency and duration of recurrent attacks. The benefits of these antiviral agents may outweigh any theoretic risk.

Prevention
Patients should be examined closely for genital lesions in the third trimester and at delivery. Cultures for cervicovaginal shedding in patients with chronic recurrent herpes are of limited use late in the third trimester.

In women with confirmed primary HSV infection within 6 weeks of delivery, cesarean section should be considered because of the prolonged period of viral shedding and lack of maternal antibody. Women with frequent herpes recurrences should receive antiviral medications in the final months of pregnancy to reduce risk of recurrences and viral shedding.

Newborn infants from infected mothers should be isolated and examined for 12 to 14 days for the development of herpetic infection.

Infants inadvertently exposed to HSV at delivery should have urine, stool, eye, and throat cultures sent for HSV isolation. If a culture becomes positive, the child should be treated with acyclovir. Close observation for clinical symptoms and signs should be performed.

Syphilis
Background
Treponema pallidum, the etiologic agent of syphilis, is transmitted through sexual contact.
- In recent years, the incidence of primary and secondary syphilis in the United States has increased with a concomitant increase in congenital infection (39).
- The syphilis rate among women increased from 1.1/100,000 cases in 2007 to 1.5/100,000 in 2008.
- Infections are transmitted readily from the mother to fetus.

Diagnosis
Physical Examination
- The chancre of primary syphilis is usually found on vaginal and cervical membranes. Chancres also occur extragenitally, most often in oral and anal regions. The lesions begin as nontender papules and subsequently ulcerate. Healing occurs within 3 to 6 weeks. Clinical features of primary syphilis are infrequently seen in pregnancy.
- Manifestations of secondary syphilis appear 2 to 12 weeks after the primary chancre and include skin rashes of various types (e.g., macular, papular, pustular, bullous), which often occur on the palms and soles; condylomas in perigenital areas; alopecia; generalized adenopathy; and low-grade fever. Condyloma latum is the most commonly observed lesion of secondary syphilis in pregnancy.

Testing
- Using dark-field microscopy, the diagnosis is established by identifying *T. pallidum* in specimens from suspicious lesions.
- In the absence of a positive dark-field examination, a presumptive diagnosis is made by detecting antibody to reagin (a cardiolipin–lecithin antigen) with the Venereal Disease Research Laboratory (VDRL) or rapid plasma reagin card (RPRC) test.
- Because false-positive results occur with these tests, positive results are confirmed with the fluorescent treponemal antibody absorption test (FTA-ABS) or the microhemagglutination assay (MHATP) for antibodies to *T. pallidum.* The diagnostic accuracy of the FTA-ABS or MHATP test is nearly 100% in cases of secondary syphilis, and the rate of false-positive results is less than 1%.

Clinical Findings
- The manifestations of congenital syphilis may occur at birth, but more often they appear in the first weeks of life.
- The most common clinical findings are skin eruptions of the type and distribution observed in adults, osteitis of nasal bones resulting in characteristic saddle nose deformities, periostitis and osteochondritis of long bones, hepatosplenomegaly, frontal bossing, notched incisors, mulberry molars, eighth nerve deafness, and neurosyphilis.

Prognosis
Mother. The morbidity of primary and secondary syphilis is the same in pregnant and nonpregnant women.

Fetus. If the mother is not treated
- Twenty-five percent of fetuses will die in utero.
- Twenty-five percent to thirty percent will die shortly after birth.
- Forty percent of survivors will acquire syphilis after the 3rd week of life.

Treatment
Management
- Treat pregnant patients with primary, secondary, or tertiary syphilis with 1 to 3 weekly injections of 2.4 million units IM of benzathine penicillin G.
- Patients allergic to penicillin should have their penicillin allergy confirmed. If they are truly allergic to penicillin, they should be desensitized before each dosage of penicillin (Table 23-8).

Table 23-8	Oral Desensitization Protocol for Women with Penicillin Allergy and Syphilis[a]			
Penicillin V suspension dose[b]	Dose strength (U/mL)[c]	Measured dose (mL)[c]	Total dose (units)	Cumulative dose (units)
1	1000	0.1	100	100
2	1000	0.2	200	300
3	1000	0.4	400	700
4	1000	0.8	800	1500
5	1000	1.6	1600	3100
6	1000	3.2	3200	6300
7	1000	6.4	6400	12,700
8	10,000	1.2	12,000	24,700
9	10,000	2.4	24,000	48,700
10	10,000	4.8	48,000	96,700
11	80,000	1.0	80,000	176,700
12	80,000	2.0	160,000	336,700
13	80,000	4.0	320,000	656,700
14	80,000	8.0	640,000	1,296,700

[a]Observe 30 min for allergic signs or symptoms before parenteral administration of penicillin. Then observe for at least 1 h after injection or infusion for signs of urticaria, angioedema, or anaphylaxis.
[b]Interval between doses: 15 min; elapsed time, 3 h, 45 min.
[c]Undiluted penicillin V suspension is 80,000 units/mL. The penicillin V suspension is first diluted to 1000 or 10,000 units/mL and then administered orally in 30 mL of water.

- If the serologic titer as measured by serial quantitative VDRL tests does not decrease, a second course of therapy is indicated. Patients with a history of treatment of syphilis should be retreated if doubts exist regarding the adequacy of therapy.
- Patients with suspected treatment failure or who are infected with HIV or who have an antibody titer greater than 1:32 should have consideration of a lumbar puncture to ascertain the presence of neurosyphilis (40).
- Adequate treatment of infected mothers before the 16th week of gestation prevents congenital syphilis, whereas treatment after the 16th week cures the infection but may not prevent the stigmata of congenital syphilis (41).

Prevention
Pregnant women should be tested serologically for syphilis at their first prenatal examination.

Gonorrhea

Background
Gonococcal infections are epidemic in the United States, with nearly 400,000 individuals infected annually and a prevalence of 0.5% to 0.7% (42). Infections are transmitted primarily through sexual contact.

Diagnosis
- Gonorrhea is an asymptomatic infection in 80% of women. Pain and tenderness in the pelvic region, cervical discharge, dysuria, and fever are the most common findings in patients with symptomatic infection. Pustular skin lesions, migratory arthralgias, and tenosynovitis culminating in a monoarticular septic arthritis indicate disseminated infection.
- The diagnosis is established by demonstrating gram-negative diplococci within polymorphonuclear leukocytes from vaginal and cervical exudates. The microscopic impression is confirmed by culturing the exudates on the Thayer-Martin media. Newer laboratory techniques using nucleic acid hybridization permit rapid detection of gonococci in infected urogenital specimens and the identification of *Neisseria gonorrhoeae* isolated from culture. These techniques also allow detection of *N. gonorrhoeae* and *Chlamydia trachomatis* in the same specimen.
- Gonococci can be cultured from pharyngeal and rectal swabs, blood, septic joints, and skin pustules.

Prognosis
Mother
- Women who become infected during the last 20 weeks of gestation or in the puerperium have an increased incidence of gonococcal arthritis.
- Women who harbor gonococci in the genital tract may have a flare-up of their latent disease during labor or immediately postpartum. There may be an increased risk of gonococcemia in such women.
- Abortion may occur because of premature rupture of the membranes secondary to gonococcal infection.
- Chronic pelvic inflammatory disease, secondary to gonorrhea, is an important cause of ectopic pregnancy.

Fetus
- Neonatal gonorrhea is acquired in utero or during delivery when the fetus traverses an infected birth canal.
- Infection in utero results in chorioamnionitis and subsequent neonatal sepsis.
- Infections acquired during delivery cause conjunctivitis (ophthalmia neonatorum), otitis externa, and vulvovaginitis. Gonorrhea is transmitted to 30% to 35% of newborns who pass through an infected cervix.

Treatment

The 2005 CDC recommendations for treatment of *N. gonorrhoeae* during pregnancy are as follows:

- Uncomplicated gonococcal infections of the cervix, urethra, and rectum during pregnancy.
  - Recommended regimens: cefixime, 400 mg orally in a single dose, or ceftriaxone, 125 mg IM in a single dose.
  - Alternative regimens: spectinomycin, 2 g IM in a single dose, or ceftizoxime, 500 mg IM in a single dose, or cefotaxime, 500 mg IM in a single dose, or cefotetan, 1 g IM in a single dose, or cefoxitin, 2 g IM, with probenecid, 1 g orally in a single dose.
- Uncomplicated gonococcal infection of the pharynx during pregnancy: ceftriaxone, 125 mg IM in a single dose.
- Gonococcal conjunctivitis during pregnancy: ceftriaxone, 1 g IM in a single dose, and lavage the infected eye with saline solution once.
- Disseminated gonococcal infection during pregnancy:
  - Recommended: ceftriaxone, 1 g IM or IV every 24 hours.
  - Alternatives: cefotaxime, 1 g IV q8h, or ceftizoxime, 1 g IV q8h, or spectinomycin, 2 g IM q12h.
  - All regimens should be continued for 24 to 48 hours after improvement begins, at which time therapy may be switched to cefixime, 400 mg orally bid, to complete a full week of antimicrobial therapy.
- Gonococcal meningitis and endocarditis during pregnancy: ceftriaxone, 1 to 2 g IV q12h. Therapy for meningitis should be continued for 10 to 14 days. Therapy for endocarditis should be continued for at least 4 weeks.
- Ophthalmia neonatorum prophylaxis regimens:
  - Silver nitrate, 1% aqueous solution in a single application
  - Erythromycin, 0.5% ophthalmic ointment in a single application
  - Tetracycline, 1% ophthalmic ointment in a single application

Chlamydial Infections

Background

Chlamydia trachomatis is a small bacterial microorganism that is an obligatory intracellular parasite.

- It is recognized as the most common sexually transmitted disease in the United States, and the cause of nongonococcal urethritis, lymphogranuloma venereum, epididymitis, pelvic inflammatory disease, and conjunctivitis in adults and of inclusion conjunctivitis, pneumonia, otitis media, and vaginitis in infants who are born through infected birth canals (43).
- It can be isolated from the genital tract of approximately 25% of sexually active nonpregnant women, approximately 5% of pregnant women, and fewer than 5% of women without a history of sexual contact.

Diagnosis

The CDC recommends screening at the initial intake obstetric visit for all patients, with rescreening in the third trimester for high-risk patients or for those thought to have shown poor compliance.

- In pregnant women:
  - Cervical *Chlamydia* cultures are 100% specific and 80% to 90% sensitive.
  - Direct fluorescent antibody and enzyme immunoassay tests have high specificity and sensitivity in high prevalence populations, while in groups of women with lower prevalences, culture techniques are more accurate.
  - Nucleic acid probes have greater than 98% correlation with culture in asymptomatic pregnant women.
  - Only culture is applicable to all anatomic sites and specimens (44).
- Tests of cure are recommended during pregnancy at least 3 weeks after treatment (40).

Treatment
- Treatment recommendations include first-line and alternative therapies. All sexual contacts require treatment, regardless of symptomatology.
- The 2005 CDC recommendations for the treatment of *Chlamydia* in pregnant women call for
  - Erythromycin base, 500 mg orally qid for 7 days or
  - Amoxicillin, 500 mg orally tid for 7 days
  - Alternative regimens consist of
    - Erythromycin base, 250 mg orally qid for 14 days
    - Erythromycin ethylsuccinate, 800 mg orally qid for 7 days
    - Erythromycin ethylsuccinate, 400 mg orally qid for 14 days
    - Azithromycin, 1 g orally in a single dose

Maternal–Fetal Complications
- The detection of *C. trachomatis,* especially during pregnancy, is very important because many of the women infected with this pathogen are asymptomatic.
- Untreated infection can result in spontaneous abortion, fetal death, premature rupture of membranes, preterm delivery, and postpartum endometritis–salpingitis.

Neonatal Complications
- Vertical transmission of *C. trachomatis* during vaginal delivery has been noted to occur in 50% to 70% of infants born to infected women (45).
- Initial *C. trachomatis* perinatal infection involves mucous membranes of the eye, oropharynx, urogenital tract, and rectum.
- *Chlamydia* is the most frequent identifiable infectious cause of ophthalmia neonatorum. This infection is most often recognized by conjunctivitis that develops 5 to 12 days after birth.
- *Chlamydia* is also a common cause of subacute, afebrile pneumonia with onset from 1 to 3 months of age.

Trichomonas Vaginalis
Background
- *Trichomonas vaginalis* causes approximately 25% of vulvovaginal infections.
- It is the most prevalent nonviral, sexually transmitted disease.
- Risk factors include multiple sexual partners, black race, previous history of sexually transmitted diseases, and coexistent infection with *N. gonorrhoeae.*

Evaluation
Clinical Presentation
- Symptomatic patients generally complain of a foul odor, a copious, yellow-gray or green homogeneous frothy vaginal discharge, vulvovaginal irritation, and occasionally dysuria.
- Up to 50% of infected women are asymptomatic.

Diagnosis
- Diagnosis of trichomonal infection is made by wet-mount preparation for mobile, flagellated organisms and an elevated pH level (greater than 4.5). An abundance of leukocytes usually is noted.
- Occasionally, trichomonal infection is diagnosed incidentally in asymptomatic females by Papanicolaou smear.

Treatment
Metronidazole, 2 g in a single dose orally, after the first trimester. Sexual partners should also be treated (40).

Pregnancy Complications
Trichomoniasis is associated with preterm labor, preterm delivery, low birth weight, and premature rupture of the membranes.

Fetal/Neonatal Complications
- Complications are secondary to preterm delivery.
- Vertical transmission of *Trichomonas* has been described in rare case reports but is believed to be cleared from the newborn once the maternal hormonal milieu has dissipated.

Bacterial vaginosis
Background
- Bacterial vaginosis, previously known as nonspecific vaginitis or *Gardnerella* vaginitis, is the most common cause of vaginal discharge.
- Between 9% and 41% of pregnant women will have bacterial vaginosis during pregnancy.

Diagnosis
- The patient typically complains of a gray, malodorous, fishy-smelling vaginal discharge, although a large percentage of patients will be asymptomatic.
- Diagnosis is made by demonstrating three of the following four signs:
  - Thin, dark or gray, homogeneous, malodorous discharge that adheres to the vaginal walls
  - Elevated pH level (greater than 4.5)
  - Positive KOH (whiff/amine test)
  - Presence of clue cells on wet-mount microscopic evaluation

Treatment
- Treatment recommendations include first-line and alternative therapies.
- The 2006 CDC-recommended regimen for the treatment of bacterial vaginosis in pregnancy includes
  - Metronidazole, 5000 mg orally bid for 7 days
  - Metronidazole gel 0.75%, one full applicator (5 g) intravaginally once a day for 5 days
  - Clindamycin cream 2% one full applicator (5 g) intravaginally at bedtime for 7 days
  - Alternative regimens include
    - Metronidazole, 2 g orally in a single dose
    - Clindamycin, 300 mg orally bid for 7 days
    - Clindamycin ovules 100 g intravaginally once at bedtime for 3 days

Maternal/Pregnancy Complications
Pregnant women with bacterial vaginosis are at increased risk of preterm labor, preterm premature rupture of membranes, and chorioamnionitis (46).

Fetal/Neonatal Complications
The risks are those associated with preterm delivery and chorioamnionitis.

FUNGAL INFECTION
Vulvovaginal Candidiasis
Background
- Approximately 30% of women with a healthy vaginal ecosystem harbor *Candida,* usually *Candida albicans.* These patients are asymptomatic, and yeast most likely would not be identified on wet-mount examination (47).
- The most common symptom of *Candida* infection is vulvovaginal pruritus. Also, vulvar burning, which can be exacerbated with micturition or sexual intercourse, is common, along with an increase or change in consistency of the vaginal discharge.

Diagnosis
Diagnosis is made by:
- Nonmalodorous, thick, white, "cottage cheese–like" discharge that adheres to the vaginal walls
- Presence of hyphal forms or budding yeast cells on wet-mount microscopic evaluation
- Pruritus

Treatment

The 2005 CDC-recommended regimens for the treatment of vulvovaginal candidiasis include
- Fluconazole, 150 mg orally once
- Butoconazole 2% cream, 5 g intravaginally for 3 days
- Clotrimazole 1% cream, 5 g intravaginally for 7 to 14 days
- Clotrimazole, 100-mg vaginal tablet for 7 days
- Clotrimazole, 100-mg vaginal tablet, two tablets for 3 days
- Clotrimazole, 500-mg vaginal tablet, one tablet in a single application
- Miconazole 2% cream, 5 g intravaginally for 7 days
- Miconazole, 200 mg vaginal suppository, one suppository for 3 days
- Miconazole, 100 mg vaginal suppository, one suppository daily for 7 days
- Terconazole 0.4% cream, 5 g intravaginally for 7 days
- Terconazole 0.8% cream, 5 g intravaginally for 3 days
- Terconazole, 80-mg vaginal suppository, one suppository daily for 3 days

Maternal/Pregnancy Complications

Vulvovaginal candidiasis is not associated with an untoward obstetric outcome.

Fetal/Neonatal Complications

Vulvovaginal candidiasis is not generally associated with fetal or neonatal complications. However, there have been reports of intra-amniotic fetal *Candida* infection associated with cervical cerclage and with IUDs retained during pregnancy

Recurrent Vulvovaginal Candidiasis

- Recurrent vulvovaginal candidiasis is defined as four or more episodes of symptomatic vulvovaginal candidiasis annually.
- The optimal treatment is an initial intensive regimen continued for approximately 10 to 14 days, followed immediately by a maintenance regimen for at least 6 months (40).

OTHER INFECTIONS OF IMPORTANCE IN PREGNANCY

Toxoplasmosis

Background

The causative microorganism, *Toxoplasma gondii,* is a protozoan with infectious cystic forms that are found in cat feces (oocyst) and herbivorous and carnivorous animal tissue (tissue cyst). Infection results from the ingestion of cyst-containing animal tissues or foods contaminated with cat feces and by transplacental transmission when women are infected during pregnancy.

Diagnosis

- Asymptomatic lymphadenopathy is the most common manifestation.
- More severe infections resemble infectious mononucleosis with fever, myalgias, sore throat, lymphadenopathy, macular rashes, migratory polyarthritis, and hepatosplenomegaly. It may also simulate viral pneumonia.
- Meningoencephalitis, the most severe complication, usually occurs in immunocompromised patients.
- Chorioretinitis is rare in acquired toxoplasmosis.
- The diagnosis is established by identifying the protozoa in tissue sections, smears, or body fluids or by demonstrating eightfold or greater increases in antibody titer using either the Sabin-Feldman dye test or immunofluorescent testing for IgM or IgG antibody. In cases limited to a single test, only elevated IgM antibody titers permit the diagnosis of acutely acquired toxoplasmosis (48).

Prognosis

Mother

- Maternal morbidity and mortality are unaffected by pregnancy.
- Infection increases the incidence of abortion and premature labor to 10% to 15% in women infected in the first and second trimesters of pregnancy.

Fetus
- Manifestations of congenital toxoplasmosis include chorioretinitis (often bilateral), cerebral calcification, mental retardation, convulsions, microphthalmia, hydrocephalus, and microcephaly.
- Signs of cerebral palsy and encephalitis can develop days or months after birth.
- Toxoplasmosis has also been implicated in stillbirth.
- The risk of intrauterine transmission in untreated women who develop acute toxoplasmosis varies by trimester (49):
  - Twenty-five percent in the first trimester
  - Fifty-four percent in the second trimester
  - Sixty-five percent in the third trimester

Treatment
Management
- The usual treatment of acute maternal toxoplasmosis is spiramycin, followed by pyrimethamine and sulfadiazine for confirmed fetal infections if the pregnancy is continued. Treatment with spiramycin reduces, but does not eliminate, the risk of transmission to the fetus (48).
- One management paradigm is to begin spiramycin on diagnosis of maternal infection and perform an amniocentesis for PCR.
  - A positive PCR would suggest fetal infection and would prompt a change from spiramycin to pyrimethamine and sulfadiazine.
  - A negative PCR would result in the continuation of spiramycin to reduce the incidence of subsequent fetal infection.
  - Serial ultrasounds should be considered for the remainder of the pregnancy to rule out obvious fetal involvement.

Prevention
- Prevention is of great importance, especially during pregnancy.
- Various prenatal programs throughout the world perform routine toxoplasmosis serologic testing (e.g., France, Austria, and Italy).
- Universal screening for maternal toxoplasmosis in the United States is currently not practiced secondary to the relatively low prevalence of the disease and the high false-positive rate of serologic screens in commercial labs.
- Targeted screening after finding an incidental abnormality on ultrasound consistent with toxoplasmosis infection is commonly practiced (48).
- Pregnant women should not eat raw meat products.
- If there are cats in the household, hands should be thoroughly washed after handling them, especially before eating; their litter trays should be emptied daily by someone other than the pregnant woman, as oocytes take 2 or 3 days to become infectious (50).

Malaria
Background
- Malaria, one of the most common infections of humans, causes significant morbidity and mortality in medically indigent areas of the world.
- Acute life-threatening illnesses are invariably caused by *Plasmodium falciparum,* whereas relapsing chronic infections are caused by *P. vivax* or, in selected endemic areas, *P. ovale,* or *P. malariae.*

Diagnosis
- Episodic paroxysms of high, spiking fever, headache, and myalgia distinguish malaria from virtually every other illness. Splenic enlargement is present in chronic infections.
- A history of residence in or passage through an endemic area usually is obtained.
- In the United States, the possibility of illicit intravenous drug use should be considered because malaria is transmitted by contaminated blood.

- Microscopic identification of the parasite in blood smears confirms the diagnosis.
- Chronic infections are diagnosed by demonstrating high levels of indirect fluorescent antibody in serum.

Prognosis
Mother
- Malarial attacks, especially those caused by *P. falciparum,* are particularly severe in pregnant patients.
- Abortions, prematurity, and stillbirths are increased in women who undergo malarial attacks during the first trimester of pregnancy.

Fetus
- Malarial parasites can cross the placenta in nonimmune mothers and cause fetal infection.
- Congenital malaria results in intrauterine growth retardation.
- Infected newborns have fever, jaundice, hepatosplenomegaly, seizures, and, occasionally, pulmonary edema 48 to 72 hours after delivery.

Treatment
Management
- Nonpregnant patients with infections caused by *P. vivax* and *P. ovale* should receive 26.3 mg of primaquine phosphate PO for 14 days. However, because fetal red cells are relatively deficient in glucose-6-phosphate dehydrogenase and glutathione, the fetus is at risk for intravascular hemolysis. *Therefore, primaquine is not recommended in pregnancy* (12).
- Treat pregnant women with malaria caused by *P. vivax, P. ovale,* and non–chloroquine-resistant *P. falciparum* with 1.0 g of chloroquine phosphate PO for one dose, followed by 0.5 g at 6, 24, and 48 hours.
- Relapses are treated with chloroquine.
- Primaquine is used after delivery.
- Treatment for drug-resistant strains of malaria:
  - Falciparum malaria resistant to chloroquine is treated with 650 mg of quinine sulfate PO tid for 10 days, combined with pyrimethamine, 50 mg/d PO for 3 days, followed by 500 mg of sulfadiazine PO qid for 5 days. *It should be emphasized that pyrimethamine is a highly teratogenic drug.*
  - Some experts recommend Fansidar (pyrimethamine and sulfadoxine) in combination with folinic acid to treat chloroquine-resistant *P. falciparum,* because quinine is an abortifacient in early pregnancy and can lead to premature labor in later pregnancy. Quinine has been associated with fetal auditory nerve hypoplasia, deafness, visual changes, and limb abnormalities.
  - Fansidar-resistant malaria is treated with quinine and tetracycline despite the risks of teratogenicity.

Prevention
- If travel to an endemic area is required, chloroquine is considered to be the drug for prophylaxis. It can cause retinal and cochleovestibular damage but is generally considered sufficiently safe in pregnancy to be recommended for prophylaxis.
- Chloroquine phosphate, 500 mg PO, is given 1 week before leaving and once weekly while the patient must remain in endemic areas. The drug should be continued for 6 weeks after the patient has left the endemic area.
- Fansidar is no longer recommended as prophylaxis in areas with chloroquine-resistant *P. falciparum* as a result of severe drug reactions. It is recommended that Fansidar be carried by travelers to these areas and taken therapeutically at the first sign of illness.
- Because safe, effective chemoprophylaxis is unavailable for chloroquine-resistant *P. falciparum,* nonimmune pregnant women should be discouraged from traveling to endemic areas unless absolutely necessary.

Lyme Borreliosis
Background
Lyme borreliosis is caused by *Borrelia burgdorferi,* a tick-borne spirochete (51). The organism is transmitted by the bite of *Ixodes* ticks, generally during the spring and summer.

Diagnosis
- Early infection is characterized by a distinctive rash (erythema migrans) that has advancing serpiginous borders with central clearing.
- Later disease can involve the heart, neurologic system, musculoskeletal system (arthritis), and eyes.
- The diagnosis is made clinically by noting a history of tick bite followed by a rash consistent with erythema migrans in association with a positive antibody test, with the ELISA being the preferred test. Serologic test results must be interpreted with caution because false-positive and false-negative results occur with all assays.

Prognosis
Mother
- Infection is similar in pregnant women and nonpregnant women.
- Gestational Lyme borreliosis is associated with fetal deaths and miscarriage.

Fetus
- Transplacental transmission of *B. burgdorferi* has been reported and is associated with congenital cardiac malformations and encephalitis.
- Serosurveys suggest that although *B. burgdorferi* can cause an adverse fetal outcome, it is uncommon (51,52).

Treatment
Management
- Early infection is treated with amoxicillin, 500 mg PO tid for 21 days. Doxycycline is contraindicated in pregnancy.
- Arthritis is treated with amoxicillin, 500 mg PO qid, plus probenecid, 500 mg qid, for 30 days. The alternative is ceftriaxone, 2 g IV qd for 14 days, or penicillin, 3 million units IV q4h for 14 days.
- Severe cardiac or neurologic disease is treated with ceftriaxone, 2 g IV qd for 14 days, or penicillin, 3 million units IV q4h for 14 days.

Prevention
- Avoidance of tick bites is the only method of prevention.
- There is no vaccine available.

Listeriosis
Background
- *Listeria monocytogenes* is a small facultative, anaerobic gram-positive bacillus and is the only one of its seven species that is pathogenic for humans.
- Pregnant women account for 27% of all cases and for 60% of cases among persons 10 to 40 years of age (53).
- Infection most likely occurs after ingestion of the organism in food, as many foods are contaminated with *L. monocytogenes;* it has been recovered from raw vegetables, raw milk, fish, poultry, and meats.
- The incubation period for invasive illness ranges from 11 to 70 days, with a mean of 31 days.
- *L. monocytogenes* crosses the mucosal barrier of the intestine, and once the bacillus enters the bloodstream, it may disseminate hematogenously to any site; *L. monocytogenes* has a predilection for the CNS and the placenta.
- It is generally believed that resistance to infection by *L. monocytogenes* is cell mediated, as evidenced by clinical association between listerial infection and conditions associated with impaired immunity such as lymphomas, pregnancy, AIDS, and corticosteroid-induced immunosuppression.

Diagnosis

Diagnosis requires:

- Isolation of *L. monocytogenes* from CSF, blood, joint fluid, urine, amniotic fluid, placenta, and cervix
- Identifying the organism via standard microbiologic techniques

Treatment

- For treatment of listeriosis during pregnancy, ampicillin (a 2-week course of 4 to 6 g/d in four equal doses) or penicillin is recommended. Cephalosporins are not adequate therapy against *L. monocytogenes* (54). Erythromycin has also proved to be efficacious in pregnancy (55).
- Because iron is a virulence factor for *L. monocytogenes* and iron overload states are risk factors for listerial infection, it is recommended to withhold iron replacement therapy until treatment is completed (56).

Maternal Complications

- Typical clinical syndromes among pregnant women are sepsis and a mild flu-like illness. Symptoms are often subtle and include malaise, fever, abdominal pain, gastrointestinal complaints, premature contractions, and decreased fetal movements.
- Infection can uncommonly result in maternal complications such as meningitis and endocarditis.

Fetal/Neonatal Complications

- When in utero infection occurs, the fetus may be stillborn or die within hours of a disseminated form of listerial infection known as granulomatosis infantiseptica, which is characterized by the widespread presence of microabscesses and granulomas that are prevalent in the liver and spleen (57).
- Overall perinatal mortality is widely quoted to be between 22% and 30% (53). The chances of perinatal morbidity and mortality are high when listeriosis is contracted in late gestation.
- Neonatal disease can cause both an early-onset sepsis, occurring shortly after birth, and a late-onset sepsis, occurring within the first few weeks of life.

EMERGING INFECTIONS

Avian Flu

Background

- Bird flu is an infection caused by an avian (bird) influenza virus. These viruses do not generally infect humans, but several cases of human infection including during pregnancy have been reported since 1997.
- The largest risk is for mutation of the avian influenza virus mixed with human virus in patients with human influenza. This would allow the virus to mutate and potentially spread from person to person.
- There have been no cases of avian flu reported in the United States.

Treatment

- Currently, there is no vaccine available for avian flu.
- Worldwide surveillance is taking place and travel to areas with avian flu is discouraged.

Severe Acute Respiratory Syndrome

Background

- Severe acute respiratory syndrome (SARS) is a recently recognized febrile severe lower respiratory illness caused by infection with a novel coronavirus (SARS-CoV).
- The case fatality rate approximates 10%.
- Early recognition and application of appropriate infection control measures are critical in controlling outbreaks of SARS.
- The vast majority of patients with SARS-CoV has a clear history or exposure to an SARS patient or to a setting in which it can occur and develop pneumonia.

Diagnosis

There are no currently available laboratory tests that can distinguish SARS virus from other respiratory illnesses rapidly enough to direct clinical management.

Treatment

- No specific treatment guidelines are currently in existence.
- Patients should receive supportive care and treatment with empiric therapy for community-acquired pneumonia. Infectious disease consultation is strongly recommended.

West Nile Virus

Background

West Nile virus (WNV) is a single-stranded RNS virus. It is a member of the Japanese encephalitis virus antigenic complex.

- The main route of human infection is through the bite of an infected mosquito. Mosquitoes become infected when they feed on infected birds.
- Humans, horses, and other mammals are not known to commonly develop infectious level viremias. Therefore, there is no documentation of animal-to-person transmission of WNV.
- Alternative modes of transmission include breast milk (one probable case reported) and transplacental (mother to child).

Epidemiology

- Most patients (four out of five) who are infected with WNV will not develop illness.
- Approximately 20% of patients with WNV will develop West Nile fever with the potential for severe illness.

Diagnosis

Clinical Manifestations

- Symptoms include fever, headache, tiredness, body aches, and an occasional skin rash on the trunk of the body as well as swollen lymph nodes. The symptoms of severe disease include headache, high fever, neck stiffness, stupor, disorientation, coma, tremors, convulsions, muscle weakness, and paralysis.
- The illness can be a few days to a few weeks in duration.
- Serious illness can occur in people of any age; however, people over the age of 50 or immunocompromised patients are at the highest risk for severe illness.

Treatment

Antibiotic Selection and Considerations

Except for the additional consideration of fetal toxicity, the selection of antibiotics for treatment in pregnant women is the same as for women who are not pregnant.

- Antimicrobial efficacy and toxicity are almost always unaltered in pregnancy.
- The two distinctive considerations in pregnancy are the potential toxicity for the fetus or mother of some commonly used antibiotics (e.g., sulfonamides, tetracyclines) and the occasional need for higher drug dosages because of the expanded blood volume, increased renal blood flow, and increased glomerular filtration rate, which reduce drug levels below the therapeutic range (13,47).
- Appropriate microbial smears and cultures should be obtained before therapy is initiated to identify pathogens and to determine their antimicrobial susceptibility patterns. If the smear is not helpful diagnostically, treatment is initiated on the basis of an educated guess concerning the likely pathogens for a particular infection (e.g., urinary tract infections are most often caused by *E. coli*).
- Interpretation of culture results from the female genital tract requires knowledge of the normal flora. This flora, which is unchanged by pregnancy, consists of aerobic and anaerobic bacteria and small numbers of fungi, usually *Candida* sp.

Normal Vaginal Flora of Pregnancy
- *Commonly isolated flora* include *Staphylococcus epidermidis,* * *Enterococcus faecalis,* * *Lactobacillus* sp., *Corynebacterium* sp., *Bacteroides fragilis,* * *Fusobacterium* sp., *Veillonella* sp., *Peptococcus* sp., and *Peptostreptococcus* sp.
- Occasionally isolated flora include *Staphylococcus aureus,* * *Streptococcus* sp.,* *Clostridium perfringens,* * *Candida* sp., *E. coli,* * *Proteus* sp.,* *Klebsiella* sp.,* *Gardnerella vaginalis,* *Actinomyces* sp., and *Mobiluncus* sp.
- Potential pathogens are *Pseudomonas* sp., *Streptococcus pneumoniae, Listeria monocytogenes, Neisseria gonorrhoeae, Chlamydia trachomatis, Mycoplasma hominis, Ureaplasma urealyticum,* and *Haemophilus aphrophilus.*

Effects of Selected Antibiotics and Antiviral Agents on Mother and Fetus (Table 23-9)
- **Penicillins.** Penicillins are safe in pregnancy. There is no increase in maternal toxicity and no known fetal toxicity (5,57).
- **Cephalosporins.** Cephalosporins are safe and do not cause increased fetal toxicity.
- **Carbapenems.** Imipenem is a carbapenem antibiotic related closely to the penicillins. Cilastatin is an inhibitor of a renal dehydropeptidase, which prevents rapid degradation of imipenem. Little is known about its use in pregnancy. Therefore, despite safety in animal studies, it should not be used in pregnancy when alternative therapies are available (58,59). The other carbapenem antibiotic, meropenem, was recently approved for commercial use in the United States.
- **Monobactam.** Aztreonam is a monobactam antibiotic that has only a β-lactam ring. It is considered safe in pregnancy. Patients with allergies to other β-lactam antibiotics often tolerate aztreonam (7,13).
- **Tetracyclines.** Parenteral tetracycline can cause fulminant maternal hepatitis and pancreatitis when administered during the third trimester of pregnancy. Oral tetracycline causes staining and deformity of deciduous teeth as well as inhibition of bone growth in the fetus. Tetracycline should be avoided in pregnancy unless no other appropriate antibiotic is available.
- **Sulfonamides.** Maternal toxicity does not increase with sulfonamides. Fetal toxicity occurs in the perinatal period, when the inability of the neonatal liver to conjugate sulfonamides results in hyperbilirubinemia and kernicterus caused by blockage of the binding sites necessary to conjugate bilirubin. When these drugs are used before the perinatal period, the maternal liver removes sulfonamide from the fetal bloodstream (13).
- **Chloramphenicol.** No increase in maternal toxicity occurs with chloramphenicol. Inability of the neonatal liver to conjugate chloramphenicol results in the "gray-baby syndrome," which is characterized by gray facies, generalized flaccidity, hypothermia, and cardiovascular collapse (13).
- **Aminoglycosides.** The risk of ototoxicity and nephrotoxicity secondary to use of gentamicin, kanamycin, netilmicin, streptomycin, amikacin, or tobramycin is the same in pregnant and nonpregnant women. Fetal toxicity to the eighth cranial nerve has occurred after prolonged use of streptomycin in treating TB. Streptomycin should not be used unless INH, ethambutol, or rifampin is contraindicated. These drugs may also cause nephrotoxicity in the fetus; therefore, their use should be limited as much as possible (58,59).
- **Macrolides.** Erythromycin, clarithromycin, and azithromycin are the macrolide antibiotics presently available. No increase in maternal toxicity and no known fetal toxicity occur with erythromycin. The estolate form of this drug causes transient, self-limited elevations of serum transaminases, particularly in the latter half of pregnancy, so treatment with this agent is not recommended. Clarithromycin has been associated with toxicity to the fetus in animal studies; therefore, it should not be used in pregnancy except when

---
*Significant Pathogens

Table 23-9	Antibiotics and Antiviral Agents and Pregnancy[a]			
Antimicrobial agent	Problem in pregnancy	Passes placenta	Harmful to fetus	Harmful to newborn
Acyclovir		Yes		No
Amantadine	Possible			
Amikacin	No[b]	Yes	Possible[c]	Possible[c]
Amoxicillin–clavulanate	No[b]	Yes	No[b]	
Amphotericin B	No[b]	Yes		
Ampicillin	No[b]	Yes	No[b]	No
Ampicillin–sulbactam	No[b]	Yes	No[b]	
Azithromycin	No[b]		No[b]	
Aztreonam	No[b]	Yes	No[b]	
Cefaclor	No[b]	Yes	No[b]	
Cefadroxil	No[b]	Yes	No[b]	
Cefamandole	No[b]	Yes	No[b]	No[b]
Cefazolin	No[b]	Yes	No[b]	
Cefixime	No[b]		No[b]	
Cefonicid	No[b]	Yes	No[b]	
Cefoperazone	No[b]	Yes	No[b]	
Ceforanide	No[b]	Yes	No[b]	No[b]
Cefotaxime	No[b]	Yes	No[b]	No
Cefotetan	No[b]	Yes	No[b]	
Cefoxitin	No[b]	Yes	No[b]	Possible[d]
Cefpodoxime	No[b]		No[b]	
Cefprozil	No[b]		No[b]	
Ceftazidime	No[b]	Yes	No[b]	No
Ceftizoxime	No[b]	Yes	No[b]	Possible[d]
Ceftriaxone	No[b]	Yes	No[b]	No[b,e]
Cefuroxime	No[b]	Yes	No[b]	
Cephalexin	No[b]	Yes	No[b]	
Cephradine	No[b]	Yes	No[b]	
Chloramphenicol	No[b]	Yes	No[b]	Yes
Ciprofloxacin	Yes	Yes	Possible	Yes
Clarithromycin	Possible[f]		Possible[f]	
Clindamycin		Yes		No[b]
Cloxacillin	No	Yes	No[b]	No
Dapsone	Possible	Yes	Possible	Possible
Dicloxacillin	No	Yes	No[b]	
Didanosine	No[b]	Yes	No[b]	No[b]
Doxycycline	Yes	Yes	Yes	Yes
Erythromycin		Yes	No[b]	
Ethambutol	No[b]	Yes	No[b]	
Fluconazole	Possible	Yes	Possible	Possible
Flucytosine		Yes	Possible[f]	
Foscarnet	Possible[b]		Possible	Possible
Ganciclovir	Possible	Yes	Possible	Possible[c,g]
Gentamicin	No[b]	Yes	Possible[c]	Possible[c]
Imipenem–cilistatin	No[b]			
Isoniazid	No	Yes	One report unconfirmed	No[b]
Itraconazole	Possible[f]		Possible[f]	
Kanamycin	No[b]	Yes	Possible[c]	Possible[c]
Ketoconazole		Yes	Possible[h]	Possible[h]
Lorcarbacef	No[b]		No[b]	
Methenamine mandelate				
Methicillin	No	Yes	No[b]	No

(*Continued*)

Table 23-9   Antibiotics and Antiviral Agents and Pregnancy[a] (*Continued*)

Antimicrobial agent	Problem in pregnancy	Passes placenta	Harmful to fetus	Harmful to newborn
Metronidazole	Yes[b,l]	Yes	Yes[l]	
Mezlocillin	No	Yes	No[b]	No
Minocycline	Yes	Yes	Yes	Yes
Nafcillin	No	Yes	No[b]	No
Nalidixic acid	Yes[j]	Yes	Yes[j]	Yes[j]
Netilmicin	No	Yes	Possible[c]	Possible[c]
Nitrofurantoin		Yes		Yes
Norfloxacin	Yes	Yes	Yes	Yes
Oxacillin	No[b]	Yes	No[b]	
Penicillin G	No	Yes	No[b]	
Penicillin V potassium	No			
Pentamidine				
Piperacillin	No[b]	Yes	No[b]	
Piperacillin–tazobactam	No[b]		No[b]	
Pyrazinamide				
Pyrimethamine	Yes	Yes	Yes[k]	
Rifampin	No[b]	Yes	Possible[b]	
Spectinomycin				
Streptomycin	No	Yes	Rare[b]	
Sulfonamides	No[m]	Yes	No[b,l]	Yes
Tetracycline	Yes	Yes	Yes	Yes
Ticarcillin/clavulanate	No[b]	Yes	No[b]	
Tobramycin	No[b]	Yes	Possible[c]	Possible[c]
Trimethoprim and sulfamethoxazole	Yes	Yes	Yes[l,m]	Yes
Vancomycin			Possible[c]	Possible[c]
Zalcitabine	Possible[f]		Possible[f]	
Zidovudine	Possible			

[a]Breast milk levels greater than 50% of maternal serum levels are seen with acyclovir, ampicillin, carbenicillin, chloramphenicol, erythromycin, INH, itraconazole, metronidazole, tetracycline, and sulfonamides. Breast milk levels less than 25% of maternal serum levels are seen with aztreonam, cefazolin, cefotaxime, cefoxitin, clindamycin, nalidixic acid, nitrofurantoin, methicillin, oxacillin, penicillin G, penicillin V potassium, and pyrimethamine. Blank spaces indicate information not well known.

[b]Not known to be harmful, but no adequate and well-controlled studies have been performed for pregnant women; therefore, should be used during pregnancy only if clearly needed.

[c]Ototoxicity and nephrotoxicity are potential consequences of use.

[d]Safety in infants from birth to 3 months has not yet been established. In older children, the drug's use has been associated with high incidence of increased eosinophils and elevated serum AST.

[e]Ceftriaxone should not be given to hyperbilirubinemic newborns, especially prematures.

[f]Teratogenic effects have been seen in animal studies.

[g]Ganciclovir should be used with extreme caution in newborns because of the probability of carcinogenicity.

[h]Has been shown to be teratogenic to rats in high doses (10 times maximum human doses). Has also been shown to be embryotoxic in rats during the first trimester in the same dosage. Dystocia was noted in rats receiving ketoconazole in the third trimester. It probably is excreted in breast milk; therefore, mothers who are on ketoconazole should not breast-feed their children.

[i]A potential carcinogen.

[j]Increased CNS side effects in newborns.

[k]Significant teratogenic effect in the first and probably the second trimesters. Safe in the third trimester if clinically warranted. Used for treatment of toxoplasmosis.

[l]If given in large doses shortly before delivery, hyperbilirubinemia and kernicterus may occur in the newborn.

[m]Not recommended; trimethoprim is a folate antagonist.

no alternative therapy is available. Conversely, azithromycin has been shown to be safe to the fetus in animal studies. Although data in humans are limited, azithromycin appears to be a safe agent in pregnancy.

- **Clindamycin.** Maternal or fetal toxicity is not known to increase with clindamycin. Its most common obstetric indication is for postpartum endomyometritis. It is also the drug of choice for group B streptococcal prophylaxis in the penicillin-allergic patient.
- **Trimethoprim–sulfamethoxazole.** Maternal toxicity does not increase with trimethoprim and sulfamethoxazole, but folic acid antagonists may increase anemia. Although unproved clinically, trimethoprim has the potential for teratogenicity; therefore, this drug should not be used unless absolutely indicated (13).
- **Vancomycin.** Vancomycin given either intravenously or orally can be associated with fetal ototoxicity or nephrotoxicity. It is the drug of choice for *C. difficile*–induced pseudomembranous colitis (13,58).
- **Fluoroquinolones.** Ciprofloxacin and ofloxacin cause chronic arthrosis deformans in animal studies. Therefore, quinolones are contraindicated in pregnant or lactating women (58).
- **Metronidazole.** Although the data suggesting teratogenic effects of metronidazole are equivocal, it is recommended for use only in the second and third trimesters (58).
- **Anti-tuberculosis agents.** These agents include INH, rifampin, ethambutol, streptomycin, pyrazinamide, ethionamide, and cycloserine. Treatment with INH, rifampin, and ethambutol represents a smaller risk to a woman and her fetus than does untreated disease. Congenital malformation rates are not increased. Streptomycin is not recommended for use in pregnancy, and the teratogenicity of other agents is unclear. Their use should be avoided during pregnancy (58,59).
- **Pyrimethamine.** Although no increase in maternal toxicity is known, pyrimethamine should not be used in the first or second trimester because it is potentially teratogenic. If absolutely necessary, pyrimethamine can be used in the third trimester.
- **Antiherpetic agents.** Three oral therapies for the treatment of genital HSV infections are available in the United States: acyclovir, famciclovir, and valacyclovir. Animal studies and use in humans suggest their use is safe.
- **Antiretroviral agents.** Drug registry information has failed to reveal an increase in malformations in children born to mothers taking ZDV, but animal studies have suggested an increase in embryo resorption as well as an increase in development of cancer in the offspring born to pregnant mice treated with high doses of ZDV during pregnancy. Data regarding the safety and efficacy of the newer antiretroviral agents suggest that they are safe especially in the second and third trimesters of pregnancy. One exception is Sustiva (efavirenz), which has been shown to be teratogenic in the first trimester and should be avoided. In managing a pregnant HIV-positive woman, it is important to treat the patient as someone who is HIV positive rather than someone who is pregnant. There is no justification for withholding antiviral or prophylactic therapies to the mother for fear of harming the child because lack of treatment of the mother may increase fetal risk (60).
  - **Reverse transcriptase inhibitors** (nucleoside analog and nonnucleoside). These agents include ZDV, didanosine (ddI), zalcitabine (ddC), lamivudine (3TC) (the nucleoside analogs), and nevirapine (nonnucleoside). Once the HIV enters the CD4 cell, the HIV converts its single-stranded RNA genetic information into complementary double-stranded DNA before replication. This requires the viral enzyme reverse transcriptase. The nucleoside analogs (ZDV, ddI, ddC, 3TC) as well as the NNRTIs (nevirapine) inhibit this step of replication (12,61).
  - **Protease inhibitors.** These agents include saquinavir, ritonavir, indinavir, and nelfinavir. Once DNA is transcribed from the HIV RNA, it is inserted into cell DNA and instructs the cell to begin making new HIV copies. The viral particles must then "bud" through the host cell wall in order to infect new cells, thereby propagating the infection. The protease inhibitors work at this step by preventing the virus from leaving the host cell (12,57,61).

Causes of Antibiotic Failure

- **Human factors**
  - Incorrect diagnosis
  - Treatment initiated too late
  - Antibiotic not given or taken improperly because of prescription error or lack of compliance
- **Drug factors**
  - Inadequate dose or inappropriate dose interval. (Pregnant women may require higher doses than nonpregnant women because of altered pharmacokinetics.)
  - Inadequate course of therapy.
  - Wrong route of administration.
  - Failure of drug to reach the site of infection.
- **Pathogen factors**
  - Microbial resistance
  - Bacteria in dormant state
  - Superinfection
- **Host factors**
  - New, unrelated infection elsewhere in the body
  - Rapid degradation of the antibiotic (e.g., acetylation of INH)
  - Failure to institute appropriate supportive measures (e.g., surgical drainage, debridement, or dilation and curettage)
  - Impaired host defenses resulting from underlying illness or immunosuppressive therapy

Immunization During Pregnancy

- Pregnancy is considered a contraindication for immunization with live attenuated virus vaccines in nonepidemic settings. A nonpregnant woman of childbearing age receiving a live virus vaccine should avoid pregnancy during the subsequent 3 months.
- Use of inactivated virus vaccines is considered safe and acceptable in pregnancy.
- The specifics of immunization are given in Table 23-9.

Patient Education

For the latest and most accurate updates on worldwide infectious diseases and vaccinations, the reader should log onto http://www.cdc.gov

REFERENCES

1. American College of Obstetricians and Gynecologists. Antimicrobial therapy for obstetric patients. *ACOG Educ Bull.* 1998:245.
2. Goodrum LA. Pneumonia in pregnancy. *Semin Perinatol.* 1997;21:276–283.
3. Riley L. Pneumonia and tuberculosis in pregnancy. *Infect Dis Clin North Am.* 1997;11:119–132.
4. Starke JR. Tuberculosis: an old disease but a new threat to the mother, fetus, and neonate. *Clin Perinatol.* 1997;24:107–127.
5. Casey BM, Cox SM. Chorioamnionitis and endometritis. *Infect Dis Clin North Am.* 1997;11:203–218.
6. Phares CR, Lynfield R, Farley MM, et al. Epidemiology of invasive group B streptococcal disease in the United States, 1999–2005. *JAMA.* 2008;299(17):2056–2065.
7. ACOG Committee Opinion. Prevention of early-onset group B streptococcal disease in newborns. *Int J Gynecol Obstet.* 1996;54:197–205.
8. Special Medical Reports: CDC issues recommendations for the prevention of perinatal group B streptococcal disease. *Am Fam Physician.* 1996;54:1787–1793.
9. Lindsay MK, Nesheim SR. Human immunodeficiency virus infection in pregnant women and their newborns. *Clin Perinatol.* 1997;24:161–180.
10. Centers for Disease Control and Prevention. *HIV/AIDS Surveillance Report Volume 15, 2003.* Atlanta: U.S. Department of Health and Human Services, Centers for Disease Control and Prevention.

11. Bulterys M, Lepage P. Mother-to-child transmission of HIV. *Curr Opin Pediatr.* 1998;10: 143–150.

12. Dattel BJ. Antiretroviral therapy during pregnancy: beyond AZT (ZDV). *Obstet Gynecol Clin North Am.* 1997;24:645–657.

13. Cooper ER, Charurat M, Mofenson L, et al. Combination antiretroviral strategies for the treatment of pregnant HIV-1-infected women and prevention of perinatal HIV-1 transmission. *J Acquir Immune Defic Syndr.* 2002;29(5):484–494.

14. Centers for Disease Control and Prevention (CDC). Global measles mortality, 2000–2008. *MMWR Morb Mortal Wkly Rep.* 2009;58(47):1321–1326.

15. Siston AM, Rasmussen SA, Honein MA, et al. Pandemic 2009 influenza A(H1N1) virus illness among pregnant women in the United States. *JAMA.* 2010;303(15):1517–1525.

16. Ali ME, Albar HM. Measles in pregnancy: maternal morbidity and perinatal outcome. *Int J Gynecol Obstet.* 1997;59:109–113.

17. Nies BM, Lien JM, Grossman JH. TORCH virus-induced fetal disease. In: Reece EA, Hobbins JC, Mahoney MJ, eds. *Medicine of the fetus and mother.* Philadelphia: JB Lippincott, 1992. Chapter 25.

18. Reef SE, Redd SB, Abernathy E, et al. The epidemiological profile of rubella and congenital rubella syndrome in the United States, 1998–2004: the evidence for absence of endemic transmission. *Clin Infect Dis.* 2006;43 (Suppl 3):S126–S132.

19. Gibbs RS. Fetal infections from non-TORCH viruses. In: Reece EA, Hobbins JC, Mahoney MJ, eds. *Medicine of the fetus and mother.* Philadelphia: JB Lippincott, 1992. Chapter 26.

20. Cherry JD. Enteroviruses. In: Remington JS, Klein JO, eds. *Infectious diseases of the fetus and newborn infant,* 3rd ed. Philadelphia: WB Saunders, 1990:325–366.

21. Glantz JC, Mushlin AI. Cost-effectiveness of routine antenatal varicella screening. *Obstet Gynecol.* 1998;91:519–528.

22. Skve DV. Varicella in pregnancy. *WMJ.* 1997;96:44–47.

23. Nathwani D, Maclean A, Conway S, et al. Varicella infections in pregnancy and the newborn: a review prepared for the UK advisory group on chickenpox on behalf of the British Society for the Study of Infection. *J Infect.* 1998;36(suppl 1):59–71.

24. Katz VL, Kuller JA, McMahon MJ, et al. Varicella during pregnancy: maternal and fetal effects. *WMJ.* 1995;163:446–450.

25. Birthistle K, Carrington D. Fetal varicella syndrome—a reappraisal of the literature: a review prepared for the UK Advisory Group on Chickenpox on behalf of the British Society for the Study of Infection. *J Infect.* 1998;36(suppl 1):25–29.

26. Kenneson A, Cannon MJ. Review and meta-analysis of the epidemiology of congenital cytomegalovirus (CMV) infection. *Rev Med Virol.* 2007;17(4):253–276.

27. Nigro G, Adler SP, La Torre R, et al. Passive immunization during pregnancy for congenital cytomegalovirus infection. *N Engl J Med.* ;353(131):1350–1362.

28. Lipitz S, Yagel S, Shalev E, et al. Prenatal diagnosis of fetal primary cytomegalovirus infection. *Obstet Gynecol.* 1997;89:763–767.

29. Hagay ZJ, Biran G, Ornoy A, et al. Congenital cytomegalovirus infection: a long-standing problem still seeking a solution. *Am J Obstet Gynecol.* 1996;174:241–245.

30. Whitley RJ, Kimberlin DW. Infections in perinatology: treatment of viral infections during pregnancy and the neonatal period. *Clin Perinatol.* 1997;24:267–283.

31. Carroll ED, Campbell ME, Shaw BNJ, et al. Congenital lobar emphysema in congenital cytomegalovirus infection. *Pediatr Radiol.* 1996;26:900–902.

32. Revello MG, Zavattoni M, Sarasini A, et al. Human cytomegalovirus in blood of immunocompetent persons during primary infection: prognostic implications for pregnancy. *J Infect Dis.* 1998;177:1170–1175.

33. Mandelbrot L. Vertical transmission of viral infections. *Curr Opin Obstet Gynecol.* 1998;10: 123–128.

34. Zeldis JB, Crumpacker CS. Hepatitis. In: Remington JS, Klein JO, eds. *Infectious diseases of the fetus and newborn infant,* 3rd ed. Philadelphia: WB Saunders, 1990:574–600.

35. Ohto H, Terazawa S, Sasaki N, et al. Transmission of hepatitis C virus from mothers to infants. *N Engl J Med.* 1994;330:744–750.

36. Arvin AM, Yeager AS. Other viral infections of the fetus and newborn. In: Remington JS, Klein JO, eds. *Infectious diseases of the fetus and newborn infant*, 3rd ed. Philadelphia: WB Saunders, 1990.

37. Brown KE, Young NS. Parvovirus B 19 in human disease. *Annu Rev Med.* 1997;48:59–67.

38. Brandenberg H, Los FJ, Cohen-Overbeek TE. Short communication: a case of early intrauterine parvovirus B19 infection. *Prenat Diagn.* 1996;16:75–77.

39. Centers for Disease Control and Prevalence (CDC). Congenital syphilis—United States, 2003–2008. *MMWR Morb Mortal Wkly Rep.* 2010;59(14):413–417.

40. Centers for Disease Control and Prevention. 1998 guidelines for treatment of sexually transmitted diseases. *MMWR Morb Mortal Wkly Rep.* 1998;47(RR-1):1–116.

41. Fiumara NJ. The diagnosis and treatment of infectious syphilis. *Compr Ther.* 1995;21:639–644.

42. Wendel PJ, Wendel GD Jr. Sexually transmitted diseases in pregnancy. *Semin Perinatol.* 1993;17:443–451.

43. Centers for Disease Control and Prevention. *Chlamydia trachomatis* genital infections—United States, 1995. *MMWR Morb Mortal Wkly Rep.* 1997;46(9):193–198.

44. Mou SM. Bacterial infections. In: Willett GD, ed. *Laboratory testing in OB/GYN.* London: Blackwell Scientific Publishing, 1994.

45. Adair CD, Gunter M, Stovall TG, et al. *Chlamydia* in pregnancy: a randomized trial of azithromycin and erythromycin. *Obstet Gynecol.* 1998;91:165–168.

46. MacDermott RIJ. Review: bacterial vaginosis. *Br J Obstet Gynaecol.* 1995;102:92–94.

47. ACOG Technical Bulletin. Vaginitis. *Int J Gynecol Obstet.* 1996;54:293–302.

48. Bader TJ, Macones GA, Asch DA. Prenatal screening for toxoplasmosis. *Obstet Gynecol.* 1997;90:457–464.

49. Zargar AH, Masoodi SR, Laway BA, et al. Seroprevalence of toxoplasmosis in women with repeated abortions in Kashmir. *J Epidemiol Community Health.* 1998;52:135–136.

50. Gordon N. Toxoplasmosis: a preventable cause of brain damage. *Dev Med Child Neurol.* 1993;35:567–573.

51. Steere AC. Lyme disease. *N Engl J Med.* 1989;321:586–596.

52. MacDonald AB. Gestational Lyme borreliosis: implications for the fetus. *Rheum Dis Clin North Am.* 1989;15:657–677.

53. Craig S, Permezel M, Doyle L, et al. Perinatal infection with *Listeria monocytogenes. Aust N Z J Obstet Gynaecol.* 1996;36:286–290.

54. Schuchat A. A guest editorial: listeriosis and pregnancy: food for thought. *Obstet Gynecol Surv.* 1997;52:721–722.

55. Dimpfl T, Gloning KP. Listeriosis in pregnancy: letter to the editor. *Int J Gynecol Obstet.* 1994;45:284–285.

56. Lorber B. Listeriosis: state of the art clinical article. *Clin Infect Dis.* 1997;24:1–9.

57. Millar LD, Cox SM. Urinary tract infections complicating pregnancy. *Infect Dis Clin North Am.* 1997;11:13–26.

58. Dashe JS, Gilstrap LC III. Antibiotic use in pregnancy. *Obstet Gynecol Clin North Am.* 1997;24:617–629.

59. Duff P. Antibiotic selection in obstetric patients. *Infect Dis Clin North Am.* 1997;11:1–12.

60. Kotler DP. HIV in pregnancy. *Gastroenterol Clin North Am.* 1998;27:269–280.

61. Andiman WA. Medical management of the pregnant woman infected with human immunodeficiency virus type I and her child. *Semin Perinatol.* 1998;22:72–86.

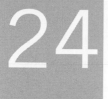

Neurologic Complications

Jennifer Cavitt and Reena Shah

SEIZURES IN THE PREGNANT PATIENT

Key Points

- Pregnancy is not contraindicated in women with epilepsy (WWE).
- Greater than 90% of WWE have favorable pregnancy outcomes.
- In most cases, antiepileptic drugs (AED) should be continued during pregnancy.
- Both seizures and AED are associated with increased risk of adverse outcomes of pregnancy.
- Goal for treatment in pregnancy is seizure freedom with the lowest effective AED dose.
- Avoid AED polytherapy when possible.
- Valproic acid (VPA) exposure during pregnancy is associated with significantly greater risks than other AED exposures.
- Folic acid supplementation is recommended prior to conception and during pregnancy.
- Pregnant WWE should be managed jointly by their neurologist and obstetrician.

Background

Definitions

- A *seizure* is a sudden, abnormal synchronous electrical discharge of cerebral neurons.
  - Seizures may be provoked (toxic, metabolic, infectious, etc.) or unprovoked.
  - Symptoms vary depending on the area of brain involved.
    - Brief change in awareness and/or behavior
    - Abnormal movement: tonic posture, clonic jerking, myoclonic jerks, loss of muscle tone, etc.
    - May be followed by postictal confusion
- **Epilepsy** is defined as ≥2 unprovoked seizures greater than 24 hours apart.
  - **Focal seizures** (aka **partial seizures**) begin in a localized area of the brain and may or may not spread to involve other regions of the brain. Focal seizures may occur *with or without impairment of consciousness or awareness*; *with observable motor or autonomic components*, such as twitching or jerking, flushing, or automatic behaviors called automatisms (e.g., lip smacking or picking); or *involving subjective sensory or psychic phenomena only* (also called an "aura"). Focal seizures may spread to diffuse brain involvement, leading to a convulsion, such as a tonic–clonic seizure (1).
  - **Generalized seizures** involve nearly all of the brain at onset and include *generalized tonic–clonic (GTC), tonic or atonic* ("drops"), *myoclonic,* and *absence* seizure types (1).

Risk Factors

- Some epilepsy syndromes have a genetic component.
- Other epilepsy risk factors include traumatic brain injury, stroke, brain tumor or other cerebral structural abnormality, congenital or developmental neurologic disorder, or degenerative disorder.

Epidemiology

- Epilepsy affects approximately 1% of the population (2).
- Greater than 1 million WWE of reproductive age in the United States give birth to greater than 24,000 infants each year (3).

Evaluation
History
- Proper evaluation of a woman with epilepsy should begin prior to pregnancy.
- Essential information includes
  - Certainty of the diagnosis of epilepsy—is further diagnostic evaluation required?
  - Is the woman followed regularly by a neurologist?
  - The seizure type, frequency, intensity, and duration should be assessed.
  - Identify current AED treatment:
    o Evaluate compliance, efficacy, and adverse effects.
    o Is she a candidate to discontinue AED *prior* to conception?
  - Are there any other associated neurologic disorders?
  - Does she have any complications related to seizures or AED that occurred in prior pregnancies?
  - Is she taking supplemental folic acid?
- Is pregnancy desired or planned, or is the woman already pregnant?
  - If pregnancy is *not* desired, what (if any) is the method of contraception?
  - If pregnancy *is* desired (or possible), is she taking supplemental folic acid?
  - If the woman *is pregnant*
    o What is the stage of gestation?
    o Has she continued her AED treatment?
    o Has there been any change in seizure frequency or intensity?
    o Is she taking supplemental folic acid?

Diagnosis
- In women with a well-established epilepsy diagnosis, the diagnosis is ordinarily not an issue for the obstetrician. However, certain important scenarios make diagnosis an issue.
  - In patients with well-established epilepsy, the appearance of clinical spells different from the patient's usual seizures may indicate another disorder.
  - A few patients will experience new-onset seizure disorder during pregnancy.
- The *differential diagnosis* of seizures includes many other kinds of clinical "spells" including: syncope, panic attacks, psychogenic nonepileptic seizures, episodic vertigo, paroxysmal movement disorders, and others. These attacks are sometimes difficult to distinguish from epileptic seizures, and expert consultation may be needed.
- Correct diagnosis is important:
  - Nonepileptic events are not effectively treated with AEDs.
  - Use of AED for nonepileptic events exposes the mother and baby to risks of AED therapy with no concomitant benefit.
  - Treatment for the correct diagnosis will be delayed.
- If the obstetrician observes an attack, it is important to obtain as detailed a description as possible. Particular attention should be paid to the onset of the attack, its clinical characteristics, its duration, and any postattack symptoms.
- If a woman develops a seizure disorder during pregnancy, a complete evaluation should be performed by a neurologist to establish a diagnosis and search for an underlying cause.

Treatment
General Principles
- Every effort should be made to maintain seizure control during pregnancy and delivery.
- Most WWE require continuing AED treatment prior to, during, and after pregnancy and delivery.
- The best AED for a given patient is an AED appropriate for the patient's seizure type, which provides best seizure control at the lowest dose and with the fewest side effects.

Risks

WWE taking AED are at greater risk of adverse pregnancy outcomes related to teratogenicity, cognitive effects in the children exposed in utero to AED, seizures during pregnancy, and possibly increased rates of some obstetrical complications.

Major Congenital Malformations

- The vast majority of WWE will have babies with no malformations.
- The most common major congenital malformations (MCM) occurring in infants of WWE on AED include congenital heart disease, cleft lip/palate, neural tube defects, and urogenital defects (3).
- The overall risk of MCM in WWE taking AED is approximately 3% to 9%, or approximately two to four times the risk in the general population (3).
  - Approximately 2% to 8% risk of MCM with any first-trimester monotherapy AED exposure (3)
  - Approximately 6.5% to 19% risk of MCM with any first-trimester polytherapy AED exposure (3)
  - MCM risk is significantly higher with first-trimester monotherapy or polytherapy including VPA compared to other monotherapy AED exposure or polytherapy without VPA (3).
  - First-trimester topiramate (TPM) exposure is associated with a greater risk of cleft lip (4).
  - Greater risk of MCM is associated with higher first-trimester VPA, lamotrigine (LTG), and phenobarbital (PB) doses.
    - VPA doses above approximately 1000 mg/d or levels greater than 70 μg/mL (5)
    - LTG doses ≥300 mg/d (6)
    - PB doses ≥150 mg/d (6)

Cognitive Outcomes in Children of Women with Epilepsy

- In utero exposure to VPA is associated with reduced cognitive abilities measured in children at ages 3, 4.5, and 6 years, and the effect is dose dependent (7–9).
- In utero VPA exposure is associated with significantly increased absolute risk (4.4%) of autism spectrum disorders in children compared with those not exposed to VPA (2.4%) (10).
- Use of periconceptional folic acid by WWE on AED is associated with significantly higher IQ scores in their children at age 6 years (7).

Obstetrical Complications and Perinatal Outcomes

- Rigorous literature reviews have raised concern for possible increased obstetrical complications and adverse perinatal outcomes in WWE.
  - There may be a modestly increased risk (up to 1.5 times expected) of cesarean delivery for WWE on AED (11).
  - An increased risk (greater than 2 times expected) of premature contractions and premature labor and delivery (L&D) in WWE who smoke has also been reported (11).
  - Insufficient evidence exists to support or refute increased risk of preeclampsia, pregnancy-related hypertension (HTN), or miscarriage (11).
  - WWE taking AED are at increased risk of having small for gestational age neonates, approximately 2 times expected rate (5).
  - There is probably no substantially increased risk (greater than 2 times expected) of perinatal death in newborns of WWE (5).

Vitamin K Supplementation

- There is insufficient evidence to support or refute increased risk of neonatal hemorrhagic complications in newborns of WWE on AED or decreased risk when these women are treated with *prenatal* vitamin K supplementation (12).
- Newborns of WWE taking enzyme-inducing AED (EIAED) (phenytoin [PHT], carbamazepine (CBZ), PB, primidone [PRM]) routinely receive vitamin K at delivery, as do all newborns.

Effect of Maternal Seizures on the Fetus
- GTC seizures pose a risk to the fetus, as well as to the mother.
  - Maternal and fetal hypoxia and acidosis (3).
  - Fetal intracranial hemorrhage, miscarriage, prolonged fetal heart rate (HR) depression (greater than 20 minutes), and stillbirths have been reported following GTC seizures (3).
- Effects to the fetus from nonconvulsive seizures are less clear.
- There are case reports of fetal HR decelerations (3).
- There is risk of trauma with multiple seizure types, potentially leading to perinatal complications.

Seizure Frequency During Pregnancy
- Most WWE (64%) have unchanged seizure frequency during pregnancy (3).
  - Sixteen percent have fewer seizures in pregnancy compared to baseline.
  - Seventeen percent have an increase in seizure frequency during pregnancy.
- Studies observing seizure frequency in pregnant WWE have not included a control group of nonpregnant WWE with seizure frequency data for comparison. Thus, the influence of pregnancy on seizure frequency is unclear (11).
- Seizure freedom ≥9 months prior to conception is associated with high likelihood (84% to 92%) of seizure freedom during pregnancy (11).
- There is insufficient evidence to support or refute increased risk of status epilepticus (SE) in pregnancy (11).

Laboratory Tests
- AED levels can provide important guidance in managing AED therapy before, during, and after pregnancy. However, physicians should
  - Evaluate seizure control, not an AED level, to determine AED effectiveness
  - Be cognizant that drug toxicity is a clinical diagnosis, which may or may not correlate with "toxic" blood levels

Contraceptive Management
- Oral contraceptives (OC) per se have no effects on seizure frequency.
- Estrogen may lower serum levels of LTG up to 50%, potentially leading to breakthrough seizures (13,14).
- EIAED, including PHT, PB, PRM, CBZ, felbamate (FBM), clobazam (CLB), and rufinamide (RUF), may reduce hormone levels, leading to contraceptive failure. Oxcarbazepine (OXC) greater than 1200 mg/d and TPM greater than 200 mg/d have a similar effect. It has been recommended WWE taking these agents should take OC with ≥50 μg estradiol or its equivalent, though no studies have determined whether this improves the risk of contraceptive failure in the setting of EIAED. Transdermal patch and vaginal ring formulations and intramuscular (IM) medroxyprogesterone also have higher failure rates. An 8- to 10-week dosing interval for IM medroxyprogesterone in the setting of EIAED has been suggested, though whether this improves efficacy has not been established (3,14).
- Perampanel (PMP) reduces levonorgestrel levels by up to 40% (see Table 24-1).

Prepregnancy Management
- Any uncertainty about the diagnosis of epilepsy should be resolved. Consultation with a neurologist should be obtained and continued through pregnancy.
- If seizure free greater than 2 years on AED with normal imaging, electroencephalography (EEG), and exam, consider whether the patient is a candidate to wean off AED under care of neurologist, dependent on epilepsy syndrome diagnosis. If electing to wean AED, counsel regarding risk of seizure recurrence. This should be accomplished ≥6 months prior to conception.
- Consider changing to an alternative to VPA therapy, if possible prior to conception (5).

Table 24-1	Antiepileptic Drug Therapy in Women						
Antiepileptic drug name	Abbreviation	Common brand name(s)	Pregnancy class	Interaction with HC[a]	Weight gain or loss	Bone loss association	Protein binding	Elimination
Carbamazepine	CBZ	Tegretol, Tegretol XR, Carbatrol	D	Yes	Gain	Yes	70%–80%	Hepatic
Clobazam	CLB	Onfi	C	Yes			80%–90%	Hepatic
Clonazepam	KLO	Klonopin	D	No			85%	Hepatic
Ethosuximide	ESX	Zarontin	C	No	Loss		N/A	Hepatic
Ezogabine	EZG	Potiga	C	No	Gain		80%	Hepatic/renal
Felbamate	FBM	Felbatol	C	Yes	Loss		25%	Hepatic/renal
Gabapentin	GBP	Neurontin	C	No	Gain		<3%	Renal
Lacosamide	LCM	Vimpat	C	No			<15%	Hepatic/renal
Lamotrigine	LTG	Lamictal, Lamictal XR	C	Yes[b]			44%	Hepatic
Levetiracetam	LEV	Keppra, Keppra XR	C	No			<10%	Renal
Lorazepam	LRZ	Ativan	D	No			85%	Hepatic/renal
Oxcarbazepine	OXC	Trileptal, Oxtellar XR	C	Yes >1200 mg/d			40%	Hepatic
Perampanel	PMP	Fycompa	C	[c]	Gain		95%	Hepatic
Phenobarbital	PB	Luminal	D	Yes		Yes	50%	Hepatic
Phenytoin	PHT	Dilantin, Phenytek	D	Yes		Yes	90%	Hepatic
Pregabalin	PGB	Lyrica	C	No	Gain		Low	Renal
Primidone	PRM	Mysoline	D	Yes		Yes	50%–60%	Hepatic
Rufinamide	RUF	Banzel	C	Yes			34%	Hepatic/renal
Tiagabine	TGB	Gabitril	C	No			96%	Hepatic
Topiramate	TPM	Topamax	D	Yes >200 mg/d	Loss	Yes	15%–40%	Renal > hepatic
Valproic acid	VPA	Depakote, Depakote ER, Depacon, Depakene	D	No	Gain		90%	Hepatic
Zonisamide	ZNS	Zonegran	C	No	Loss		40%	Hepatic > renal

HC, hormonal contraceptive

[a]HC levels may be reduced greater than 50% in the presence of estrogen-based contraceptives, leading to risk of increased seizures when HC is added.
[b]LTG does not appear to significantly affect efficacy of HC.
[c]PMP reduces levonorgestrel levels by up to 40%.

- Consider converting from polytherapy to monotherapy prior to conception if possible (5).
- Due to high risk of unplanned pregnancy, all women of childbearing age on AED should be given supplemental folate. The ideal dose is unclear due to lack of rigorous evidence with respect to dosing. Current guidelines from the American Academy of Neurology recommend a minimum of 0.4 mg daily prior to conception and during pregnancy, but other experts, including the American and Canadian Obstetricians and Gynecologists organizations, have recommended higher doses, up to 4 to 5 mg/d (3).

Management During Pregnancy

- Once pregnancy is established, there is little or no benefit, and some risk, of changing an established treatment regimen.
  - The fetus has already been exposed to the current AED, during at least part of the most sensitive stage of gestation, prior to the patient's seeking medical attention.
  - A change in medication may increase the risk of maternal seizures.
  - Overlapping two AEDs during the change exposes the fetus to the risks of a second AED and added risk of polytherapy.
  - Physicians should suggest that their patients register with the North American Antiepileptic Drug Pregnancy Registry (www.aedpregnancyregistry.org).
- Compliance with AED and supplemental folic acid should be encouraged.
- Maternal serum screening, ultrasound imaging, and other appropriate studies to identify MCM should be considered.
- Normal L&D can be anticipated.
  - Some WWE may have other neurologic disorders, which may complicate L&D.
  - One percent to two percent of WWE experience seizures during L&D; another 1% to 2% experience seizures within 24 hours of delivery. Idiopathic generalized epilepsy has been associated with greater risk (12.5%) of seizures during L&D (3).
- Emergency cesarean delivery may be needed for WWE with refractory seizures during labor.

Antiepileptic Drug Levels During Pregnancy

- The effect of pregnancy on AED levels is complex:
  - Total levels of AED typically decline during pregnancy due to
    - Increased blood volume
    - Increased hepatic and renal clearance of most AED
  - For some AED with high protein binding, non–protein-bound drug levels ("free levels") may remain constant or increase due to decreased plasma protein binding. Free levels reflect the active fraction of the drug (Table 24-1) (3).
    - PHT free levels decrease 15% to 40% in the third trimester.
    - CBZ free levels do not significantly change during pregnancy.
    - VPA free levels increase in the second and third trimesters.
    - PB free levels decrease 50% in pregnancy.
  - LTG clearance increases by 65% to 230% during pregnancy with significant variability between patients. Decreasing LTG concentration in pregnancy has been associated with increased seizure frequency (12).
  - The active metabolite of OXC, monohydroxy derivative, decreases 36% to 61% during pregnancy, and WWE on OXC may be at greater risk for convulsive seizures (3).
  - Levetiracetam (LEV) concentrations may decrease by 60% in the third trimester (3).
- AED levels should be measured
  - Prior to conception (baseline)
  - At the beginning of each trimester
  - During the last 4 weeks of pregnancy
  - Additional monitoring may be needed if there is a change in seizure frequency or if clinical side effects appear.

- More frequent monitoring of certain AED levels may be indicated when a greater magnitude of change from baseline is expected or observed; dosage adjustment to maintain levels similar to prepregnancy baseline may be considered.
- Non–protein-bound ("free") drug levels should be obtained when available.

Postpartum Management
Antiepileptic Drugs
- AED levels may rise rapidly in the weeks after delivery due to decreasing blood volume, decreased hepatic/renal clearance, and altered protein binding, resulting in possible toxicity in the absence of appropriate dosing adjustments (3).
- Most AED levels return to baseline within 10 weeks after delivery (3).
- Drug levels and clinical response should be followed closely.
- LTG levels increase more rapidly following delivery as LTG clearance returns to baseline within 2 to 3 weeks. Careful dosing adjustment and monitoring for toxicity beginning within several days postpartum are suggested (3).
- Drug withdrawal may occur in babies exposed to PB during gestation.
- Neonates exposed to EIAED in utero should be observed for clotting disorders.

Breast-feeding
- All AEDs are present in breast milk to some extent.
  - Highly protein-bound AED will be present at lower concentrations than others (see Table 24-1).
  - The benefits of breast-feeding are considered to outweigh the relatively small risk of AED adverse effects in infants (3).
  - Newborns have immature drug elimination systems, and infants should be observed for signs of drug intoxication (lethargy, poor feeding, irritability, etc.).
  - One large study examining cognitive outcomes in children of WWE following in utero CBZ, LTG, PHT, and VPA exposure found no adverse effect of breast-feeding on IQ at age 3 for all AED combined or for each of the four individual AED groups (15).

Child Care and Seizure Precautions
- Recommend close supervision by another adult for WWE when bathing infant, or give sponge bath.
- Changing/dressing infant on pad on the floor is safer than using a changing table.
- WWE who have uncontrolled seizures with loss of awareness or falls should consider use of a sling or small lightweight stroller when moving about the house with baby.
- For WWE with uncontrolled seizures, it may be safest to have another adult present to ensure safety of mother and infant, depending on seizure type and frequency.

COMPLICATIONS
Status Epilepticus
- SE is defined as continuous seizure activity for ≥30 minutes or repeated seizures over a ≥30-minute period without full recovery between attacks.
- A *presumptive diagnosis* of SE is made when seizures last ≥5 minutes or when two or more discrete seizures occur without return to baseline in between.
  - SE is a medical emergency and requires prompt diagnosis and treatment.
    - Mortality in SE ranges from 3% to 32% and depends largely on the underlying cause, severity of the seizures, and SE duration (16).
    - Mortality in uncomplicated SE is approximately 3% (16).
    - Control of SE becomes increasingly difficult as its duration increases.
- Management of SE requires multiple measures, carried out virtually simultaneously:
  - Protect the patient from injury; avoid mechanical restraints
  - ABCs—airway, breathing, circulation: O_2, IV, cardiopulmonary resuscitation (CPR), and intubation if required

- Consider thiamine 100 mg + 50 mL D50% IV
- Assess the likely causes of SE:
  - Withdrawal of anticonvulsant drugs (including noncompliance)
  - Withdrawal from drugs or alcohol
  - Metabolic derangements (e.g., electrolyte or glucose abnormalities)
  - Eclampsia (see Chapter 11)
  - Central nervous system (CNS) infections, head trauma, etc.
- Obtain blood specimen for glucose, electrolytes (including Ca, Mg, phosphorus), complete blood count (CBC), liver function test (LFTs), AED levels, arterial blood gas (ABG), troponin, and toxicology studies.
- Lumbar puncture is indicated only when meningitis is suspected, and empiric antibiotic therapy should be started immediately.
- Imaging studies should be delayed until the seizures are controlled.
- Continuous EEG is indicated to aid in diagnosis and management.
- Drug treatment of SE
  - For continuous or nearly continuous seizures, lorazepam IV in 2-mg increments every 2 minutes while seizure is ongoing up to maximum dose 0.1 mg/kg is the drug of choice. If rapid IV access is not available, give midazolam 10 mg IM, fosphenytoin (**not phenytoin**) IM, or diazepam 20 mg per rectum (PR).
  - For ongoing or intermittent seizures, or following termination of SE with benzodiazepines, use fosphenytoin 20 mg/kg PE (phenytoin equivalent) IV at 100 to 150 mg/min with BP and EKG monitoring. If necessary, additional fosphenytoin, up to 10 mg/kg, can be given.
  - If fosphenytoin fails to control seizures, reasonable options include
    - LEV 1000 mg IV over 15 minutes, repeat × 1 if still seizing.
    - PB 20 mg/kg IV at 50 mg/min.
    - Initiate continuous IV infusion with midazolam, pentobarbital, or propofol, or give inhalation anesthesia if seizures persist. Few controlled comparison studies are available.
    - Intubation and ventilator support will probably be needed.
    - Monitor closely for hypotension.
  - Advice and/or consultation from a neurologist or specialist in critical care medicine should be obtained as soon as possible.
  - SE due to eclampsia should be managed as outlined in Chapter 11.

NEW-ONSET SEIZURES

- Occasionally, patients experience their first seizures during pregnancy (other than as part of eclampsia syndrome). Urgent issues facing the physician and patient include
  - Was the event an epileptic seizure or a nonepileptic event?
  - What is the likelihood of recurrence?
  - Is there an associated medical or neurologic disorder?
  - Is anticonvulsant drug treatment needed?
- Evaluation
  - Consider neurological consultation.
  - Differential diagnosis for new-onset seizure includes nonepileptic events such as hypoglycemia, hyperventilation, panic attack, syncope, and psychogenic nonepileptic seizure, as well as epileptic seizure.
    - Obtain as detailed a description of the event as possible. Features typical of epileptic seizures include
      - Abrupt onset and offset.
      - Brief duration (a few minutes or less).
      - Motor activity (if present) is not purposeful.

- – Little or no recall for the details of the attack.
- – Postictal confusion and lethargy.
- ◦ Was the attack truly a *first* seizure?
  - – Is there a prior history of staring spells, transient loss of awareness, or childhood seizures?
  - – Is there a history of unexplained nocturnal incontinence, tongue biting, or other injury?
- • Is there evidence for any underlying medical or neurologic disorder?
  - ◦ Evaluate with detailed history, physical and neurologic examinations.
    - – Computed tomography (CT) or magnetic resonance imaging (MRI) can be done safely during pregnancy if necessary (17).
  - ◦ The need for laboratory studies, toxicology screening, etc. should be determined by the clinical setting.
  - ◦ EEG is often helpful.
- • Is AED treatment needed?
- • In the case of a single seizure for which no cause is identified, in an otherwise healthy patient with normal imaging and EEG, AED treatment should be deferred.
- • If a specific medical cause for the seizure is identified, the underlying cause should be treated.
- • In the case of recurrent seizures, or in cases where evaluation suggests a high likelihood of recurrent seizures, anticonvulsant treatment should be initiated.
- • For all patients, regardless of whether or not treatment is started
  - ◦ Patients should be counseled about the risks of recurrent seizures and the risks of AED to them and to their babies.
  - ◦ Patients should be counseled about safety measures to reduce the risk of injury if additional seizures occur.
  - ◦ Three- to six-month seizure freedom prior to returning to driving is typically required, but state laws vary.

Patient Education
- • Reassure patients that the vast majority of women with seizures have healthy babies, even when treated with AED during pregnancy and even if they have seizures during pregnancy, labor, or delivery.
- • Women with seizures should be strongly encouraged to meet with their physicians at least 6 months prior to a planned pregnancy so that any needed alterations to their seizure management can be completed before pregnancy begins.
- • Women should be advised to take folic acid prior to, during, and after pregnancy.
- • Women should be encouraged to continue their AED in the event of an unplanned pregnancy. Sudden withdrawal of AED is much more likely to be harmful than beneficial, both to the mother and to the baby.
- • Mothers should be encouraged to promptly report any change in the frequency, character, or intensity of their seizures to their obstetrician and to their neurologist.

HEADACHES (HA) IN THE PREGNANT PATIENT
Key Points
- • All headaches (HA) should be taken seriously, since even medically "benign" HA may cause severe distress and disability.
- • Physicians should be especially alert to HA of recent onset or a sudden change in the character of a previously stable HA syndrome.
- • In patients with chronic HA, a realistic goal of management is 50% reduction in the frequency and severity of HA. Cure of the HA is rarely achieved.

Background

- HA management, especially in pregnant patients, is often difficult and frustrating for both physicians and patients.
  - HA pain (like all pain) is subjective, with no objective criteria to measure the success or failure of treatment.
  - Many of the standard agents used in the prophylaxis and treatment of HA are at least relatively contraindicated in pregnancy.
  - The goal of treatment is often satisfactory management of a chronic condition rather than cure of an acute condition.
  - Treatment often includes chronic use of medications with high abuse potential.

Pathophysiology

- Head pain may originate from either intracranial or extracranial sources.
  - Pain-sensitive structures within the skull include the meninges and the larger blood vessels at the base of the brain. The brain itself is largely insensitive to pain. Pain may result from increased intracranial pressure, from distortion or traction of the meninges or blood vessels, or from irritation of the meninges.
  - Pain-sensitive structures outside the skull include the muscles of the face and scalp, the blood vessels of the face and scalp, the mucosal lining of the sinuses, and the skin and subcutaneous tissues of the face and scalp.
- Head pain is often referred, and patients often cannot distinguish the source of their pain. Pain perceived by the patient as coming from deep inside the head may in fact be coming from an extracranial source.

Evaluation of the Patient with Headache

History

- Is there a prior history of HA? If so, is the current HA problem consistent with the previous HA syndrome or is it a new problem?
- Obtain a description of the HA: location, intensity, frequency, character (steady, throbbing, stabbing, squeezing, etc.). Is the HA provoked or relieved by activity, position, medications, time of day, etc?
- Are there any premonitory symptoms, such as changes in vision, numbness or weakness of the extremities, etc., before the HA begins?
- Are there associated symptoms, such as nausea and vomiting, photophobia, phonophobia, blurred vision, visual loss or hallucinations, focal neurologic symptoms, etc?
- Is the HA pattern stable, worsening, or improving? Does the HA pattern seem to be acute, subacute, or chronic (see below)?

Physical Examination

- In the majority of patients (especially those with "benign" disease), the physical and neurologic examinations are often normal.
- A careful neurologic examination should be carried out in all pregnant patients with complaint of HA.

Laboratory Studies

- For patients with well-established HA syndromes (e.g., migraine or tension type), routine laboratory and imaging studies, such as CT and MRI scanning, are usually not needed.
- For patients with new-onset HA or those who have a substantial change in the frequency, severity, or clinical features of a previously stable HA pattern, the "worst headache" of their lives (particularly if abrupt in onset), an abnormal neurologic examination, a progressive or new daily persistent HA, EEG evidence of a focal abnormality, or a comorbid partial seizure, a full diagnostic evaluation, including imaging studies, lumbar puncture, or other laboratory studies, may be needed (see below) (18).

ACUTE HEADACHE SYNDROMES

Background

- Acute HA syndromes develop over a short period of time, usually hours to days. Acute HA syndromes raise the greatest concern regarding severe or life-threatening disease.
- An acute HA may be the first attack of migraine or tension HA, which is usually associated with chronic HA syndromes.
- In patients with chronic HA syndromes (see below), an abrupt change in the character of the HA may indicate the development of a new acute HA syndrome.

Subarachnoid Hemorrhage

- Half of all cerebrovascular diseases during pregnancy are caused by subarachnoid hemorrhage (SAH).
- SAH is most often due to rupture of an aneurysm of one of the large blood vessels at the base of the brain ("berry aneurysm"); less often from leakage from an arteriovenous malformation or other vascular anomaly. Approximately 10% occur without any identified cause.
- The risk of SAH is increased in late pregnancy and in the puerperium.
- The initial hemorrhage may be catastrophic or fatal for both mother and fetus. The maternal mortality from the initial hemorrhage is approximately 50%.
- Symptoms of SAH include
  - *Abrupt* onset HA, usually severe (not always "worst headache of my life").
  - Nausea, vomiting, photophobia, stiff neck, confusion, and lethargy are common.
  - Physical findings may include retinal hemorrhages, elevated blood pressure, fever, stiff neck, or focal neurologic signs, but the exam may be entirely normal.
- CT scanning is diagnostic in greater than 90% of patients with good technique and experienced radiologists. A negative CT scan does not rule out SAH; if the diagnosis is suspected and CT is negative, lumbar puncture is mandatory.
- Major hemorrhages are sometimes preceded by less severe or even minor "sentinel" hemorrhages; prompt recognition and aggressive treatment may prevent subsequent catastrophe. There is a high risk of rebleeding (and death) within a few weeks following the initial hemorrhage. Urgent referral to a neurosurgeon is indicated, and treatment should not be delayed (19).
- If SAH is present, urgent referral to a neurologist or neurosurgeon is indicated. Evaluation and management should not be delayed.
- Cesarean delivery may be indicated if the mother is critically ill, if symptomatic vascular malformation is diagnosed at term, or if the patient has had surgical treatment within the last 8 days. Otherwise, route of delivery should be determined based on obstetric indications (20).

MENINGITIS

- Acute bacterial meningitis is a true medical emergency; untreated, there is virtually 100% mortality for both the mother and the fetus. Viral meningitis usually carries a much less ominous prognosis, and spontaneous recovery is likely.
- The most common causative agent of bacterial meningitis is *Streptococcus pneumoniae*, most often preceded by otitis or sinusitis. The second most common causative agent is *Listeria monocytogenes*. In teens and young adults, *Neisseria meningitidis* is a common cause. Death, miscarriage, stillbirth, and neonatal death are possible complications.
- The classic clinical triad of HA, fever, and stiff neck is not always present; worsening HA associated with fever should always suggest the diagnosis. Malaise, nausea and vomiting, and lethargy and confusion are often present.
- CT and MRI can rule out structural lesions but are not helpful in the diagnosis of acute meningitis.

- If meningitis is suspected, *urgent* lumbar puncture is *mandatory.*
- If lumbar puncture cannot be carried out immediately, empiric antibiotic treatment should be started immediately. Empirical therapy should cover *S. pneumonia, L. mono-cytogenes,* and *N. meningitidis.* Adjunctive treatment with dexamethasone may also be appropriate. *Treatment should not be delayed* waiting for imaging studies, lumbar puncture, etc.
- Recommendations for antibiotic treatment of meningitis are frequently revised. The consultation from an expert in infectious diseases should be obtained (21).

HYPERTENSIVE ENCEPHALOPATHY

- Hypertensive encephalopathy (HE) is characterized by severe HA, impaired consciousness (which may progress to coma), seizures (including SE), and visual field deficits (including cortical blindness), in patients with severe HTN.
- Focal neurologic signs are usually mild and transient; prominent focal signs suggest ischemic stroke or intracerebral hemorrhage (ICH) (see below).
- CT imaging is often normal, but MRI may demonstrate extensive areas of edema, especially in the white matter of the parietal and occipital lobes. In this case, the syndrome is also referred to as posterior reversible encephalopathy syndrome (PRES), posterior leukoencephalopathy syndrome (PLES), and other synonyms.
- The underlying pathology in PRES is vasogenic edema. Elevation of blood pressure exceeds the autoregulatory capability of the brain vasculature resulting in endothelial damage, increased permeability, and hydrostatic edema. While the posterior circulation is most susceptible to inadequate autoregulation, other areas, such as the brain stem, cerebellum, basal ganglia, and frontal lobes, can also be involved.
- Treatment consists of aggressive management of severe HTN and seizures (see above and below and Chapters 4 and 11).
- The prognosis is generally good, with most patients making a full recovery. However, deaths and permanent neurologic sequelae may result.
- A similar picture may be seen in patients with HTN related to eclampsia, acute glomerulonephritis, and in those treated with cytotoxic or immunosuppressive drugs (22).

Preeclampsia/Eclampsia

- The International Classification of Headache Disorders-II definition of HA attributable to preeclampsia or eclampsia includes the criteria for preeclampsia or eclampsia (see Chapter 11) and also specifies that
  - The HA must be bilateral, pulsating, or aggravated by physical activity
  - The HA must develop during episodes of HTN and resolve within 7 days of effective HTN treatment (23)

Post–Lumbar Puncture Headache

- HA may occur after inadvertent dural puncture in patients receiving epidural anesthesia or after spinal anesthesia. Smaller spinal needle size, the use of noncutting spinal needles, and orienting the needle parallel to the longitudinal dural fibers decrease the risk of post–lumbar puncture HA.
- Patients who have not had dural puncture may still develop low-pressure HA, possibly secondary to dural tears from labor-related pushing.
- The HA is usually worsened by upright posture and promptly relieved by recumbency (especially the Trendelenburg position).
- The HA typically begins within 24 to 48 hours postpuncture. It is typically throbbing, in the fronto-occipital regions.
- Post–dural puncture HA may be severe and virtually incapacitating and may make it difficult or impossible for the new mother to care for her baby. If severe, the HA may be accompanied by neck stiffness, nausea, vomiting, and photophobia.

- Rupture of the bridging veins as the brain retracts from the dura can result in a subdural hematoma.
- Treatment includes bed rest and hydration. In refractory cases, an epidural blood patch (usually performed by an anesthesiologist) may give dramatic relief in 85% to 90% of patients within 1 to 24 hours (24).

Pituitary Disorders
- Pituitary adenoma
  - The pituitary gland enlarges by 136% by the end of pregnancy.
  - Pregnancy is associated with accelerated growth of certain tumors such as meningiomas and pituitary adenomas.
  - Patients with macroadenomas (greater than 10 mm) should be seen monthly to assess for symptoms such as HA or visual changes and each trimester for visual field testing.
  - If there is evidence of tumor enlargement during pregnancy, bromocriptine should be restarted and titrated up quickly. If no response, alternative dopamine agonists, transsphenoidal surgery, or delivery (if appropriate) should be considered.
- Pituitary apoplexy is the sudden destruction of the pituitary tissue by infarction or hemorrhage of the pituitary gland.
  - Presenting signs and symptoms include fever, acute HA, nausea, vomiting, signs of meningeal irritation, visual impairment, ophthalmoplegia, hemiplegia, and decreased level of consciousness.
  - It can be caused by rapid expansion of an adenoma. Other predisposing factors include head trauma, sudden changes in arterial or intracranial pressure, anticoagulation or bleeding disorders, diabetes, and postpartum hemorrhage.
  - Urgent surgery may be required to preserve vision. Corticosteroids may be critical to treat acute adrenal insufficiency (25,26).

OTHER CAUSES OF ACUTE HEADACHE
- *Vascular disease.* HA is a common symptom in patients with stroke, cerebral vein thrombosis or occlusion, etc. (see below).
- *Vasospasm* can occur in the setting of preeclampsia, PRES, or postpartum (postpartum cerebral angiopathy) (27).
- *Sheehan syndrome* (necrosis of the anterior pituitary). Rare in developed nations, but potentially lethal. Symptoms include hypotension, tachycardia, failure to lactate, hypoglycemia, fatigue, nausea, and vomiting.

SUBACUTE HEADACHE SYNDROMES
Background
- Subacute HA syndromes usually develop over a period of a few weeks to a few months. A pattern of increasingly frequent, severe, and prolonged HA is especially worrisome.
- Important diagnostic considerations are intracranial masses, chronic meningitis, or idiopathic intracranial hypertension.

Increased Intracranial Pressure
- Intracranial masses such as primary or metastatic malignant tumors, benign tumors (such as meningiomas), subdural hematomas, brain abscesses, etc. may cause increased intracranial pressure.
  - Clinical symptoms are nonspecific. They include worsening HA, nausea and vomiting, lethargy, and altered personality or behavior.
  - Neurologic examination may reveal papilledema or focal findings.
  - If the history suggests an intracranial mass, CT or MRI is indicated, even if the physical examination is negative. MRI is preferred.
  - If a mass is present, referral to a neuro-oncologist or neurosurgeon is indicated.

- Subacute or chronic meningitis may be due to infectious or noninfectious causes.
  - Infections may be due to fungi (e.g., *Cryptococcus*), mycobacteria, viruses (e.g., HIV), spirochetes (e.g., syphilis and Lyme disease), and others.
  - Noninfectious causes include sarcoidosis, autoimmune disorders, metastatic tumors, etc.
  - Diagnosis requires lumbar puncture, but the findings are frequently nonspecific; special serologies, DNA probes, cerebrospinal fluid (CSF) cytology, or other special studies may be needed. Consultation from a neurologist or infectious disease expert is advised.
  - Treatment and prognosis depend on the specific diagnosis.

IDIOPATHIC INTRACRANIAL HYPERTENSION (PSEUDOTUMOR CEREBRI)

- The syndrome is characterized by persistent elevation of intracranial pressure. It is presumably related to an abnormality of CSF drainage, but the specific cause is often obscure. Some medications, including tetracycline, vitamin A, and Norplant can cause pseudotumor cerebri.
- Patients typically present with steadily worsening HA, sometimes with vomiting or with episodes of transient loss of vision (usually lasting for only a few seconds).
- The neurologic examination reveals papilledema and may reveal abducens nerve palsies with double vision but is otherwise normal.
- Imaging studies are usually normal but may show flattening of the posterior sclera and/ or an empty or partially empty sella turcica.
- Lumbar puncture reveals increased CSF pressure, greater than 25 cm H_2O, but the CSF is normal.
- The prognosis is generally good, with spontaneous resolution sometimes possible with discontinuation of an offending agent or weight loss. Weight gain should be limited to 20 pounds in pregnant individuals. Drug treatment may include acetazolamide (after 20 weeks), corticosteroids, and diuretics.
- During pregnancy, patients should be evaluated and followed closely by an ophthalmologist for both funduscopic exam and visual field testing at least every 2 to 3 months because permanent visual loss can occur. Threatened visual loss may require surgical intervention (optic sheath fenestration or lumbar–peritoneal shunt) (28).

CHRONIC HEADACHE SYNDROMES
Background

- Chronic HA syndromes are characterized by a long history, often over years or decades. Although typically due to non–life-threatening or "benign" disorders, such HA may have serious effects on a woman's ability to work, care for her home or children, or enjoy life.
- Chronic HA may vary in their frequency, intensity, and duration in response to life events, changes in medication, concurrent illness, or for no discernable reason.
- Patients are likely to seek medical attention at times when their HA have increased in frequency or intensity. A careful history may be needed to distinguish such variations in chronic HA syndromes from evolving acute or subacute HA syndromes.
- The two most common chronic HA syndromes are migraine and tension-type HA (TTH).
  - Migraine HA affects about 18% of women and is particularly common during the childbearing years.
  - TTH affects up to 88% of women.
  - Approximately 62% of women with migraines will also have TTH.
  - Patients with a history of migraine have a 1.8-fold increased risk of preeclampsia. Overweight women with migraine have a 12-fold increased risk of preeclampsia compared to lean women without migraine (29).

Evaluation

- The diagnosis of the chronic HA syndromes depends almost entirely on the clinical history. The physical and neurologic examinations are generally normal; any abnormal finding should suggest another diagnosis.
- In patients who meet the diagnostic criteria for migraine or TTH, imaging studies and other laboratory studies are usually not required. Further study should be considered if there is any substantial change in the HA character or if unexpected symptoms develop.

Diagnosis

- The International Headache Society has developed diagnostic criteria for TTH and for migraine HA with and without aura.
- Detailed diagnostic criteria have been developed for a wide variety of other HA syndromes as well (30).

Treatment

General Considerations

- Treatment of both TTH and migraine syndromes can be very challenging for physicians, patients, and patients' families. "Cure" of chronic HA is unlikely; a more realistic goal is to obtain a meaningful reduction in the frequency and intensity of the attacks.
- As noted previously, it is important that these patients be taken seriously and that the severity of their distress is recognized.
- It is important to avoid over medication and polypharmacy in a vain attempt to achieve "complete" control of HA. Many patients use large amounts of over-the-counter medications or may obtain pain medications from several different physicians. Overuse of such medications can cause rebound HA. A detailed medication history is thus crucial.
- Patients often benefit when multiple redundant medications are eliminated and their treatment regimens are simplified (see Table 24-2).
- Fortunately, many women with migraines (60% to 70%) will experience significant reduction in their HA during pregnancy, especially during their second and third trimesters (31).

Tension-Type Headache

- Nonpharmacologic treatment
  - Physical therapy, regular exercise, ice, and massage are helpful for many patients.
  - Biofeedback and relaxation training may be helpful for some patients.
- Pharmacologic treatment
  - Acetaminophen can be used with good effect and is generally safe for use in pregnancy. Nonsteroidal anti-inflammatory drugs (NSAIDS) are generally recommended to be avoided during pregnancy, especially during third trimester.
  - For occasional use, butalbital (present in many proprietary HA preparations) is acceptable. Care must be taken to avoid overuse.
  - Benzodiazepines (mostly category D) and narcotics should generally be avoided for chronic use because of their high abuse potential. Short-term or occasional use of narcotics for HA treatment in pregnancy may be reasonable.
- If significant depression is present, effective depression treatment may also relieve HA.

Migraine Headache

- Women with migraine HA are more likely to suffer from gestational hypertension and have an increased risk for preeclampsia.
- Clomiphene, used in some infertility regimens, may increase the risk of migrainous infarction.
- Women with migraine without aura and with menstrual-related migraines are more likely to improve with pregnancy than those with migraine with aura or migraines unrelated to menstruation.

Table 24-2	Selected Drugs Used for the Acute and Prophylactic Treatment of Migraine			
Drug	**Pregnancy category**	**Maternal effects**	**Fetal effects**	**Breast-feeding**
Tylenol	B/C	Hepatotoxicity	Premature constriction of ductus (third trimester use, case reports)	Compatible
NSAIDS	C/D	Inhibits implantation	Premature closure of ductus, oligohydramnios, small increased risk of spontaneous abortion	Compatible
Aspirin	D	Increased bleeding, decreased uterine contractions	Premature closure of ductus, increased bleeding, neonatal acidosis, IUGR, mortality, salicylate intoxication	Caution
Opioids	B/C	Overuse/abuse	Cleft palate, inguinal hernia, withdrawal, respiratory depression	Compatible/caution
Triptans	C	Triptan sensation, vasoconstriction	Unknown	Caution
Ergotamines	X	Reduced placental blood flow	Fetal growth retardation	Not recommended
Beta-blockers	C/D	Hypotension, bradycardia	IUGR, bradycardia, hypoglycemia, respiratory distress, cardiovascular defect	Caution
Calcium channel blockers	C	Constipation, hypotension	Bradycardia, heart block, hypotension	Not recommended
Antiepileptics		See Table 24-1		
Tricyclic Antidepressants	C/D	Anticholinergic	Limb deformities, developmental delay	Caution

- As with TTH, nonpharmacologic treatments are helpful for many patients.
- If HA are not better by the end of the first trimester, they are unlikely to improve and pharmacologic treatment may be needed (23).
- Symptomatic treatment
  - Acetaminophen may be effective in some cases. NSAIDS can be considered for brief, infrequent use in pregnancy but should be avoided during the third trimester.
  - Morphine, hydromorphone, codeine, and meperidine are in pregnancy category C. All should be used with caution to avoid overuse and dependency.
  - For severe nausea and vomiting, metoclopramide (category B), promethazine, or prochlorperazine (category C) and similar agents can be used.
  - Very severe and prolonged migraines may respond to corticosteroids such as prednisone.
  - Sumatriptan and the other "triptan" agents, which have revolutionized the treatment of migraine in nonpregnant women, are currently classified in pregnancy category C. The few available data regarding their effects on pregnancy show no evidence of teratogenesis but do suggest increased risk of preterm birth. Only naratriptan, rizatriptan, and sumatriptan have pregnancy registries, and the information currently available from them is not sufficient for ruling out a mild increased risk of teratogenicity (32).
  - The ergot alkaloids ergotamine and dihydroergotamine are in category X because of their oxytocic and teratogenic effects and should not be used in women who are or who may become pregnant.
- Prophylactic treatment
  - Since prophylactic treatment requires daily exposure to medication, it should be avoided if possible.
  - If the frequency and severity of HA mandates prophylactic treatment, propranolol, a category C drug, is probably safest. Amitriptyline is also category C but may be associated with neonatal withdrawal. Topiramate and valproate are category D and should be avoided.
  - Botulinum toxin A, which is approved for treatment of chronic migraine, has not been studied for safety in pregnant women. In one survey of almost 400 physicians, only 12 reported using it during pregnancy, all for causes other than migraine. All but 2 of the 16 treated women went to term, and there were no fetal malformations reported.

Patient Education
- Women should be encouraged to report the development of any severe and persistent HA during pregnancy to their physicians and not assume HA is a normal part of pregnancy.
- Women with chronic HA (migraine and TTH) should be encouraged to report any abrupt change in the frequency, intensity, or character of their HA to their physician.
- Women with chronic HA (migraine and TTH) should be encouraged to discuss their HA management with their obstetrician and other treating physicians prior to pregnancy.
  - All women on symptomatic treatment not planning pregnancy should be encouraged to use contraception and at least 0.4 mg of folate.
  - Medication discontinuation should be pursued prior to conception. Patients can begin trying to conceive immediately after stopping their medications.
- Women with chronic HA who have an unplanned pregnancy should immediately stop using prophylactic medications and other HA treatments unless specifically approved by their obstetricians.

Arnold-Chiari Malformation in Pregnancy
- Arnold-Chiari malformation is the downward displacement of the cerebellar tonsils through the foramen magnum. Depending on the type (I–IV), it may be associated with other anatomic malformations.
- HA is typically occipital and occurs after exertion, coughing, or laughing. Other associated symptoms include weakness and numbness of the extremities, imbalance, nystagmus, and syncope.

- There is a lack of data regarding the optimal management of Arnold-Chiari during pregnancy or precautions needed during labor or for use of regional anesthesia.
- Spinal anesthesia is typically avoided to prevent further downward shift of cerebellar tonsils/herniation should the dura be inadvertently punctured. While it is not clear that pushing during labor or uterine contractions worsen the condition, patients with uncorrected Arnold-Chiari malformation typically undergo cesarean delivery under general anesthesia (33).

CEREBROVASCULAR DISORDERS IN PREGNANT WOMEN

Key Points
- Stroke is a rare but potentially devastating complication of pregnancy.
- Stroke may result from a wide variety of underlying medical causes. Prompt diagnosis and treatment of the underlying cause may reduce the risk of recurrent stroke.
- Some "traditional" treatments for acute stroke (anticoagulation, rapid blood pressure control, etc.) have been found to be of little benefit and may worsen outcome.

Background
Definitions
- Cerebrovascular disorders in pregnant women include ischemic stroke, ICH, and cerebral venous thrombosis (CVT).
- The term *stroke* is properly used to indicate a focal (localized) injury to the nervous system that occurs as a disruption of the brain blood supply.
  - Arterial or venous channels may be affected.
  - Used in this way, the term stroke does *not* include global or generalized brain injury resulting from cardiac arrest or severe hypotension (anoxic–ischemic encephalopathy) or diffuse cerebral injury due to SAH.
- *Ischemic stroke* results from occlusion of the arterial blood supply.
- *Transient ischemic attack (TIA)* occurs when transient occlusion of arterial blood supply results in focal neurological deficits lasting less than 24 hours without acute cerebral infarction (34).
- *Intracerebral hemorrhage* results from bleeding into the brain parenchyma, either as the primary event or as a result of secondary bleeding into a region of the brain previously damaged as a result of an ischemic stroke.
- *Cerebral venous thrombosis* is caused by thrombosis of the venous sinuses, cerebral veins, or jugular veins.

Pathophysiology
- Pregnancy and the postpartum period comprise a hypercoagulable state related to prothrombotic changes during pregnancy that persist several weeks postpartum, and which are made worse following delivery due to hemoconcentration. Thus, pregnancy increases risk of ischemic stroke, TIA, and CVT (17,35).
- Ischemic stroke
  - Brain cells are uniquely dependent on constant and stable perfusion; failure of perfusion for only a few seconds results in failure of neuronal function. With rapid reperfusion, recovery is also rapid, and any neurologic deficit may recover.
  - If reperfusion is delayed longer than a few minutes, permanent damage is likely.
  - Ischemic stroke is characterized by a region of neuronal death (*infarction*), surrounded by an *ischemic penumbra,* a zone where perfusion is at least partially preserved, and which may recover normal function if perfusion is restored.
- ICH
  - Bleeding into the brain parenchyma may result in local destruction of brain neurons, disruption of nerve fiber pathways, local mass effect and herniation syndromes, hydrocephalus, and increased intracranial pressure.

- CVT
  - Thrombosis and occlusion of cerebral veins or venous sinuses may result in localized cerebral edema, parenchymal hemorrhage, or infarction.
  - Obstruction of venous drainage may cause increased intracranial pressure.

Etiology
- Ischemic strokes may be either *thrombotic* or *embolic*. These may be difficult to distinguish based on clinical criteria alone.
  - Thrombotic strokes result from in situ occlusion of a blood vessel. Important causes include (among others)
    - Preeclampsia and eclampsia
    - Reversible cerebral vasoconstriction syndrome (RCVS), that is, postpartum angiopathy
    - Atherosclerosis of large arteries
    - Small vessel disease
    - Arterial dissection (spontaneous or traumatic).
    - Thrombophilic disorders (e.g., antiphospholipid syndrome, lupus, sickle cell disease, etc.)
    - Intrinsic vasculopathies (e.g., vasculitis, moyamoya, CADASIL, etc.)
    - Vasospasm (e.g., cocaine, severe migraine, etc.)
  - Embolic strokes result from blood clots or other embolic debris migrating to cerebral vessels from another source (often cardiac). Important causes include
    - Cardiac valve disease (including infectious endocarditis).
    - Atrial fibrillation.
    - Myocardial infarction.
    - Cardiomyopathy, including peripartum cardiomyopathy.
    - Amniotic fluid embolus.
    - Intracardiac shunts may allow "paradoxical" embolization from systemic venous circulation to enter arterial circulation, potentially causing stroke.
    - *Patent foramen ovale*, a common congenital anomaly, has received much attention as a potential cause of stroke in young people, but its true significance remains unknown (17,36,37).
- ICH may result from
  - Degenerative changes in brain blood vessels due to hypertension or diabetes.
  - Aneurysms, either congenital or mycotic. Other vascular anomalies include arteriovenous malformations, cavernous hemangiomas, etc.
  - Vascular injury from vasculitis, eclampsia, or severe preeclampsia.
  - Coagulopathies.
  - RCVS, aka postpartum angiopathy.
- CVT may result from
  - A hypercoagulable state associated with pregnancy
  - Other clotting disorders (including Leiden factor V mutation, sickle cell disease, etc.)
  - Dehydration, polycythemia, or hyperviscosity syndromes

Epidemiology
- Estimates of pregnancy-related stroke incidence vary from 3.8 to 18 per 100,000 deliveries (36).
- CVT comprises 0.5% to 1% of all strokes and approximately 2% of pregnancy-related strokes (35).
  - One case per 2500 to 10,000 deliveries (35).
  - Pregnancy-related CVT most often occurs in the third trimester or postpartum (35).
- Estimates of the incidence of pregnancy-related ICH (including SAH) vary from 6.1 to 25.4 per 100,000 deliveries (36).

- It is unclear whether the risk of ischemic stroke is increased during pregnancy, but there is an increased risk in the peripartum period and up to 2 weeks postpartum (36).
- ICH risk is increased during pregnancy and further increased postpartum (36).

Risk Factors
- Age greater than 35 years increases risk of pregnancy-related stroke and ICH twofold (36).
- Ethnicity
  - 1.5 times greater risk of pregnancy-related stroke in African Americans (36).
  - The risk of pregnancy-related ICH may be higher in Asian women (36).
- Medical conditions associated with an increased risk of pregnancy-related stroke include migraine, hypercoagulable disorders, valvular heart disease, sickle cell disease, hypertension, diabetes, lupus, and tobacco use (36).
  - Hypertension in pregnancy: 6 to 9 times increased stroke risk (36).
  - Complications of pregnancy and delivery are linked to greater stroke risk (36).
    - Preeclampsia and eclampsia
    - Hyperemesis gravidarum
    - Anemia
    - Thrombocytopenia
    - Postpartum hemorrhage
    - Transfusion of blood and blood products
    - Fluid, electrolyte, and acid–base disorders
    - Infection
    - Peripartum cardiomyopathy (17,37)
    - Amniotic fluid embolus (17,37)
    - Metastatic choriocarcinoma (37)
- Risk factors for CVT also include hypertension, infections, dehydration, thrombophilias, advanced maternal age, cesarean delivery, and hyperhomocysteinemia (35).
- Cesarean delivery may be a risk factor for peripartum stroke due to CVT (36).
- ICH risk factors include preeclampsia and eclampsia, cerebrovascular malformations, metastatic choriocarcinoma, and alcohol and methamphetamine abuse (36).
- Severe preeclampsia and eclampsia may lead to
  - *Reversible posterior leukoencephalopathy syndrome* (at times associated with vasogenic edema or ICH), typically presenting with agitation, confusion, seizures, visual hallucinations, or vision loss.
  - *Reversible cerebral vasoconstriction syndrome*, aka postpartum angiopathy (severe recurrent HA ± focal neurologic deficits and reversible segmental narrowing of intracranial arteries on angiography).
    - Associated with infarcts and hemorrhages (17).
    - Felt to be relatively common and underrecognized (17).
    - May be confused with vasculitis (17).
    - May occur without preeclampsia/eclampsia (17).
    - Long-acting calcium channel blockers may be helpful (17).
  - Both may present primarily with HA and visual scotomata (17,36,37).

Evaluation
- Stroke should be seen as the final outcome of a multitude of different clinical syndromes. Accordingly, the diagnostic evaluation should seek not only to confirm and characterize the diagnosis of stroke but also to determine the underlying cause(s).

History and Physical Examination
- The initial diagnosis of ischemic stroke and ICH is usually straightforward. The characteristic clinical presentation is the abrupt onset of a focal neurological deficit.
  - The neurologic deficits usually reach their maximum severity within minutes of onset, although a stuttering or progressive course may be seen.

- HA is common.
- Seizures and alteration of consciousness may occur.
- There are no reliable clinical criteria to distinguish ischemic stroke from ICH.
- CVT typically presents with severe and progressing HA, evolving focal deficits, seizures, and progressive impairment of consciousness.
  - HA alone may be the only symptom of CVT in 25% of cases (35).
  - CVT presents with ICH in 30% to 40% of cases (35).
- In women with suspected or confirmed stroke, ICH, or CVT, the history should evaluate for the presence of hypertension, known vascular malformations, diabetes, clotting disorders, heart disease, connective tissue disease, preeclampsia, and other pregnancy complications.
- Detailed physical and neurological examinations should be performed. The neurological examination should be repeated at regular intervals to monitor the patient for signs of progressive impairment of consciousness.

Laboratory Studies
- Routine lab studies in patients with stroke often include CBC/differential, sedimentation rate, platelet count, blood glucose and electrolytes, lipids, and prothrombin time (PT)/international normalized ratio (INR) and partial thromboplastin time (PTT).
- Additional studies may include hypercoagulable workup, such as anticardiolipin antibodies, Leiden factor V mutation, protein C and protein S assays, antinuclear antibody, blood cultures (if infection or bacterial endocarditis is suspected), etc.
- Lumbar puncture is not indicated in evaluation of patients with suspected stroke or CVT.

Imaging Studies
- CT scanning (without contrast) is virtually diagnostic for ICH but much less sensitive and specific for ischemic stroke or CVT. Fetal radiation exposure with maternal head CT is very low, less than 1 rad. Risk of childhood leukemia following in utero ionizing radiation exposure is estimated 1 in 2000 compared to 1 in 3000 background (17).
- MRI with diffusion-weighted imaging is highly sensitive for acute stroke and CVT. It is recommended to avoid gadolinium contrast, which crosses the placenta. Otherwise, 1.5 T MRI appears safe in all trimesters (17).
- Magnetic resonance angiography (MRA) or CT angiography may identify focal arterial occlusion, atheromatous disease, aneurysms, or arterial dissection.
- MRV can confirm the diagnosis of CVT.
- Consultation with a neurologist or radiologist may help guide selection of the most appropriate studies.
- Echocardiography may identify likely sources of cardiogenic embolism. Transesophageal echocardiography (TEE) may be more sensitive in detecting potential sources of cardiogenic emboli in selected patients.

Cardiac monitoring
- Cardiac monitoring to screen for arrhythmia is recommended for the first 24 hours after ischemic stroke (38).

Differential Diagnosis
- Focal seizures:
  - Typically present with "positive" symptoms, such as involuntary movements, paresthesias, automatisms, etc. Stroke is more often characterized by "negative" symptoms, such as paralysis, loss of sensation, aphasia, etc.
  - May be followed by transient focal neurologic symptoms, sometimes lasting several hours or more, making diagnosis difficult.
  - Seizures may occur in patients with stroke.

- Migraine:
  - Focal migraine symptoms, when present, typically evolve slowly over 15 to 20 minutes and then resolve slowly. The onset of stroke symptoms is typically abrupt.
  - Stroke-like symptoms may occur with or without HA, but when migraine HA is present, focal symptoms typically resolve before the HA.
  - Patients with migraine-associated neurologic symptoms will usually have a prior history of similar attacks.
- HE and eclampsia are characterized by depressed consciousness and seizures but usually not by focal neurologic signs.

Treatment
General Measures
- ABCs:
  - Airway support/ventilator assistance for bulbar dysfunction or impaired consciousness (38)
  - Supplemental O_2 for hypoxia (38)
- Blood pressure is commonly elevated in patients with acute stroke and ordinarily should *not* be lowered. *Cautious* treatment is appropriate when
  - Other medical conditions, such as angina or heart failure, require urgent treatment.
  - Blood pressure is *markedly* elevated (systolic greater than 220 mm Hg or diastolic greater than 120 mm Hg) (38).
  - In patients with ICH, current recommendations suggest that *mean* arterial pressure be kept below 130 mm Hg (39).
  - See Chapter 4 for appropriate management of hypertension.
- Hypotension is uncommon but should be treated and a cause sought (38).
- Blood glucose should be maintained at normal levels (38).
- Fever should be reduced (38).
- Anticonvulsants are indicated only if seizures occur (35).
- Steroids are of no value in the treatment of stroke, ICH, or CVT (35).
- Patients should be kept NPO until safe swallowing is assured.
- Prophylaxis for venous thromboembolism should be started.
- Physical therapy, occupational therapy, and speech therapy, if needed, should be initiated as soon as is practical.
- The delivery method should be determined by usual obstetric criteria. In patients with elevated intracranial pressure, such as with large ischemic stroke, ICH, or CVT, C-section may reduce the risk of further increases in intracranial pressure associated with Valsalva.

Thrombolytic Therapy
- In selected nonpregnant patients with acute ischemic stroke, systemic thrombolysis with IV tissue plasminogen activator (tPA) may result in significantly improved neurological outcome. There is increased risk of ICH (6%) but no increase in overall mortality.
  - tPA does not cross the placenta, is pregnancy class C, but pregnancy is a relative contraindication for its use (36).
  - Case reports of successful use of IV and intra-arterial tPA in pregnant women suggest tPA may be a reasonable option in select patients with careful assessment of risks and benefits. However, no randomized studies of tPA use in pregnancy exist, and overall safety is not established (36).
    - Possibly greater ICH risk (8%) when used for stroke in pregnancy (17)
  - IV tPA is contraindicated at the time of delivery and postpartum because of the risk of catastrophic hemorrhage.

Anticoagulation
- Anticoagulation is not routinely indicated in patients with acute ischemic stroke, but it is indicated in acute treatment of CVT.

- Anticoagulation with unfractionated heparin (UFH) or low molecular weight heparin (LMWH) appears to improve CVT outcomes, even with ICH (35).
- Anticoagulation for 3 months with UFH or LMWH followed by antiplatelet therapy (in the nonpregnant state) is advised in acute management of CVT. There are case reports of their successful use in pregnant women (34).
- Warfarin crosses the placenta and is pregnancy category D for patients with mechanical heart valve and pregnancy category X for all other patients.
- LMWH (pregnancy category B) and UFH (pregnancy category C) do not cross the placenta. Both agents are commonly used in pregnancy.
- Little or no data regarding safety in pregnancy are available for the thrombin inhibitors argatroban and dabigatran or factor Xa inhibitor rivaroxaban (37).
  - Dabigatran and rivaroxaban are pregnancy category C.
  - Argatroban is pregnancy category B.

Antiplatelet Therapy
- Aspirin (ASA) is pregnancy category D.
- Low-dose ASA is considered safe in the second and third trimesters, but safety in the first trimester is not established (37). However, low-dose ASA is commonly used in pregnancy and is recommended in pregnancy for some conditions such as antiphospholipid antibody syndrome.
- Little data are available regarding use of other antiplatelet agents in pregnancy (37).
  - Clopidogrel is pregnancy category B.
  - ASA–dipyridamole is pregnancy category D.

Intracerebral Hemorrhage
- There are no clear guidelines for the management of this condition in pregnancy.
- While drugs typically used in nonpregnant patients with ICH may have risks in pregnancy (e.g., mannitol), benefits may outweigh risks in the critically ill patient (36).
- Surgical treatment of ruptured aneurysms during pregnancy appears to lower maternal and fetal mortality (36).
- Cesarean delivery does not appear to improve outcome over vaginal delivery in women with most vascular anomalies (36).

Complications
- Stroke per se has little effect on L&D. Obstetric management can be determined by standard criteria.
- A pregnancy-related stroke case fatality rate of 4.1% has been reported or mortality rate of 1.4 per 100,000 deliveries, lower than the case fatality rate for stroke at any age (24%) or stroke in young adults (4.5% to 24%) (36).
- Pregnancy-related cerebrovascular complications may contribute 25% to all maternal deaths (17).
- ICH is associated with highest pregnancy-related stroke mortality (20.3%) (36).
- Limited data are available regarding postpregnancy-related stroke morbidity (36).
  - Thirty-three percent of women with ischemic stroke had minimal disability.
  - Fifty percent of women with ICH had mild to moderate residual deficits.
  - Nine percent to twenty-two percent are discharged to a facility other than home.
  - Some of those who do go home may require substantial assistance with care.
- One study of 37 women with first pregnancy-related stroke found no recurrent strokes in 24 subsequent pregnancies, suggesting pregnancy-related stroke does not contraindicate subsequent pregnancy. Counseling regarding specific risk factors is indicated (36).

Prevention
Recommendations
- American Heart Association/American Stroke Association Guidelines:

- When antiplatelet therapy would be indicated outside of pregnancy for women at increased risk of stroke, consider UFH or LMWH in the first trimester and low-dose ASA after the first trimester (34).
- For pregnant women with stroke or TIA and high-risk thromboembolic conditions (e.g., hypercoagulable state, mechanical heart valves), consider UFH in all trimesters; LMWH in all trimesters; or UFH or LMWH until week 13, followed by warfarin until midway third trimester, followed by UFH or LMWH until delivery (34). Consultation with a perinatologist for counseling regarding risks and benefits of warfarin in pregnancy is recommended prior to initiating this therapy in carefully selected patients.
- For women with venous thromboembolism history and known high-risk thrombophilia, consider LMWH or UFH during pregnancy and warfarin anticoagulation postpartum (36).
- For pregnant women with antiphospholipid antibody syndrome, no history of venous thromboembolism, and recurrent pregnancy loss, treat with UFC or LMWH + baby ASA throughout pregnancy and the postpartum period (36).
- LMWH use in pregnancy for women with mechanical heart valves is controversial due to reports of maternal and fetal death (17).
- Risks associated with ASA treatment in pregnancy include maternal or fetal bleeding and premature closure of fetal ductus arteriosus (17,36).
- LMWH may increase epidural hematoma risk when used proximate to the time of administration of regional anesthesia (36).

PERIPHERAL NERVE AND MUSCLE DISORDERS
Idiopathic Facial Nerve Palsy (Bell Palsy)
Background
- Bell palsy is characterized by partial or complete paralysis of one side of the face of unknown cause.
- The pathophysiology remains obscure but appears to involve a localized injury to the facial nerve as it passes through the facial canal. Infection with *Herpes simplex* virus (HSV) has been proposed as a mechanism in some cases.
- The incidence of Bell palsy is increased in late pregnancy and the puerperium from 17 per 100,000 per year in the general population to 38 to 45 per 100,000 pregnant women per year.
- A higher rate of gestational hypertension and preeclampsia has been reported in pregnant women afflicted by Bell palsy.

Evaluation
- The usual clinical presentation is abrupt (up to 48 hours) onset of partial or complete paralysis affecting both the upper and lower portions of the face on one side. Additional symptoms may include pain, usually behind the ear on the affected side, hyperacusis on the affected side, reduced tearing on the affected side, and sometimes a metallic taste.
- Physical examination reveals weakness of the affected side of the face. There should be no disturbance of vision, no loss of sensation, or other cranial nerve deficit. The remainder of the neurologic examination should be normal.
- In a patient with "typical" Bell palsy presentation, laboratory and imaging studies (CT or MRI) can safely be deferred.

Diagnosis
- In most cases, clinical diagnosis is straightforward. Weakness confined to the lower half of the face on the affected side, deficits in other cranial nerve functions, or neurologic deficits affecting other body parts are *not* seen in Bell palsy and should prompt full neurologic evaluation.

Treatment
- The prognosis (without treatment) is excellent; 85% of patients recover normal or near-normal function spontaneously.
- Most recent evidence-based guidelines put forth by the American Academy of Neurology suggest that steroids are highly likely to be effective and should be offered to increase the chances of recovery of function of the facial nerve. If steroids are used, prednisone 1 mg/kg/d for 10 days is "reasonable." The use of antiviral agents (for presumed HSV) in addition to steroids may provide a modest benefit, though the true benefit has not been well established. Acyclovir was considered only "possibly" effective in one recent review (40).
- Patients with severe facial weakness are often unable to fully close the eye on the affected side and risk drying of the eye, corneal abrasion, and severe eye injury. Artificial tears, patching, or even tarsorrhaphy may be required. Consultation with an ophthalmologist should be sought early if there is persistent burning, itching, pain, or other symptoms in the affected eye (41).

Carpal Tunnel Syndrome
Background
- Carpal tunnel syndrome is characterized by pain, paresthesias, and sometimes sensory loss or muscle weakness in the distribution of the median nerve in the hand.
- The syndrome is commonly attributed to compression or entrapment of the median nerve as it passes under the transverse ligaments on the ventral side of the wrist.
- Carpal tunnel syndrome is common in pregnancy, particularly in late pregnancy, possibly as a result of fluid retention and swelling. The rates of preeclampsia, HTN, and edema are higher in symptomatic pregnant women (42).

Evaluation
- Patients report tingling, numbness, and sometimes pain involving especially the thumb and first two or three fingers of the affected hand.
  - In many cases, the whole hand is involved, or the little finger may be spared.
  - Symptoms are commonly present on awakening and initially may be relieved by changing position, shaking the hand, etc. The discomfort may become more severe and persistent with time.
- The physical examination may reveal decreased sensation over the affected areas. Tinel and Phalen signs may be present. There may be weakness of the abductor pollicis brevis muscle of the affected thumb, but this may be difficult to detect.
- Electrodiagnostic studies, such as electromyography (EMG), and nerve conduction studies (NCS) may be diagnostic but are often normal, especially in mild or early cases.

Diagnosis
- Diagnosis is usually straightforward and depends on recognition of the characteristic symptoms. As noted above, the physical examination and electrodiagnostic studies may be negative. In patients with mild symptoms, no further diagnostic study is needed.
- Differential diagnosis includes more proximal injury to the median nerve or injury to the brachial plexus or cervical spinal roots. EMG/NCS may be helpful in localizing the lesion.

Treatment
- In pregnant patients, the syndrome is usually self-limited, and symptoms will resolve spontaneously within 2 weeks of delivery. Electrodiagnostic abnormalities may persist well beyond symptom relief.
- Conservative management with wrist splint(s) and edema control may relieve the discomfort.
- Steroid injections may also provide temporarily relief.
- If symptoms persist after delivery, or if weakness of hand muscles develops, more aggressive treatment, including surgical decompression, may be needed (43,44).

MERALGIA PARESTHETICA

Background

- Meralgia paresthetica is characterized by pain, paresthesias, and sometimes by sensory loss over the anterolateral thigh, in the distribution of the lateral femoral cutaneous nerve. The nerve is purely sensory, and there are no motor signs.
- The syndrome is attributed to entrapment or compression of the nerve at the level of the inguinal ligament but may occur with no evident structural lesion.
  - The cause is often unknown.
  - Meralgia paresthetica may occur as a complication of diabetes.
  - The nerve may be compressed by the abdomen in pregnant women. The syndrome has also been attributed to obesity, tight undergarments, and local trauma.

Evaluation

- Pain and paresthesias often begin abruptly, without evident cause. Symptoms can be quite severe and distressing. Patients may complain of subjective weakness due to their discomfort.
- Physical findings include diminished sensation over the anterolateral thigh, corresponding to the cutaneous nerve distribution. There is no true muscle weakness, and reflexes are normal. There may be local tenderness at the site of nerve compression by the inguinal ligament.

Diagnosis

- Diagnosis ordinarily presents no difficulty and is obvious once the syndrome is recognized. NCS may be helpful but are rarely needed and may be technically difficult, especially in obese patients.
- Differential diagnosis includes femoral neuropathy (see below), lumbar radiculopathy from disc herniation, and iliac crest tumor.

Treatment

- The condition is self-limited and gradually resolves in most cases.
- Drug treatment is limited. Analgesics are usually of little benefit. Gabapentin or amitriptyline (category C) may be helpful, and CBZ (category D) has been used as well. Pregabalin (category C), approved for the treatment of painful diabetic neuropathy, may prove helpful in some patients.
- Local anesthetic block with bupivacaine followed by recurrent steroid block may be helpful as can topical capsaicin or lidocaine.
- In patients with very severe and persistent pain, surgical decompression of the nerve can be attempted (45).

FEMORAL NEUROPATHY

Background

- Femoral neuropathy is characterized by isolated weakness of the quadriceps and sometimes iliopsoas muscles, with or without sensory loss over the anteromedial thigh. It results either from localized femoral nerve injury in the retroperitoneal space or as it exits the abdomen.
- Femoral neuropathy is not usually a complication of pregnancy per se but may occur after vaginal delivery, cesarean, or pelvic surgery. The cause is usually unclear, but the nerve may be injured by obstetric or surgical procedures or prolonged posture in the lithotomy position. Femoral neuropathy is often idiopathic but may occur as a complication of diabetes.

Evaluation

- Femoral neuropathy may be painless and may first become evident when the patient tries to stand and walk following delivery and finds that her knee(s) buckle(s) and she is unable to support her weight.

- Physical examination reveals isolated weakness of the quadriceps and sometimes the ilio-psoas muscles. As noted above, there may be sensory loss over the anteromedial thigh. The knee reflex is absent, and one or both sides may be affected.
- EMG/NCS are not helpful in the acute phase but may be useful after 2 to 3 weeks if spontaneous recovery does not occur. If there is other clinical evidence for a retro-peritoneal process (e.g., retroperitoneal bleeding), appropriate imaging studies should be obtained.

Diagnosis
- As with other mononeuropathies, in patients with typical symptoms, the diagnosis usu-ally is clinically obvious, and further studies are not needed.
- Differential diagnosis includes meralgia paresthetica (see above), lesions of the lumbar roots, and lumbosacral plexus lesions.

Treatment
- Spontaneous recovery is expected and may ensue over the first 2 to 8 weeks. However, full recovery may take up to 6 months. If weakness is severe, patients may require addi-tional assistance at home. If spontaneous recovery does not occur, a neurologist should be consulted (46).

OBTURATOR NEUROPATHY
Background
- Injury to the obturator nerve causes weakness of the adductor muscles of the thigh and, sometimes, sensory loss over the upper medial thigh.
- As with femoral neuropathy, the cause may be unknown or the nerve may be injured in the course of vaginal delivery, cesarean, or pelvic surgery.

Diagnosis and Treatment
- Similar to femoral neuropathy (see above).
- Spontaneous recovery is expected.

PERONEAL NEUROPATHY
Background
- Injury to the peroneal nerve causes weakness of muscles of the anterior compartment of the lower leg, resulting in weakness of dorsiflexion of the foot (foot drop) and, some-times, sensory loss over the dorsum of the foot.
- The peroneal nerve is a branch of the sciatic nerve. It emerges behind the knee and passes across the fibula just below the knee. The nerve is easily palpated through the skin. Because of its superficial location and the underlying bone, it is easily injured by local compression. Potential causes include pressure from stirrups, prolonged bed rest, pressure from bed rails, patient hand positioning during labor, etc. Many cases are idiopathic.

Diagnosis
- Diagnosis is based on the clinical findings of isolated foot drop and weakness of eversion of the foot, with or without sensory impairment over the dorsum of the foot.
- Differential diagnosis includes injury to the sciatic nerve (often resulting in weakness of the posterior calf muscles as well) or lumbosacral root lesions.
- EMG/NCS are not helpful in the acute phase but may be useful after 2 to 3 weeks.

Treatment
- Spontaneous recovery is the rule.
- An ankle brace (ankle-foot orthosis) may be helpful to facilitate walking until spontaneous recovery occurs.

GUILLAIN-BARRÈ SYNDROME (ACUTE INFLAMMATORY DEMYELINATING POLYRADICULONEUROPATHY, AIDP)

Background
- Acute inflammatory demyelinating polyradiculoneuropathy (AIDP) is characterized by acute, progressive muscle weakness that usually begins in the lower extremities and may spread rapidly to involve the trunk, the upper extremities, and the face. If the respiratory muscles are affected, the disease can be life threatening.
- Caused by an immune-mediated attack on peripheral nerve myelin, leading to focal demyelination and sometimes to injury of the nerve axons.
- About two-thirds of cases are preceded by an infectious illness; a multitude of viral agents have been implicated, and there is a close association with *Campylobacter jejuni* infection.
- There is no significant increase in the frequency or severity of AIDP during pregnancy. However, it is important that obstetrics and gynecology (OB/GYN) physicians be aware of the illness since they frequently serve as primary care physicians for pregnant patients and may be the first contacted regarding symptoms of this disorder.

Evaluation
- The key to early diagnosis and treatment is recognition of the clinical syndrome by an alert physician. In most cases, the diagnosis is based on the clinical presentation.
- Patients usually complain of progressive weakness beginning in the lower extremities and spreading upward. Sensory symptoms (paresthesias and pain) often precede the weakness by a day or so but may not be prominent.
- The weakness may gradually worsen over several weeks or may progress rapidly, leading to generalized paralysis and respiratory failure in less than 24 hours.
- The physical examination reveals symmetrical weakness, usually most severe in the lower extremities. A hallmark of the disease is diffuse reduction or absence of stretch reflexes, even in muscles that do not appear weak.
- Laboratory studies are usually of little help. The CSF protein may be elevated without a concomitant increase in cells, but this is unreliable very early in the course.

Treatment
- If AIDP is suspected, urgent evaluation in an emergency department is necessary. Patients should be hospitalized with careful monitoring of respiratory function. A neurologist or critical care specialist should be consulted.
  - Approximately 25% of patients will require ventilator support.
  - In patients with severe disease, urgent treatment with plasma exchange or intravenous immune globulin (IVIG) may substantially shorten the duration of ventilator dependence (if needed) and the course of the disease. Either treatment can be used safely during pregnancy (47).
  - Corticosteroids are not helpful.
  - Autonomic dysfunction (hypotension or hypertension, bradycardia or tachycardia, etc.) may occur and require expert management.

Complications
- AIDP has no effect on the progress or outcome of pregnancy, and pregnancy has no effect on the course or outcome of AIDP.
- There is no effect on uterine contractions. The mode of delivery can be determined by standard obstetric criteria.
- Because of prolonged immobility, patients are at high risk for pulmonary embolism, pneumonias, urinary tract infections, etc.
- Prognosis is generally favorable, with 75% to 80% of patients achieving a good functional recovery; the remainder may be left with some degree of permanent weakness. Mortality is 3% to 8%.

MYASTHENIA GRAVIS

Background

- Myasthenia gravis (MG) is characterized by variable weakness affecting both bulbar (cranial nerve) and skeletal muscles. The weakness is often worsened by activity of the affected muscles and relieved by rest.
- MG is an autoimmune disease, characterized by antibodies directed against the acetylcholine receptors (AChR) on muscle cells, partially or completely blocking neuromuscular transmission.
- Nearly 15% of patients with MG have thymomas. Sixty percent to eighty percent present with hyperplastic thymus.
- MG is quite rare but approximately twice as common in women as in men.
- Maternal mortality is highest when pregnancy occurs in the first year after MG diagnosis and lowest 7 years after disease onset. It is recommended that women delay childbirth for 2 years after diagnosis.
- Approximately one-third of women will have increased weakness during pregnancy or the puerperium. The highest risk for exacerbation is during the first trimester and following delivery.
- Women with MG should be managed in cooperation with their neurologists before, during, and after their pregnancies.

Evaluation

- Patients typically present with a history of fluctuating muscle weakness.
  - In most cases, extraocular muscles and facial muscles are affected early; patients present with transient and variable double vision, ptosis of the eyelids, facial weakness, and difficulty with chewing or swallowing.
  - Muscles of the trunk and limbs are affected in 85% of patients.
  - The neurologic examination reveals weakness of the affected muscles; sensation and reflexes are normal.
- The diagnosis can be confirmed by detection of elevated serum titers of antibodies against AChR and by EMG/NCS. Appropriate diagnostic studies should be chosen by a neurologist.

Treatment

- Patients with thymoma or hyperplasia of the thymus should undergo thymectomy. Complete remission of MG has been seen in up to 45% of patients following thymectomy. The risk of exacerbation during pregnancy and the risk of neonatal MG are lower in those who have undergone thymectomy. Thus, patients planning pregnancy should be advised to undergo thymectomy prior to pregnancy (48).
- Anticholinesterase drugs (pyridostigmine or neostigmine) often provide symptomatic relief. These agents can be safely continued during pregnancy.
- In many patients, chronic immunosuppression is required. Prednisone, azathioprine, and cyclosporine, alone or in combination, may be effective. These agents appear to be reasonably safe and well tolerated during pregnancy. Patients should be informed that prednisone carries an increased risk of cleft palate when used in the first trimester. Azathioprine may be associated with intrauterine growth restriction and low birth weight. A study in renal transplant patients showed a higher risk of preterm delivery and low birth weight in those patients on cyclosporine. Mycophenolate mofetil and methotrexate, also used in the treatment of MG, are teratogenic and should not be used during pregnancy. Mycophenolate mofetil is also associated with increased risk of first-trimester miscarriage (49,50).
- Severe exacerbations of myasthenia may be associated with respiratory failure. Plasma exchange or high-dose immune globulins may be used effectively and safely if needed.

Complications

- MG has no effect on the course or outcome of pregnancy, and pregnancy has no effect on the course or outcome of MG.
- MG has no effect on uterine contractions and L&D usually proceeds normally. Mothers with severe generalized weakness may require assisted vaginal delivery. Cesarean delivery is typically reserved for standard obstetric indications (51).
- Women with MG may be very sensitive to inhalation anesthetics, neuromuscular blocking agents, aminoglycoside antibiotics, magnesium sulfate, and other drugs. Physicians are advised to carefully assess the safety profile of any drug to be used in myasthenic women. Because inhalation anesthetics may cause exacerbation, epidural anesthesia is preferred.
- About 10% to 20% of babies born to myasthenic women will be affected with neonatal myasthenia due to placental transfer of AChR antibodies. Clinical weakness may be evident at birth or within 3 days after delivery. These children may require treatment with anticholinesterase drugs. The disorder is self-limited and usually resolves within 3 weeks of birth. It does not imply an increased risk of myasthenia later in life.
- Maternal MG is a rare cause of arthrogryposis multiplex congenita in the neonate. This congenital disorder probably results from lack of movement in utero and is characterized by multiple joint contractures and other anomalies. In the worst case, intrauterine or neonatal death can occur.
- MG is not a contraindication to breast-feeding. Women treated with prednisone and low doses of anticholinesterase medications may also breast-feed safely. Women on high doses of anticholinesterase agents and women taking azathioprine and cyclosporine are advised not to breast-feed (52,53).

MULTIPLE SCLEROSIS
Background

- Multiple sclerosis (MS) is an immune-mediated disease characterized by focal areas of inflammation and demyelination in the CNS.
- The cause of MS remains unknown despite extensive research. Genetic factors affect susceptibility to the disease, but MS is not a heritable disease.
- MS is relatively common; the prevalence in the United States is 1 per 1000. The disease is roughly twice as common in women as in men, and the peak age of onset is between 20 and 40 years. Approximately 10% of cases begin during pregnancy (54).
- In approximately 85% of cases, MS is characterized by a course of intermittent relapses and remissions, with gradual accumulation of neurologic deficits of varying severity. This is called relapsing remitting MS (RRMS). Even after 15 years of MS, the majority of patients remain ambulatory and 40% continue working.
- Frequency of relapses decreases during pregnancy and increases 3 months postpartum.

Evaluation

- The diagnosis of MS is based on the clinical history, the neurological examination, and laboratory and imaging studies. There is no definitive "test" for MS, and many of the clinical features of MS may be mimicked by other conditions.
  - Stroke, migraine, transverse myelitis, optic neuritis, lupus, cerebral vasculitis, Lyme disease, sarcoidosis, and other conditions can cause clinical symptoms, physical findings, and imaging findings that can be confused with MS.
  - MRI scans of the brain, obtained for other indications, may reveal white matter lesions that cannot be easily distinguished from those of MS. A radiologist's report of "possible" MS or "cannot exclude MS" may lead to an erroneous diagnosis and cause considerable distress for patients and their families.
- All patients with suspected MS should be evaluated by a neurologist.

Treatment

- There is no definitive or curative treatment for MS. Many patients with MS utilize various alternative treatments for their disease, sometimes without medical supervision. Physicians should ask their patients whether they are using such therapies.
- Until recently, injectable immunomodulating agents, interferon beta 1a (Avonex, Rebif), interferon beta 1b (Betaseron), and glatiramer acetate (Copaxone), were the mainstay of treatment, shown to reduce the frequency and severity of MS exacerbations. There are limited data on the safety of these medications during pregnancy.
  - Interferons:
    - Abortifacient in animals at high doses.
    - Use during the first trimester was thought to increase the risk of fetal loss and low birth rate (55). More recently, a prospective study of over 600 pregnant females using interferon beta 1a showed that most births to these women were normal. There was no increase in the rate of spontaneous abortion or major congenital anomalies (56).
    - Interferon use immediately prior to beginning pregnancy (within 2 weeks) was not associated with increased risk of fetal loss or low birth weight (57).
  - Glatiramer acetate:
    - Exposure does not appear to affect gestational age, birth weight, or length (58).
  - Given the insufficient data available, it is currently recommended that treatment with interferon or glatiramer be discontinued prior to pregnancy in most cases (59). However, it may be reasonable to continue these drugs in select patients with active disease (i.e., if benefits appear to outweigh potential risks) (60).
  - Males fathering children while undergoing treatment with interferon or glatiramer do not appear to cause increased fetal or neonatal risks (61).
- Three oral medications are now FDA approved for the treatment of MS: fingolimod (Gilenya), teriflunomide (Aubagio), and dimethyl fumarate (Tecfidera) (62–65).
  - Fingolimod:
    - Teratogenic effects have been observed in animal studies. Pregnancy should be avoided for 2 months after discontinuation of treatment.
  - Teriflunomide:
    - Based on animal data, teriflunomide may cause major birth defects and is contraindicated in pregnant women or women of childbearing potential who are not using reliable contraception.
    - As this drug may stay in the serum for 2 years, an accelerated drug elimination procedure using cholestyramine or activated charcoal powder has been devised. Pregnancy should be avoided until undetectable serum concentrations are achieved via this method. If pregnancy occurs during treatment, therapy should be discontinued and the accelerated elimination procedure initiated.
    - Teriflunomide is present in semen. Men who wish to father a child should discontinue therapy and undergo the accelerated elimination procedure.
  - Dimethyl fumarate:
    - Adverse events have been reported in animal reproductive studies.
- Natalizumab, a humanized monoclonal antibody, is used in the treatment of those with highly active disease. While highly effective, it is considered second line secondary to the risk of progressive multifocal leukoencephalopathy.
  - Animal studies showed an increased risk of abortion and possible hematologic abnormalities postnatally, though there have been case reports of normal neonatal outcome in patients incidentally treated with natalizumab during pregnancy.
  - Patients planning pregnancy should stop the drug 3 months prior to conception (66–68).
- IVIG may be considered as second- or third-line therapy in RRMS if injectable or oral therapies are not tolerated or in pregnancy when other therapies may not be used (69).

- Corticosteroids (prednisone and methylprednisolone) are used in the treatment of acute exacerbations of MS and appear to be reasonably safe during pregnancy. However, there is an increased risk of oral cleft when used during the first trimester.
- Azathioprine is sometimes used in the treatment of patients with progressive MS and may be continued with reasonable safety during pregnancy.
- Methotrexate and cyclophosphamide should be avoided during pregnancy (54).

Complications

- MS has no effect on pregnancy or L&D in most cases. Typically, the mode of delivery, anesthesia, etc. can all be determined by standard obstetric indications (54). In some populations of women with MS, however, a higher risk of small for gestational age, preterm birth, lower mean birth weights, and need for cesarean delivery have been reported (70–73).
- Pregnancy and L&D have no effect on the long-term course of MS and no effect on eventual disability (if any).
  - Regional anesthesia has no effect on MS.
  - Multiple studies indicate a reduced risk of exacerbations of MS during pregnancy. This is balanced by a comparable increase in risk during the postpartum period.
  - Corticosteroids (74) and perhaps IVIG (75) may reduce the risk of postpartum exacerbations, but further studies are required.

Patient Education

- Women with MS can be reassured they can expect a normal pregnancy and L&D.
- Women can be reassured that pregnancy will have no effect on the long-term course or long-term disability (if any) from their MS.
- Treatment with disease modifying therapy should be discontinued prior to pregnancy or as soon as possible after pregnancy begins.

REFERENCES

1. Berg AT, Berkovic SF, Brodie MJ, et al. Revised terminology and concepts for organization of seizures and epilepsies: report of the ILAE Commission on Classification and Terminology, 2005–2009. *Epilepsia.* 2010;51(4):676–685.
2. Kobau R, Luo YH, Zack MM, et al. Epilepsy in adults and access to care—United States, 2010. *MMWR.* 2012;61(45):909–913.
3. Pennell PB. Treatment of epilepsy during pregnancy. In: *Wyllie's treatment of epilepsy.* 5th ed. Philadelphia: Lippincott Williams & Wilkins, 2011:557–568.
4. Hernandez-Diaz S, Smith CR, Shen A, et al. Comparative safety of antiepileptic drugs during pregnancy. *Neurology* 2012;78:1692–1699.
5. Harden CL, Meador KJ, Pennell PB, et al. Practice parameter update: management issues for women with epilepsy—focus on pregnancy (an evidence-based review): teratogenesis and perinatal outcomes: report of Quality Standards Subcommittee of American Academy of Neurology and American Epilepsy Society. *Neurology.* 2009;73(2):133–141.
6. Tomson T, Battino D, Bonizzoni E, et al. Dose-dependent risk of malformations with antiepileptic drugs: an analysis of data from the EURAP epilepsy and pregnancy registry. *Lancet Neurol.* 2011;10(7):609–617.
7. Meador KJ, Baker GA, Browning N, et al. Fetal antiepileptic drug exposure and cognitive outcomes at age 6 years (NEAD study): a prospective observational study. *Lancet Neurol.* 2013;12(3):244–252.
8. Meador KJ, Baker GA, Browning N, et al. Effects of fetal antiepileptic drug exposure: Outcomes at age 4.5 years. *Neurology.* 2012;78(16):1207–1214.
9. Meador KJ, Gus A Baker GA, et al. Cognitive function at 3 years of age after fetal exposure to antiepileptic drugs. *N Engl J Med.* 2009;360:1597–1605.
10. Christensen J, Grønborg TK, Sørensen MJ, et al. Prenatal valproate exposure and risk of autism spectrum disorders and childhood autism. *JAMA.* 2013;309(16):1696–1703.

11. Harden CL, Hopp J, Ting TY, et al. Practice parameter update: management issues for women with epilepsy—focus on pregnancy (an evidence-based review): obstetrical complications and change in seizure frequency: report of Quality Standards Subcommittee of AAN and AES. *Neurology.* 2009;73:126–132.
12. Harden CL, Pennell PB, Koppel BS, et al. Practice parameter update: management issues for women with epilepsy—focus on pregnancy (an evidence-based review): vitamin K, folic acid, blood levels, and breast feeding: report of the Quality Standards Subcommittee of AAN and AES. *Neurology.* 2009;73(2):142–149.
13. Sabers A. Pharmacokinetic interactions between contraceptives and antiepileptic drugs. *Seizure.* 2008;17(2):141–144.
14. Johannessen SI, Landmark CJ. Antiepileptic drug interactions—principles and clinical implications. *Curr Neuropharmacol.* 2010;8(3):254–267.
15. Meador KJ, Baker GA, Browning N, et al. Effects of breastfeeding in children of women taking antiepileptic drugs. *Neurology.* 2010;75(22):1954–1960.
16. Goodkin HP, Riviello JJ. Status epilepticus. In: *Wyllie's treatment of epilepsy.* 5th ed. Philadelphia: Lippincott Williams & Wilkins, 2011:469–485.
17. Sidorov EV, Feng W, Caplan LR, et al. Stroke in pregnant and postpartum women. *Expert Rev Cardiovasc Ther.* 2011;9(9):1235–1247.
18. Silberstein SD. Headaches in pregnancy. *Neurol Clin.* 2004;22(4):727–756.
19. Karnad DR, Guntupalli KK. Neurologic disorders in pregnancy. *Crit Care Med.* 2005;33 (10 suppl):S362–S371.
20. Riviello C, Ammannati F, Bordi L. Pregnancy and subarachnoid hemorrhage: a case report. *J Matern Fetal Neonatal Med* 2004;16:245–246.
21. Adriani KS, Brouwer MC, van der Ende A, et al. Bacterial meningitis in pregnancy: report of six cases and review of the literature. *Clin Microbiol Infect.* 2012;18(4):345–351.
22. Fujiwara Y, Higaki H, Yamada T, et al. Two cases of reversible posterior leukoencephalopathy syndrome, one with and the other without pre-eclampsia. *J Obstet Gynaecol Res.* 2005;31(6):520–526.
23. Loder E. Migraine in pregnancy. *Semin Neurol.* 2007;27(5):425–433.
24. Spencer HC. Postdural puncture headache: what matters in technique. *Reg Anesth Pain Med.* 1998;23:374–379.
25. Jassal DS, McGinn G, Embil JM. Pituitary apoplexy masquerading as meningoencephalitis. *Headache.* 2004;44:75–78.
26. Iuliano S, Laws ER. Management of pituitary tumors in pregnancy. *Semin Neurol.* 2011;31(4):423–428.
27. Lele A, Lyon T, Pollack A, et al. Intra-arterial nicardipine for the treatment of cerebral vasospasm in postpartum cerebral angiopathy: a case study and review of literature. *Int J Neurosci.* 2011;537–542, 2011.
28. Evans RW, Friedman DI. The management of pseudotumor cerebri during pregnancy. *Headache.* 2000;40:495–497.
29. Adeney KL, Williams MA, Miller RS, et al. Risk of pre-eclampsia in relation to maternal history of migraine headaches. *J Matern Fetal Neonatal Med.* 2005;18(3):167–172.
30. Headache Classification Committee. The International Classification of Headache Disorders. 2nd ed. *Cephalalgia.* 2004;24:1–160.
31. Menon R, Bushnell CD. Headache and pregnancy. *Neurologist.* 2008;14(2):108–119.
32. Soldin OP, Dahlin J, O'Mara DM. Triptans in pregnancy. *Ther Drug Monit.* 2008;30(1):5–9.
33. Sicuranza GB, Steinber P, Figueroa R. Arnold chiari malformation in a pregnant woman. *Obstet Gynecol.* 2003102(5 Pt 2):1191–1194.
34. Furie KL, Kasner SE, Adams RJ, et al. Guidelines for the prevention of stroke in patients with stroke or transient ischemic attack. A guideline for healthcare professionals from the American Heart Association/American Stroke Association. *Stroke.* 2011;42:227–276.
35. Saposnik G, Barinagarrementeria F, Brown RD, Jr. Diagnosis and management of cerebral venous thrombosis: a statement for healthcare professionals from the American Heart Association/American Stroke Association. *Stroke.* 2011;42:1158–1192.
36. Tate J. Pregnancy and stroke risk in women. *Womens Health (Lond Engl).* 2011;7(3):363–374.

37. Tettenborn B. Stroke and pregnancy. *Neurol Clin.* 2012;30:913–924.
38. Adams HP Jr, del Zoppo G, Alberts MJ, et al. Guidelines for the early management of adults with ischemic stroke: a guideline from the American Heart Association/American Stroke Council, and the atherosclerotic peripheral vascular disease and quality of care outcomes in RSCH Working Groups. *Circulation.* 2007;115:478–534.
39. Morgenstern LB, Hemphill JC III, Anderson C, et al. Guidelines for the management of spontaneous intracerebral hemorrhage: a guideline for healthcare professionals from the American Heart Association/American Stroke Association. *Stroke.* 2010;41:2108–2129.
40. Gronseth G, Paduga R. Evidence-based guideline update: steroids and antivirals for Bell palsy. Report of the Guideline Development Subcommittee of the American Academy of Neurology. *Neurology.* 2012;79(22):2209–2213.
41. Kovo M, Sagi Y, Lampl Y, et al. Simultaneous bilateral Bell's palsy during pregnancy. *J Matern Fetal Neonatal Med.* 2009;22(12):1211–1213.
42. Voitk AJ, Mueller JC, Farlinger DE. Carpal tunnel syndrome in pregnancy. *Can Med Assoc J.* 1983;128(3):277–281.
43. Finsen V, Zeitlmann H. Carpal tunnel syndrome during pregnancy. *Scand J Plast Reconstr Surg Hand Surg.* 2006;40:41–45.
44. Ablove RH, Ablove TS. Prevalence of carpal tunnel syndrome in pregnant women. *WMJ.* 2009;108(4):194–196.
45. Harney D, Patijn J. Meralgia paresthetica: diagnosis and management strategies. *Pain Med.* 2007;8:669–677.
46. Pierce C, O'Brien C, O'Herlihy C. Post partum femoral neuropathy following spontaneous vaginal delivery. *J Obstet Gynaecol.* 2010;30(2):203–204.
47. Mabie W. Peripheral neuropathies during pregnancy. *Clin Obstet Gynecol.* 2005;48:57–66.
48. Hoff JM, Daltveith AK. Myasthenia gravis in pregnancy and birth: identifying risk factors, optimizing care. *Eur J Neurol.* 2007;14(1):38–43.
49. Batocchi AP, Majolini L, Evoli A, et al. Course and treatment of myasthenia during pregnancy. *Neurology.* 1999;8:447–452.
50. Ferrero S, Pretta S, Nicoletti A, et al. Myasthenia gravis: management issues during pregnancy. *Eur J Obstet Gynecol Reprod Biol.* 2005;121:129–138.
51. Stafford IP, Dildy GA. Myasthenia gravis and pregnancy. *Clin Obstet Gynecol.* 2005;48:48–56.
52. Chaudry SA, Vignarajah B, Koren G. Myasthenia gravis during pregnancy. *Can Fam Physician.* 2012;58(12):1346–1349.
53. Kalidindi M, Ganpot S, Tahmesebi F, et al. Myasthenia gravis and pregnancy. *J Obstet Gynaecol.* 2007;27(1):30–32.
54. Bennett KA. Pregnancy and multiple sclerosis. *Clin Obstet Gynecol.* 2005;48:48–56.
55. Boskovic R, Wide R, Wolpin J. The reproductive effects of beta interferon therapy during pregnancy: a longitudinal cohort. *Neurology.* 2005;65:807–811.
56. Sandberg-Wollheim M, Alteri E, Moraga MS. Pregnancy outcomes in multiple sclerosis following subcutaneous interferon beta-1a therapy. *Mult Scler.* 2011;17(4):423–430.
57. Sandberg-Wolheim M, Frank D, Goodwin T, et al. Pregnancy outcomes during treatment with interferon beta-1a in patients with multiple sclerosis. *Neurology.* 2005;65:807–811.
58. Giannini M, Portacciol E, Ghezz A, et al. Pregnancy and fetal outcomes after Glatiramer Acetate exposure in patients with multiple sclerosis: a prospective observational multicentric study. *BMC Neurol.* 2012;12:124.
59. Hellwig K, Gold R. Glatiramer acetate and interferon-beta throughout gestation and post-partum in women with multiple sclerosis. *J Neurol.* 2011;258:502–503.
60. Salminen H, Leggett J, Boggild M. Galteramer acetate exposure in pregnancy: preliminary safety and birth outcomes. *J Neurol.* 2010;257:2020–2023.
61. Hellwig K, Haghikia A, Gold R. Parenthood and immunomodulation in patients with multiple sclerosis. *J Neurol.* 2010;257(4):580–583.
62. Gold R, Kappos L, Arnold DL, et al. Placebo-controlled phase 3 study of oral BG12 for relapsing multiple sclerosis. *N Engl J Med.* 2012;367(12):1098–1107.
63. New drugs for relapsing multiple sclerosis. *Med Lett Drugs Ther.* 2012;54(1403):89–91.

64. FDA approves new multiple sclerosis treatment Aubagio, [Online]. Available at: www.fda. gov/NewsEvents/Newsroom/PressAnnouncements/ucm319277.htm. Accessed September 13, 2012.

65. Gold R. Oral therapies for multiple sclerosis. A review of agents in phase III development or recently approved. *CNS Drugs*. 2011:37–52.

66. Bayas A, Penzien J, Hellwig K. Accidental natalizumab administration to the third trimester of pregnancy in an adolescent patient with multiple sclerosis. *Acta Neurol Scand*. 2011;124:290–292.

67. Hoevenaren L, de Vries L, Rijnders R, et al. Delivery of healthy babies after natalizumab use for multiple sclerosis: a report of two cases. *Acta Neurol Scand*. 2011;123:430–433.

68. Hellwig K, Haghikia A, Gold R. Pregnancy and natalizumab: results of an observational study in 35 accidental pregnancies during natalizumab treatment. *Mult Scler J*. 2011;958–963.

69. Elovaaraa I, Apostolskib S, van Doorn P. EFNS guidelines for the use of intravenous immunoglobulin in treatment of neurologic diseases. Members of the Task Force. *Eur J Neurol*. 2008;15:893–908.

70. Dahl J, Myhr K, Daltveit A, et al. Pregnancy, delivery, and birth outcome in women with multiple sclerosis. *Neurology*. 2005;65:1961–1963.

71. Dahl J, Myhr K, Daltveit A, et al. Pregnancy, delivery and birth outcome in different stages of maternal multiple sclerosis. *J Neurol*. 2008;255:623–627.

72. Dahl J, Myhr K, Daltveit A, et al. Planned vaginal births in women with multiple sclerosis: delivery and birth outcome. *Acta Neurol Scand*. 2006;183(suppl):51–54.

73. Chen Y, Lin H, Lin H. Does multiple sclerosis increase risk of adverse pregnancy outcomes? A population-based study. *Mult Scler* 2009;15L:606–612.

74. de Seze J, Chapelotte M, Delelande S, et al. Intravenous corticosteroids in the postpartum period for reduction of acute exacerbations in multiple sclerosis. *Mult Scler*. 2004;10:596–597.

75. Achiron A, Kishner I, Dolev M, et al. Effect of intravenous immunoglobulin treatment on pregnancy and postpartum-related relapses in multiple sclerosis. *J Neurol*. 2004;251:1133–1137.

25 Dermatologic Complications

Brett Blake, Kalyani Marathe and David M. Pariser

KEY POINTS

- The skin is significantly affected by the profound endocrine, metabolic, psychological, and immunologic changes that occur with pregnancy.
- A thorough review of all the dermatologic complications of pregnancy would be beyond the scope of this chapter. This is a summary of the most common and important conditions.
- Four broad categories of pregnancy-related skin changes are reviewed:
  - Physiologic skin changes of pregnancy
  - Skin diseases specifically related to pregnancy
  - Cutaneous tumors and dermatoses influenced by pregnancy
  - Infections affecting pregnancy

PHYSIOLOGIC SKIN CHANGES OF PREGNANCY

Pigmentation Changes

Background
- Localized hyperpigmentation is a common skin finding in pregnancy, occurring in up to 90% of pregnant women (1).
- Common manifestations are darkening of the nipples, areolae, linea alba, inner thighs, and external genitalia.
- Nevi, freckles, and recent scars may darken during pregnancy.
- Pigmentary change is related to elevated levels of melanocyte-stimulating hormone, estrogen, and possibly progesterone.
- Most of these pigment changes regress postpartum, rarely requiring treatment.

Melasma

Background
- Melasma (also known as chloasma or the mask of pregnancy) is an acquired, symmetric, hypermelanosis of the forehead, cheeks, and sometimes the upper lip.
- Melasma is an extremely common condition, having been reported in up to 70% of pregnant women (2). It is also associated with the use of oral contraceptives.
- Increased levels of serum estrogen, progesterone, and melanocyte-stimulating hormone are thought to be responsible for this condition.
- The hyperpigmentation usually fades after delivery in lightly pigmented individuals, but dyspigmentation may persist for darker complected women (3). Continued exposure to the UVB rays may allow the condition to persist following pregnancy.

Treatment
- Sun avoidance and the judicious use of sunscreens are essential not only to successful treatment of this condition but also for maintenance of remission.
- Bleaching agents such as hydroquinone and topical retinoids have been shown to be efficacious in treating this condition. Both classes of medications are pregnancy category C and should be avoided until parturition (4).

Hair
Background
- The physiologic state of pregnancy affects hair by prolonging the anagen (growing) phase. In some people, this results in excessive hair growth, predominantly on the face, and less often on the arms, legs, and back.

Treatment
- Excessive hair growth usually spontaneously resolves after delivery.
- An additional effect of prolonging the anagen phase during pregnancy is delaying the telogen (resting) phase of the hair. As a result, 3 months following pregnancy, the major portion of the scalp hair is cycled into the telogen phase often leading to mass shedding called telogen effluvium. This resolves in 1 to 5 months but can last for as long as 15 months postpartum (1).
- If severe hirsutism occurs, the possibility of androgen-secreting tumors of the ovary, lutein cysts, luteomas, or polycystic ovary disease should be investigated.

Nails
- Nail changes in pregnancy include brittleness, transverse grooving, and distal onycholysis. The pathogenesis behind these changes is not clear.

VASCULAR CHANGES
Palmar Erythema
- Palmar erythema appears on the palms in a diffuse or localized distribution generally between the 2nd and 5th months of pregnancy. There are no symptoms, and resolution is generally seen within 3 months following delivery. This condition is often seen in conjunction with spider telangiectasias.

Spider Telangiectasias
- Spider telangiectasias appear as a red papule with multiple radiating vessels emerging from the central papule, approximately 2 to 10 mm in diameter.
  - They are seen in approximately two-thirds of pregnant women, most often in areas drained by the superior vena cava such as the periocular region. Resolution without treatment often occurs within 3 months following delivery; however, 20% to 50% of these lesions persist.
  - Treatment is not necessary, but electrosurgical destruction and laser therapy are viable options.

Striae Distensae
- Striae distensae or "stretch marks," appear in up to 90% of pregnant women (2). Initially, they are slightly erythematous, linear, atrophic bands appearing most commonly in the breasts, abdomen, and hips. Following pregnancy, the erythema fades, but the lesions persist.
  - Striae are thought to be a risk factor for lacerations during vaginal delivery and for the development of pelvic relaxation and clinical prolapse (5,6).
  - No uniformly satisfactory treatment of striae exists; however, treatment with topical tretinoin and/or laser may help improve the appearance.

SKIN DISEASES SPECIFICALLY RELATED TO PREGNANCY
Intrahepatic Cholestasis of Pregnancy
Background
- Intrahepatic cholestasis of pregnancy (ICP) is characterized by pruritus in the absence of preceding skin lesions. Skin lesions are caused by scratching. The disease commonly presents itself in the third trimester of pregnancy (7).

Etiology
- The cause is multifactorial including hormonal, genetic, environmental, and likely alimentary factors. Estrogens inhibit glucuronyl transferase, which produces a cholestatic effect by reducing bile acid uptake into hepatocytes (8). This results in increased levels of circulating bile acids.
- Some evidence exists for a genetic predisposition to this condition, with several gene mutations linked to ICP risk.

Epidemiology
- The incidence of ICP varies from 2% to 28% of pregnancies depending on ethnicity (9).

Evaluation
Laboratory Findings
- Fasting serum bile acid elevation is the most sensitive marker of ICP, and liver function abnormalities are commonly found (8).
  - Jaundice is rare but can be complicated by steatorrhea and subsequent vitamin K deficiency and prolonged prothrombin time (8).
  - Skin biopsy is nonspecific (10).

Treatment
- Mild ICP may respond to symptomatic treatment with emollients and topical antipruritics.
- Ursodeoxycholic acid is the mainstay of treatment of ICP (8).

Complications
- ICP is associated with preterm birth in 20% to 60% of patients, fetal distress in 20% to 30% of cases, and fetal death in 1% to 2% of patients (11).

Polymorphic Eruption of Pregnancy
Background
Definition
- Polymorphic eruption of pregnancy (PEP) (previously known as pruritic and urticarial papules and plaques of pregnancy or PUPP) is a dermatosis, most commonly of primigravid women, consisting of pruritic papules and plaques that develop suddenly over the abdomen. PEP generally occurs in the third trimester of pregnancy (12).

Epidemiology
- PEP is the most common gestational dermatosis, affecting between 1 in 130 and 1 in 300 pregnancies (13).

Evaluation
Clinical Manifestations
- PEP is a polymorphous eruption but usually consists of small 1 to 2 mm juicy erythematous papules that coalesce to form urticarial plaques.
- The initial lesions appear in the abdominal striae distensae in half the patients. Subsequently, the eruption generally becomes widespread, involving the trunk, proximal extremities, and infrequently the hands and feet. Periumbilical sparing is a classic finding (9).
- Despite extreme pruritus, excoriations are rarely found.

Laboratory Findings
- No distinct abnormalities have been found.
- Biopsy is often nonspecific (8).

Treatment
Management
- Treatment is symptomatic with topical emollients, antihistamines, and corticosteroids.
- Severe cases may require systemic corticosteroids and, rarely, early delivery.

Course and Prognosis
- Most lesions resolve about 4 to 6 weeks after initial onset (14).
- Fetal morbidity and mortality have not been reported, and there is usually no recurrence in subsequent pregnancies (10).

Pemphigoid Gestations (PG)
Background
Definition
- Pemphigoid gestation (PG) is the rarest but most well-defined dermatosis of pregnancy. PG is more common in multigravid women in the third trimester.

Etiology
- The blistering is initiated by the presence of immunoglobulin (IgG1) directed against an epidermal basal lamina protein.
  - This is the same immunoglobulin that causes the disease bullous pemphigoid (11).
  - Although rare, transplacental transfer of these antibodies can occur, causing fetal disease.
- PG has also been associated with autoimmune diseases, particularly Graves disease.
- The disease typically regresses postpartum, but recurrence may occur in subsequent pregnancies, with menses or with use of oral contraceptives.

Epidemiology
- The incidence is estimated to be between 1 in 10,000 to 1 in 50,000 pregnancies (8).

Evaluation
Clinical Presentation
- Skin disease presents with pruritic urticarial plaques, which become annular or polycyclic, and subsequently develops into vesicles or bulla located on the extremities, abdomen, and buttocks.
- The face, mucous membranes, palms, and soles are generally spared.

Laboratory Tests
- A biopsy is generally helpful, revealing a subepidermal vesicle with perivascular lymphocytes and eosinophils.
- Direct immunofluorescence of perilesional skin reveals a linear deposition of C3 with or without IgG at the basement membrane zone.
- Serum ELISA reveals circulating IgG antibodies against NC16A domain of BP180 (8).

Treatment
Management
- Mild cases may respond to treatment with oral antihistamines and topical steroids.
- Most patients will require oral prednisone, responding to doses of 0.5 mg/kg/d.
- Doses above 80 mg/d are rarely necessary.
  - Due to the frequent postpartum flare, it is recommended that steroids be continue until after delivery, tapering as the disease allows.

Course and Prognosis
- Resolution usually occurs within 3 months following delivery.
- Exacerbation at delivery or immediately postpartum occurs in approximately 75% of cases (1).
- There are no maternal medical risks associated with PG.
- Immunoglobulin may cross the placental barrier causing mild, self-limited disease in the fetus.
- Studies have shown a tendency for small-for-gestational-age infants as well as prematurity, neither of which is altered by the use of systemic steroids. Despite this, there is no increase in fetal morbidity or mortality.
- PG tends to recur during subsequent pregnancies, generally presenting with an earlier onset and more severe manifestations.

Impetigo Herpetiformis (IH)
Background
- Impetigo herpetiformis (IH) is a rare variant of pustular psoriasis. Women usually have no family or personal history of psoriasis. IH can present at any time during pregnancy; however, the onset is typically in the last trimester (2).

Evaluation
Clinical Manifestations
- IH has been associated with malaise, chills, fever, diarrhea, vomiting, and sometimes tetany.
- Skin lesions first appear symmetrically in the inguinal folds and axillae and consist of large erythematous patches studded with grouped pustules.
- Pustules tend to coalesce and dry while new ones appear toward the periphery of the expanding erythematous areas.
- The face, hands, and feet are generally spared, while the mucous membranes are occasionally involved.

Laboratory Tests
- Serologic findings include leukocytosis and elevated erythrocyte sedimentation rate.
- Occasionally, hypocalcemia or decreased vitamin D levels secondary to hypoparathyroidism are found.
- Histopathologic findings mimic those of pustular psoriasis.

Treatment
Management
- Underlying metabolic disturbances should be corrected.
- Prednisone 15 to 30 mg daily is generally sufficient to control the disease (1).
- Superinfection should be treated with systemic antibiotics.
- Postpartum, the disease may be controlled with oral retinoids or PUVA.

Course and Prognosis
- With the use of corticosteroids and antibiotics, maternal mortality is low; however, associated placental insufficiency and stillbirth risk have been reported.
- Antepartum fetal surveillance is recommended in patients with IH.

ATOPIC ERUPTION OF PREGNANCY (AEP)
Background
Pathophysiology
- Because of extensive clinical overlap, pruritic folliculitis of pregnancy and prurigo of pregnancy are now referred to as atopic eruption of pregnancy (15). Presentation usually occurs in the first or second trimester of pregnancy (9).

Epidemiology
- Atopic eruption of pregnancy (AEP) is the most common pruritic condition in pregnancy (15).

Evaluation
Clinical Manifestations
- AEP is characterized by pruritic, eczematous papules.
- The lesions are usually covered with hemorrhagic crust or excoriations.
- Scabies, arthropod bites, and drug eruptions should be excluded (12).

Laboratory Evaluation
- Serum elevations of IgE may be found.
- Histopathologic findings are nonspecific.
- Direct immunofluorescence is negative.

Treatment
Medications
- Treatment is directed at alleviating the pruritus through the use of oral antihistamines and topical corticosteroids.

Course and Prognosis
- Recurrence in subsequent pregnancies is variable.
- Neonatal birth weights are unaffected, and fetal and maternal prognosis is excellent.

IMMUNOLOGIC DERMATOSES INFLUENCED BY PREGNANCY
Systemic Lupus Erythematosus (SLE)
Background
- Pregnancy is usually well tolerated by mothers who have been in remission for at least 3 to 6 months before conception. Patients with systemic lupus may have a mild increase in cutaneous flares and arthritis, but overall worsening of the disease during pregnancy is still debated (16,17). Renal or cardiac involvement indicates a less favorable outlook. If systemic lupus erythematosus (SLE) is active during conception, half of those patients will worsen during pregnancy, and permanent renal damage or death may occur. Postpartum remission and successful subsequent pregnancies occur in over two-thirds of cases.

Treatment
- Systemic corticosteroids and antimalarials should be continued during pregnancy so that an acute flare may be avoided.

Complications
- Up to 30% of infants of mothers with circulating anti-Ro (SS-A) antibodies will develop neonatal lupus with congenital heart block (18).
- Premature birth occurs in 16% to 39% of pregnancies, and there is also an increased risk of spontaneous abortion, intrauterine growth restriction, stillbirth, and neonatal death (19,20).

Systemic Sclerosis
- The effects of pregnancy on progressive systemic sclerosis are not well established, and both improvements and exacerbations of the disease have been reported. Although retrospective studies do show an increased risk of prematurity and infants that are small for gestational age, overall maternal and fetal outcomes are favorable (21).

Pemphigus
Background
- All forms of this disease may worsen, especially during the first trimester. In one study, 10% of the pregnancies ended in fetal loss and up to half of mothers had a postpartum flare (22).

Evaluation
- Immunofluorescence studies are necessary to distinguish this from PG. IgG antibodies may cross the placenta to the fetus.

Complications
- Blisters that may occur upon delivery usually resolve within a few weeks postpartum, but an increased incidence in fetal mortality and morbidity is seen (23).

Rheumatoid Arthritis (RA)
Background
- While most patients with rheumatoid arthritis (RA) have some improvement in their symptoms during pregnancy, approximately a quarter of patients continue to have active disease or worsening of the disease, requiring treatment through pregnancy. This improvement in arthritis during pregnancy tends to be short-lived, and most patients

who improve tend to relapse in the postpartum period. Possible causes for flare-up during the postpartum period may include a decrease in anti-inflammatory steroid levels and increased prolactin levels.

Complications
- Although RA has been shown to be associated with an increased risk of preterm labor (24), it does not appear to adversely affect fetal outcome, and overall, most women have an uneventful pregnancy (25).

Dermatomyositis/Polymyositis
Background
- A flare with proximal muscle weakness and a heliotrope rash may occur in half of affected mothers.

Complications
- Flares may be associated with neonatal death in more than half of cases (19,26).

Psoriasis
Background
- Chronic plaque psoriasis is the most common type of psoriasis affected by pregnancy, although pustular psoriasis may occasionally be seen. Psoriasis more often improves during pregnancy, but psoriatic arthritis has been noted to develop or worsen. In a recent study, psoriasis was not associated with increased risk of cesarean section, preeclampsia, or spontaneous abortion, although an association with preterm birth and low birth weight were noted (27).

Treatment
- Calcipotriol, tar, and topical corticosteroids are safe to use during pregnancy. Cyclosporine may be used for severe flares.
- Biologic medications (TNF-α and IL-2 and 23 inhibitors) are available for the treatment of psoriasis and psoriatic arthritis; the majority of which are pregnancy category B.

METABOLIC DISTURBANCES INFLUENCED BY PREGNANCY
Porphyria Cutanea Tarda (PCT)
Background
- This disorder is characterized by accumulation and excretion of uroporphyrin and coproporphyrins. Pregnancy may exacerbate the cutaneous lesions of porphyria cutanea tarda (PCT), particularly during the first trimester.

Evaluation
- Newborns should be tested for the disorder during the neonatal period, and genetic counseling is recommended (28).

Acrodermatitis Enteropathica (AE)
Background
- Acrodermatitis enteropathica (AE) may be exacerbated during pregnancy, resulting in a decreased zinc level, but responds well to zinc sulfate therapy. This disease should be considered in the differential diagnosis of unresponsive bullous dermatoses occurring during pregnancy (29,30).

CONNECTIVE TISSUE DISORDERS INFLUENCED BY PREGNANCY
Pseudoxanthoma Elasticum (PXE)
Background
- Pseudoxanthoma elasticum (PXE) is a rare hereditary disease characterized by systemic degeneration of elastic tissue.

Complications
- Vascular complications of PXE may be aggravated during pregnancy, with gastrointestinal bleeding and hypertension being the most common complications. Epistaxis and congestive heart failure with arrhythmias have also been reported. There appears to be minimal risk to the fetus during pregnancy (31).

Ehlers-Danlos Syndrome (EDS)
Background
- Patients with type II (mitis) and X (fibronectin) Ehlers-Danlos syndrome (EDS) tend to have a favorable outcome of pregnancy, but those with types I (gravis) and IV (vascular) EDS have increased risk of complications (32).

Complications
- Patients with EDS are prone to postpartum bleeding, and those with the vascular type are at risk for uterine or major blood vessel rupture (32). Bladder and uterine prolapse may also occur, and these patients tend to have poor wound healing. Type IV (vascular) EDS has a high maternal mortality rate from 11.5% to 25% for each pregnancy (29,33).

INFLAMMATORY DERMATOSES INFLUENCED BY PREGNANCY
Acne Vulgaris
Background
- Acne may worsen during pregnancy, secondary to increased sebaceous gland activity.

Treatment
- Topical antibiotics, azelaic acid, and some oral antibiotics, including penicillins, cephalosporins, and erythromycin (except the estolate form) may all be used during pregnancy (34).
- Most topical retinoids are pregnancy category C with the exception of tazarotene, which is pregnancy category X.

Urticaria
Background
- Urticaria are well circumscribed, elevated, and erythematous wheals formed by edema resulting from mast cell degranulation and histamine release. This response may be triggered by exposure to allergic, chemical, infectious, or emotional stimuli. Avoidance of these triggers is the mainstay of prevention. Chronic urticaria may worsen during pregnancy.

Treatment
- First-generation antihistamines may provide symptomatic relief, while systemic steroids may be needed for more aggressive treatment.

TUMORS INFLUENCED BY PREGNANCY
Pyogenic Granuloma
Background
- Also called granuloma gravidarum, pyogenic granuloma is a nodular proliferation of capillaries that frequently occurs within the gingiva during the 2nd to 5th month of pregnancy (35).

Treatment
- Postpartum shrinkage occurs spontaneously; however, surgical removal may be undertaken for cosmesis.

Skin Tag (Acrochordon)
Background
- These small, fleshy, pedunculated papules may occur during the later months of pregnancy and often disappear after delivery. They vary in color and size and may be found on the face, neck, and chest or beneath the breasts.

Treatment
- If lesions should become irritated or tender, they can easily be removed by clipping the base with surgical scissors and applying a styptic solution. The specimen should then be sent for pathologic review.

Melanocytic Nevi
- Nevi may develop, darken, or enlarge during pregnancy. An increase in progesterone and estrogen receptors may be an explanation for the pigmentary changes that can occur. A mild degree of cellular atypia may also be seen on histopathology.

Malignant Melanoma
- Melanoma is the third most common cancer diagnosed in pregnancy (36). Prognosis is determined by tumor thickness. Some studies have found melanomas that develop during pregnancy tend to be diagnosed at a more advanced stage, leading to a shorter disease-free survival period (37). Other studies have shown that while melanomas diagnosed during pregnancy are thicker, they do not have a less favorable prognosis. Women with a previously diagnosed melanoma do not have an increased risk of tumor recurrence as a result of pregnancy (38,39).

Dermatofibroma, Neurofibroma, and Keloid
Background
- These lesions may develop and grow rapidly during pregnancy.

Complications
- There are rare cases of dermatofibromas becoming disseminated during pregnancy. Patients with neurofibromatosis may also have vascular complications, such as renal artery rupture and severe hypertension.

INFECTIONS AFFECTING PREGNANCY
- A decrease in cell-mediated immunity, neutrophil function, and impairment of antibody response may increase the incidence of various infections (40).

Herpes Virus
Background
- Genital herpes simplex virus (HSV) infection is common, but not exacerbated by pregnancy. However, acquisition of the virus by the newborn has potentially serious consequences. Varicella zoster (VZV or chickenpox) is another herpes virus that can adversely affect the newborn infant.

Complications
- Maternal–neonatal transmission is approximately 50% with primary HSV genital infection, while the risk with recurrent genital infection is 5% or less. Neonatal infection may result in severe neurologic sequelae or death. Varicella zoster can result in severe neonatal infection, maternal pneumonitis, maternal death, or congenital varicella syndrome if the primary infection occurs during the first trimester (41,42). In pregnant women with known genital herpes infection, acyclovir prophylaxis is recommended after 36 weeks of gestation (43). While this does decrease the risk of maternal recurrence, its impact on vertical transmission leading to neonatal herpes infection is still unknown (44).

Human Papilloma Virus (HPV)
Background
- Human papilloma virus (HPV) is one of the most common sexually transmitted diseases (STD) in the world. HPV causes genital warts and is etiologically linked to cervical cancer.

Complications
- Genital warts may cause a number of problems during pregnancy. Hormonal changes may cause enlargement of warts, making urination difficult. If the warts are on the vaginal wall, they may decrease vaginal elasticity and cause obstruction during delivery. Rarely, infants born to women with genital warts develop laryngeal papillomatosis. Although rare, it can be a potentially life-threatening condition for the child, requiring frequent laser surgery to prevent obstruction of the airway. Due to the rarity of this condition, the presence of genital warts does not warrant the use of cesarean section to attempt to prevent fetal exposure to HPV. Data suggest that while HPV can be transmitted vertically, the neonates appear to clear the infection by 6 months of age. This suggests temporary inoculation rather than true infection (45).

Treatment
- Interferon therapy in combination with laser surgery may show promise in slowing the course of the disease. Photodynamic therapy has also been shown to be effective in early studies (46). HPV vaccines are now available for prevention of HPV infection.

Candida

Background
- Candidal vaginitis may be seen in over 60% of pregnant women and may be cultured from up to 50% of newborns of infected mothers (40,47). Pregnancy may depress T-lymphocyte proliferation, which can lead to a decreased ability to resist Candida infection. Furthermore, a rise in circulating hormone levels increases the glycogen content of vaginal cells, which can stimulate yeast growth.

Treatment
- During pregnancy, topical polyene, or imidazole antifungals are effective in the treatment of acute vulvovaginal candidiasis, although use of the shorter courses of therapy can lead to incomplete eradication of symptoms.
- The imidazoles are not recommended during the first trimester of pregnancy.
- Oral antifungals are not recommended as first-line therapy for localized disease in pregnant patients.

Patient Education
Skin changes in pregnancy are common and varied. Increasing size of benign lesions should not be a cause for alarm. However, patients who experience significant changes in the skin, changes in pigmented lesions, pruritus unresponsive to conservative measures, or vesicular or bullous eruptions, should receive consultation from a dermatologist.

REFERENCES

1. Kroumpousos G, Cohen L. Dermatoses of pregnancy. *J Am Acad Dermatol.* 2001;45:1–19.
2. Vaughan-Jones S, Munro Black M. Pregnancy dermatoses. *J Am Acad Dermatol.* 1999;40 (2 Pt 1):233–241.
3. Bolognia JL, Jorizzo JL, Schaffer JV, eds. *Dermatology.* St. Louis: Elsevier, 2012:1052–1054.
4. Pandya A, Guevara I. Disorders of hyperpigmentation. *Dermatol Clin.* 2000;18:91–98, ix.
5. Wahman AJ, Finan MA, Emerson SC. Striae gravidarum as a predictor of vaginal lacerations at delivery. *South Med J.* 2000;93:873–876.
6. Salter SA, Batra RS, Rohrer TE, et al. Striae and pelvic relaxation: two disorders of connective tissue with a strong association. *J Invest Dermatol.* 2006;126:1745–1748.
7. Sasseville D, Wilkinson RD, Schnader JY. Dermatoses of pregnancy. *Int J Dermatol.* 1981;20:223–241.
8. Kroumpouzos G, Cohen LM. Specific dermatoses of pregnancy: an evidence-based systematic review. *Am J Obstet Gynecol.* 2003;188:1083–1092.
9. Warshauer E, Mercurio M. Update on dermatoses of pregnancy. *Int J Dermatol.* 2013;52:6–13.

10. Hanno R, Saleeby ER, Krull EA. Pruritic eruptions of pregnancy. *Dermatol Clin.* 1983;4:553–570.

11. Lammert F, Marschall HU, Glantz A, et al. Intrahepatic cholestasis of pregnancy: molecular pathogenesis, diagnosis and management. *J Hepatol.* 2000;33:1012–1021.

12. Aronson IK, Bond S, Fiedler VC, et al. Pruritic urticarial papules and plaques of pregnancy: clinical and immunopathologic observations in 57 patients. *J Am Acad Dermatol.* 1998;39:933–939.

13. Roger D, Vaillant L, Fignon A, et al. Specific pruritic diseases of pregnancy. A prospective study of 3192 pregnant women. *Arch Dermatol.* 1994;130:734–739.

14. Beckett MA, Goldberg NS. Pruritic urticarial plaques and papules of pregnancy and skin distention. *Arch Dermatol.* 1991;127:125–126.

15. Ambros-Rudolph CM. Dermatoses of pregnancy—clues to diagnosis, fetal risk and therapy. *Ann Dermatol.* 2011;23(3):265–275.

16. Faussett M, Branch D. Autoimmunity and pregnancy loss. *Semin Reprod Med.* 2000;18:379–392.

17. Stojan G, Baer AN. Flares of systemic lupus erythematosus during pregnancy and the puerperium: prevention, diagnosis and management. *Expert Rev Clin Immunol.* 2012;8(5):439–453.

18. Schachner L, Hansen R, eds. *Pediatric dermatology.* St. Louis: Elsevier, 2003:566–578.

19. Sairam S, Costeloe K. Prospective risk of stillbirth in multiple-gestation pregnancies: a population-based analysis. *Obstet Gynecol.* 2002;100:638–641.

20. Smyth A, Oliveira GH, Lahr BD, et al. A systematic review and meta-analysis of pregnancy outcomes in patients with systemic lupus erythematosus and lupus nephritis. *Clin J Am Soc Nephrol.* 2010;5(11):2060–2068.

21. Lidar M, Langevitz P. Pregnancy issues in scleroderma. *Autoimmun Rev.* 2012;11(6–7): A515–A519.

22. Daneshpazhooh M, Chams-Davatchi C, Valikhani M, et al. Pemphigus and pregnancy: a 23-year experience. *Indian J Dermatol Venereol Leprol.* 2011;77(4):534.

23. Kardos M, Levine D, Gürcan HM, et al. Pemphigus vulgaris in pregnancy: analysis of current data on the management and outcomes. *Obstet Gynecol Surv.* 2009;64(11):739–749.

24. Langen ES, Chakravarty EF, Liaquat M, et al. High rate of preterm birth in pregnancies complicated by rheumatoid arthritis. *Am J Perinatol.* 2013. [Epub ahead of print].

25. Xu B, Pekkanen J, Jarvelin M. Obstetric complications and asthma in childhood. *J Asthma.* 2000;37:589–594.

26. Chopra S, Suri V, Bagga R, et al. Autoimmune inflammatory myopathy in pregnancy. *Medscape J Med.* 2008;10(1):17.

27. Lima XT, Janakiraman V, Hughes MD, et al. The impact of psoriasis on pregnancy outcomes. *J Invest Dermatol.* 2012;132(1):85–91.

28. Loret de Mola J, Muise K, Duchon M. Porphyria cutanea tarda and pregnancy. *Obstet Gynecol Surv.* 1996;51:493–497.

29. Winton G. Skin diseases aggravated by pregnancy. *J Am Acad Dermatol.* 1989;20:1–13.

30. Pérez-Maldonado A, Kurban AK. Metabolic diseases and pregnancy. *Clin Dermatol.* 2006;24(2):88–90.

31. Bercovitch L, Leroux T, Terry S, et al. Pregnancy and obstetrical outcomes in pseudoxanthoma elasticum. *Br J Dermatol.* 2004;151:1011–1018.

32. Chetty SP, Shaffer BL, Norton ME. Management of pregnancy in women with genetic disorders, Part 1: Disorders of the connective tissue, muscle, vascular, and skeletal systems. *Obstet Gynecol Surv.* 2011;66(11):699–709.

33. Pepin M, Schwarze U, Superti-Furga A, et al. Clinical and genetic features of Ehlers-Danlos type IV, the vascular type. *N Engl J Med.* 2000;342:673–680.

34. Kamangar F, Shinkai K. Acne in the adult female patient: a practical approach. *Int J Dermatol.* 2012;51(10):1162–1174.

35. Krishnapillai R, Punnoose K, Angadi PV, et al. Oral pyogenic granuloma—a review of 215 cases in a South Indian Teaching Hospital, Karnataka, over a period of 20 years. *Oral Maxillofac Surg.* 2012;16(3):305–309.

36. Wu X, Groves F, McLaughlin C, et al. Cancer incidence patterns among adolescents and young adults in the United States. *Cancer Causes Control.* 2005;16:309–320.

37. Reintgen DS, McCarty KS Jr, Vollmer R, et al. Malignant melanoma and pregnancy. *Cancer.* 1985;55:1340–1344.

38. Driscoll M, Jorgensen C, Grant-Kels J. Does pregnancy influence the prognosis of malignant melanoma? *J Am Acad Dermatol.* 1993;29:619–630.

39. Broer N, Buonocore S, Goldberg C, et al. A proposal for the timing of management of patients with melanoma presenting during pregnancy. *J Surg Oncol.* 2012;106(1):36–40.

40. Cline M, Bailey-Dorton C, Cayelli M. Maternal infections: diagnosis and management. *Prim Care.* 2000;27:13–33.

41. Shrim A, Koren G, Yudin MH, et al.; Maternal Fetal Medicine Committee. Management of varicella infection (chickenpox) in pregnancy. *J Obstet Gynaecol Can.* 2012;34(3):287–292.

42. Lamont RF, Sobel JD, Carrington D, et al. Varicella-zoster virus (chickenpox) infection in pregnancy. *BJOG.* 2011;118(10):1155–1162.

43. Guerra B, Puccetti C, Cervi F. The genital herpes problem in pregnancy. *G Ital Dermatol Venereol.* 2012;147(5):455–466.

44. Hollier LM, Wendel GD. Third trimester antiviral prophylaxis for preventing maternal genital herpes simplex virus (HSV) recurrences and neonatal infection. *Cochrane Database Syst Rev.* 2008;(1):CD004946.

45. Park H, Lee SW, Lee IH, et al. Rate of vertical transmission of human papillomavirus from mothers to infants: relationship between infection rate and mode of delivery. *Virol J.* 2012;9:80.

46. Yang YG, Zou XB, Zhao H, et al. Photodynamic therapy of condyloma acuminata in pregnant women. *Chin Med J (Engl).* 2012;125(16):2925–2928.

47. Parveen N, Munir AA, Din I, et al. Frequency of vaginal candidiasis in pregnant women attending routine antenatal clinic. *J Coll Physicians Surg Pak.* 2008;18(3):154–157.

26 Substance-Related and Addictive Disorders in Pregnancy

James W. Van Hook

KEY POINTS

- Chemical dependence or abuse is not an uncommon complication of pregnancy.
- Abuse or addiction behaviors generally do not directly impair fertility. Behaviors associated with addiction or abuse may lead to unplanned pregnancy.
- Chemical use or addiction may lead to significant adverse effects on the mother and developing child.
- Addiction is a brain disorder.
- Treatment of addiction may be successful, although success is not a certainty.
- Substitution therapy improves overall outcome in pregnant opioid addicts.

BACKGROUND

Definition

- Table 26-1 lists common agents of abuse and addiction.
- Substance-related disorders:
  - A mental disorder resulting from use of a legal or illicit substance
  - Examples (partial list):
    - Alcohol
    - Tobacco
    - Sedative–hypnotics
    - Stimulants
    - Psychotropic agents
    - Over-the-counter medicines
- Background—diagnostic criteria:
  - Recently (2013), The American Psychiatric Association (APA) revised diagnostic categorization for what are now called Substance-Related and Addictive Disorders (1).
    - Dependence and abuse have been replaced with a vernacular that recognizes the dynamic spectrum of substance use disorders.
- Continuum Classification
  - Disorders based upon a number of individual criteria—basic list (more extensive criteria for specific diagnosis for a particular substance)
    - Tolerance—the need to use larger and larger amounts of the substance in order to obtain an effect
    - Withdrawal—adverse physical or psychological manifestations from discontinuation of the substance
    - Increased usage
    - Ineffective self-efforts to cut down on use
    - Drug-seeking behaviors (going to multiple pharmacies, theft of medication)
    - Important social, recreational, or occupational activities discontinued in order to consistently facilitate the use of the substance (abandonment of children, repeated loss of job)

Table 26-1	Common Drugs of Abuse and Addiction				
Agent	Classification	Effect	Physical dependence[a]	Psychological dependence[b]
Tobacco (nicotine)	Stimulant	Nicotinic adrenergic stimulation	Yes	Yes
Ethanol	CNS depressant	Mixed	Yes	Yes
Marijuana (cannabis)	Anxiolytic Hallucinogenic Antiemetic	Specific receptor	Uncertain	Yes
Cocaine (benzoylecgonine)	CNS and peripheral stimulant	Dopamine Norepinephrine	Yes	Yes
Amphetamine Methamphetamine	CNS and peripheral stimulant	Dopamine Norepinephrine	Yes	Yes
Methylenedioxy- methamphetamine (MDMA)	CNS and peripheral stimulant Hallucinogenic	Dopamine Norepinephrine Serotonin	No	Yes
Lysergic acid diethylamide (LSD)	Hallucinogenic	Serotonin	No	Uncertain
Opiates	CNS Depressant Analgesic	Endorphin	Yes	Yes

[a]Physical dependence, evidence suggestive of at least some physical effects or systems after abrupt discontinuation of chemical use.
[b]Psychological dependence, evidence suggestive of at least some desire of altered neurobehavior, or host neurochemistry after chronic use.
CNS, central nervous system
Data referenced in text.

- Continued use of substance despite known physical or mental problems resulting from the substance (smoking despite the diagnosis of emphysema, drinking in the face of hepatic cirrhosis)
- Specific diagnosis criteria for a particular substance should be specifically referenced through the Diagnostic and Statistical Manual of Mental Disorders.
- "Addiction" operationally implies loss of control and increased use of the agent(s) despite overwhelming reasons not to.
- Instead of classification as abuse or dependence, classification based upon severity:
  - Mild disease—presence of two to three criteria or symptoms
  - Moderate disease—presence of four to five symptoms
  - Severe disease—presence of six or more symptoms
- Environment and duration of remission are important.
  - Early remission—criteria for full diagnosis no longer present for 3 to 12 months
  - Sustained remission—criteria for full diagnosis no longer present for greater than 12 months
  - Specify if in a controlled environment (treatment facility, incarceration, etc.)
- Substance use disorder in pregnancy:
  - Involves substance abuse or dependence in the periods immediately prior to conception, during pregnancy, or postdelivery

Pathophysiology

- The pathophysiology of dependence is complex. Addiction, like other disease processes, requires the following interactions (2,3):
  - Agent or substance of abuse:
    ○ Availability of an agent may affect its use.
      - Cost may affect use habits (crack cocaine availability and cost reduced the financial burden necessary to be exposed to cocaine).
    ○ Societal influences:
      - Acceptability of social drinking makes alcohol widely available.
      - Negative implications of illegal use of drugs of abuse.
    ○ Psychoactive efficacy:
      - Greater pleasurable efficacy increases the addictive potential of an agent.
      - Onset of action and cerebral bioavailability.
        * Rapid onset of action and cerebral bioavailability increases the addictive potential of an agent (e.g., crack cocaine, intravenous fentanyl).
  - Host susceptibility
    ○ Genetic influences:
      - Genetic differences may exist with agent absorption, brain receptor susceptibility to the effects of an agent, or the remodeling of brain receptors caused by exposure to a substance.
    ○ Familial host vulnerability:
      - Chemical exposure.
    ○ Comorbidity with other psychiatric disorders has been shown to occur.
      - The cause-and-effect relationship between other psychiatric disorders and addiction is not fully established.
  - Environmental effect
    ○ Occupations that allow less structured exposure to a given substance may increase the likelihood of abuse or dependence (e.g., bartenders, anesthesiologists, those with solitary unstructured jobs, sex trade industry worker).
    ○ Peer group influences may affect exposure and choice of the agent.
      - An alcoholic spouse increases the chance that his or her mate is an alcoholic.
    ○ Cultural perspective and perceptions may affect the mechanisms of and types of substance exposure (4).
    ○ Social instability may increase both the population exposure to a substance and may reduce social disincentives to abuse or become dependent.
- Substance use and dependence in women often exhibit specific pathophysiologic manifestations:
  - Chemically dependent women are more likely to have other concurrent psychiatric diagnoses than women without addiction disorder (5).
  - Spousal abuse, domestic violence, and prostitution are seen more frequently in women with chemical dependence (6,7).
  - A smaller circulatory volume of distribution gives women, on average, a greater exposure, effect, and abuse liability than men given a similar substance use history (8).
    ○ The progression of addiction, with the inevitable deterioration of the dependent patient, frequently occurs much more rapidly in women than in men (9).

Epidemiology

- The prevalence of substance abuse or dependence during pregnancy is not precisely defined.
  - More than 10 years ago, the National Institute on Drug Abuse (NIDA) surveyed 2613 women (10).
    ○ 20.4% of women smoked cigarettes during pregnancy.

- ○ 18.8% of women used alcohol during pregnancy.
- ○ 5.5% of pregnant women used illicit drugs during pregnancy.
- A more recent assessment (11) of substance abuse among women during and after childbirth indicates
  - ○ Alcohol, tobacco, and illicit substance use was higher in nonpregnant adult women.
  - ○ Pregnancy use declines as pregnancy progresses.
  - ○ Resumption of intemperate use often occurs within the first 3 months after childbirth.
- Despite conventionally held wisdom to the contrary, socioeconomic and ethnic differences were not noted in at least one large study (12).
- Substance abuse and dependence disorders are more common in males than in females; however, trends in usage may be changing (13).
  - ○ In a recent survey of 12- to 17-year-olds, comparable rates of alcohol, tobacco, cocaine, and heroin use were found among males and females (14).
  - ○ Tobacco use during pregnancy for women 18 and 19 years of age was higher than that of any other age range (15).
  - ○ Adolescent girls and women greater than 35 years of age have greater rates of abuse and dependence on psychotherapeutic drugs than men (16).

EVALUATION
Laboratory Tests
- Drug screen testing
  - Most illicit substances and prescription drugs may be detected in maternal body fluids (16).
  - Factors affecting performance of testing include
    - ○ Volume of distribution and elimination of specific agents
      - – Ethanol is difficult to effectively screen for more than a few hours after ingestion, and urine testing is not reliable (17,18).
      - – Agent persistence makes marijuana and long-acting benzodiazepines detectable for several weeks after exposure.
    - ○ Tissue or body fluid analyzed
    - ○ Time from last exposure until testing performed
    - ○ Cumulative dose of agent ingested by host
    - ○ Performance characteristics of specific testing methodology
    - ○ Cross-positive results from legitimately administered substances (e.g., testing of the postoperative patient may demonstrate positive test results secondary to anesthetic or analgesic agents legitimately prescribed)
  - Drug screen testing involves several ethical and legal issues (19,20):
    - ○ Consent:
      - – Depending on the locale, general "consent for diagnosis and treatment" versus specific permission for drug testing may be required.
    - ○ Chain of custody issues (21):
      - – In most hospital emergency departments, clinical laboratories, or clinic reference labs, testing is evidentiary in a general sense (not unlike other hospital lab tests).
      - – Chain of custody testing generally implies specific relevance insofar as the legal system and employment are concerned.
    - ○ Chain of custody testing usually requires specific consent from the screened individual.
  - Clinical testing policy:
    - ○ Selective toxicology testing is the testing of patients based on an increased, perceived risk of abuse or dependence.
    - ○ Universal toxicology testing is blanket testing of all pregnant patients presenting for care.

○ Selective testing is less intrusive, while universal testing is more sensitive for detection in a mixed or less rigorously screened population.
○ Universal testing is more costly than selective testing.
• Types of drug testing:
  ○ Blood
  ○ Urine
  ○ Salivary
  ○ Hair
  ○ Amniotic fluid or meconium
    – May detect fetal exposure for some time after maternal exposure (22)

DIAGNOSIS
Clinical Manifestations
• The clinical diagnosis of addiction is made based upon diagnostic criteria previously described (refer to the definitions in the substance abuse and substance dependence sections).
• Frequently, substance abuse and substance dependence in women are seen in association with several other comorbid conditions and psychosocial cofactors (7):
• Domestic violence
• Poor general health
• Sexually transmitted diseases
• Sexual exploitation, maternal incest, or sexual victim history
• Obstetric conditions that may be associated with substance abuse or dependence include
  ○ Intrauterine growth restriction
  ○ Preterm labor or preterm birth
  ○ *Abruptio placentae*
• As evidenced by the broad socioeconomic prevalence of substance abuse and dependence in pregnancy:
  ○ Medical and social comorbidities often do not become clearly apparent until fairly late in the natural progression of addiction.
  ○ Behavioral signs or symptoms in the early-stage disease may be confused with other factors such as noncompliance with care.
• Continued tobacco use (smoking) during pregnancy, without apparent efforts to reduce use, is evident more frequently in those with other abuse or dependence disorders (11,22,23).
• Psychiatric comorbidity is seen more commonly in women than in men with the diagnosis of chemical abuse or dependence.
  ○ One in five women with alcohol abuse or dependence also fulfill the diagnostic criteria for depression (four times more common than in males) (22,24).
  ○ Anxiety disorders are the most common group of psychiatric disorders in women (7).
  ○ The most common psychiatric disorders in addicted pregnant women are personality—the diagnosis may not be accurate secondary to inherent inaccuracy in codiagnosis of addition and personality disorders (7,25).
  ○ Women with borderline personality disorder diagnosis frequently have an associated history of childhood or partner sexual trauma.
• For alcohol abuse and dependence assessment, several interview-based screens have been validated for use in pregnancy (26):
  ○ T-ACE (27)
    – *T*olerance
    – *A*nnoyed
    – Need to *c*ut down
    – *E*ye opener (morning drinking)

- o TWEAK (28)
  - – *T*olerance
  - – Others *w*orried about your drinking
  - – *E*ye opener
  - – *A*mnesia
  - – Need to (*K*) cut down
  - o NIAAA Questionnaire (Table 26-2) (29)
- General substance screening in pregnant women may not only identify addictive behavior but may also identify maternal at-risk behavior and fetal exposure–directed intervention.
  - o Use of the 4P + screen is a good general screen for all illicit substances (30).
  - o Composite scales that result in a screening profile score may be useful for screening in a diverse pregnant population (31).

TREATMENT
General Principles
- There are currently no singularly effective treatments for chemical dependence.
  - There are currently no Food and Drug Administration–approved pharmacologic treatments for chemical dependence in pregnancy.
    - o Medical treatment of chemical dependence during pregnancy involves the balancing of the known risks to the mother and fetus from the use of the agent, with the possible or unknown effects from use of a medication to treat detoxification or help manage recovery.
- Pregnancy notwithstanding, pharmacotherapy regimens are available for dependence disorders of the following agents:
  - o Alcohol
  - o Tobacco
  - o Narcotics (opiates)
- Detoxification and withdrawal management are different from recovery treatments.
  - o Detoxification and withdrawal treatment involves the short-term management of acute cessation of regular use of the agent of dependence.
    - – Detoxification is stopping the use of the agent of addiction.
  - o Recovery treatment involves initiation of the process of managing the addiction itself, with the goal of therapy being long-term abstinence from the use of the agent and elimination or reduction of the behaviors associated with the addiction.

Table 26-2	NIAAA Alcohol Dependence Screening Questionnaire
Question	**Score**
1. Do you drink?	1 point for Yes
2. Do you use drugs?	1 point for Yes
3. On average, how many drinks per week do you drink?	Men: 1 point if >14 drinks Women: 1 point if >7 drinks
4. What is the maximum number of drinks you have had on anyone occasion during the past month?	1 point for each of maximum number
Positive Score (at risk for abuse or addiction)	Men: >4 Women: >3

From National Institute on Alcohol Abuse and Alcoholism (NIAAA). *Helping patients with alcohol problems: a health practitioner's guide.* NIAAA, 2003.

- – Recovery treatment is increasing the likelihood of the dependent individual not wanting and not starting the use of the agent again.
- Because addiction is a medical–psychological–social disease, pharmacotherapy alone is rarely successful.
- Additional nonpharmacologic treatments of dependence disorders include
  - ○ Twelve-step programs
  - ○ Treatment of medical complications of addiction
  - ○ Treatment of psychiatric comorbidity
  - ○ Family therapy
- Detoxification and/or pharmacologic management of detoxification/withdrawal of the pregnant addict should generally be a multidisciplinary process, with comanagement by a(n)
  - ○ Obstetrician
  - ○ Addiction medicine specialist
  - ○ Maternal–fetal medicine specialist
  - ○ Medical specialist

ALCOHOL
Scope and Significance
- Maternal alcoholism ranks as one of the leading causes of newborn neurodevelopmental disorders (32).
  - Up to 1 in 500 live newborns meet the diagnostic criteria for Fetal Alcohol Syndrome (FAS) (33,34).
- More than 2.5 million women in the United States are estimated to be alcohol dependent (14).

Mechanism of Action
- The neurochemistry of alcohol intoxication and dependence is relatively complex and involves activation or modification of the following neurotransmitter pathways (35):
  - Gama-aminobutyric acid (GABA)
  - Serotonin
  - Dopamine
  - Norepinephrine
  - Endorphin (opioid)
  - Glutamate
- Seizure activity from alcohol withdrawal occurs due to chronic alcohol-induced up-regulation of excitatory neurotransmitters (36,37).
  - Delirium tremens (DTs) are the most serious manifestation of acute alcohol withdrawal.
    - ○ Risk of both maternal and fetal mortality may be appreciable from uncontrolled DTs.
    - ○ A major goal of alcohol withdrawal management is prevention of DTs.

Detoxification Treatment (22,35)
- Benzodiazepines are standard therapy for seizure prevention.
  - Long-acting agents generally perform better than do short-acting agents and may have a lower predilection for cross addiction.
  - The teratogenic effects of benzodiazepines are uncertain.
  - Benzodiazepines may themselves produce a withdrawal syndrome.
- Other medications used for acute withdrawal therapy include
  - Carbamazepine
  - Valproic acid
  - Clonidine

- Adjunctive management of detoxification includes
  - Nutritional therapy
  - Prevention of Wernicke encephalopathy (22,35,36) from administration of thiamine (100 mg IV) during initiation of treatment and as a continued supplement for several days thereafter

Recovery Pharmacotherapy
- Naltrexone
  - Opioid antagonist—attenuates opioid-mediated reinforcement initiated by alcohol consumption
  - Naltrexone nonpregnant subjects—reduces drinking associated with relapse—not as successful for maintenance of abstinence (38)
  - Limited data in pregnancy consistent with safety (39–41)
- Disulfiram
  - Induces physical illness with alcohol consumption via alcohol dehydrogenase inhibited production of excessive acetaldehyde metabolites.
  - Although data are not conclusive, disulfiram should probably not be used during pregnancy (13).

TOBACCO
Scope and Significance
- From 1990 to 2003, the rate of smoking reported by pregnant women decreased from 18.4% to 11% (23,42).
- Smoking is associated with several pregnancy-related risks (23):
  - Intrauterine growth delay
  - Abruptio placentae
  - Placenta previa
  - Ectopic pregnancy
  - Poor newborn outcome

Mechanism of Action
- The primary addictive agent in tobacco products is nicotine.
  - Delivery system chosen by the user offers ritualistic reinforcement of nicotine use.
- Nicotine's central nervous system (CNS) effects are complex (43).
  - At low doses, nicotine causes sympathetic activation (mild CNS stimulant).
  - At higher doses, ganglionic activation occurs and may produce mild anxiolytic effects.
  - Addictive reinforcement is mediated by both the low-dose stimulation and the high-dose reduction in anxiety.
  - Continued tobacco use (without attempts to quit or modulate consumption) may be indicative of increased risk of alcohol or illicit drug use during pregnancy (23).
- Dosing kinetics and reinforcement kinetics of nicotine are formidable (44).

Pharmacotherapy
- Nicotine substitution systems
  - Provide controlled dosing of nicotine without, or perhaps with less, ritualistic reinforcement.
  - Allow use of nicotine without harmful inhalation or ingestion of other components of tobacco (e.g., "tar," carbon monoxide, etc.).
  - Large-scale clinical trials not performed in pregnancy (23).
    - Short-term results not suggestive of hemodynamic effects in mother or fetus and found to demonstrate less overall total nicotine use (45)
    - Safety of use data not presently conclusive

○ Evidence still insufficient to show efficacy, although nicotine substitution in pregnancy is only therapy yet studied via a randomized controlled trial
- Efficacy of nicotine replacement (gum) evidenced by (46):
  ○ Small but significant increase in smoking cessation
  ○ Small but statistically significant increase in newborn birth weight
- If the nicotine patch is used, some suggest removing the patch at bedtime to reduce overall exposure of the fetus to nicotine (23).
- Bupropion
  - Adrenergic antidepressant that inhibits neuronal uptake of norepinephrine and dopamine.
    ○ Precise mechanism of action in smoking cessation not certain
  - Effectiveness (nonpregnant smokers)—approximately two and a half times more effective than nontreated controls after 1 year of initiation of abstinence (25% to 30% without tobacco use).
  - Effectiveness in pregnancy less well studied:
    ○ Ten of 22 smokers (45%) with successful abstinence in comparison to 14% in the control group (47)
  - Safety is not conclusively established in pregnancy.
    ○ One recent trial of 136 exposures to bupropion without increased rate of malformations (48)
  - Maternal side effects include (uncommon) risk of medication-induced seizures.

Other Treatments
- Brief intervention ("Ask, Advise, Assess, Assist, Arrange") may be somewhat effective in smoking cessation during pregnancy (49).
- Multiple resources are available via phone self-help lines and online (23).
  - http://www.surgeongeneral.gov/tobacco
  - http://www.americanlegacy.org

OPIATE (NARCOTICS)
Scope and Significance
- Although not as common as alcohol addiction, opiate addiction is a significant problem for both the mother and the unborn fetus.
- Opiate addiction may be through illicit use of prescription narcotics or use of heroin or other "street" narcotics, which is generally parenteral.
- Use of prescription narcotics and abuse/dependence are on the rise in the United States.
- Illicit use carries concomitant risks associated with how the drug is taken and high-risk behaviors associated with drug seeking.

Mechanism of Action
- Narcotics act centrally by binding opioid receptors that are present throughout the CNS (50).
  - Activation of endorphin psychoactive and analgesic pathways produces the euphoria associated with narcotic use.
  - Rebound from chronic administration-mediated receptor down-regulation induces withdrawal.
    ○ Alcohol withdrawal may be fatal while opioid withdrawal *feels* fatal to otherwise healthy adults (51).
    ○ Withdrawal in pregnancy may precipitate preterm labor (13).
    ○ A specific neonatal withdrawal syndrome may occur in newborns of opioid-dependent gravidas (25).

Detoxification Treatment
- It is very difficult for the opiate addict to abstain from narcotic use.
  - Most addicts who abstain after withdrawal return to illicit use of opiates within 1 year of initial discontinuation.
  - Pregnant narcotic (heroin) addicts have better outcomes if enrolled in structured methadone maintenance regimens than if treated via abstinence or drug reduction therapy (50,51).
  - The goal of detoxification treatment is usually to attenuate acute withdrawal by substitution of the addictive opiate of choice with an equivalent cross-tolerant dose of a medically controlled, long-acting narcotic.

Recovery Pharmacotherapy
- As mentioned previously, it is recommended that long-acting opioid agonists are used for maintenance treatment of opiate-dependent pregnant patients (see subsequent section on agents used).

Agents Used for Opiate Dependence Treatment
- Methadone
  - Long-acting opioid agonist receptor saturation attenuates withdrawal and pleasurable effects from use.
  - Most effective treatment for established narcotic addicts (50,51).
  - Use in pregnancy demonstrated to be effective.
  - Most authorities do not recommend discontinuation during pregnancy:
    - Fetal withdrawal risk present.
    - Maternal relapse occurs more frequently.
  - Formerly thought to produce a dose-related risk of neonatal addiction—association not currently thought to be clear secondary to increased relapse risk and use of street drugs and methadone together at lower doses (52,53).
  - Use and dose adjustment management should occur in conjunction with the addiction specialist.
    - Requirements may be increased during pregnancy—80 to 150 mg/d or higher is not uncommon.
  - Fetal effects and risk from methadone use during pregnancy difficult to discern from effects of other substance use or lifestyle risks from addiction (13)
- Buprenorphine
  - Buprenorphine is a mixed opioid agonist–partial antagonist used in the United States since 2002 as a treatment of opiate dependence (54).
  - Restrictions on use are far less than with methadone.
    - Goal of introduction of buprenorphine was to allow wider availability of treatment for narcotic addiction.
  - Patients may be started on buprenorphine de novo or converted from methadone.
    - Because buprenorphine is a mixed agonist–antagonist agent, patients on high doses of methadone (pure agonist) should not be converted to buprenorphine because of the risk of precipitation of withdrawal.
  - Some data show effectiveness of buprenorphine equivalent to methadone at dose-for-equivalent dose (55).
    - Neonatal withdrawal is possible, however.
    - Neonatal withdrawal possibly less likely.
    - Use during pregnancy should be in comanagement with an addiction specialist.

ADJUNCTIVE TREATMENT
Pharmacotherapy
- Many agents and medications are used for adjunctive therapy of addiction (35), management of complications, or treatment of comorbidities. Examples include, but are not limited to

- Clonidine—treatment of autonomic instability and/or hypertension
- Antidepressants—treatment of comorbid psychiatric diagnoses
- Mood stabilizers—treatment of comorbid psychiatric diagnoses
- Beta-adrenergic–blocking agents—treatment of hypertensive complications
- Adjunctive pharmacotherapy is not used to treat drug dependence directly. Rather, such treatments are for control of symptoms or for therapy of other conditions that may affect outcome.
- Use of adjunctive treatments during pregnancy must be determined on a case-by-case basis, with the balance of potential benefit of treatment with possible or unknown risk to the pregnancy or the mother.

Recovery Treatment

- Because addiction is a disease that results in "collateral damage" to one's family, friends, finances, employment, and spirituality, most feel that successful treatment of addiction requires whole person and family therapy for long-term success.
- Completion of predetermined recovery milestones appears to have a positive effect on duration of recovery (56).
- Women, and in particular, pregnant women, have faced difficulty in accessing long-term inpatient or outpatient comprehensive treatment for chemical dependence, albeit the current trend is one of increased specific availability of gender-sensitive treatments (57).
- As with many other diseases, an eventual desire to recover is crucial to long-term success.
  - Forced treatment (medical or legal) is generally not successful for long-term results (58).
- Because of the high social comorbidity associated with the pregnant dependent patient, multidisciplinary treatment for the addict and her family are necessary for success.
  - Despite the challenges inherent in the treatment of the pregnant addict, there is tremendous potential for creating positive influences on the lives of several people for each female addict who is successfully treated (the patient, her fetus, other family members). It is to society's advantage to increase the resources available to addicted pregnant patients.

Twelve-Step Program Recovery

- The prototype of 12-step recovery is Alcoholics Anonymous (AA) (59).
  - Empiric spirituality-based program of recovery.
    - Program started more than 70 years ago by a recently sober alcoholic stockbroker (Bill W.) and an alcoholic physician (Dr. Bob)
  - Only requirement for membership is "a desire to stop drinking."
    - No dues or fees required to participate
  - Twelve-step process is followed through use of sponsor, attendance at group meetings, and helping fellow alcoholics.
  - Program is available worldwide and is not religious based.
  - Information for health professionals on AA available (60).
  - Open gender meetings are the norm for AA, although women-only meetings are available.
- In addition to AA, 12-step programs are now present for many other chemical and social addictions. Examples include (but are not limited to)
  - Narcotics Anonymous
  - Cocaine Anonymous
  - Overeaters Anonymous
  - Debtors Anonymous
- Most medical treatment programs of addiction are based, at least in part, on a 12-step format.

- Efficacy of 12-step recovery programs for the treatment of chemical dependency in pregnancy has not been definitively studied.
  - In general, long-term participation in 12-step recovery is a positive predictor for long-term (frequently lifetime) recovery (61).

COMPLICATIONS

Fetal Alcohol Syndrome

- Alcohol is a known teratogen. Postnatal manifestations of prenatal maternal exposure to alcohol are characterized broadly as fetal alcohol effect(s) (FAE) (62).
- FAS is the most significant manifestation of maternal alcohol use in pregnancy.
- Complete expression of FAS is characterized by (63)
  - Intrauterine growth delay
  - Microcephaly
  - Micropthalmia
  - Neurobehavioral manifestations (mental retardation, developmental delay, etc.)
  - Dysmorphic facies:
    - Thin upper lip
    - Short palpebral fissures
    - Flattened philtrum and nasal bridge
- FAS is the leading preventable cause of mental retardation in the United States (64).
- Incomplete manifestation of FAS is subcharacterized as FAE (65).
  - Genetic and environmental factors appear to play a part in expression of FAS and FAE.
  - A safe threshold for alcohol consumption in pregnancy has not been established—it is recommended that women who are pregnant or who plan to become pregnant abstain from alcohol.
- Prenatal screening of the fetus for FAE or FAS is not generally possible—intrauterine growth delay may be a relatively nonspecific finding (or it may be caused by other comorbidities such as tobacco use or poor nutrition).

Effects of Tobacco Use in Pregnancy

- Effects on pregnancy from maternal smoking are far more pronounced than the apparent short-term maternal complications of use.
- Smoking during pregnancy increases the rate of the following complications (23,46,49):
  - Intrauterine growth delay
  - Abruptio placentae
  - Placenta previa and accreta
  - Spontaneous abortion
  - Preterm labor
  - Stillbirth—rate in smokers at 10 per 1000 (66)
  - Risk particularly increased in smoking women with concurrent pregnancy diagnosis of fetal intrauterine growth restriction
- Cigarette use during pregnancy does not appear to increase the risk of the following (13,67):
  - Congenital malformations (identifiable at birth)
  - Preeclampsia
    - May be a function or effect of smoking on gestational age at delivery (preterm birth)
- Possible postnatal effects of cigarette use during pregnancy (or postnatal exposure to the newborn from continued maternal use) may include
  - Increased risk of sudden infant death syndrome (68)
  - A possible association with neurodevelopmental outcome (69)
    - Postnatal outcome data may be confounded by other substance exposures.
- Perinatal effects from smoking may be attenuated in those who cannot stop during pregnancy by modulation (reduction) of use while pregnant (23).

- Intrauterine growth delay risk increased by 53% in those who smoked less than one pack per day as compared to 130% in those who smoked more than one pack per day (66).
- Patients should be advised to reduce use of tobacco during pregnancy even if they are unable to abstain completely.

Effects of Other Substances of Abuse or Dependence in Pregnancy

- Marijuana (Cannabis)
  - Marijuana is the most common illicit drug used in pregnancy (13).
  - Current evidence does not suggest an association with cannabis use and intrauterine growth delay, in the absence of concomitant tobacco use (70).
  - No consistent association with congenital malformation and maternal marijuana use in pregnancy.
  - Recent data may suggest an increased risk of childhood depression in children of prenatal cannabis users (71).
  - Additional investigation is needed to evaluate fetal risk from maternal marijuana use.
- Cocaine
  - Cocaine functions as a central and peripheral adrenergic agonists.
    - Vasoconstriction is a common feature.
    - Maternal morbidity and mortality are related to increased blood pressure and resulting cardiovascular, CNS, and uteroplacental effects from vasoconstriction, loss of autoregulation, and vascular bed ischemia.
  - Cocaine in powdered, injectable, or inhaled ("crack") delivery systems is a powerfully addictive substance.
    - Principle active ingredient of cocaine is benzoylecgonine.
    - In those who chronically use cocaine during pregnancy, accumulation of the drug occurs in the fetal compartment (72).
      - Cocaine's pK_a is alkaline, so the lower fetal pH enhances concentration in the fetal compartment.
      - Demethylation metabolism, which occurs in the liver, is much slower in the fetus due to hepatic immaturity.
  - Short-term pregnancy effects from maternal cocaine use include (73)
    - Increased perinatal mortality
    - Preterm labor
    - Preeclampsia
    - Abruptio placentae
    - Fetal cerebral hemorrhage (74)
    - Increased risk of spontaneous abortion
  - Teratogenic risk from maternal cocaine use is less clear and may be related to the cocaine itself or correlates of cocaine use (64).
  - Postdelivery developmental effects on the offspring of pregnant women who used cocaine during pregnancy are not as clearly defined as once thought.
    - Many authorities feel that previously observed cocaine-induced effects on childhood neurodevelopmental performance may be related to fetal exposure to chaotic environmental influences during childhood or prenatal alcohol or tobacco use in conjunction with illicit cocaine use (75,76).
    - Definitive data on offspring effects from prenatal cocaine exposure are not presently conclusive.
- Methamphetamines and other related CNS stimulants:
  - Although the receptor-mediated mechanism of action is different than with cocaine, other CNS stimulants produce similar effects and maternal risk profiles.

- Crystal methamphetamine ("ice" or "crank") is a rapidly growing drug of addiction or abuse.
- Direct fetal risks from maternal CNS stimulant use in pregnancy are similar to those risks found with cocaine use (77).
- Data are presently inconclusive regarding long-term neurodevelopmental or teratogenic effects from noncocaine CNS stimulants (78).
- Hallucinogenic agents:
  - Lysergic acid diethylamide (LSD), psilocybin, peyote (mescaline), and phencyclidine (PCP) do not demonstrate consistent newborn or developmental effects in offspring of reported users (79).
  - PCP and MDMA may exhibit appreciable sympathomimetic or anticholinergic effects—fetal risk is at least potentially similar to other CNS stimulants (80).
    - Maternal risk from MDMA use may include anticholinergic crisis and dehydration.
  - Conclusive data regarding pregnancy-related risk from the use of hallucinogens are lacking.
  - MDMA use during pregnancy is associated with differences in 1 year of life neurodevelopmental scores in exposed offspring (81).
- Volatile solvents and inhalants:
  - Inhalation of industrial solvents are associated with a variety of teratogenic and fetal neurodevelopmental effects (82,83).
    - Maternal and/or fetal hypoxia, electrolyte disturbances, and heart rate abnormalities may occur as a result of solvent inhalation.
    - Long-term maternal hepatic or CNS dysfunctions are tragic consequences of chronic solvent inhalation.
    - A particular toluene embryopathy has been described in the offspring of pregnant women who inhaled the agent during gestation.
      - The effects are similar to those seen with FAS—embryologic pathophysiology appears to be similar (84).
- Dextromethorphan (DM):
  - DM is a common ingredient in over the counter cough and cold remedies.
  - In supernormal doses, DM has become popular as a "club drug" of abuse.
  - Euphoric effects of DM are similar to MDMA.
  - Ingestion of a recreational dose of DM may lead to significant metabolic consequences (85)
    - Acid–base disorders
    - Autonomic instability
    - Seizures
  - Inconclusive data regarding normal (nonrecreational) use of DM in pregnancy are not suggestive of a consistent pattern of malformations (86).
  - Data on the recreational use of DM during pregnancy are limited.

PATIENT EDUCATION

- Provider recognition and discussion of substance use and chemical dependence are crucial to both moderation of abusive use and self-recognition of addiction by the dependent patient.
- Brief intervention may be effective in abuse and low level dependence of alcohol.
- Smoking intervention (previously described) and resources enhance the medical treatment of smoking cessation.
- Several US government and other foundation resources are available to patients wanting more information about substance abuse/addiction and to those who wish to cease addictive behavior (Table 26-3).

Table 26-3	Resources for Patients
Smoking	Surgeon General U.S. Department of Health and Human Services http://www.surgeongeneral.gov/tobacco/prenatal.pdf 800-358-9295. American Legacy Foundation http://www.americanlegacy.org/866-66-START
Alcohol	National Institute on Alcohol Abuse and Alcoholism (NIAAA) http:\\www.niaaa.nih.gov/faqs/general-english/default.htm http:\\www.thecoolspot.gov
Illicit substances	National Institute on Drug Abuse (NIDA) http:\\www.nida.nih.gov/students.html
Twelve-step recovery	Alcoholics Anonymous http:\\www.alcoholics-anonymous.org Narcotics Anonymous http:\\www.na.org Cocaine Anonymous http:\\www.ca.org

REFERENCES

1. American Psychiatric Association. *Diagnostic and statistical manual of mental disorders*. 5th ed. DSM-V. Washington, DC: American Psychiatric Association, 2013.
2. Leshner AI. Science-based views of drug addiction and its treatment. *JAMA*. 1999; 282:1314–1316.
3. Barthwell AG, Brown L. The treatment of drug addiction: an overview. In: Ries RK, Fiellin DA, Miller SC, et al., eds. *Principles of addiction medicine*. 4th ed. Philadelphia: Lippincott Williams & Wilkins, 2009:349–360.
4. Vaillant GE. *Natural history of alcoholism revisited*. Cambridge: Harvard University Press, 1995.
5. Kessler RC, McGonagle KA, Zhao S, et al. Lifetime and 12 month prevalences of DSM IIIR psychiatric disorders in the United States. *Arch Gen Psychiatry*. 1994;52:1048–1060.
6. Rand MR, Strom K. *Violence-related injuries treated in hospital emergency departments*. (Bureau of Justice Statistics Special Report NCJ-156921). Washington, DC: Bureau of Justice, 1997.
7. Zweben JE. Special issues in treatment: women. In: Rice RK, Fiellin DA, Miller SC, et al., eds. *Principles of addiction medicine*. 4th ed. Philadelphia: Lippincott Williams & Wilkins, 2009:465–478.
8. Mumenthaler MS, Taylor JL, O'Hara R, et al. Gender differences in moderate drinking effects. *Alcohol Res Health*. 1999;23:55–64.
9. National Institute on Alcohol Abuse and Alcoholism. *10th Special Report to the U.S. Congress on Alcohol and Health*. Rockville: U.S. Department of Health and Human Services, 2000.
10. Office of Applied Studies. *Substance use among women during pregnancy and following childbirth*. NSDUH Report. Rockville: Substance Abuse and Mental Health Services Administration, 2009.
11. National Institute on Drug Abuse. *Topics in brief: prenatal exposure to drugs of abuse—May 2011*. (National Institute on Drug Abuse web site). Rockville: U.S. Department of Health and Human Services, 2011. Available at: http://www.drugabuse.gov/publications/topics-in-brief/prenatal-exposure-to-drugs-abuse. Accessed April 03, 2013.
12. Chasnoff IJ, Landress HJ, Barrett ME. The prevalence of illicit drug or alcohol use during pregnancy and discrepancies in mandatory reporting in Pinellas County, Florida. *N Engl J Med*. 1990;322:1202–1206.
13. Rayburn WF, Bogenschutz MP. Pharmacotherapy for pregnant women with addictions. *Am J Obstet Gynecol*. 2004;191:1885–1897.

14. Substance Abuse and Mental Health Services Administration. *Summary of findings from the 2000 National Household Survey on Drug Abuse. Publication SMA 01-3549.* Rockville: U.S. Department of Health and Human Services, 2001.

15. National Center for Health Statistics. *Health, United States, 2004: with chart book on trends in the health of Americans.* Hyattsville: National Center for Health Statistics, 2004. Available at: http://www.cdc.gov/nchs/data/hus/hus04.pdf. Accessed October 16, 2005.

16. American Congress of Obstetricians and Gynecologists. *Nonmedical use of prescription drugs.* ACOG Committee Opinion No. 538. American Congress of Obstetricians and Gynecologists, 2012.

17. Verstraete A. Detection times of drugs of abuse in blood, urine, and oral fluid. *Ther Drug Monit.* 2004;26:200–205.

18. Maurer H. Position of chromatographic techniques in screening for detection of drugs forensic toxicology and/or doping control. *Clin Chem Lab Med.* 2004;42:1310–1324.

19. Willette R. The role of the substance abuse professional. In: Graham A, Schultz T, Mayo-Smith M, et al., eds. *Principles of addiction medicine.* 3rd ed. Chevy Chase: American Society of Addiction Medicine, 2003:993–1000.

20. American Congress of Obstetricians and Gynecologists. *Substance abuse reporting and pregnancy: the role of the obstetrician-gynecologist.* ACOG Committee Opinion No. 473. American Congress of Obstetricians and Gynecologists, 2011.

21. Erlich L. *A textbook of forensic addiction medicine and psychiatry.* Springfield: Charles C. Thomas, 2001.

22. Wunsch MJ, Weaver MF. Alcohol and other drug use during pregnancy: management of the mother and child. In: Ries RK, Fiellin DA, Miller SC, et al., eds. *Principles of addiction medicine.* 4th ed. Philadelphia: Lippincott Williams & Wilkins, 2009:1111–1124.

23. American Congress of Obstetricians and Gynecologists. *Smoking cessation during pregnancy.* ACOG Committee Opinion No. 316. American Congress of Obstetricians and Gynecologists, 2005.

24. Sonderregger T. *Perinatal substance abuse.* Baltimore: Johns Hopkins University Press, 1992.

25. Hoegerman G, Schnoll SH. Narcotic use in pregnancy. *Clin Perinatol.* 1991;18:51–76.

26. American Congress of Obstetricians and Gynecologists. *At-risk drinking and illicit drug use: ethical issues in obstetric and gynecologic practice.* ACOG Committee Opinion No. 294. American Congress of Obstetricians and Gynecologists, 2004.

27. Sokol RJ, Martier SS, Ager JW. The T-ACE questions: practical prenatal detection of risk drinking. *Am J Obstet Gynecol.* 1989;160:863–868.

28. Chan AW, Pristach EA, Welte JW, et al. Use of the TWEAK test in screening for alcoholism/heavy drinking in three populations. *Alcohol Clin Exp Res.* 1993;17:1188–1192.

29. National Institute on Alcohol Abuse and Alcoholism (NIAAA). *Helping patients with alcohol problems: a health practitioners guide.* Rockville: U.S. Department of Health and Human Services, 2003.

30. Chasnoff IF, Wells AM, McGourty RF, et al. Validations of the 4P's Plus screen for substance use in pregnancy validation of the 4P's Plus. *J Perinatol.* 2007;12:744–748.

31. Yonkers KA, Gotman N, Kershaw T, et al. Screening for prenatal substance use: development of the substance use risk profile-pregnancy scale. *Obstet Gynecol.* 2010;116:827–833.

32. Hoyme HE, May PA, Kalberg WO, et al. A practical clinical approach to diagnosis of fetal alcohol spectrum disorders: clarification of the 1996 Institute of Medicine criteria. *Pediatrics.* 2005;115:39–47.

33. Bertrand J, Floyd LL, Weber MK. Guidelines for identifying and referring persons with fetal alcohol syndrome. *MMWR Recomm Rep.* 2005;54(RR-11):1–14.

34. May PA, Gossage JP. Estimating the prevalence of fetal alcohol syndrome: a summary. *Alcohol Res Health.* 2001;25:159–167.

35. Hillemacher T. Biologic mechanisms in alcohol dependence—new perspectives. *Alcohol Alcohol.* 2011;46:224–230.

36. Gordon AJ. *Physical illness and drugs of abuse. A review of the evidence.* Nyack, NY: Cambridge University Press, 2010.

37. Kumar N. Neurologic presentation of nutritional deficiencies. *Neurol Clin.* 2010;28:107–170.

38. Gastfriend DR. Intramuscular extended release naltrexone. Current evidence. *Ann N Y Acad Sci.* 2011;1216:144–166.

39. Hulse GK, O'Neill G, Pereira C, et al. Obstetric and neonatal outcomes associated with maternal naltrexone exposure. *Aust N Z J Obstet Gynaecol.* 2001;41:424–428.

40. Hulse GK, Arnold-Reed DE, O'Neil G. Naltrexone implant and blood naltrexone levels over pregnancy. *Aust N Z J Obstet Gynaecol.* 2003;43:386–388.

41. Jones HE. Acceptance of naltrexone by pregnant women enrolled in comprehensive drug addiction treatment: an initial survey. *Am J Addict.* 2012;21:199–201.

42. Hamilton BE, Martin JA, Sutton PD. Births: preliminary data for 2003. Centers for Disease Control and Prevention, National Center for Health Statistics. *National Vital Stat Rep.* 2004;53(a):1–17.

43. Harmey D, Griffin PR, Keney PJ. Development of novel pharmacotherapeutics for tobacco dependence: progress and future directions. *Nicotine Tob Res.* 2012;14:1300–1318.

44. Wynn WP III, Stroman RT, Almgren MM, et al. The pharmacist "toolbox" for smoking cessation: a review of methods, medicines, and novel means to help patients along the path of smoking reduction to smoking cessation. *J Pharm Pract.* 2012;(6):591–599.

45. Oncken CA, Hatsukami DK, Lupo VR, et al. Effects of short-term use of nicotine gum in pregnant smokers. *Clin Pharmacol Ther.* 1996;59:654–661.

46. Coleman T, Chamberlain C, Davey MA, et al. Pharmacological interventions for promoting smoking cessation during pregnancy. *Cochrane Database Syst Rev.* 2012;(9):CD010078.

47. Chan B, Einarson A, Koren G. Effectiveness of Bupropion for smoking cessation during pregnancy. *J Addict Dis.* 2005;24:19–23.

48. Chun-Fai-Chan B, Koren G, Fayez I, et al. Pregnancy outcome of women exposed to Bupropion during pregnancy: a prospective comparative study. *Am J Obstet Gynecol.* 2005;192:932–936.

49. Fiore MC, Bailey WC, Cohen SJ, et al. *Treating tobacco use and dependence. Clinical practice guideline.* Rockville: U.S. Department of Health and Human Services, Public Health Service, 2000.

50. Rahimi-Movaghar A, Amin-Esmaeili M, Hefazi M, et al. Pharmacological therapies for maintenance treatments of opium dependence. *Cochrane Database Syst Rev.* 2013;(1):CD007775.

51. National Consensus Development Panel on Effective Medical Treatment of Opiate Addiction. Effective medical treatment of opiate addiction. *JAMA.* 1998;280:1936–1943.

52. Sharp C, Kuschel C. Outcomes of infants born to mothers receiving methadone for pain management in pregnancy. *Arch Dis Child Fetal Neonatal Ed.* 2004;89:33–36.

53. Berghella V, Lim P, Hill M, et al. Maternal methadone dose and neonatal withdrawal. *Am J Obstet Gynecol.* 2003;189:312–317.

54. U.S. Department of Health and Human Services. Substance abuse and mental health services administration center for substance abuse treatment. *Buprenorphine.* Rockville: U.S. Department of Health and Human Services, 2005. Available at http://buprenorphine.samhsa.gov/about.html. Accessed October 30, 2005.

55. Jones HE, Kaltenbach K, Heil SH, et al., Neonatal abstinence syndrome after methadone or buprenorphine exposure. *N Engl J Med.* 2010;363:2320–2331.

56. Greenfield L, Burgdorf K, Xiaowu C, et al. Effectiveness of long term residential substance abuse treatment for women: findings from three national studies. *Am J Drug Alcohol Abuse.* 2004;30:537–550.

57. Grella C, Greenwell L. Substance abuse treatment for women: changes in the setting where women received treatment and types of services provided, 1987—1998. *J Behav-Health Serv Res.* 2004;31:367–383.

58. Jones H, Svikis D, Rosado J, et al. What if they do not want treatment? Lessons learned from intervention studies of non-treatment-seeking, drug-using pregnant women. *Am J Addict.* 2004;13:342–357.

59. Alcoholics Anonymous. *Alcoholics Anonymous.* 4th ed. New York: Alcoholics Anonymous World Service, Inc., 2002.

60. Alcoholics Anonymous. *AA as a resource for the medical profession.* New York: Alcoholic Anonymous World Service, Inc., 1982.

61. McCrady B, Tonigan S. Recent research into twelve step programs. I. In: Ries RK, Fiellin DA, Miller SC, et al., eds. *Principles of addiction medicine.* 4th ed. Philadelphia: Lippincott Williams & Wilkins, 2009:923–938.

62. Pruett D, Waterman EH, Caughey AB. Fetal alcohol exposure: consequences, diagnosis and treatment. *Obstet Gynecol Surv.* 2013;68:62–69.

63. Jones KL, Smith DW. Recognition of the fetal alcohol syndrome in early infancy. *Lancet.* 1973;302:999–1001.

64. Pagliaro L, Pagliaro A. Drugs as human teratogens and fetotoxins. In: Pagliaro L, Pagliaro A, eds. *Problems in pediatric drug therapy.* 4th ed. Washington: American Pharmaceutical Association, 2002.

65. Smitherman C. The lasting impact of fetal alcohol syndrome and fetal alcohol effect on children and adolescents. *J Pediatr Health Care.* 1994;8:121–126.

66. ACOG Practice Bulletin No. 102: management of stillbirth. *Obstet Gynecol.* 2009;113(3):748–761.

67. Hammoud AO, Bujold E, Sorokin Y, et al. Smoking in pregnancy revisited: findings from a large population-based study. *Am J Obstet Gynecol.* 2005;192:1856–1862.

68. Wisborg K, Kesmodel U, Henriksen TB, et al. A prospective study of smoking during pregnancy and SIDS. *Arch Dis Child.* 2000;83(3):203–206.

69. Clifford A, Lang L, Chen R. Effects of maternal cigarette smoking during pregnancy on cognitive parameters of children and young adults: a literature review. *Neurotoxicol Teratol.* 2012;34:560–570.

70. English D, Hulse GK, Milne E, et al. Maternal cannabis use and birth weight: a meta-analysis. *Addiction.* 1997;92:1553–1560.

71. Gray K, Day N, Leech S, et al. Prenatal marijuana exposure: effect on child depressive symptoms at ten years of age. *Neurotoxicol Teratol.* 2005;27:439–448.

72. Scanlon J. The neuroteratology of cocaine: background, theory, and clinical implications. *Reprod Toxicol.* 1991;5:89–98.

73. Cain MA, Bormick P, Whiteman V. The maternal, fetal, and neonatal effects of cocaine exposure in pregnancy. *Clin Obstet Gynecol.* 2013;56:124–132.

74. Gieron-Korthals M, Hedal A, Martinez C. Expanding spectrum of cocaine induced central nervous system malformations. *Brain Dev.* 1994;16:253–256.

75. Messinger D, Bauer C, Das A, et al. The maternal life type study: cognitive, motor, and behavioral outcomes of cocaine-exposed and opiate-exposed infants through three years of age. *Pediatrics.* 2004;113:1677–1685.

76. Mansoor E, Morrow CE, Accomero VH, et al. Longitudinal effects of prenatal cocaine use on mother-child interactions at ages 3 and 5 years. *J Dev Behav Pediatr.* 2012;33(1):32–41.

77. Pagliaro A, Pagliaro L. *Substance use among women.* Philadelphia: Brunner/Mazel, 2000.

78. Wouldes T, LaGasse L, Sheridan J, et al. Maternal methamphetamine use during pregnancy and child outcome: what do we know? *NZ Med J.* 2004:U1180.

79. Pagliaro L. Pharmacopsychology updates: psychotropic teratogens. *Psymposium.* 1995;6:18–19.

80. Tabor B, Smith-Wallace T, Yonekura M. Perinatal outcome associated with PCP versus cocaine use. *Am J Drug Alcohol Abuse.* 1990;16:337–348.

81. Singer LT, Moore DG, Min MO, et al. One year outcomes of prenatal exposure to MDMA and other recreational drugs. *Pediatrics.* 2012;130:407–413.

82. Hannigan JH, Bowen SE. Reproductive toxicology and teratology of abused toluene. *Syst Biol Reprod Med.* 2010;56:184–200.

83. Arnold G, Kirby R, Langendoerfer S. Toluene embryopathy: clinical delineation and developmental follow-up. *Pediatrics.* 1994;93:216–220.

84. Pearson MA, Hoyme H, Seaver L, et al. Toluene embryopathy: delineation of the phenotype and comparison with fetal alcohol syndrome. *Pediatrics.* 1994;93:211–215.

85. Forrester MB. Dextromethorphan abuse in Texas, 2000–2009. *J Addict Dis.* 2011;30:243–247.

86. Martinez-Frias M, Rodriguez-Pinilla E. Epidemiologic analysis of prenatal exposure to cough medicines containing dextromethorphan: no evidence of human teratogenicity. *Teratology.* 2001;63:38–41.

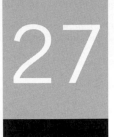

Gynecologic Complications

Kellie Flood-Shaffer

KEY POINTS

- Pregnancy does not prevent or protect a woman from developing common gynecologic problems and complications.
- Untreated gynecologic problems can adversely affect obstetric care and exacerbate obstetric complications.
- Treatment of gynecologic problems is frequently the same for the pregnant and the nonpregnant patient with some notable exceptions.

EXTERNAL GENITALIA

Careful inspection of the external genitalia before pregnancy, as well as at the initial prenatal visit, is crucial to the patient's health. Counseling about the signs and symptoms of external genital infections, as well as the risks of transmission with exposure to infectious organisms, should also be discussed.

Bartholin Abscess

Background
- Bartholin cysts are a common occurrence in the reproductive age female, and pregnancy can exacerbate their symptoms.
- Although asymptomatic cysts need not necessarily be treated, an abscess of the Bartholin gland usually requires immediate treatment.

Diagnosis
- A Bartholin gland abscess typically causes significant pain and inflammation. The diagnosis can often be made based solely on the patient's complaints.
- Patients will complain that they feel a large tender "bump" on their labia and have severe pain with standing, walking, or sitting.
- Although the symptoms are fairly classic, a thorough examination and evaluation must be performed (1,2).

Treatment
- Drainage via an incision on the mucosal side of the gland is appropriate when the area is fluctuant. Otherwise, warm sitz baths are recommended until the abscess is ready for drainage.
- Cultures obtained at the time of initial drainage are useful, as gonococcus is often the etiologic agent, and when suspected, antibiotics are appropriate.
- Once the abscess is incised, a Word catheter is placed for 4 to 6 weeks to allow adequate epithelialization of a drainage tract. Packing the incised abscess pocket with narrow gauze is also acceptable.
- Recurrent infection or development of recurrent symptomatic cysts warrants subsequent marsupialization (surgical exteriorization of the cyst for drainage). Removal of the gland is not recommended in pregnancy and should be deferred until the puerperium is complete.

Human Papillomavirus and Condylomata Acuminata
Background
- Condylomata acuminata or genital warts are very common in both men and women.
- They are caused by the human papillomavirus (HPV) of which there are more than 100 subtypes. More than 40 of these subtypes can infect the genital area. Genital warts are usually caused by HPV types 6 and 11 (3,4).
- Reinfection and persistent infection are common.

Diagnosis
- Condyloma acuminatum has a classic "cauliflower-like" appearance and can protrude from the skin on stalks. The lesions appear fleshy and may cause some minor itching but are not painful.
- The clinician must clinically distinguish the very common condylomata acuminata (genital warts) from the *rare, wart-like growths* of condyloma latum, which is caused by *Treponema pallidum* (1,2).
- During pregnancy, genital warts may proliferate, rapidly enlarge, and become friable and can obstruct the vaginal canal.
- HPV, in rare cases, may be transmitted to the newborn, resulting in laryngeal papillomas with respiratory complications. However, delivery by cesarean section is not indicated to prevent fetal intrapartum exposure.

Treatment
- Outpatient treatment of genital warts during pregnancy can be safely achieved by
  - Cryotherapy (liquid nitrogen application or nitrous oxide cryoprobe).
  - Carbon dioxide laser therapy.
  - Topical application of 50% to 80% trichloroacetic acid solution.
  - Imiquimod cream has been used with some success but should be used with caution and only when benefits outweigh risks, as it is a category C drug in pregnancy and may be associated with fetal toxicity.
- Podophyllin, podofilox, and sinecatechins are currently not advised for use in pregnancy because of the risks of birth defects, fetal death, stillbirth, and maternal toxicity.
- Removal of condyloma via electrocautery or laser therapy is an alternative that may require general or regional anesthesia (see Chapter 3).
- Both cryotherapy and carbon dioxide laser therapy appear to be highly effective when used to treat condyloma in pregnancy, with no significant fetal, neonatal, or maternal morbidity.
- The recurrence rate of genital warts appears to be the lowest when treated in the third trimester.
- Genital warts are not considered an indication for cesarean delivery unless they are so large as to constitute physical obstruction or significant risk for vaginal/cervical lacerations.
- There are currently two U.S. Food and Drug Administration (FDA)–approved vaccines shown to be effective in preventing HPV infection in adolescents and young adults. Inadvertent administration of these vaccines during pregnancy has shown no harmful fetal effect, but women with known pregnancy should not be vaccinated (3).

Genital Herpes Simplex (See Chapter 23)
VAGINITIS (5)
Background
- Vaginal infections are among the most common reasons for urgent gynecologic office visits.
- Speculum examination and microscopic study are essential in the evaluation of pregnant women complaining of vaginal discharge. Both physiologic secretions and rupture of membranes may be misdiagnosed as vaginitis.

- Although most vaginal infections are easily treated, these infections may be associated with more serious obstetric complications such as maternal and neonatal infection, preterm premature rupture of membranes (PPROM), or preterm labor.

Candidiasis
Background
- Candida accounts for approximately 35% of vaginal infections. However, a "yeast infection" is not a sexually transmitted disease. It is a result of the overgrowth of fungal organisms that are present in the normal vaginal flora.
- The most common fungal organism is *Candida albicans*. Other important pathogens include *Monilia*, *Candida tropicalis*, and *Candida glabrata*.
- Several factors may predispose a patient to vaginal candidiasis including pregnancy, diabetes, immunosuppressive disorders, use of oral contraceptives or oral corticosteroids, or recent use of broad-spectrum antibiotics.

Diagnosis
- Typical symptoms include itching, burning, dysuria, an erythematous vulva, and curd-like ("cottage cheese") discharge, which tends to adhere to the vaginal mucosa. The vaginal pH remains normal at less than 4.2. The vulva and groin may also exhibit "satellite lesions" or erythematous papules that often cause intense pruritus.
- Confirmation of the diagnosis is made with the microscopic observation of hyphae and budding yeast in a 10% potassium hydroxide wet preparation.
- Pregnant women, especially those previously infected, are at increased risk for candida vulvovaginitis. The signs, symptoms, and method of diagnosis are the same as for the nonpregnant patient.

Treatment
- Clotrimazole and miconazole nitrate topical (intravaginal) treatments are more effective than is nystatin and require fewer treatment days. Because small amounts of these drugs may be absorbed from the vagina, they should be used with caution in the first trimester. Topical azole treatments, applied for 7 days, are the first line for symptomatic candidiasis in pregnancy.
- Fluconazole oral medication has been used anecdotally in pregnancy, but caution should be exercised with benefits outweighing risks as it is also a category C drug in pregnancy.

Trichomoniasis
Background
- Trichomoniasis accounts for approximately 20% to 25% of vaginal infections. The causative agent is the protozoan *Trichomonas vaginalis*.
- Trichomoniasis is a highly contagious, sexually transmitted infection and is more often seen in young, single patients with multiple sexual partners.
- There is evidence that *T. vaginalis* has been associated with obstetric complications (6).

Diagnosis
- Typical signs and symptoms of this venereally transmitted protozoan include an often malodorous, frothy, yellow-green discharge accompanied by intense pruritus and dysuria.
- In 25% of cases, there may be red subepithelial abscesses and punctuate hemorrhages noted on the cervix and in the vaginal fornices giving the cervicovaginal epithelium a "strawberry" appearance.
- The diagnosis is confirmed microscopically with the observation of motile trichomonads in a wet preparation with normal saline. Vaginal pH is elevated, usually ≥4.5 (1).

Treatment
- Metronidazole is the preferred treatment for both the nonpregnant and the pregnant patient. It is administered as either

- Single 2-g oral dose or 250 mg orally three times daily for 7 to 10 days.
- Topical metronidazole is not recommended for treatment of trichomoniasis.
- The patient's partner(s) must be referred for treatment. One must suspect, with recurrent infections, that the patient's partner(s) has failed to receive therapy.
- Many studies have examined mother–infant pairs exposed to metronidazole throughout pregnancy with conflicting results.
  - Metronidazole is known to increase the fetotoxicity and teratogenicity of alcohol in mice, which may be a confounding factor in humans as well.
  - There are conflicting data regarding a potential increase in facial abnormalities in fetuses exposed to metronidazole in the first trimester. This has led to the recommendation by some experts that its use should probably be avoided early in gestation. Symptomatic treatment such as a dilute povidone–iodine douche or vaginal clotrimazole suppositories, therefore, may be helpful for the first-trimester patient. The Centers for Disease Control and Prevention (CDC), however, recommends that all symptomatic pregnant women with trichomoniasis should be considered for treatment regardless of stage of pregnancy (CDC Sexually Transmitted Treatment Guidelines, 2010; www.cdc.gov).
  - There are no data to date suggesting any poor outcomes from the use of metronidazole in the second and third trimesters. The manufacturer recommends against using single-dose therapy in pregnancy (1,6); however, CDC-recommended treatment is a single 2-g oral dose in pregnancy.

Bacterial Vaginosis
Background
- Previously named for the presence of *Gardnerella vaginalis,* bacterial vaginosis (BV) is now understood to be a polymicrobial vaginal infection resulting from the disruption of normal vaginal flora and is comprised of anaerobes, *Mobiluncus, Gardnerella,* and mycoplasma organisms.
- BV in pregnant women has been associated with preterm labor and delivery, PPROM, and maternal and neonatal infections; therefore, treatment is essential to a healthy pregnancy (7).

Diagnosis
- Typically, the patient complains of a profuse, thin, grayish-white, yellow, or greenish discharge with a fishy odor. Most patients complain that the odor is worse after intercourse, but they typically do not complain of pruritus. Vaginal pH is ≥4.5 (1,7).
- Microscopically, squamous cells studded with coccobacilli ("clue cells"), as well as a decrease or absence of lactobacilli, make this diagnosis.
- When vaginal secretions are mixed with a drop of 10% potassium hydroxide solution, the characteristic amine odor (spoiled fish) is released. This is the so-called whiff test and can also help to confirm the diagnosis.

Treatment
- Metronidazole, 250 mg orally three times daily or 500 mg orally twice daily for 7 days, is the most effective therapy. Ampicillin has been used with some success but is not recommended for first-line treatment.
- Clindamycin is effective but may be more expensive and may cause diarrhea. It may be used as an alternative first-line agent in place of metronidazole. The dose for treatment of BV in pregnancy is 300 mg orally twice daily for 7 days (CDC Sexually Transmitted Treatment Guidelines, 2010; www.cdc.gov).
- As noted previously, metronidazole may be avoided in the first trimester for asymptomatic patients. It is commonly recommended that symptomatic infections with BV should be treated in pregnancy because of its association with preterm labor and delivery and PPROM. Data are inconsistent regarding the benefit of treating asymptomatic cases of BV in pregnancy.

- Treatment of the sexual partner is not usually recommended but may be considered in recurrent or persistent infections (1,7).

CERVICAL DISEASES

Cervical Intraepithelial Neoplasia

Background

Pregnancy represents an opportunity to screen a wide range of women for preinvasive disease who might otherwise not seek routine exams. Abnormal cervical cytology is encountered in up to 3% of all pregnancies, with severe dysplasia present in 1.3 per 1000 pregnancies. The vast majority of all cervical dysplasias (greater than 99%) are directly associated with the HPV. The American Society for Colposcopy and Cervical Pathology (ASCCP) and American College of Obstetricians and Gynecologists (ACOG) have revised evaluation and treatment guidelines in 2013, and although there is not a large amount of data specific to pregnancy, these guidelines are the standard of care nationally (4,8,9).

Diagnosis

- Nonpregnant evaluation of abnormal cervical cytology in pregnancy differs little from that in the nonpregnant woman.
- The most notable exception in the 2013 ASCCP Treatment Guidelines is that LGSIL (low-grade squamous intraepithelial lesion) in pregnant women may be evaluated by colposcopy during pregnancy *or* colposcopy may be deferred to the postpartum period (4).
- Eversion of the transformation zone in the pregnant patient may make colposcopic examination of the cervix somewhat easier. If a lesion appears suspicious by presence of dense acetowhite changes, thickened edges, or the presence of atypical vessels, directed biopsies must be done to rule out invasive cancer.
- Endocervical curettage is omitted to avoid stimulation of prostaglandin release in the endocervical canal and the theoretical risk of spontaneous abortion in the first trimester or PROM (premature rupture of membranes) or PTL (preterm labor) in the second or third trimesters.
- Cone biopsies are not routinely performed in pregnancy because of the risks of spontaneous abortion and hemorrhage. Occasionally, a cone biopsy will be indicated if the full extent of the disease is not seen or if the directed biopsy shows microinvasion. When possible, the cone biopsy should be performed during the second trimester, when the risk for spontaneous abortion is less (10). A prophylactic cerclage may be placed immediately before the cone biopsy, both for assistance with hemostasis and prevention of cervical incompetence; however, there is considerable ongoing controversy as to the obstetric benefits of cerclage in this situation (4,9).

Cervical Cancer

Although invasive cervical carcinoma has become less prevalent as a result of cytologic screening and eradication of precursor lesions, a large percentage of women with the disease are of reproductive age.

- Cervical carcinoma is the most common gynecologic malignancy encountered during pregnancy, occurring in approximately 1 per 2200 pregnancies. Three percent of all cervical carcinomas occur during pregnancy (11).
- Pregnancy does not affect the growth of cervical cancer, and stage for stage, survival is the same as for nonpregnant women.
- HPV is known worldwide to be a carcinogen for cervical cancer (4,12).

Microinvasive Carcinoma

- Patients with microinvasive carcinoma (depth of penetration not greater than 3 mm) by cervical biopsy should have a cone biopsy performed to rule out frank invasion as well as possibly providing definitive therapy (10).

- Microinvasive carcinoma by cone biopsy with negative margins and no lymphovascular space invasion may be managed expectantly throughout the pregnancy with periodic Papanicolaou tests and colposcopic exams.
- Vaginal delivery can be planned, with cesarean delivery reserved for obstetric indications. Definitive treatment can then be pursued postpartum as indicated.

Invasive Cervical Carcinoma
Diagnosis
- The diagnosis is based on biopsy, either colposcopically directed or obtained directly from suspicious exophytic lesions. The diagnosis should be considered in any women with unexplained vaginal bleeding, especially if the bleeding occurs after sexual intercourse (11).

Treatment
- Treatment recommendations depend largely on the gestational age of the pregnancy at diagnosis.
  - For stage IB or IIA disease up to 20 weeks, the patient can be treated with radiation therapy (which usually results in a spontaneous abortion) or primary radical hysterectomy with pelvic lymphadenectomy (with the fetus left in situ or evacuated by hysterotomy at the time of the hysterectomy). Surgical therapy may be preferred, especially in younger women, in order to preserve ovarian function.
  - After 20 weeks, consideration may be given to several cycles of platinum-based chemotherapy, which has shown no adverse fetal effects in the treatment of patients with ovarian cancer (11), while time is gained to permit additional fetal maturation. The fetus can then be delivered by cesarean section, followed by radical hysterectomy with pelvic lymphadenectomy, or radiation therapy.
- Radiation therapy is recommended for stage IIB to IIIB disease, again dependent on the gestational age with regard to timing of delivery. After 24 weeks of gestation, steroid administration for fetal lung maturation may be undertaken followed by cesarean section prior to the start of radiation therapy. Ideally, if the health of the mother is not in jeopardy, prolonging the pregnancy as long as possible is preferred for best fetal outcome.
- Although no data have consistently shown an increased risk from vaginal delivery through a small stage I or II tumor, one multivariate analysis did find a trend toward worse outcomes after vaginal delivery (11,13). Implants of squamous and adenocarcinoma have also been reported in episiotomy scars.

DISEASE OF THE UTERUS
Abnormalities of Position
- **Anterior sacculation of the uterus**
  - Severe anteflexion of the uterus caused by poor abdominal muscle tone or diastasis recti in the late third trimester may result in abnormal presentation and lack of engagement of the presenting part. This abnormality is seen almost exclusively in the grand multiparous but is not uncommon in African American females.
  - Correction of the abnormal orientation of the fetus with abdominal pressure provided by a well-fitting girdle or other binding support may allow for more effective pushing in the second stage of labor.
- **Retroflexion**
  - Retrodisplacement of the uterus is common in early pregnancy, but the enlarging uterus nearly always assumes a more anteverted position by 12 weeks of pregnancy. Rarely, the retroflexed enlarging uterus may become incarcerated in the hollow of the sacrum, with resulting edema from venous obstruction, marked pain, and, notably, an inability to void because of urethral "kinking" and obstruction.

- Patients with an incarcerated, retroflexed uterus should be placed in the knee–chest position, and the anterior lip of the cervix should be grasped and pulled with a ring forceps. Simultaneously, the posterior surface of the uterus is pushed ventrally by exerting pressure through the posterior fornix. This procedure is painful and typically requires anesthesia.
- **Prolapse**
  - Complete prolapse of the uterus is rare in pregnancy. With partial prolapse, a ring (with or without support), Smith-Hodge, or Gellhorn pessary may provide relief of symptoms. The pessary should be removed and washed with mild soap and water daily to prevent infection.
- **Torsion of the uterus**
  - This rare complication of pregnancy is almost always associated with a pathologic condition of the uterus such as leiomyomata or adhesions from previous uterine surgery.
  - The clinical picture is that of an abdominal catastrophe, with severe abdominal pain or shock, and may be confused with the picture of abruptio placentae. The patient has acute abdominal findings and requires laparotomy. Detorsion may be attempted in early pregnancy. Cesarean section followed by hysterectomy is often required near term.
  - Fetal morality is very high, with maternal mortality as high as 50%.

Leiomyomata Uteri
Background

Uterine fibroid tumors are usually asymptomatic in pregnancy but may interfere with conception and may cause early spontaneous abortion. Later in gestation, they may predispose the fetus to abnormal presentation, obstruct labor, and occasionally lead to preterm labor, placental separation, or postpartum hemorrhage. Infarction or degeneration of fibroids may occur, leading to acute abdominal pain, often with fever, leukocytosis, and uterine tenderness.

Treatment

- Treatment for symptomatic uterine fibroids in pregnancy is limited to analgesics in most cases. Acute pain associated with degenerating fibroid may be treated with a short course of nonsteroidal antiinflammatory agent. Laparotomy is avoided unless the diagnosis is uncertain.
- Fibroid tumors that obstruct labor may necessitate cesarean section. The uterine incision may be difficult or impossible to repair in the presence of massive leiomyomata, and cesarean hysterectomy is occasionally necessary. Hysterectomy may also be indicated for intractable postpartum hemorrhage caused by submucous leiomyomata or severe uterine atony. Under these circumstances, typed and cross-matched blood is to be immediately available in the operating room.

DISEASE OF THE FALLOPIAN TUBE
Acute Salpingitis
Background
- Acute or chronic pelvic inflammatory disease (PID) is very rare in pregnancy.
- Other conditions are far more common and should be considered before a diagnosis of PID is entertained.
- When PID does occur during pregnancy, it is associated with a high risk for septic abortion or fetal loss; therefore, hospitalization for treatment is recommended (1,2).

Diagnosis
- The diagnosis is difficult to make and easily confused with other entities, such as appendicitis, torsion of the adnexa, threatened abortion, and ectopic pregnancy. All of these conditions should be excluded before considering a diagnosis of PID.
- Laparoscopy or laparotomy should be performed if the suspicion for appendicitis, torsion, or ectopic pregnancy is high.

- In many cases, infection may have been present before conception. One theory holds that pathogenic organisms may be able to ascend from the cervix to the upper tract early in pregnancy, contrary to the thought that the conceptus acts as a barrier to the development of salpingitis. The presence of gonococcus or *Chlamydia* should be confirmed by cervical culture.

Treatment

- PID during pregnancy should be treated with gentamicin and clindamycin to avoid potential fetal effects of the other treatment regimens recommended by the CDC.
- Gonococcal infections worldwide have become increasingly resistant to antibiotic therapy, and CDC guidelines should be regularly referenced for optimal therapeutic management (1).
- In subclinical disease, vaginal delivery puts the fetus at risk for contracting gonococcal or chlamydial ophthalmia or chlamydial pneumonia if the mother is not treated prior to delivery.

Torsion of the Fallopian Tube

Background

- Torsion of the fallopian tube has been described in pregnancy and should be included in the differential diagnosis of abdominal pain during pregnancy.
- The patient presents with pain, generally sudden in onset, located in the quadrant of the involved tube and perhaps radiating to the flank or thigh. Tenderness usually is present, but signs of peritoneal irritation are variable. Other symptoms include nausea, vomiting, and bladder or bowel irritability. Maternal temperature, white blood cell count, and erythrocyte sedimentation rate usually are normal or only slightly elevated.

Diagnosis

- Differential diagnosis includes
  - Torsion or degeneration of an ovarian cyst
  - Torsion or degeneration of a uterine leiomyoma
  - Ureteral or renal colic
  - Acute appendicitis
  - Placental abruption
  - Inflammatory peritoneal processes
  - Intraperitoneal bleeding

Treatment

- Therapy is surgical.
  - If the affected tube is beyond recovery, it is excised. There is no reason to remove a normal ovary.
  - If torsion is incomplete or recent, and if tissue distal to the torsion remains viable, detorsion of the tube with stabilization by suture may be considered.

DISEASES OF THE OVARIES

The Pelvic Mass in Pregnancy (14)

The most important issue in any woman with a pelvic mass is the possibility of a malignant ovarian neoplasm.

- Functional cysts are usually less than 8 cm in diameter and should resolve spontaneously by the beginning of the second trimester.
- Cystic masses of 8 cm or larger, smaller masses that increase in size or persist, and solid adnexal masses require surgical exploration, ideally in the early second trimester.
- Adnexal masses of any kind may precipitate torsion of the mass or the entire adnexa, resulting in acute symptoms and signs, which may be intermittent but may necessitate exploration either during pregnancy or in the puerperium.
- Rarely, ovarian masses may obstruct labor, making cesarean section necessary, at which time the neoplasm can be addressed.

CANCER

Malignant diseases of the gynecologic organs may occur in pregnancy, most commonly including breast cancer, ovarian cancer, and cervical cancer.

Ovarian Cancer

Background
- A malignant ovarian neoplasm is encountered one in every 20,000 to 30,000 deliveries.
- Of the three types of ovarian cancer (epithelial, stromal, and germ cell), there seem to be a disproportionate number of germ cell tumors in pregnant compared to nonpregnant women, although this difference may partially result from reporting bias.
- Fortunately, early-stage, low-grade tumors are the most common (15).

Treatment
- Early consultation with a gynecologic oncologist is strongly encouraged.
- Thorough surgical staging of the disease is desirable.
- There are special considerations for stage IA tumors:
  - Unilateral salpingo-oophorectomy in women who desire future childbearing may be justified if the tumor is unilateral and localized (stage IA).
  - Further adjuvant therapy may be required for stage IA malignant germ cell tumors.
  - Unilateral pelvic and para-aortic lymphadenectomy is recommended for correct evaluation of apparently stage IA dysgerminomas because of their propensity for lymphatic dissemination.
- Cancers other than stage IA are treated as in the nonpregnant patient, except in the third trimester (16).
- When ovarian cancer is suspected in the third trimester, therapy may be delayed until fetal pulmonary maturity is demonstrated. Cesarean section is then performed along with definitive surgery and staging for the neoplasm (13).

Breast Cancer

Background
- The incidence of breast cancer is approximately 1 in 3500 to 10,000 deliveries. Approximately 1.5% to 4.0% of breast cancers coexist with pregnancy, making it an uncommon, but not rare, event (17).
- The glandular hyperplasia of the breast that accompanies pregnancy makes recognition of suspicious breast masses difficult. Therefore, breast cancer is often recognized at a later stage than would occur in the nonpregnant state.

Diagnosis
- The diagnosis relies on a physical exam because mammograms are not routinely obtained during pregnancy.
- The suspicious breast lump is evaluated in the same manner in the pregnant and nonpregnant patient. Tissue diagnosis is obtained by fine needle aspiration of fluid, by tissue core, or by open biopsy.
- The role of mammography remains controversial because of the radiographic density of the breast in younger women and during pregnancy (18,19). The radiation dose is negligible, however, and mammography can be used safely, if necessary, especially after the first trimester.

Treatment
- Debate continues about the best form of therapy in the nonpregnant state, but modified radical mastectomy appears to be the most common choice during pregnancy. Simple lumpectomy with radiation treatment is less desirable because of fetal radiation exposure.
- The role of adjuvant chemotherapy remains controversial because of the potential risks of fetal teratogenesis and mutagenesis.

- When matched for age and stage, there is no difference in survival rates between pregnant and nonpregnant women. It has been suggested that breast cancer has a worse prognosis when diagnosed in pregnancy; however, this opinion probably reflects the tendency to find more advanced stage cancers and/or a higher proportion of high-grade and estrogen receptor–negative cancers in pregnant women.
- Survival is not improved by pregnancy termination, but it may be recommended to avoid the risk of fetal exposure to either chemotherapy or radiation therapy (20).

PATIENT EDUCATION

- Women should understand that they can expect to experience most of the same gynecologic problems during pregnancy that they would when not pregnant.
- Women with PID and endometriosis can be informed that they will likely experience an improvement or disappearance of their symptoms during pregnancy.
- Pregnant women should receive information about the continued risk for breast and cervical cancer during pregnancy, along with the need to receive appropriate evaluation of any abnormal breast findings or Papanicolaou test/cervical biopsy results.

REFERENCES

1. Update to the Centers for Disease Control and Prevention-Sexually transmitted diseases treatment guidelines 2010. *MMWR Morb Mortal Wkly Rep.* 2010;59(RR-12):21–22.
2. Sweet RL, Gibbs RS. *Infectious diseases of the female genital tract.* 5th ed. Philadelphia: Wolters Kluwer/Lippincott Williams and Wilkins, 2009.
3. American College of Obstetricians and Gynecologists. Human Papillomavirus vaccination. ACOG Committee Opinion No. 467. *ACOG Obstet Gynecol.* 2010;116:800–803.
4. Massad LS, Einstein MH, Huh WK, et al. 2012 updated consensus guidelines for managing abnormal cervical cancer screening tests and cancer precursors. *J Low Genit Tract Dis.* 2013;17(5):S1–S27.
5. American College of Obstetricians and Gynecologists. ACOG Practice Bulletin No. 72: vaginitis. *Obstet Gynecol.* 2006;107:1195–1206.
6. Cotch, MF, Pastorek JG II, Nugent RP, et al. Trichomonas vaginalis associated with low birth weight and preterm labor. *Sex Transm Dis* 1997;24(6):353–360.
7. Nelson DB, Macones G. Bacterial vaginosis in pregnancy: current findings and future directions. *Epidemiol Rev.* 2002;24(2):102–108.
8. American College of Obstetricians and Gynecologists. ACOG Practice Bulletin No. 131: screening for cervical cancer. *Obstet Gynecol.* 2012;120(5):1222–1238.
9. American College of Obstetricians and Gynecologists. ACOG Practice Bulletin No. 99: management of abnormal cervical cytology and histology. *Obstet Gynecol.* 2008, reaffirmed 2010;112(16):1419–1444.
10. Demeter A, Sziller I, Csapo Z, et al. Outcome of pregnancies after cold-knife conization of the uterine cervix during pregnancy. *Eur J Gynaecol Oncol.* 2002;23:207–210.
11. Nevin J, Soeters R, Dehaeck K, et al. Cervical carcinoma associated with pregnancy. *Obstet Gynecol Surv.* 1995;50:228–239.
12. Walboomers JM, Jacobs MV, Manos MM, et al. Human papillomavirus is a necessary cause of invasive cervical cancer worldwide. *J Pathol.* 1999;189:12–19.
13. Arment F. Gynecologic cancers in pregnancy. *Lancet.* 2012;379.
14. American College of Obstetricians and Gynecologists. ACOG Practice Bulletin No. 83: management of adnexal masses. *Obstet Gynecol.* 2007, reaffirmed 2011;110(1):201–214.
15. American College of Obstetricians and Gynecologists. ACOG Committee Opinion number 280: the role of the generalist obstetrician-gynecologist in the early detection of ovarian cancer. *Obstet Gynecol.* 2002;100(6):1413–1416.
16. Malfetano JH, Goldkrand JW. Cis-platinum combination chemotherapy during pregnancy for advanced epithelial ovarian carcinoma. *Obstet Gynecol.* 1990;75:545–547.

17. American College of Obstetricians and Gynecologists. ACOG Committee Opinion Number 186: role of the obstetrician-gynecologist in the diagnosis and treatment of breast disease. *Int J Gynaecol Obstet.* 1997;59(2):162–163.
18. Sukumvanich P. Review of current treatment options for pregnancy-associated breast cancer. *Clin Obstet Gynecol.* 2011;54(1):164–172.
19. Barthelmes L, Davidson LA, Gaffney C, et al. Pregnancy and breast cancer. *BMJ.* 2005;330:1375–1383.
20. National Cancer Institute: Breast Cancer Treatment and Pregnancy(PDQ). www.cancer. gov. 2012.

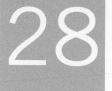

28 Surgical Problems and Trauma
Hope M. Cottrill and Susan C. Modesitt

TRAUMA IN OBSTETRICS
Key Points
- The pregnant patient with trauma should undergo evaluation, treatment, and care for her injuries similar to the nonpregnant patient.
- While the well-being of the unborn fetus is always important, it should be considered only after the pregnant woman has undergone necessary assessment to allow appropriate stabilization and treatment efforts to begin.
- The coordinated care of the pregnant trauma patient and her fetus depends on gestational age as well as maternal and fetal status.
- Fetal viability is currently accepted as equal to or greater than 23 to 24 weeks' gestation.

Background
Definition
- Trauma is damage to the body caused by an external force.
- Trauma can result in fracture, dislocation, sprain, intracranial injuries, internal injuries of chest or pelvis, open wound, blood vessel injury, contusion, crush injury, burn, nerve, and spinal cord injury, and it can be caused by a variety of sources:
  - Forces of nature: lightning strikes, animal bites
  - Mechanical forces: motor vehicle collisions (MVCs) or assault
  - Self-inflicted: attempted suicide

Etiology/Epidemiology
- Trauma occurs commonly in pregnancy:
  - The leading cause of death for women of childbearing age is unintentional injury (accidents) with the majority being MVCs (1).
  - Falls affect 27% of pregnancies (2).
  - Women aged 18 to 35 have the highest incidence of intimate partner violence with the risk of physical abuse being 1% to 20% during pregnancy (1,3,4).

Evaluation
History and Physical Exam
- MVC
  - Nature of MVC: Car, motorcycle, direction of collision, vehicle rollover, ejection from vehicle, etc
  - Speed of MVC: High speed, low speed, stationary
  - Patient's location in vehicle and role as passenger or driver
  - Patient restrained or unrestrained
  - Loss of consciousness
  - Alcohol or drugs involved
- Physical abuse
  - Routine screening is recommended at first prenatal visit, then in each trimester, and at postpartum visit.
    - Consider use of a questionnaire.

o Ask the patient about violence away from the partner.

o Document statements in quotations.

• Document any injuries in detail, including diagrams and/or photos.

• Assess safety and notify law enforcement officials of suspected abuse.

• Falls: Circumstances, area of body struck, and loss of consciousness

• Obstetric information: gestational age, obstetric history, and complications

Initial Management

• Primary survey (ABCs [airway, breathing, circulation])

• Airway

o Clear foreign bodies and suction as necessary.

o Establish airway with head tilt (cervical spine must be evaluated prior to moving head) and jaw thrust. Apply cricoid pressure prior with positive pressure ventilation and with endotracheal tube placement to decrease aspiration (5).

o Consider inserting an artificial airway device early in resuscitation to decrease the risk of aspiration keeping in mind that a smaller endotracheal tube may be needed for the pregnant patient due to edema (5).

o If no other airway can be obtained, a cricothyroidotomy should be performed (6).

• Breathing

o Consider mouth-to-mouth resuscitation or intermittent positive pressure ventilation.

o Supplemental oxygen and monitoring of oxygenation status are standard for the trauma patient until evaluation is complete (6):

   - Maintain maternal pulse oxygen at ≥95% for pregnancies that are ≥23 to 24 weeks' gestation (fetal viability).

   - If the exact gestational age is not known, then the presumption should be that the fetus is viable until proven otherwise.

o If inadequate ventilation is noted, the differential diagnosis includes tension pneumothorax, massive hemothorax, or flail chest with pulmonary contusion (6). These are emergent situations and require immediate intervention.

• Circulation

o Control obvious external hemorrhage.

o Obtain intravenous access.

o Modification to basic life support technique at ≥20 weeks' gestation: Manually displace the gravid uterus to the left *or* position the patient with a wedge under the right hip *or* place the woman in a modified left lateral position to prevent compression of inferior vena cava. Perform chest compressions slightly above the center of the sternum to allow for increased abdominal contents and elevated diaphragm (5).

o Advanced cardiopulmonary life support: No additional modification.

• Shock

o Physiologic changes of pregnancy alter normal vital sign parameters and can mask hemorrhage (see below).

o Volume resuscitation should be based on other parameters (peripheral perfusion, mental status changes, diaphoresis, pallor, fetal heart rate decelerations) as well as vital signs changes.

o Pneumatic antishock garment may be utilized, but the abdominal portion should not be inflated in pregnancies with fetal viability.

o The underlying etiology of reversible causes of cardiac arrest in the pregnant patient may be related to cardiac disease (myocardial infarction, aortic dissection), iatrogenic magnesium sulfate toxicity, pulmonary embolism, preeclampsia/eclampsia, amniotic fluid embolism, and anesthetic complication (high spinal) (5).

• Secondary survey

• Further evaluation: Complete the history and physical exam (including bimanual pelvic/speculum exam, exclusion of obvious rupture of membranes, and rectal exam), laboratory values, and radiographic evaluation.

- Assessment of fetal status:
  - Fetal heart tones
  - Ultrasound to evaluate
    - Intra-abdominal hemorrhage and organ damage
    - Fetal cardiac activity
    - Fetal number
    - Fetal position
    - Gestational age
    - Placental location and status
    - Amniotic fluid volume
  - Prolonged electronic monitoring of the fetal heart rate and uterine activity should be performed for the viable fetus when the mother is stable. The length of time necessary for reassurance will vary with the type and severity of the trauma, but the recommended minimum time is 4 hours (7).
- Perimortem cesarean section:
  - If maternal chest compressions do not produce a pulse, consider emptying the uterus to improve resuscitation.
  - The suggested time frame to initiate perimortem cesarean section is 4 minutes. Maternal neurologic damage occurs 6 minutes after cerebral blood flow ceases. Therefore, the goal is to initiate cesarean section in 4 minutes, complete evacuation of the uterus in 5 minutes, and achieve cerebral blood flow in 6 minutes (8).
  - If the maternal injuries are fatal and there is a chance the fetus will survive, proceed with cesarean delivery (9).

Laboratory Tests
- Complete blood count.
- Comprehensive metabolic panel (electrolytes, liver function, and renal function).
- Coagulation profile.
- Amylase.
- Lipase.
- Urinalysis.
- Urine drug screen and consider blood alcohol level.
- Urine pregnancy test in reproductive age females who are not obviously pregnant.
- Blood type and screen (or crossmatch if necessary).
- Rh status to determine if Rh immune globulin needs to be given to the patient.
- Kleihauer-Betke test may be of use, but has significant limitations (10).

Radiographic Tests
- Evaluation of the pregnant patient should utilize the same tests as the nonpregnant patient, but radiation exposure to the fetus should be considered.
  - Focused abdominal sonography for trauma (FAST) has been shown to be efficacious in pregnant patients (11).
  - Magnetic resonance imaging (MRI) has no radiation exposure or known adverse fetal effects (12).
  - X-ray and computed tomography (CT) techniques have associated radiation exposure, and parents should be appropriately counseled if time permits (Table 28-1).
- The fetus is at greatest risk at 8 to 15 weeks' gestation for teratogenic effects from radiation exposure (13).
  - Exposure to less than 5 rad has not been shown to increase fetal loss or anomalies (14).
  - The pregnant uterus should be shielded whenever possible.

Diagnosis
Differential Diagnosis
- The differential diagnosis depends on the nature of the injury, examination of the patient, further history, and observation. For example, someone found unconscious and

Table 28-1	Estimated Fetal Exposure from Radiologic Procedures (13)
Procedure	**Mean fetal exposure (mGy)[b]**
Ultrasound	0
MRI	0
Chest x-ray	<0.01
Abdominal film (single view)	1.4
Pelvis x-ray	1.1
CT[a] scan of head or chest	<0.06
CT scan of lumbar spine	2.4
CT scan of abdomen	8.0
CT scan of abdomen	8.0
CT scan of pelvis	25

[a]CT, computed tomography.
[b]10 mGy = 1 rad
Modified from Gabbe SG, Niebyl JR, Simpson JL, et al. *Obstetrics: normal and problem pregnancies*. 6th ed. Philadelphia: Elsevier Saunders, 2012:140–165.

obtunded may have had a stroke, head injury, or overdosed on medication as just the most obvious possibilities.
• Blunt abdominal trauma.
  • Etiology is frequently MVC, assault, and falls.
  • Maternal injury.
    ○ Intra-abdominal hemorrhage due to acceleration/deceleration injury with rupture or laceration of
      – Aorta, vena cava, or other vessels
      – Solid organs
      – Uterus
    ○ Fetal injury
      – Includes skull fracture, splenic rupture, and intracranial hemorrhage (15).
      – Most cases of fetal demise are related to placental abruption (7).
    ○ Placental injury:
      – Frequently due to shearing force of abrupt deceleration
      – Laceration
      – Abruption or complete separation
      – Fetal–maternal hemorrhage
• Penetrating abdominal trauma.
  • Etiology is frequently gunshots or stab wounds.
  • Mother or fetus may be injured by penetrating trauma.
  • Uterus and/or solid organs may be penetrated, lacerated, or destroyed leading to intra-abdominal hemorrhage and/or disrupted anatomy.
  • The criteria and decisions regarding proceeding with surgery are the same as in a non-pregnant female.

Clinical Manifestations
• Gestational age
  • At 12 weeks' gestation, the uterus is well protected by the bony pelvis.
  • Before the fetus is viable, the mother's health is the major concern.
  • When the fetus is viable, rapid intervention may be necessary to save the mother, fetus, or both (see below).
• Type of trauma
  • Motor vehicle accidents, falls, and assaults can present with minor injuries or multiple injuries involving multiple organ systems including the uterus, placenta, and fetus.

- Burns, electrical shock, and lightning strikes occur in pregnancy.
  - ○ Due to changes of pregnancy, aggressive and early fluid resuscitation is recommended (16).
  - ○ Carbon dioxide is readily bound by fetal hemoglobin, and therefore, supplemental oxygenation should be provided (17).
  - ○ Pregnant patients with these injuries should be treated the same as the nonpregnant patient.

Treatment
Medications
- Only medications safe in pregnancy should be administered if the fetus may survive.
- Advanced cardiac life support (ACLS) protocols and techniques do not require any dose modifications because of pregnancy.

Procedures
- Any radiologic evaluation or surgical procedure deemed necessary for treatment of the pregnant patient should be undertaken (see above).
- Surgical procedures should be performed as indicated for both fetal and maternal well-being (see section on Surgery).

Referrals/Counseling
- Obstetrician should be involved with the assessment of the mother and the fetus.
- Maternal–fetal medicine specialty consultation may be helpful in assessment and further management.
- Neonatologists may be helpful if delivery is necessary, especially in the preterm or compromised fetus.
- Involvement of other specialists is dictated by the nature of the injuries and further treatment: orthopedics, general surgery, trauma surgery, and neurosurgery, among others.

Risk Management
- As with any patient care, documentation and informed consent are paramount.

Complications
- Maternal death is uncommon (18).
- Fetal death can complicate up to 16% of pregnant trauma patients hospitalized at a level 1 trauma center (19).
- Pelvic fracture does not interfere with subsequent vaginal delivery:
  - Seventy-nine percent (27/34) of women with a history of pelvic fractures (including 12 with displaced fractures) successfully delivered vaginally (20).
- Worse outcomes are typical of the pregnant trauma patient who is delivered at the time of admission due to trauma, with increased risk of maternal death, fetal death, uterine rupture, and placental abruption (18).

Patient Education
Prevention of trauma requires educating pregnant women to take specific protective measures.
- Seat belt use:
  - Always wear seat belts.
  - Use three-point restraint belts.
  - Lap belt should be at the hips, not over the fundus.
  - Improper seat belt use is a major risk factor for adverse outcomes in MVCs (21).
- Fire safety:
  - Smoke detectors:
    - ○ At least one on each floor of the home is recommended.
    - ○ More than 90% of those surveyed in the United States report having smoke detectors, but fewer than 20% check every 3 months to see if they work (22).
  - Fire extinguisher: Only 71% of homes have a fire extinguisher (22).

• Burn prevention:
  • Keep hot water heaters set at no greater than 120°F and measure the tap water temperature (22).
  • Wear sunscreen and protective clothing.
• Carbon monoxide: Only about 30% of those surveyed have carbon monoxide detectors (22).

Resources
• Seat belt use—National Highway Traffic Safety Administration: 1-888-327-4236
• Fire safety—U.S. Fire Administration: 1-301-447-1000
• Intimate partner violence
  • Local, state, national, and international resources exist.
  • Specialized groups target minorities and those for whom English is a second language.
  • Domestic violence hotlines
    ○ National Domestic Violence Hotline: 1-800-799-SAFE (7233)
    ○ American Domestic Violence Crisis Line: 1-866-USWOMEN
    ○ The Coalition for Family Harmony: 1-800-300-2181

SURGICAL PROBLEMS IN OBSTETRICS
Key Points
• Pregnant women will present with processes that require surgical treatment.
• Recognition of surgical emergencies (i.e., acute abdomen) can be more difficult in pregnancy.
• Coordination of all the members of the surgical team (anesthesia, obstetrics, and surgery) is imperative to correctly diagnose and treat surgical events while minimizing both maternal and fetal morbidity.
• Delay of necessary surgical intervention can increase both maternal and fetal morbidity.
• "Elective" or nonemergent surgeries should be scheduled in the second trimester, if feasible, but again, there should be NO delay for emergent cases.

Background
Definition
• Nonobstetric surgery will be required in about 1 in 500 pregnancies (23) or a total of 75,000 pregnant women each year (24).
• Pregnancy poses several challenges to the surgeon:
  • Pregnancy may disguise or obscure classic diagnostic features of surgical conditions.
  • Physiologic changes in pregnancy may require modification of standard surgical and diagnostic procedures.
  • Unique ethical issues may be encountered as treatment decisions must balance the well-being of both the mother and the fetus.

Pathophysiology
Pregnancy causes multiple changes in maternal physiology that may hinder appropriate and timely diagnosis of surgical situations:
• Pregnancy-associated symptoms can also imply other disease processes:
  • Headache
  • Syncope
  • Nausea and vomiting
  • Abdominal discomfort and pain
• Normal hemodynamic parameters are altered in pregnancy.
  • Diastolic blood pressure can be lower.
  • Maternal pulse increases by 7 weeks' gestation and may increase up to 20% in late pregnancy.
  • Blood volume increases by 50%.
  • Supine hypotension may occur due to compression of the vena cava by the gravid uterus.
• Normal abdominal anatomy may be displaced or distorted by the gravid uterus.
  • For example, the appendix moves progressively cephalad as pregnancy progresses and will be at the level of the iliac crest by 6 months' gestation.

Etiology/Epidemiology
- Acute abdomen
  - This refers to the symptoms and signs of acute intraperitoneal disease. This may or may not be due to obstetrical causes.
  - Surgical exploration is usually required to rule out major causes of maternal and fetal morbidity, establish the diagnosis, and proceed with treatment.
  - The most common entities diagnosed in pregnancy (23,25):
    - Appendicitis (1 in 1500 pregnancies)
    - Ectopic pregnancy (1 in 100; see Chapter 7)
    - Cholecystitis (1 in 1600 pregnancies)
      - Asymptomatic cholelithiasis occurs in about 3.5% of pregnancies.
    - Bowel obstruction (1 in 1500 to 3000 pregnancies)
      - Most commonly secondary to adhesions (60% to 70%).
      - Less likely causes are volvulus (25%) and intussusception (5%).
    - Inflammatory bowel disease (1 in 1000 pregnancies)
    - Ovarian torsion (rare)
    - Spontaneous hepatic rupture (rare)
- There are other processes in the differential for acute abdomen that may require only medical management (Table 28-2):
  - Gastroenteritis
  - Nephrolithiasis
  - Pyelonephritis
  - Pancreatitis
  - Peptic ulcer disease
  - Pneumonia
- Other diseases that potentially require surgery during pregnancy:
  - Solid/complex adnexal masses
  - Cervical intraepithelial neoplasia
  - Malignant diseases
    - Breast
    - Ovarian
    - Cervical
    - Melanoma
    - Bone cancer
  - Nonurgent trauma (see prior section of chapter)
  - Cardiac disease that is surgically correctable and has failed medical management during pregnancy
  - Neurosurgical emergencies such as aneurysms or arteriovenous malformations

Evaluation
History and Physical Exam
- The history should focus on a thorough evaluation of the history of the present illness, past medical history, and current obstetric history.
- The physical exam should be thorough and include all maternal systems as well as evaluation of fetal well-being.

Laboratory Tests
- Pregnant women should receive the same laboratory tests that would normally be used to evaluate a nonpregnant woman with an acute abdomen.
- However, pregnancy is accompanied by physiologic adaptations that may alter the normal ranges of commonly used laboratory tests:
  - A relative state of anemia (Hgb 10 to 13 g/dL, hematocrit over 30%)
  - A mild leukocytosis (up to 16,000/uL)

Table 28-2	Differential Diagnosis of Abdominal Pain in Pregnancy

Gastrointestinal causes
Surgical
Appendicitis
Cholecystitis/cholelithiasis
Bowel obstruction/perforation
Hepatic rupture
Nonsurgical
Biliary colic
Gastroenteritis
Gastroesophageal reflux
Hepatitis
Pancreatitis
Inflammatory bowel disease
Irritable bowel syndrome
Peptic ulcer disease
Acute mesenteric adenitis
Acute porphyria
Sickle cell crisis
Obstetric causes
Surgical
Trauma
Ectopic pregnancy
Placental abruption
Nonsurgical
HELLP syndrome
Hyperemesis gravidarum
Round ligament syndrome
Preterm contractions and/or labor
Chorioamnionitis
Urinary causes
Surgical
Acute ureteral obstruction
Nonsurgical
Pyelonephritis
Nephrolithiasis
Gynecologic causes
Surgical
Ovarian or fallopian tube torsion
Ectopic pregnancy
Nonsurgical
Endometriosis
Uterine leiomyoma
Pelvic inflammatory disease
Ovarian cyst rupture
Miscellaneous
Pneumonia

Radiographic Tests
- Radiologic tests appropriate for the nonpregnant patient should be used in pregnancy if their omission would delay or adversely affect diagnosis.
- Ultrasound is usually the first imaging study of choice as there are no fetal contraindications.

- MRI may be the backup imaging study of choice as it affords excellent anatomic detail, no radiation exposure, and diagnostic accuracy in pregnant women with abdominal pain (26).
- CT scan is the third choice, due to fetal radiation exposure. However, if a CT scan is indicated or necessary for assessment, then it should be performed.
- Use of the minimum x-ray exposure, avoidance of redundant studies, and shielding of the fetus are advisable. (Refer to Table 28-1 for fetal exposures.)

Diagnosis
Acute Abdomen Differential Diagnoses That Require Surgery
- Acute appendicitis
- Cholecystitis
- Ovarian torsion
- Bowel obstruction

Clinical Manifestations
- Most common symptoms of acute abdomen in pregnancy (27)
  - Abdominal pain (82%)
  - Tachycardia (82%)
  - Fever (75%)
  - Nausea or vomiting (63%)
- Acute appendicitis (23,25,27–31)
  - Suspected appendicitis is the most common indication for surgery in pregnancy.
  - Majority (80%) will present with right lower quadrant pain although it can be epigastric or periumbilical (28).
  - Pain is typically colicky.
  - Nausea and/or vomiting.
  - Leukocytosis (but can be elevated in pregnancy regardless).
  - Fever.
  - Rebound and guarding.
- Acute cholecystitis (23,25,32,33)
  - Nausea and vomiting.
  - Acute abdominal pain, usually colicky.
  - Pain is located in the midepigastrium and right upper quadrant and may radiate to the back.
  - Murphy sign (pain below the right costal margin) may be present.
  - Fever.
  - Tachycardia.
  - Tachypnea.
  - May have increased serum bilirubin level, liver enzymes, and serum alkaline phosphatase, but these can also be falsely elevated in pregnancy.
  - Ultrasound is 95% sensitive for gallstones even in pregnancy (25).
- Ovarian/fallopian tube torsion
  - Acute onset of pain, usually lower abdominal
  - May have fever or leukocytosis (but normal values do not exclude the diagnosis)
  - May have mass or enlarged ovary
  - May have loss of ovarian blood flow on Doppler ultrasound
- Bowel obstruction (23,25,34)
  - Abdomen is usually distended with potentially high-pitched bowel sounds.
  - Symptoms include nausea, vomiting, and crampy abdominal pain that is poorly localized.
  - Fever and leukocytosis are usually present.
  - Do not confuse this with hyperemesis, especially in the second and third trimester.

Treatment

Decision for Surgery During Pregnancy
- Once a surgical acute abdomen has been diagnosed, surgery is necessary to reduce the risk of both maternal and fetal complications.
  - In these situations, the patient and family should receive as much counseling as possible about the surgery, the potential courses of action, and the risks and benefits.
  - Counseling may be less than complete since time may be of the essence and delay for counseling may have dire consequences.
- Some procedures, due to complexity or the need for patient directions, may require more extensive counseling among the patient, her family, the obstetrician, the anesthesiologist, and the surgeon to discuss risks and benefits of surgery during pregnancy.
- For nonemergent problems (e.g., an adnexal mass), a thorough discussion with the patient must be undertaken to discuss the risks and benefits of immediate surgery compared to waiting for either fetal viability or delivery.

Preoperative Management
- Timing of surgery
  - Determined more by the severity and acuity of the surgical illness than by gestational age.
  - Delay of an indicated surgical procedure to allow for fetal maturity or delivery should not occur if the delay is likely to have an adverse maternal impact.
  - Elective surgery should be postponed until after delivery.
  - Surgery that is not emergent, but that should not be delayed until the postpartum period, is best performed in the second trimester when the risk of spontaneous abortion is the least.
  - The highest risk of pregnancy loss and/or premature delivery is in the third trimester.
- Deep venous thromboembolism (DVT) risks (35–37)
  - Pregnancy is considered to be a hypercoagulable state.
  - Surgical procedures during pregnancy further increase the risk for thromboembolic events.
  - Other risk factors for DVT include
    - Age over 40
    - Surgical procedure lasting longer than 30 minutes
    - Major orthopedic or pelvic surgery
    - Previous myocardial infarction
    - Previous thromboembolic event
    - Malignant disease
    - Prior stroke
  - DVT prophylaxis in pregnancy
    - Prophylaxis with pneumatic compression stockings and/or heparin should be strongly considered for any surgical procedure in a pregnant woman.
    - For women with other risk factors (personal or based on surgical risk), low molecular weight heparin is the prophylactic agent of choice because of once-daily dosing and lower risk of bleeding complications.
    - Unfractionated heparin, 5000 units subcutaneously given 2 hours preoperatively and then every 12 hours until the patient is ambulatory, may be used.
- Informed consent should be obtained from the patient when a surgical procedure is anticipated and should contain the following components:
  - A discussion of the risks of spontaneous abortion/premature labor.
  - External fetal heart rate monitoring is appropriate for viable pregnancies before, during, and after surgery.
  - If the risk of premature delivery is significant, arrangements for neonatal intensive care services should be made.

Anesthesia Considerations (24,38)
- Prevention of aspiration. Pregnancy causes a delay in gastric emptying as well as an increase in reflux, so the following steps should be implemented to prevent aspiration:
  - Preoperative administration of antacids (e.g., 30 mL of 0.3 M sodium citrate)
  - Use of cricothyroid pressure during induction
  - Rapid sequence induction
  - Intraoperative nasogastric suctioning
- Intraoperative monitoring issues in pregnancy
  - Must maintain the best physiologic condition for the mother to ensure adequate perfusion for the fetus.
  - Hyperventilation should be avoided due to the fact that the resting CO_2 in pregnancy is already lowered and further respiratory alkalosis can shift the oxyhemoglobin dissociation curve to the left impairing fetal oxygenation.
  - Intraoperative monitoring of the woman should include vital signs, oxygen saturation, end tidal carbon dioxide, fetal heart rate (if indicated), and uterine activity (if indicated).
- Choice of anesthetic
  - Essentially, every drug or inhalation anesthetic is teratogenic to some species under certain conditions.
  - No anesthetic drug has been found to be a definitive human teratogen (38).
  - Regional anesthesia is considered preferable as local anesthetics have not been associated with birth defects and little drug enters the fetal circulation. Maternal hypotension can be due to peripheral vasodilation if the woman is not volume resuscitated adequately before induction.
  - General anesthetic agents considered to be safe in the second and third trimesters include thiopental, muscle relaxants, narcotics, nitrous oxide, and low-dose inhalational agents such as halothane, enflurane, and isoflurane.

Medications
- For pain relief and antibiotic coverage, every effort should be made to utilize drugs appropriate for pregnancy (preferably class A or B agents).
- See anesthesia considerations above.
- Intravenous narcotics appear to be safe in pregnancy for short periods of time. The use of patient-controlled analgesia is appropriate in the pregnant patient.
- Epidural analgesia can be used intraoperatively and for postoperative pain control with appropriate monitoring for respiratory depression and hypotension.
- Codeine has been associated with a modest increased risk of birth defects, and use is optimally limited to after the first trimester.
- Nonsteroidal anti-inflammatory medications should be avoided secondary to concerns regarding constriction of the ductus arteriosus in utero and platelet dysfunction leading to a hemostatic disorder.
- Acetaminophen appears safe as an analgesic and antipyretic.

Procedures
- Patient positioning
  - The patient should be supine but rotated thirty degrees to the left with a hip roll.
  - This position maximizes blood flow to the fetus.
- Fetal surveillance (38,40)
  - Prior to 23 weeks' gestation, fetal heart tones need only be documented prior to and after the surgery. Intraoperative fetal monitoring is not necessary since the fetus is not viable and not a candidate for emergency intervention.
  - After fetal viability, intraoperative fetal monitoring may be indicated when the following conditions are met. If these are NOT met, would simply document fetal heart tones before and after the procedure:
    - The fetus is viable.
    - It is physically possible to perform intraoperative monitoring.

- ○ An obstetrically qualified practitioner is available and willing to intervene DURING surgery for fetal indications.
- ○ The woman has given informed consent for an emergent C-section.
- ○ The planned surgery can be interrupted safely to perform a C-section.
- Route of surgery
  - Minimally invasive surgery
    - ○ If technically feasible, laparoscopy can be performed. To date, there are limited reports of robotic surgery (outside of cerclage placement) during pregnancy (39).
    - ○ See Table 28-3 for updated Society of American Gastrointestinal and Endoscopic Surgeons (SAGES) guidelines for laparoscopy in the pregnant patient (40).
    - ○ Laparoscopy results in shorter hospital stays, decreased pain, and a quicker return to normal activity compared to open procedures and can be safely employed at any point in pregnancy (40–42).
    - ○ Appendectomy, cholecystectomy, or salpingo-oophorectomy can usually be accomplished using minimally invasive procedures:
      - – Outcomes initially appeared to be equivalent for laparotomy and laparoscopic appendectomy, but a 2012 meta-analysis concluded that the laparoscopic route "might be associated with a greater risk of fetal loss" (30).
      - – Laparoscopic cholecystectomy may decrease risk of spontaneous abortion and preterm labor (32,33).
      - – Laparoscopic BSO is the method of choice if necessary during pregnancy (40,42).
      - – Adnexal masses complicate 1% to 4% of pregnancies and only require removal if greater than 10 cm, are torsed, or have features suggestive of malignancy (42).
  - Laparotomy
    - ○ Used in emergent situations.
    - ○ A midline vertical incision enables the surgeon to deal with any diagnosis.
    - ○ Preferred if the size of the uterus precludes laparoscopy, an abscess is suspected, or malignancy is suspected and full evaluation cannot be performed with minimally invasive surgery.

Complications

Spontaneous Abortion
- Baseline miscarriage rates in the first trimester range between 8% and 16% of recognized pregnancies and 2% and 4% of second-trimester pregnancies. It is unclear if surgery increases this in any appreciable way (43–45).
- Certain conditions (e.g., appendicitis) may increase the spontaneous abortion rate, and this is likely due to underlying conditions rather than the required surgical intervention.
- Older data from dentists and dental assistants with high exposure to anesthetic gases (especially nitrous oxide) do demonstrate a twofold increased risk of abortion (46).

Teratogenesis
- The first trimester has the highest risk for teratogenesis because of ongoing organogenesis.
- The majority of recent studies have not demonstrated increased risks of congenital abnormalities in offspring of women who had surgery during pregnancy (24,44,45,47,48).
- One registry study of 2252 women undergoing surgery during the first trimester of pregnancy showed a small but significant increase in neural tube defects. However, causality could not be determined (49).
- Advances in anesthesia equipment reduce anesthetic gas leakage into the operating room and decrease exposure and risk.

Preterm Delivery
- Preterm delivery (PTD) is increased with intraperitoneal surgeries and disease processes.
- Delay in surgical intervention with appendicitis and bowel obstruction may increase the risk of PTD (25,27,29,43).

Table 28-3	Guidelines for Diagnosis, Treatment, and Use of Laparoscopy in Pregnancy

Imaging techniques
1. Ultrasound during pregnancy is safe and useful to evaluate etiology of acute abdominal pain in pregnancy.
2. Expeditious and accurate diagnosis takes precedence over risk of ionizing radiation exposure to fetus. Limit cumulative radiation doses to less than 5 rads during pregnancy.
3. CT has a low radiation dose and may be used when clinically indicated.
4. MRI without gadolinium can be performed at any stage in pregnancy.
5. Use of radionuclide for diagnostic studies is generally safe for the mother and fetus.
6. Intraoperative cholangiography has minimal exposure and may be used selectively with lower abdominal shielding.

Surgical techniques
7. Diagnostic laparoscopy is generally considered safe in pregnancy.
8. Laparoscopic treatment of acute abdominal disease has the same indications for pregnant and nonpregnant patients.
9. Laparoscopy can be safely performed in any trimester.
10. Gravid patients should be placed in left lateral decubitus position to minimize vena cava compression.
11. Initial port placement can be done with any technique *IF* location is adjusted according to fundal height and previous incisions.
12. CO_2 insufflation of 10–15 mm Hg is safe.
13. Intraoperative CO_2 monitoring by capnography should be used in the pregnant patient.

Venous thromboembolic prophylaxis
14. Intraoperative and postoperative pneumatic compression devices and early postoperative ambulation are recommended.

Specific surgical-type recommendations
15. Laparoscopic cholecystectomy is the treatment of choice in the pregnant patient, regardless of trimester.
16. Choledocholithiasis during pregnancy may be managed with preoperative ERCP with sphincterotomy followed by laparoscopic cholecystectomy or bile duct exploration.
17. Laparoscopic appendectomy may be performed safely in pregnant patients.
18. Laparoscopic adrenalectomy, nephrectomy, and splenectomy are safe in pregnancy.
19. Laparoscopy is safe and effective in gravid women with symptomatic cystic masses, and observation is acceptable for asymptomatic masses provided ultrasound/tumor markers are not concerning for malignancy.
20. Laparoscopy is recommended for both diagnosis and treatment of adnexal torsion unless clinical severity warrants laparotomy.

Fetal heart monitoring/care during surgery
21. Fetal heart monitoring should occur pre- and postoperatively in the setting of urgent abdominal surgery during pregnancy.
22. Obstetric consultation can be obtained pre- and postoperatively based on the disease, gestational age, and consultant availability.
23. Tocolytics should not be used prophylactically but can be considered perioperatively when signs of preterm labor are present.

Modified from the Society of American Gastrointestinal Endoscopic Surgeons, 2007. http://www.sagescms.org

- In a study of 778 patients with appendicitis in pregnancy, the increased risk of PTD was limited to the first week after surgery (31):
  - Appendicitis was also associated with decreased birth weight and increased risk of neonatal death.
- PTD risk does not appear to differ between laparoscopic and open abdominal procedures; however, a recent meta-analysis of appendicitis cases suggested that laparoscopic appendectomy may have a greater risk of fetal loss (RR 1.91, CI 1.31–2.77) (30).
- Routine postoperative tocolytics are no longer recommended; however, the following options are available if preterm labor is suspected (38):
  - Tocolytic options for documented uterine contractions
    - Indomethacin
    - Magnesium sulfate intravenously
    - Terbutaline subcutaneously or IV
    - Nifedipine orally

Neonatal Death
- A large registry linked surgery during pregnancy with increased neonatal deaths (within the first 7 days of life) but the causality is unclear (47).
- Other studies with appendicitis and acute abdomen also demonstrate an increased rate of neonatal death (27,31).
- While an association exists, it is unclear whether the increased rate of neonatal death is secondary to the surgery itself or the underlying condition that necessitated surgery.

Maternal Mortality/Morbidity
- Overall, maternal mortality is incredibly low and is primarily due to sepsis related to delay in diagnosis.
- In appendicitis, maternal mortality is now rare, and appendiceal perforation usually occurs secondary to marked delay in time to surgical intervention (25,30,43).
- Delay in surgical intervention in women with acute abdomen results in increased maternal morbidity as marked by increased admissions and lengths of hospital stay (27).
- Bowel obstruction is marked by higher maternal mortality rate (6% in 66 cases) and 26% fetal mortality (34).

Patient Education
- Pregnant women should be encouraged to not delay seeking evaluation for potential surgical symptoms or problems just because they are pregnant.
- Surgical consent during pregnancy requires a definitive explanation and discussion of the risks to both the pregnancy/fetus and the mother from both surgery and delay of surgery.
- When fetal viability is present, the patient and family should meet with neonatal intensive care unit (NICU) personnel to discuss the implications of PTD at that gestational age.

REFERENCES

1. Center for Disease Control, Office of Women's Health. 2009. Available at: http://www.cdc.gov/women/lcod/. Accessed April 22, 2013.
2. Dunning K, Lemasters G, Bhattacharya A. A major public health issue: the high incidence of falls during pregnancy. *Matern Child Health J.* 2010;14:720–725.
3. Catalano SM. Intimate partner violence, 1993–2010. *National Criminal Justice Reference Service.* 2012:1–17.
4. Gazmararian JA, Lazorick S, Spitz AM, et al. Prevalence of violence against pregnant women. *JAMA.* 1996;275:1915–1920.
5. Vanden Hoek TL, Morrison LJ, Shuster M, et al. 2010 American Heart Association guidelines for cardiopulmonary resuscitation and emergency cardiovascular care science Part 12.3: cardiac arrest associated with pregnancy. *Circulation.* 2010;122:S829–S861.

6. Townsend CM, Beauchamp RD, Evers BM, et al. *Sabiston textbook of surgery: the biological basis of modern surgical practice, 19th edition. Chapter 18: management of acute trauma.* Philadelphia: Elsevier Saunders, 2012:430–470.

7. Brown HL. Trauma in pregnancy. *Obstet Gynecol.* 2009;14;147–160.

8. Katz V, Balderston K, DeFreest M. Perimortem cesarean delivery: were our assumptions correct? *Am J Obstet Gynecol.* 2005;192:1916–1821.

9. Warraich Q, Esen U. Perimortem cesarean section. *J Obstet Gynaecol.* 2009;29:690–693.

10. Dhanraj D, Lambers D. The incidences of positive Kleihauer-Betke test in low-risk pregnancies and maternal trauma patients. *Am J Obstet Gynecol.* 2004;190:1461–1463.

11. Ornsby EL, Geng J, McGahan JP, et al. Pelvic free fluid: clinical importance for reproductive age women with blunt abdominal trauma. *Ultrasound Obstet Gynecol.* 2005;26:271–278.

12. Chen MM, Coakley FV, Kaimal A, et al. Guidelines for computed tomography and magnetic resonance imaging use during pregnancy and lactation. *Obstet Gynecol.* 2008;112:333–340.

13. Gabbe SG, Neibyl JR, Simpson JL, et al. *Obstetrics: normal and problem pregnancies. Chapter 8: occupational and environmental hazards.* Philadelphia: Elsevier Saunders, 2012:140–165.

14. ACOG Committee in Obstetric Practice. ACOG Committee Opinion 299: guidelines for diagnostic imaging during pregnancy. *Obstet Gynecol.* 2004;104(3):647–651.

15. El Kady D. Perinatal outcomes of traumatic injuries during pregnancy. *Clin Obstet Gynecol.* 2007;50:582–591.

16. Guo SS, Greenspoon JS, Kahn AM. Management of burn injuries in pregnancy. *Burns.* 2001;27:394–397.

17. Gabbe SG, Neibyl JR, Simpson JL, et al. *Obstetrics: normal and problem pregnancies. Chapter 25: trauma and related surgery in the pregnant patient.* Philadelphia: Elsevier Saunders, 2012:581–591.

18. Kady D, Gilbert WM, Anderson J, et al. Trauma during pregnancy: an analysis of maternal and fetal outcomes in a large population. *Am J Obstet Gynecol.* 2004;190:1661–1668.

19. Petrone P, Talving P, Brawder T, et al. Abdominal injuries in pregnancy: a 155-months sturdy at two level 1 trauma centers. *Injury.* 2011;42:47–49.

20. Madsen LV, Jensen J, Christensen ST. Parturition and pelvic fracture: follow-up of 34 obstetric patients with a history of pelvic fracture. *Acta Obstet Gynecol Scand.* 1983;62:617–620.

21. Mendez-Figueroa J, Dahlke JD, Vress RA, et al. Trauma in pregnancy: an updated systemic review. *Am J Obstet Gynecol.* 2013;209(1):1–10.

22. Runyan CW, Johnson RM, Yang J, et al. Risk and protective factors for fires, burns, and carbon monoxide poisoning in the U.S. households. *Am J Prev Med.* 2005;28:102–108.

23. Coleman MT, Trianfo VA, Rund DA. Nonobstetric emergencies in pregnancy: trauma and surgical conditions. *Am J Obstet Gynecol.* 1997;177:497–502.

24. Kuczkowski KM. Nonobstetric surgery during pregnancy: what are the risks of anesthesia? *Obstet Gynecol Surv.* 2003;59:52–56.

25. Sharp HT. The acute abdomen during pregnancy. *Clin Obstet Gynecol.* 2002;45:405–413.

26. Birchard KR, Brown MA, Hyslop WB, et al. MRI of acute abdominal and pelvic pain in pregnant patients. *AJR Am J Roentgenol.* 2005;184:452–458.

27. El-Amin AM, Yahia Al-Shehri M, Zaki ZM, et al. Acute abdomen in pregnancy. *Int J Gynaecol Obstet.* 1998;62:31–36.

28. Mourad J, Elliott JP, Erickson L, et al. Appendicitis in pregnancy: new information that contradicts long-held clinical beliefs. *Am J Obstet Gynecol.* 2000;182:127–129.

29. Horowitz MD, Gomez GA, Santiesteban R, et al. Acute appendicitis during pregnancy. *Arch Surg.* 1995;120:1362–1367.

30. Wilasrusmee C, Sukrat B, McEvoy M, et al. Systematic review and meta-analysis of safety of laparoscopic versus open appendicectomy for suspected appendicitis in pregnancy. *Br J Surg.* 2012;99:1470–1479.

31. Mazze RI, Kallen B. Appendectomy during pregnancy: a Swedish registry study of 778 cases. *Obstet Gynecol.* 1991;77:835–840.

32. Graham G, Baxi L, Tharakan T. Laparoscopic cholecystectomy during pregnancy: a case series and review of the literature. *Obstet Gynecol Surv.* 1998;53:566–574.

33. Barone JE, Bears S, Chen S, et al. Outcome study of cholecystectomy during pregnancy. *Am J Surg.* 1999;177:232–236.
34. Perdue PW, Johnson HW, Stafford PW. Intestinal obstruction complicating pregnancy. *Am J Surg.* 1992;164:384–388.
35. Daskalakis G, Antsaklis A, Papageorgiou I, et al. Thrombosis prophylaxis after treatment during pregnancy. *Eur J Obstet Gynecol Reprod Biol.* 1997;74:165–167.
36. Greer IA, Nelson-Piercy C. Low-molecular-weight heparins for thromboprophylaxis and treatment of venous thromboembolism in pregnancy: a systematic review of safety and efficacy. *Blood.* 2005;106:401–407.
37. Robertson L, Greer I. Thromboembolism in pregnancy. *Curr Opin Obstet Gynecol.* 2005;17:113–116.
38. American College of Obstetricians and Gynecologists. Committee opinion No. 474: Nonobstetric surgery during pregnancy. *Obstet Gynecol.* 2011;117:420–421.
39. Walsh TM, Borahay MA, Fox KA, et al. Robotic-assisted, ultrasound guided abdominal cerclage during pregnancy: overcoming minimally invasive surgery limitations? *J Minim Invasive Gynecol.* 2013;20(3):398–400.
40. Society of American Gastrointestinal Endoscopic Surgeons: Guidelines for diagnosis, treatment and used of laparoscopy for surgical problems during pregnancy (2007). Accessed on 5/8/2013 at http://www.sages.cms.org
41. Chohan L, Kilpatrick CC. Laparoscopy in pregnancy: a literature review. *Clin Obstet Gynecol.* 2009;4:557–569.
42. Horowitz NS. Management of adnexal masses in pregnancy. *Clin Obstet Gynecol.* 2009;54:519–527.
43. Cohen-Kerem R, Railton C, Oren D, et al. Pregnancy outcome following non-obstetric surgical intervention. *Am J Surg.* 2005;190:467–473.
44. Brodsky JB, Cohen EN, Brown BW Jr, et al. Surgery during pregnancy and fetal outcome. *Am J Obstet Gynecol.* 1980;138:1165–1167.
45. Duncan PG, Pope WD, Cohen MM, et al. Fetal risk of anesthesia and surgery during pregnancy. *Anesthesiology.* 1986;64:790–794.
46. Cohen EN, Gift HC, Brown BW, et al. Occupational disease in dentistry and chronic exposure to trace anesthetic gases. *J Am Dent Assoc.* 1980;101:21–31.
47. Mazze RI, Kallen B. Reproductive outcome after anesthesia and operation during pregnancy: a registry study of 5405 cases. *Am J Obstet Gynecol.* 1989;161:1178–1185.
48. Czeizel AE, Pataki T, Rockenbauer M. Reproductive outcome after exposure to surgery under anesthesia during pregnancy. *Arch Gynecol Obstet.* 1998;261:193–199.
49. Kallen B, Mazze RI. Neural tube defects and first trimester operations. *Teratology.* 1990;41:717–720.

PART IV

Fetal Assessment

29 Genetics, Genetic Counseling, and Genetic Risk Assessment
Selman I. Welt

GENETIC COUNSELING
Key Points
- All pregnant women should receive a basic genetic risk evaluation and assessment as part of prenatal care.
- All pregnant women should be offered serum analyte screening for fetal aneuploidies, neural tube defects (NTD), and von Willebrand Disease (VWD). This may be combined with ultrasound evaluation of fetal nuchal translucency and nasal bone if available. Cell-free DNA testing for fetal aneuploidy should be offered in specific circumstances of increased genetic risk.
- Invasive testing for fetal aneuploidies and chromosomal deletion syndromes by amniocentesis, chorionic villus sampling (CVS), or cord blood sampling should be offered to women who have a risk that meets or exceeds specific criteria.
- Follow-up counseling and care should be available for any woman with abnormal karyotype results or evidence of fetal anomalies that are significant or incompatible with life.
- Women with inherited genetic abnormalities or diseases should be offered fetal testing if it is possible and should receive appropriate medical management and prenatal care.

Background
Our understanding of the scientific basis of genetics has advanced with increasing rapidity over the past century and a half, since Gregor Mendel's groundbreaking studies of the pea plant. With the definition of the human genome, genetics has assumed a key position in clinical medicine. Many of our future diagnostic and therapeutic options will be based on or derived from the principles of genetics, making it important for clinicians to have a thorough understanding of the science (1).

Before the explosion of information in molecular genetics, the terminology of clinical genetics was based in the concepts of the gene as the basic, smallest, unit of inheritance. An understanding of the definitions cogent to these clinical terms remains important in communications regarding clinical genetics; they should be clearly understood. Some of the terms that should be familiar are genetics, heredity, counseling, phenotype, genotype, gene, allele, locus, trait, autosomal, sex-linked, heterozygote, homozygote, pedigree, crossing-over, and syndrome (2).

MENDELIAN INHERITANCE
Background
Single-gene inheritance follows the mendelian principles of unitary inheritance, allelic segregation, and independent assortment. It is elucidated by following parents and their progeny and observing distinct patterns emerge: A specific locus is passed, intact, to the offspring. The gene is passed by each of the parents. Therefore, there are two copies. When the appropriate number of copies is present in an individual, an abnormal trait may be identified. This is the basic concept; however, there are variations on this theme (3).

Evaluation
Genetics
- Autosomal dominant: These genetic traits are inherited in the presence of only one dominant gene.
  - More than half of the approximately 5000 mendelian conditions behave in an autosomal dominant fashion.
  - The specific phenotype appears in every generation, and every affected individual has an affected parent (with exceptions discussed later in this chapter).
  - A child of an affected parent has a 50% chance of inheriting the abnormal gene, and, conversely, the phenotypically normal family member does not transmit the phenotype to his or her offspring.
  - Men and women are equally likely to pass the phenotype to their children of either sex.
  - Apparent exceptions to these rules are either the result of new mutations in the germ cells (sperm and ova) or situations in which, despite the presence of the abnormal gene, the disease is not expressed in the individual.
  - Two copies of abnormal dominant genes (homozygosity) are generally lethal.
  - Common examples of autosomal dominant disorders are achondroplasia, Huntington disease, Marfan syndrome, and neurofibromatosis (4).
- Autosomal recessive: These genetic traits require the presence of two paired genes for expression of the abnormality. These traits are generally biochemical abnormalities.
  - An autosomal recessive disease is not seen more than once in a pedigree, outside of the siblings of an affected member of the family; the risk of occurrence of the disease for each sibling of the affected individual is 25%.
  - An unaffected sibling of an affected individual has a two-thirds chance of being a carrier (heterozygote).
  - When the gene is rare, the parents of an individual with such an autosomal recessive condition will be close relatives of each other.
  - Male and female offspring are equally likely to be affected.
  - Autosomal recessive disorders (and some sex-linked recessive disorders) involving single biochemical changes, used to be referred to as "inborn errors of metabolism." Examples are Tay-Sachs disease, phenylketonuria (PKU), and maple syrup urine disease.
- Sex-linked dominant and recessive
  - The dominant forms require only a single gene on the X chromosome to express the abnormality.

- The recessive forms require only one gene on the X chromosome in males but one gene on each of two X chromosomes in females.
  - The incidence of X-linked recessive conditions is much more common in male than in female offspring.
  - Phenotypically normal daughters of affected men (the recessive form) have a 50% chance of passing the abnormal gene to their sons, who will demonstrate the trait. An affected man, however, never has an affected son.
  - Heterozygous women (carriers of the recessive form) are generally unaffected.
  - In the more rare X-linked dominant conditions, affected men have no affected sons and no normal daughters. Both male and female offspring of female carriers have a 50% chance of inheriting the phenotype.
- Not all women who inherit either a single dominant gene or a pair of recessive genes will phenotypically express their genotype, as explained by the Lyon hypothesis (see discussion below) (5).
- Factors influencing the phenotype in mendelian inheritance–based genotypes:
  - Penetrance: Occasionally, an individual with a specific inherited trait or disease (especially autosomal dominant) may not demonstrate the typical phenotype. This may be secondary to the age of the individual (dies before manifestation of the phenotype) or the influence of another gene or the environment. This is referred to as *diminished penetrance*, where there is a lower-than-expected incidence of the phenotype in the genotypic population.
  - Expressivity: When the phenotype varies in the same genotype (not so much in the same family, but in other families), the condition is considered to have greater variability of expression. This can vary from minor to severe expressions and may be due to sex-influenced or limited expression. In some autosomal dominant disorders, the phenotypic manifestation differs between males and females.
  - Anticipation: The term for the situation when a dominant condition appears to present at a younger age in each subsequent generation or when the severity of the disease or trait is increased with each subsequent generation. This may be related to conditions where there is additional expansion of triplets in the genetic code, which is discussed later in this chapter.
  - The Lyon hypothesis: This hypothesis holds that whenever there is more than one X chromosome in the genome, one may be randomly inactivated, existing as inactive chromatin (the *Barr body*). Since the process is random, the percentage of cells with one or the other active X chromosome will vary within specific organ systems and within the individual as a whole. If an abnormal allele is on one of the X chromosomes, its affect may either be unopposed or absent in a percentage of cells, creating a situation in which a heterozygote may express the abnormal allele to varying degrees. It is now believed that this effect is caused by an X-inactivation–specific transcript gene on the long arm of the X chromosome (5,6).
  - Pleiotropy: Although each abnormal gene has one direct effect for which it is identified, there may be secondary or tertiary effects from that same gene on other aspects of an individual's physiology. This has to do with different characteristics of use of the RNA product and subsequent protein product of the gene. Each of these phenotypic effects is believed to be the pleiotropic result of an abnormal protein as transcribed and translated from the specific gene. Pleiotropy may be seen in Marfan syndrome and in the abnormalities of the fibroblast growth factor gene.
  - Codominance: Certain phenotypic traits demonstrate codominance, in which both traits are expressed, either from alleles in the same locus or from alleles at separate loci dictating a phenotypic appearance. Examples are hemoglobinopathies and blood types.
- A compilation of information on mendelian inherited disorders may be found updated with references online: http://www.ncbi.nlm.nih.gov/entrez/query.fcgi?db = OMIM (7).

Diagnosis
Clinical Manifestations
- Chromosomal disorders
  - General rules
    - Chromosomes can be seen only during the stage of the cell cycle when the genetic material within the nucleus condenses to become microscopically (cytogenetically) visible.
    - New staining techniques create bands on chromosomes. Each technique develops a distinctive banding pattern so that minute areas of the chromosome may be visibly distinguished and compared. With high-resolution karyotyping, chromosomes can be subdivided into hundreds of subbands, with an average length of about 3.5 million base pairs (8).
    - One set of 23 chromosomes is inherited from each parent. A pair of chromosomes is called a homolog (e.g., the two number 1 chromosomes). They have a similar cytogenetic appearance and carry "matching" genetic material down to the locus of each gene and the DNA code itself.
    - The two types of cell division, mitosis and meiosis, result in the daughter cells with the appropriate number of chromosomes and the correct amount of genetic material. Mitosis results in two cells with equal genetic material. Meiosis results in four gametes in men and one in women, each with a haploid complement of chromosomes (the other three gametes in women are usually lost).
    - Chromosomal disorders are primarily the result of a deficiency or excess of a significant amount of genetic material.
    - The presence of an extra chromosome or chromosome segment can result in a distinctive genetic condition or a peculiar phenotype.
    - Collectively, chromosome disorders are more common than are single-gene disorders and affect 6 to 10 out of 1000 liveborn infants.
    - Aneuploidies are chromosomal disorders relating to abnormal numbers of chromosomes. One extra chromosome is called a trisomy (three of one chromosome), and one less chromosome is called a monosomy (one of the chromosome instead of two). An additional set of 23 chromosomes is referred to with the suffix of "ploidy" (69 chromosomes, triploidy; 92 chromosomes, tetraploidy).
    - Rearrangements (recombination of the genetic material) occur both in somatic mitosis and gametic meiosis. Cell division errors can and do occur. From a cytogenetic standpoint, the most error-prone step in meiosis is anaphase I of the first division of meiosis. When the chromosomes do not segregate to the opposite poles of the dividing cell, the resulting gametes can have an extra chromosome or be deficient for the nonsegregating chromosome. This is called nondisjunction. Fertilization of these gametes produces an individual with an abnormal number of chromosomes (Fig. 29-1).
    - Abnormalities in the arms of the chromosomes (i.e., deletions, additions, inversions) are referred to by the letters *p* for the short arm and *q* for the long arm of the chromosome. Such abnormalities and crossing-over of genetic materials generally occur during meiosis in the germ cells. This is demonstrated at http://www.accessexcellence. org/RC/VL/GG/comeiosis.html (Accessed March 29, 2013).
    - Chromosomal terminology is established by international conferences and published on a regular basis. Some basic terminology is needed to interpret laboratory reports (9).
  - Chromosomal syndromes
    - Aneuploidy: abnormal numbers of chromosomes
      - Monosomy: 45 chromosomes
        * Autosomal monosomy is generally lethal.
        * X chromosome monosomy is referred to as Turner syndrome.
      - Trisomy: 47 chromosomes

NONDISJUNCTION

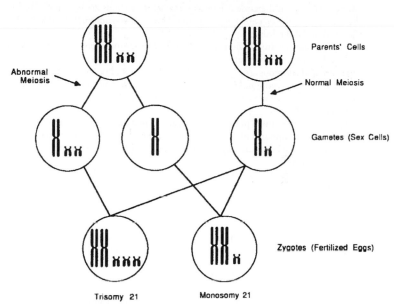

Figure 29-1. Nondisjunction resulting from an abnormal meiotic division yields an aneuploidy gamete and zygote (6).

* Trisomy 21 is Down syndrome. It has an incidence of 1 in 800 to 1000 newborns. Ninety-five percent of cases of Down syndrome result from maternal nondisjunction, and 5% result from translocations and mosaicisms.
* Trisomy 18 is Edwards syndrome. It has an incidence of 1 in 8000 newborns. Eighty-five percent of fetuses with this syndrome die between 10 and 40 weeks of gestation.
* Trisomy 13 is Patau syndrome. This syndrome affects 1 in 20,000 newborns. Median survival is 3 days, and 90% die by 1 month of age.
* XXY is Klinefelter syndrome. This genetic disorder gives rise to infertile, tall males.
* XXX syndrome: Females with variable intelligence; some develop mental problems.
* XYY syndrome: Tall phenotypically normal males, with learning disabilities and aggressiveness.
* Other trisomies are rare except as mosaicisms or partial trisomies secondary to additions.
  ○ Polyploidy
    - Partial hydatidiform mole (69 chromosomes) occurs when the extra set of chromosomes is paternal.
    - Intrauterine growth restriction of fetus and placenta (69 chromosomes) occurs when the extra set is of maternal origin.
    - Higher number ploidies are generally lethal.
  ○ Deletions and additions; copy number variations (CNV)
    - Deletion of 4p is Wolf-Hirschhorn syndrome.

- Deletion of 5p is cri-du-chat syndrome.
- Microdeletion of 22q11.2 is Shprintzen syndrome and DiGeorge syndrome, which are two extremes of the same deletions, or current methods are too inexact to further distinguish the deletion site. Note that Shprintzen syndrome is also known as velocardiofacial syndrome.
- Ring chromosomes are deletions at each end of the chromosome that "heal" with both ends stuck to each other.
- Deletions and additions are now generally detected in molecular genetics by microarray comparative genomic hybridization with fluorescence, probe amplification, or quantitative polymerase chain reaction (PCR) (10,11).

  o Translocations
  - Reciprocal: Breaks at two points with transfer of material before healing.
  - Balanced: Equal amounts of genetic materials are exchanged. One-quarter of gametes are normal, one-half are duplications and deletions, and one-quarter are translocation carriers.
  - Robertsonian: Only occurs with acrocentric chromosomes 13, 14, 15, 21, and 23. Central fusion translocation is the most common form of translocation.
  - Isochromosomes: Either two long arms (q) or two short arms (p) are fused into a new chromosome.

  o Inversions
  - Breaks occur at two points, and the material inverts before healing.
  - Paracentric: The breaks occur away from the centromeres and may be balanced or unbalanced.
  - Pericentric: The breaks include the centromere.

  o Mosaicisms
  - There are two or more cell lines in the body made up of different chromosomal complements but from the same zygote (e.g., 46XX, 45X, the loss of an X chromosome during early mitotic divisions).
  - The phenotype of the mosaic individual depends on the location and percentage of abnormal cells in the various organ systems.
  - Mosaicism in the trophoblast and placenta is relatively common.
  - Gonadal mosaicism may explain spontaneous mutations occurring more frequently than expected in a sibship.

  o Chimerism
  - There are two cell lines in the body made up of different chromosomal complements from two different zygotes.
  - Fraternal twins with exchange of hematopoietic stem cells may lead to an individual with two different DNAs on blood testing (11).
  - Commonly seen in animals but exceedingly rare in humans, the fusion of two fertilized ova may cause an individual with two separate cell lines in some organ systems (12).

NONMENDELIAN INHERITANCE
Background
A number of nonclassic patterns have been described that differ from the established patterns of inheritance. Developments in molecular genetics have allowed these unusual patterns of inheritance to be more clearly defined.

Evaluation
Genetics
- Triplet repeats in DNA: In this situation, a region of DNA exhibits repetitive repeats of a triplet nucleotide sequence (e.g., CGG at Xq27 in fragile X or Martin-Bell syndrome). During crossing-over in meiosis, sister chromatids may exchange some DNA, which

may lengthen the section of the triplet nucleotide sequence. When this happens and the sequence attains a certain length, methylation may occur and damage or inactivate the DNA, causing the specific abnormal trait. Characteristic findings with this are as follows:

- Increasing severity of the abnormal trait with subsequent generations.
- Cytogenetic techniques are not preferable for detection.
- Restriction endonuclease digestion and Southern blot analysis for nucleotide triplets and DNA methylation are the preferred detection methods (13,14).
- This situation may explain some of the cases of penetrance and varied expressivity in phenotypes with the same genetic disorders.
- Examples of disorders associated with recurrent nucleotide sequences include fragile X syndrome, myotonic dystrophy, Huntington disease, Friedrich ataxia, X-linked spinal and bulbar muscular atrophy (Kennedy disease), spinocerebellar ataxia types 1 and 2, dentatorubral-pallidoluysian atrophy, and Machado-Joseph disease (2,16):
  - Fragile X syndrome is transmitted as an X-linked disorder.
    - The number of CGG repeats varies in four classifications:
      * Unaffected (less than 45 triplets)
      * Intermediate (45 to 54 triplets)
      * Premutation (55 to 200 triplets)
      * Full mutation (greater than 200 triplets)
    - The *American College of Obstetricians and Gynecologists (ACOG)* Committee on Genetics recommends that women with a family history of fragile X–related disorders, unexplained mental retardation or developmental delay, autism, or premature ovarian insufficiency are candidates for genetic counseling and fragile X premutation carrier screening (the FMR1 DNA mutation should also be performed after genetics counseling) (15).
- Mitochondrial inheritance: The mitochondrion, the site of oxidative phosphorylation within the somatic cell, carries its own genetic information.
  - Mitochondrial DNA (mtDNA) exists as a circular chromosome within the mitochondrion.
  - During cell division, the mitochondria are thought to be randomly distributed to the daughter cells.
  - Variable expression is commonly seen in mitochondrial diseases because the phenotypic trait relates to the proportions of normal and abnormal mitochondria.
  - Peculiar to mitochondrial inheritance is its maternal inheritance pattern. A mother transmits some of her mitochondria to her eggs and offspring. A father (through his sperm) transmits none. Recurrence risks can be substantial.
  - Examples of mtDNA inheritance are myoclonic epilepsy with ragged red fibers, Leber hereditary optic neuropathy, Leigh syndrome, and pigmentary retinopathy (2,16).
- Imprinting: Some of the genetic code is inherited in a nonactive form from one parent and is only turned on or made active by a gene from the other parent. This appears to be sex specific in the offspring.
  - The best studied demonstration of imprinting is in the Prader-Willi/Angelman syndrome complex. It is linked to a cytogenetically demonstrable or molecularly identified microdeletion in the long arm of chromosome 15. When inherited from the father, it is the Prader-Willi syndrome. Angelman syndrome has a completely different phenotype when inherited with the identical Prader-Willi microdeletion but from the mother (2,16).
  - The parental origin of the genetic material appears to have a profound effect on clinical expression and phenotype (11).
  - Imprinting exerts its effect on the phenotype essentially by controlling the dosage of gene effect, making a biallelic trait monoallelic in some situations. The reason for such a mechanism has not yet been elucidated.

- Uniparental disomy exists when both members of one pair of chromosomes are inherited from the same parent. This may occur from other mechanisms, but the most common mechanism may be "trisomic rescue." Most often, there is no consequence of this phenomenon except for chromosomes 6, 7, 11, 14, and 15. Isodisomy is the term when both chromosomes in a pair are from the same single chromosome in a parental pair (3,13).

MULTIFACTORIAL AND POLYGENIC INHERITANCE
Background
Multifactorial disorders generally result from the complex interaction between genes and environment. The underlying cause may be compound, and the role of the environment may have a multifaceted involvement in the expression of the genetic material.

Evaluation
Genetics
- Multifactorial defects fail to show the classic mendelian inheritance patterns seen for single-gene defects; therefore, recurrence risks are primarily based on empirical data.
  - Multifactorial defects are obviously familial, but there is no distinctive pattern of inheritance within a family (16).
  - Risk to first-degree relatives is approximately the square root of the populational risk.
  - The risk for second-degree relatives decreases sharply from that for first-degree relatives but declines less rapidly with more distant kinship.
  - Recurrence risk is higher when more family members are affected.
  - The more serious the defect, the higher the recurrence risk.
  - Several loci are involved in creating the phenotypic trait.
  - The loci act in concert in an additive fashion, each adding or subtracting a small amount from the phenotype.
  - The environment interacts to varying degrees to produce the final phenotype (e.g., vitamin deficiency, excess hormone production).
  - The frequency of similarly affected co-twins is higher among monozygotic than among dizygotic twins.
- A number of different conditions fall into the category of multifactorial inheritance, including cleft lip with or without cleft palate, isolated cleft palate, congenital dislocation of the hip, pyloric stenosis, isolated NTD (including anencephaly and spina bifida), and isolated congenital heart defects (recurrence risks of 2% to 4%) (Table 29-1).
- For these conditions, empirical data suggest that the recurrence risk is significantly higher within a family than the general population risk, but the patterns of inheritance differ from the classic mendelian autosomal or sex-linked models.
  - Most affected children have normal parents. This is true for diseases and for quantitative traits such as intelligence; children with both very superior and extremely low intelligence quotients are born to parents with average intelligence quotients.
  - Recurrence risk increases with the number of affected children in a family and with the severity of the defect. More severely affected parents are more likely to produce a more severely affected child.
  - Consanguinity slightly increases the risk for having an affected child.
  - If the two parents have a different probability of being affected, the parent with the least probability is the one most likely to produce an affected child.
- Genetic counseling for multifactorially or polygenically inherited conditions can be difficult and depends, in large part, on diagnostic clarity and empirical data.
- Although frequently used to describe malformation disorders, multifactorial inheritance and polygenic inheritance have been implicated in such common abnormalities as some forms of cancer and predisposition to coronary artery disease, diabetes, and alcoholism.
- Categorization of polygenic and multifactorially inherited conditions (4).

Table 29-1	Common Congenital Malformations with Multifactorial Inheritance

Malformations	Population incidence per 1000 (approx.)
Cleft lip with/without cleft palate	0.4–1.7
Cleft palate	0.4
Congenital dislocation of the hip	2 per 1000 males only
Congenital heart defects	4–8
Ventricular septal defect	1.7
Patent ductus arteriosus	0.5
Atrial septal defect	1.0
Aortic stenosis	0.5
Neural tube defects	2–10
Anencephaly	Variable
Spina bifida	Variable
Pyloric stenosis	1 per 1000 females
	5 per 1000 males

From Thompson MW, McInnes RR, Willard HF. *Thompson & Thompson Genetics in Medicine.* 5th ed. Philadelphia: W.B. Saunders, 1991.

- Variable traits have a normal distribution in the general population and are measurable or quantitative traits. In these traits, the statistical principle of regression to the mean governs the bell-shaped curve without further extension of the extremes (9).
- Threshold traits are phenotypic traits that do not appear until a critical threshold is met. As such, they are an all-or-none phenomenon with greater likelihood of achieving the threshold within families and with the same environmental impacts. Some of these traits have a sex predilection (likely an environmental effect) (16).
- Complex disorders or traits involve the presence of multiple genes, the environment, and other unknown factors with familial tendencies. They may include obesity, diabetes, hypertension, and some cancers.
- Pharmacogenetics: The effects of medications and their degradation are different in different people; this is genetically based. Enzymes encoded by genes with polymorphic alleles may have different catabolic rates and routes that lead to different reactions to medications.
  - Malignant hyperthermia: mutations in the ryanodine receptor protein (16)
  - Serum pseudocholinesterase deficiency: demonstrates variations in percentages of enzyme activities
  - Adverse reactions to drugs demonstrated on a genetic basis:
    - Coumadin
    - Isoniazid
    - Corticosteroids
- Racial differences in the efficacy of drugs and drug combinations: BiDil, a combination of drugs hydralazine and isosorbide dinitrate for heart failure in African Americans (17)

MOLECULAR BIOLOGY OF GENETICS
Background
- The gene.
  - The genetic material, encoded into packets of information called genes, forms the backbone of the cytogenetically visible chromosome. The estimated 30,000 genes within the human genome, 2 m of DNA, are strung, rather like beads on a string or railroad cars in a train, along the length of the chromosome.

- This linear array of genetic information and the corresponding linear order of the genetic material allow construction of the linear genetic map.
- Genes can be ordered with respect to one another, genetically or physically linked to one another, and physically linked to a particular chromosome (18).
- The genome. Only a small percentage of the genetic information that resides within the human genome can be currently interpreted. About 75% of the DNA is single copy, unique, with only 10% coding for proteins and the remainder being various classes of repetitive DNA (19). The goal of the Human Genome Project is to decipher and understand the human genetic code, promising a more complete understanding of the complex interaction among genes, their expression, and the environment (7).
  - The information present within the genetic material of the human is encoded within the polymeric macromolecule DNA.
  - Packaged within the double five-carbon sugar backbone are millions of nitrogen-containing bases called *pyrimidines* (thymine and cytosine) and *purines* (adenine and guanine).
  - The unwinding of the double helix allows precise duplication of the DNA so that daughter cells are given the best possible opportunity of having identical genetic information to the parent cell. However, errors do occur. A replication error in the precise matching of the base sequence of the DNA can result in a base change and therefore a mutation at that site. The mutation may have a significant effect on the daughter cell, or it may have none. Varied alleles at a specific DNA locus are likely prior mutations that have been carried on (2,19).
  - It is the precise order of the bases within a length of DNA that defines the expression of the genetic material. The structure of the DNA allows that code to be read and translated into a largely single-stranded transmission molecule, RNA. The RNA molecule, in turn, directs the production of a specific protein of specific amino acid sequence. It is, therefore, the order of the bases within the DNA backbone and the genetic code that define the protein product (http://hyperphysics.phy-astr.gsu.edu/Nave-html/Faithpathh/codelife2.html) (20).
  - The code is precise. Even a single base change can have a profound effect on the ultimate protein product and therefore on its activity and expression.
  - Mutations occur when chemical or physical agents lead to base modifications; these agents are called mutagens, and their mechanisms of action include
    - Deamination of cytosine, adenine, or guanine
    - Methylation of carbon in the nucleic acids
    - Depurination of DNA by thermal fluctuations in the cell
    - Alkylation of the nucleic acids
    - Replacement with nucleic acid analogues (e.g., 5-bromodeoxyuridine for thymine)
    - Ultraviolet light–induced thymine dimers, alterations in the covalent carbon bonds of adjacent nucleic acids in the DNA (19)
  - The gene encodes more than the information necessary for the protein product. The gene also includes the adjacent functional genetic material including the start and stop signal for RNA production and the regulatory signals for gene recruitment. The gene structure of higher organisms includes regions of genetic material transcribed to RNA and expressed into the protein product (exons), separated by intervening sequences of genetic information that is not expressed in the protein product (introns). There is also a promoter, which is a regulatory region within each gene recognized as a 5′ untranslated region upstream of the exon and a 3′ untranslated region downstream of the exon. The precise processing of the RNA product, including intron removal and splicing of the RNA product, is a crucial part of the regulatory mechanics of functional informational processing and recruitment. The product protein exists in a precursor form that must be cleaved to the final product (http://www.patentlens.net/daisy/promoters/239/g1/240.html) (21).

- Single nucleotide polymorphisms (SNPs) are the most common form of DNA variation; they represent a single base substitution or the replacement of one base (i.e., A, C, G, or T) for another base in the DNA sequence. SNP is the term used to describe such substitutions when they occur relatively frequently in the population and are not associated with a mendelian disorder. On average, SNPs are observed every 200 to 300 base pairs.
- Missense mutation: A substitution that changes the codon for one amino acid to the codon for another amino acid. The size of the mRNA and protein is not changed, but the composition and possibly the function of the protein do not change.
- Nonsense mutation: A substitution that changes a codon for an amino acid to a stop codon, leading to a premature termination of translation of the mRNA transcript and a truncated protein.
- Splice site mutation: A substitution in one of the base pairs inside or flanking the intron–exon boundaries that alters normal premRNA splicing. Such mutations can result in intron retention (either partial or complete) or exon skipping.
- Silent mutation: A change in one base that results in no change in the amino acid sequence of the protein, due to the redundancy of the genetic code (there is more than one codon for most amino acids).
- Regulatory polymorphism: A substitution that alters binding affinities of transcript-related proteins, such as transcription factors, enhancers, silencers, or insulators. Such changes result in altered rates of transcription. Though protein structure is not altered by such noncoding variants, the level of transcript production can result in altered protein production and in turn confer phenotypic variation (22).
- Most human DNA (99.8%) is identical; there are only minor differences between one person and another. These differences, called polymorphisms, usually consist of a single nucleotide change about every 200 to 500 base pairs. Most polymorphisms do not affect phenotypes, but they can be used for identification purposes and to determine inheritance of a specific DNA sequence (2).
- Specific tissues may control gene expression by methylation of the regulatory region, effectively turning off the gene (19).
- Molecular diagnostic testing.
  - Restriction endonucleases are bacterial enzymes that cut DNA. They are used to cut the DNA molecule at specific sequences of nucleotides (14). There are now hundreds of these enzymes available to cleave DNA at different locations (2,17).
  - PCR is a rapid means of creating multiple copies of specific DNA when the beginning or ending sequences are known (7).
    - Southern blot is used to separate DNA fragments (23).
    - Northern blot is used to isolate RNA (2).
    - Western blot is used to isolate proteins (2).
  - Allele-specific oligonucleotide probes (dot blot or ASO) are short nucleotide probes of 15 to 25 bases synthesized in the laboratory for a specific DNA sequence. They are designed to detect specific mutations in DNA and may be used in Southern blotting as a probe in questions of familial mutation (23). This technique is currently used for detection of single-gene disorders such as Tay-Sachs, Canavan disease, cystic fibrosis, and Gaucher disease.
  - In multiplex PCR for gene deletion analysis, multiple DNA fragment copies from PCR undergo electrophoresis to determine the presence or absence of the DNA exon.
  - Complementary DNA (cDNA) is a single strand of DNA that is produced in the laboratory from RNA using a reverse transcriptase enzyme. The nucleic acid sequence of the intended DNA must be known. Libraries of cDNA are maintained for research and diagnosis (2).
    - In linkage analysis, familial studies of linked traits can be conducted to characterize a gene that has not been characterized, but whose location is known to some degree (24).

- The criteria for linkage analysis are
  - A large family with at least two generations of individuals affected
  - DNA fragments from affected and unaffected family members
  - A pedigree that allows for study of linkage and segregation
  - Mathematical calculations of crossing-over data for distance of the linkage or segregation (3,24)
- Fluorescence in situ hybridization (FISH) is a DNA technique in which fixed metaphase chromosomes are hybridized with a fluorochrome-labeled DNA probe specific to a particular region of a chromosome. FISH can be used to
  - Identify specific chromosome numbers rapidly
  - Identify translocated chromosome regions
  - Recognize deletions and additions to chromosomes
  - Identify specific abnormal regions of chromosomes associated with a specific gene within the probe (comparative genomic hybridization) (19)
- DNA sequencing can be used to identify any animal containing DNA, and additional sequencing can identify specific individuals within a species. In humans, 13 specific regions of DNA are used to create a DNA fingerprint. Some uses of this technology include establishing paternity or other family relationships and matching organ donors with transplant recipients (25,26).
- Limitations to the accuracy of molecular testing:
  - It is dependent on an accurate clinical diagnosis.
  - Testing sensitivity is related to disease prevalence.
  - Genetic disorders may be caused by different alleles at different loci.
  - An abnormal trait may exhibit populational differences in frequency, genetic constitution, and phenotypic expression.
  - Phenotypic penetrance and expressivity may not be determined by the presence or absence of one specific mutation alone but instead may also depend on environmental factors and the presence or activity of other genes.
- In microarray technology or DNA chips, PCR and cDNA are used to screen specific DNA from patients for gene mutations or polymorphisms, using a labeled cDNA hybridization (27). These specialized oligomers of DNA are increasing in number as libraries of them are being collected and catalogued. Array comparative genomic hybridization should be performed whenever congenital anomalies in the fetus exist in the presence of normal G-banded karyotypes, when fetal demise occurs with a congenital anomaly and a standard karyotype could not be obtained, or in the situation where sonographic evidence is of a nonaneuploidy fetal syndrome (ACOG) (28).
- The main limitations of conventional karyology are low resolution of the G-banding and other techniques, the requirement for cell culture, the extended time from sampling to results, the need for subjective interpretation, the limits to high-throughput automated analysis, and the likelihood that submicroscopic deletions and duplications or other rearrangements are not commonly detectable.
- The advantages of microarray are a higher diagnostic yield with resolution of 50 to 200,000 base pairs compared with banding patterns of 3 to 10 million bases, in karyology. Also, a faster turnaround time because cell culture is not always needed and the system is more amenable to automation in the laboratory.
- The main disadvantages of the array are that the smallest CNV depends on the size, density, and genomic distribution of the DNA fragment on the array; the array only detects abnormalities of those regions that are represented on the array; the exact boundary and size of the gain and loss cannot be accurately determined; single nucleotide (point mutations) cannot be detected; balanced translocation or inversions can only be picked up if a small oligonucleotide is lost at the time of the change; chromosomal mosaicism cannot be picked up; and small marker chromosomes will be detected only if the

oligonucleotide is on the array. Triploidy will not be picked up because the chromosome numbers are balanced. Many de novo CNV may be picked up but without clinical correlation. Most of the de novo CNV are considered benign, but this is not always so (e.g., 1q21, TAR syndrome). Parental blood samples for comparison may be helpful in deciding about de novo CNV; meanwhile, CNV databases are being established (29,30).

Treatment
Genetic Counseling and Risk Assessment
- Genetic counseling is the process of providing specific information and advice to an individual or family group, which ultimately results in a plan of care.
- The indications for genetic counseling are presented in Table 29-2.
- The approach is systematic:
  - Determine the disease in question, the accuracy of the diagnosis, and the extent of the clinical presentation of the affected individual (many disorders have similar phenotypic appearance but different genotypes).
  - Determine the relationship of the individual being counseled to the affected individual. Perform the pedigree with emphasis on the immediate relatives of the affected individual. Establish the means of inheritance as completely as possible. Determine the risk for family members based on their location in the pedigree and the mode of inheritance and counsel regarding the relative risks for an unborn fetus or future pregnancy.
  - Determine if a test is available for carrier status. Address the accuracy of available testing and the limits of knowledge concerning the specific abnormality. Provide information regarding the risks and benefits of procedures for more accurately assessing risk (e.g., testing other family members, amniocentesis in pregnancy). Give information on the length of time necessary to obtain results from screening and diagnostic testing.
  - Provide nondirectional counseling that includes information on pregnancy termination options when appropriate, but that does not necessitate or encourage pregnancy termination. Make available information on selected adoption.
  - Address the psychological and social concerns of the individual requesting the consultation.

Table 29-2	Indications for Genetic Counseling Prior to or During Pregnancy

Known or suspected hereditary disease in the family
Maternal age of 35 years or greater when the baby delivers
Paternal age of 40 years or greater when the baby delivers
Some ethnic groups (see Table 29-3)
Recurrent pregnancy losses, three or more
Prior unexplained stillbirth or neonatal death
Identification of one or more abnormal findings in early pregnancy by population screening techniques or individual assessment
Self, mate, parent, child, brother, sister, uncle, aunt, or first cousin with birth defect, chromosomal abnormality, mental retardation/autism, or abnormal growth and development
Pregnant woman with metabolic disorder such as diabetes type 1, phenylketonuria, thyroid disease
Pregnant woman with some hereditary disease with risk to a fetus such as thalassemia; pregnant woman on chronic medications such as anticonvulsants, thyroid medications, chemotherapy
Mother with or sibling with cardiac disease

- Explain the main differences between genetic screening tests and the more definitive gene, chromosomal, and protein analyses for disease determination.
- Recent trends in genetic counseling and prenatal diagnosis.
  - There has been a decrease in invasive procedures. Developments in analyte screening, cell-free DNA testing, and ultrasound evaluation have led to a decrease in the need for invasive testing in many situations, which has decreased patient risk and expense (26).
  - Opposition to genetic counseling is sometimes encountered on the basis of ethical and religious principles. Appropriate counseling should be offered and documented with sensitivity to these concerns.
  - Counseling should always be nondirectional and nonjudgmental, in order to allow couples to make informed decisions that are appropriate for their own situations.

Risk Management
- Genetic risk assessment requires
  - A specific and accurate diagnosis.
    - ° Accuracy of diagnosis and risk assessment are closely linked. Without an exact diagnosis, risk assessment is difficult or impossible.
  - Complete information about the individual and the family through a comprehensive genetic evaluation (31). This includes
    - ° Verification of the diagnosis or possible diagnoses.
    - ° Review of the clinical data and supporting documentation.
    - ° Detailed medical and family history.
    - ° Thorough family pedigree.
    - ° Examination of the affected individual.
    - ° Examination of relevant family members.
    - ° Examination of any stillborn infant or fetus aborted in pregnancies with genetic issues.
    - ° Evaluation of any dysmorphic newborn by an experienced dysmorphologist.
    - ° Newborn screening programs can provide helpful information about an individual child or family members who have been screened for specific disorders or deficits (32).
  - An understanding of the characteristics of the transmission and expression of the genetic abnormality so that risk calculations can be established.
    - ° Specific mendelian risk calculations can be made for many conditions. For example, a family with a previous child diagnosed with Tay-Sachs syndrome has a recurrence risk of 1:4 or 25%.
    - ° Conditional risk calculations can be made for a number of autosomal recessive, autosomal dominant (5), and X-linked recessive conditions. These conditional calculations are based on combining classic mendelian recurrence risks with other unrelated clinical measurements (33). For example, Duchenne muscular dystrophy is an X-linked recessive condition manifesting almost exclusively in male offspring. If a woman has an affected brother and a sister with an affected son, she has a 50% risk of being a carrier for the disease. If, however, she has had five normal, nonaffected sons, the risk of her next son being affected is significantly decreased. The combination of the two independent events (the mendelian calculation and the five normal sons) is accomplished by the use of a Bayesian calculation that allows one to take known information and propose alternative solutions by using probability modifiers (34).
    - ° The third level of risk assessment involves the use of empirical calculations. Many of the more common nonmendelian disorders, such as single malformations (congenital heart disease, cleft lip, cleft palate), have been studied and assigned empirical recurrence risks. It is important to note that calculating empirical risk requires a precise and accurate diagnosis (Table 29-1) (35,36).
  - Accurate and sensitive communication of the genetic risk information to the patient and family.

- Each individual's perception of risk is relative to his or her own experiences, value system, and life goals.
- Each individual's acceptance or rejection of risk is directly linked to his or her confidence in the diagnosis and treatment options.
- Construction of a diagnostic plan and subsequent management options that are acceptable to the patient and family. Whatever the diagnostic modality or therapeutic plan envisioned, the patient's ability to choose it or an alternative plan will be enhanced by his or her understanding of the diagnosis and test implications.

Antenatal Genetic Risks and Modalities of Determination

The assessment of risk from genetic disorders with regard to reproduction is based on the use of general screening tests and specific diagnostic testing. The tests used for screening for specific diagnosis are the modalities of determination.

- Populational screening
  - Prenatal recommendations: The ACOG recommends in version 5 of its Antepartum Record that a genetic screening questionnaire should be used for all pregnancies. Specifics for the testing procedures involved in these screens are listed in Table 29-3.
- The Hardy-Weinberg equilibrium is a mathematical technique that allows one to calculate the incidence of heterozygotes (carriers) of a certain autosomal recessive trait within a population by using the incidence of abnormal homozygotes at birth.
  - The Hardy-Weinberg equilibrium was advanced before the polymorphisms of alleles were established. Thus, it does not work in situations where alleles are polymorphic.
  - There are fundamental assumptions that make the equation work, and when these are not applicable, the equation may not be used for its intended purposes. The assumptions are as follows:
    - Mating is random.
    - Mutation rate is constant.
    - There is no selection for or against a specific phenotype.
    - A large population works against random fluctuations in gene frequencies.
    - No major changes in the population have occurred by migrations (37,38).
- Maternal age.
  - It is well established that the fetal risk of aneuploidy increases with maternal age, with the primary concerns being trisomies 21 and 18. Keeping in mind the risk of the diagnostic modality (genetic amniocentesis) used to determine the presence or absence of aneuploidy, the specific maternal age can be determined at which the risk of aneuploidy exceeds the risk of the genetic amniocentesis. This establishes a risk–benefit point that justifies accepting the risk of the amniocentesis and proceeding with the procedure. This age should be considered relatively fluid based on the mother's desire (or lack thereof) for a definitive diagnosis, changes in the risk/complication rates of the diagnostic modality, and the availability of other screening tests that can modify risk assessment in an individual woman. There are numerous sources of maternal age–related risks (39).
- Paternal age.
  - There is now general agreement that advanced paternal age (greater than 40 years of age or greater than 20 years older than the mother) is associated with an increase in autosomal dominant disorders in their offspring (40). The absolute frequency of such mutations has been estimated as 0.3% (4). There may also be an effect on the X chromosome, causing mutations that are carried through the daughters to their sons; this is also known as the grandfather effect (41). There is now evidence that the combination of paternal age greater than 40 years and maternal age greater than 35 years yields a much higher incidence of pregnancy losses (42).

Table 29-3	American College of Obstetricians and Gynecologists Antepartum Record Genetic Screening Form		
Concern	**Genetics**	**Population**	**Testing**
Advanced maternal age (AMA)	Chromosomal	Varies with age	Nuchal Translucency Quad screen Invasive sampling Cell-Free DNA
Down syndrome	Chromosomal	Family history AMA	Invasive sampling As above
Thalassemia	Codominance	Italians Greeks Mediterraneans Asians	$MCV < 80 \ \mu^3$ Hemoglobin Electrophoresis
Neural tube defects	Multifactorial	General population Folate deficiency Seizure medications	Maternal serum AFP Ultrasound
Congenital heart disease	Multifactorial	General population Recurrence population Type 1 diabetes	Ultrasound
Tay-Sachs disease	Autosomal Recessive	Ashkenazi Jewish Cajuns, French Canadians	Hexosaminidase A
Canavan disease	Autosomal Recessive	Ashkenazi Jewish	Aspartoacyclase
Sickle cell trait and other	Codominance	African American	Sickle cell screen Hemoglobin
Hemoglobinopathies		Asian	Electrophoresis
Hemophilia A (classical)	X-linked recessive	Family history	Factor VIII
Muscular dystrophy	X-linked recessive	Family history	Dystrophin gene Mutation
Cystic fibrosis	Autosomal Recessive Allelic polymorphisms	Whites	CFTR gene
Huntington chorea	Triplet repeat DNA	Family history	Restriction Endonuclease Digestion and Southern blot
Fragile X syndrome	Triplet repeat DNA	Family history	Restriction Endonuclease Digestion and Southern blot DNA hybridization
Previous stillbirth	Unknown	General population	Dysmorphology X-rays Tissue samples For chromosomal studies and DNA hybridization

MCV, mean corpuscular volume; AFP, α-fetoprotein; SS, hemoglobin SS.

- Hemoglobinopathies.
  - ACOG recommends antepartum screening for hemoglobinopathies in patients of African, Southeast Asian, and Mediterranean descent.
  - If a hemoglobinopathy is diagnosed, the findings are important for both the medical management of the pregnancy and genetic risk counseling for the fetus/infant (43).
- Autosomal recessive carrier state screenings.
  - ACOG recommends screening certain populations that are at risk for carrying specific autosomal recessive biochemical abnormalities. In addition, some ethnic groups have advocated screening within their own communities:
    - Tay-Sachs disease: The enzyme hexosaminidase A is deficient in some Ashkenazi Jewish and French Canadian or Cajun peoples. Carrier testing is available (44).
    - Canavan disease: The enzyme aspartoacylase is deficient in some Ashkenazi Jewish people. Carrier testing is available (45).
    - PKU: The enzyme phenylalanine hydroxylase is deficient in some whites. Women with PKU are homozygous. During pregnancy, abnormal phenylalanine metabolism may affect the fetus and lead to microcephaly, mental retardation, or heart defects. The father should be tested for carrier status to determine if the fetus will be homozygous. If the father cannot be tested, the risk of heterozygosity can be calculated (46).
    - Cystic fibrosis is an autosomal recessive disorder that is most frequent among whites.
      * ACOG recommends that carrier screening for cystic fibrosis be offered to at-risk pregnant women.
      * Hundreds of alleles have been identified that cause the various phenotypic appearances of cystic fibrosis, but only a relatively small number can be identified with current testing techniques. Because of this, it is important to know the number of alleles a laboratory tests for and the heterozygote risks for these alleles in specific demographically defined populations. This makes it possible for the risk of homozygosity to be calculated.
- Analyte screening.
  - *Analytes* refers to chemical compounds in the blood associated with abnormal clinical findings in the fetus.
  - Alone, or in combination, the maternal serum values of these substances can be plotted against a curve of the known values measured in either a general or an abnormal population of fetuses. Then, by calculating the deviation from the median value at any gestational age, the results can be stated as multiples of the median (MOM) and used to assess the relative risk for specific disorders in that fetus. The values must be obtained and interpreted with accurate knowledge of the gestational age because the values change with gestational age. The specific sensitivities and specificities for analyte tests are not listed here because they are constantly under review and improvement in proprietary algorithms.
  - Other, extraneous factors that affect the interpretation of the analyte results are still being recognized (e.g., maternal vegetarian diet, insulin dependence, smoking, race, and in vitro conception). For a discussion of the history and use of the analytes, refer to http://info.theclinic.com/mdconsult/pdf/Ultrasound_Clinics_sample_article.pdf (47).
- Maternal serum α-fetoprotein (AFP).
  - In the early second trimester, this analyte may be used in two situations:
    - Elevations above a standard value for each gestational age (expressed as MOM) are associated with an increased risk that the fetus has an opening or defect in the skin, which allows release of AFP into the maternal circulation via the amniotic fluid. Elevations in the maternal serum AFP may be seen in numerous situations, including incorrect gestational dates, fetal death, open NTD, open ventral wall defects, and teratomas.

- Depressions below a standard (expressed as MOM) are associated with fetal aneuploidy.
- Obtaining a sample of the amniotic fluid via amniocentesis remains the mainstay of evaluation, with use of acetylcholine to differentiate the involvement of the CNS. However, many centers with sufficient expertise in ultrasound are now using invasive procedures only in those cases in which either the AFP values are too high to be otherwise explained (greater than 3.5 MOM) or the ultrasound evaluation is inconclusive.
- Quadruple screen.
  - ○ The quadruple screen combines four analytes—maternal serum AFP, β-human chorionic gonadotropin (β-hCG), estriol, and inhibin A—obtained from maternal serum in the early second trimester.
  - ○ The quadruple screen is more sensitive and specific for the identification of fetuses at risk for aneuploidy than the use of one, two, or three analytes. Thus, they have replaced the triple screen.
  - ○ The four analytes are used in conjunction in a complicated proprietary algorithm that includes maternal age, maternal weight, and other factors to create a specific risk analysis for trisomies 21 and 18.
- First-trimester analyte screening.
  - ○ Pregnancy-associated plasma protein-A (PAPP-A) and free β-hCG can be combined with measurement of fetal nuchal translucency by ultrasound at the end of the first trimester to calculate the risk of fetal aneuploidy. The nasal bone measurement, Doppler blood flow of the ductus venosus, hepatic artery Doppler, and flow across the fetal tricuspid valve are being assessed and added to the algorithm in some centers (48).
  - ○ The principles of use of these analytes are the same as those for the analytes used in the second-trimester quadruple screens.
- Second-trimester ultrasound screening.
  - ○ Although not accepted as standard of care in the United States, many other countries and many individual practitioners perform the so-called aneuploidy screen, or genetic sonogram, which is an ultrasound anatomical examination of the fetus at 18 to 20 weeks of gestation. Particular attention is given to specific "soft markers" that are known to be associated with fetal aneuploidy.
  - ○ The intrinsic risk of fetal aneuploidy as estimated from maternal age or the quadruple screen may be modified by sonographic findings that are more frequently associated with an aneuploid fetus than with a normal fetus.
- First-trimester ultrasound screening is accepted as a standard of care in the United States only for the specific indication of nuchal translucency assessment.
  - ○ Patients with a high risk of fetal aneuploidy should be offered nuchal translucency and first-trimester analyte assessment. The sensitivity and specificity of combined ultrasound and analyte first-trimester testing make this an optimal screening option for most patients (48).
  - ○ The report accuracy of first-trimester analyte and combined screening is changing rapidly. Providers should obtain regular updates on current sensitivities and specificities from their reference laboratory or genetic center (49).
- Ethnic screening.
  - ○ Specific populations are at risk because some disorders have been carried over generations. Specialized screening should be performed based upon known ethnic, racial, or place-of-origin genetic risks (Table 29-4) (50).
- Individual screening. The family pedigree, personal health, and reproductive history of each individual may indicate the need for formal genetic screening.
  - • Medical problems. The presence of an inherited disorder in the individual automatically sets the stage for fetal risk. PKU, cystic fibrosis, certain multifactorial disorders

Table 29-4	Ethnic Groups and Genetic Screenings
Group	**Screen**
African Americans	Hemoglobinopathies S and C, thalassemia
	Glucose-6-phosphate dehydrogenase
	deficiency (G6PD)
	Cystic fibrosis (carrier rate of 1/65)
Ashkenazi Jewish Americans	Bloom syndrome (carrier rate 1/100)
	Canavan disease (carrier rate 1/40)
	Cystic fibrosis (carrier rate of 1/29)
	Familial dysautonomia (carrier rate of 1/32)
	Fanconi anemia (carrier rate of 1/89)
	Gaucher disease (carrier rate of 1/15)
	Mucolipidosis IV (carrier rate of 1/127)
	Niemann-Pick disease (carrier rate of 1/90)
	Tay-Sachs disease (carrier rate of 1/30)
Asian Americans	Hemoglobinopathies E, thalassemias, and
	less common hemoglobins
	Cystic fibrosis (carrier rate of 1/90)
Cajuns or Acadian ancestry	Tay-Sachs disease
French Canadians	Familial hypercholesterolemia
Whites	Cystic fibrosis (carrier rate of 1/29)
Finnish Americans	Gyrate atrophy
Hispanic Americans	Familial dysautonomia
	hemoglobinopathies
	Cystic fibrosis (carrier rate of 1/46)
Lebanese Americans	Familial hypercholesterolemia
Mediterranean ancestry Americans	G6PD deficiency
	Hemoglobinopathies
Italians, Greeks, Southern Europeans	Thalassemias
North Africans	Thalassemias

From Cunningham FG. *Williams Obstetrics.* 23rd ed. New York: McGraw Hill, 2010. (3) and ACOG Committee on Genetics. ACOG Committee Opinion no. 442: preconception and prenatal carrier screening for genetic diseases in individuals of Eastern European Jewish descent. *Obstet and Gynecol.* 2009;114:950–953.

such as spina bifida, facial clefting, pyloric stenosis, and congenital cardiac disease require risk assessment and counseling.

- Family pedigree. Although not affected herself, the pedigree of the patient may yield information on inheritance patterns and disorders in the family. The degree of relations between individuals becomes critical in risk assessment because the risks are greater with consanguinity.
- Consanguinity (inbreeding or mating within a family group). Because of the likelihood of similar genes within the family, rare disorders may be more readily demonstrated in the pedigree of a consanguineous mating. Most Western societies prohibit marriage of cousins and incest, but in some groups, it is relatively common. By the time that the genes in common have dropped below 1% (third cousins), the risks are not genetically significant. The probability that a homozygous individual has received both of their abnormal alleles from an identical ancestral source is called the coefficient of inbreeding, or *F* (Table 29-5) (37).
- Reproductive history. Pregnancy losses have a high incidence of chromosomal abnormalities. Repetitive losses may indicate a transmitted chromosomal abnormality, a new

Table 29-5	Gene Proportions in Consanguinity	
Degree of relationships	**Proportion of genes in common**	**F**
Monozygotic twins	1	
Parent–child, 1st	0.5	0.25
Brother–sister, 1st	0.5	0.25
Brother and half-sister, 2nd	0.25	0.125
One parent the same		
Uncle–niece, Aunt–nephew, 2nd	0.25	0.125
Double first cousins, 2nd	0.25	0.125
Same grandparents, parents are siblings married to siblings		
Half uncle–niece, 3rd	0.125	0.0625
The uncle's parent is the niece's grandparent.		
First cousin, 3rd	0.125	0.0625
Same grandparents		
Half first cousins, 4th	0.0625	0.0312
One grandparent is the same.		
First cousins once removed, 4th	0.0625	0.0312
Grandparent of one and parent of the other are siblings.		
Second cousins, 5th	0.0312	0.0156
Same great-grandparents; grandparents are siblings.		

Source: Categories of identical risk and explanation of relationships. The coefficient of inbreeding, *F*, is higher when the population studies are small, isolated, or homogeneous. For instance, *F* for Canadian Roman Catholics is 0.00004–0.0007; for the Japanese, F is 0.005; and for the population of Andhra Pradesh, India, is 0.02.

mutation, or a serious balanced translocation in one of the parents. Proper evaluation, including chromosomal determination on products of conception, will aid in establishing genetic risks for future pregnancies (42,51).
• Findings on ultrasound examination. Abnormal ultrasound findings may indicate a specific genetic syndrome and the necessity for genetic counseling and genetic testing.
• Paternity testing. When determination of paternity is necessary, fetal DNA can be obtained from chorionic villi, amniocytes, or fetal blood and compared to maternal and potential paternal donor DNA. A combined paternity index (CPI) is determined, which states that the likelihood of one individual being the father is so many times more likely for the individual assigned than for a random man in the population. A second assessment is the probability of paternity. The higher the probability rating, the more accurate the result. A probability of 99% is the currently required minimum to establish paternity in most states. This means that 1 in 100 men could be the baby's father; it corresponds to a CPI of 100. Some laboratories are working to raise the minimum requirement to 99.9%, which is 1 in 1000 men and a CPI of 1000 (52).
• Specific diagnostic tests available for the purpose of definitively diagnosing genetic disorders:
  • Ultrasound.
    ○ Fetal ultrasound has reached a degree of accuracy that makes it reliable in the diagnosis of some genetic disorders. The greatest accuracy is noted in single-organ system abnormalities, which are the most common, such as NTDs, diaphragmatic hernia, intestinal atresias, facial clefting, and simple, isolated cardiac or renal abnormalities.
    ○ The finding of a fetal abnormality on ultrasound may be the impetus for a more extensive study with magnetic resonance imaging, DNA studies, or an invasive technique.

- Chorionic villus sampling.
  - CVS is essentially a biopsy of the placenta. The procedure is performed either transcervically or transabdominally. The ACOG now recommends that a microarray should always be performed when a karyotype is ordered.
  - CVS is performed late in the first trimester to obtain fetal tissue for chromosomal or biochemical assessment. Because of initial concerns regarding limb reduction defects, it is recommended that CVS be performed between 11 and 12 weeks of gestation.
  - The rate of complications from CVS, including loss of the pregnancy, is 4% for new centers versus 1% to 2% for highly experienced centers. Although the risks of CVS are higher than for genetic amniocentesis after 15 weeks' gestation, the risks are less than for early (less than 15 weeks) amniocentesis (53).
  - The likelihood of chromosomal mosaicism is also greater in the CVS specimen, and this should be taken into account by the analyst and the genetic counselor.
  - A full dose of Rh immunoglobulin (300 mg) should be administered to all unsensitized Rh-negative patients following CVS.
- Genetic amniocentesis.
  - Genetic amniocentesis is performed by transabdominal needle insertion to obtain amniotic fluid that contains fetal amniocytes. The procedure is performed under direct ultrasound guidance at 15 to 20 weeks' gestation as an outpatient procedure.
  - The timing of 15 to 20 weeks' gestation was selected for two reasons:
    - The ratio of viable to nonviable cells in the amniotic fluid allows relatively easy culture of cells and subsequent cytogenetic analysis. Other tests, such as biochemical and molecular studies, can be initiated on the same cells or supernatant fluid.
    - By this gestational age, the amniotic and chorionic membranes have fused, and the risk of rupture of the membranes and subchorionic bleeding is significantly reduced.
  - The relative safety and efficacy of genetic amniocentesis has been proven by numerous prospective studies as well as by its broad clinical application. The risk of 1:200 for pregnancy loss is commonly quoted; however, this number is based on older studies with less sophisticated ultrasound guidance. More current risk figures for experienced operators doing more than 50 to 100 procedures annually are in the range of 1:700 (45,54). The ACOG now recommended that a microarray be performed any time that a karyotype is ordered.
  - The risks of genetic amniocentesis include rupture of the membranes, infection, intrauterine bleeding, puncture of the intestines, direct fetal trauma, puncture of the cord, and total loss of the pregnancy (all of which have been reported). Vertical transmission of infection is also reported: hepatitis C, HIV, toxoplasmosis, and CMV (54,55).
  - A full dose of Rh immunoglobulin (300 mg) should be administered to all unsensitized Rh-negative patients, whether the placenta was traversed or not.
  - Amniocentesis can be performed in twins or triplets but requires a needle insertion for each fetus and placement of dye (indigo carmine is preferred over methylene blue), or sono contrast material, in the first sac to identify it. A second or third needle placement does not appear to raise the complication rate (56).
- Early amniocentesis.
  - Early amniocentesis is generally not recommended due to a greater rate of pregnancy loss than with either CVS or standard genetic amniocentesis (53).
  - It is performed as an alternative for those patients presenting too late for CVS or too early for standard genetic amniocentesis (i.e., 12 to 15 weeks' gestation). The procedure is similar to traditional amniocentesis, except that a smaller volume of amniotic fluid is removed.
  - Ultrasound guidance is imperative because the maternal bladder and bowel are more likely to be in the field, and fusion of the amnion and chorion may not have yet taken place, making membrane tenting a complication.

- ○ When counseling these patients about the risks, it should be remembered that there is a naturally higher rate of pregnancy loss at these earlier gestations (53,57).
- Fetal blood sampling.
  - ○ The ability of ultrasound to allow visualization of the umbilical cord has made fetal blood sampling and subsequent diagnostic testing and therapy feasible.
  - ○ The list of potential indications for fetal blood sampling includes cytogenetics, allo-immunization, infections, and molecular diagnoses.
  - ○ Therapeutic options include fetal transfusion and administration of medications directly to the fetus.
  - ○ Fetal loss rates approximate 1% to 2%. Some of this risk depends on the status of the fetus as part of the indication for the procedure. Umbilical artery sampling and procedures attempted in the presence of oligohydramnios are also associated with increased loss.
  - ○ Fetal blood sampling should only be attempted by an experienced team of specialists in a tertiary center with appropriate support.
- Fetoscopy and embryoscopy.
  - ○ Fetoscopy and embyroscopy are techniques for visualizing the fetus that are performed research protocol in limited tertiary facilities.
  - ○ By using fiberoptic scopes placed into the intrauterine cavity either transabdominally (fetoscopy) or transvaginally (embryoscopy), specific embryonic or fetal structures may be identified in families with a specific increased genetic risk.
  - ○ In studies with fetoscopy, fetal blood sampling and biopsy of fetal skin, liver, and muscle have been accomplished under direct ultrasound guidance (58). Fetoscopy with laser is now a standard in the treatment of twin to twin transfusion syndrome and TRAP.
- Placental biopsy.
  - ○ If necessary, placental tissue can be obtained after 13 weeks of gestation for culture and karyotype or biochemical studies.
  - ○ The procedure is similar to genetic amniocentesis, except that the needle is inserted into the placenta and placental tissue is aspirated rather than amniotic fluid.
- Two new techniques with the potential to revolutionize genetic testing and diagnosis have recently become commercially available:
  - ○ The identification of fetal DNA in the maternal circulation (cell-free DNA, cfDNA), even in volumes of 1% to 3% of the maternal plasma sample, may now be performed using new techniques to align and map clonally amplified DNA fragments (58). Next-generation sequencing techniques allow miniaturization and automation to sequence hundreds of millions of DNA fragments in parallel using small volumes of reagents. Massively parallel shotgun sequencing (MPSS) and massively parallel genomic sequencing (MPGS) techniques sequence all of the cfDNA. Quantification can then occur, and proprietary algorithms are applied to read the threshold of samples expected to be of fetal origin (59). Digital analysis of selected regions (DANSR) uses created loci, which have sequences specific for the target chromosomes (60). The algorithm fetal-fraction optimized risk of trisomy evaluation (FORTE) uses a mathematical model assuming a disomic fetal DNA to model the trisomy risk. Commercial tests are now available to test for aneuploidies involving the 13, 18, 21, X, and Y chromosomes (Table 29-6). Newly reported is an assessment of specific chromosomal microdeletions using NATOS (Next-Generation-Aneuploidy Testing Using SNPs) (www.panorama,com/how-it-works/) (79). Additional research is under way to look at those clinical conditions that may increase the percentage of cfDNA in maternal plasma. Already implicated are the clinical conditions of preeclampsia, hyperemesis gravidarum, placenta accreta, and HELLP syndrome (61–64).
  - ○ Preimplantation diagnosis for in vitro fertilization preimplanted embryos is carried out on one or two blastomeres that are microsurgically removed from the embryo on day 3 of the culture; studies are completed rapidly so the embryo may be frozen or implanted

Table 29-6	Considering the Use of Cell-Free Fetal DNA Testing

Maternal age 35 years or older at delivery
Prenatal ultrasonographic findings indicating an increased risk of aneuploidy
Prior pregnancy with a trisomy
Screening test result demonstrating increased risk for aneuploidy, including first trimester, sequential, or integrated screen, or a quadruple screen
Parental balanced robertsonian translocation with increased risk of fetal trisomy 13 or trisomy 21
Failure to obtain the first-trimester combined genetic screen or fetal amniotic fluid cells for technical reasons[a]
When NOT to use cell-free fetal DNA testing
Multiple gestation including vanishing twin or triplet
Maternal somatic mosaicism
Prior to 10 weeks gestational age[b]

[a]Recommendations from the author's clinical practice.
[b]Simpson, JL Contemporary OBGyn.net 2013 (59).
Recommendations are from ACOG Committee Opinion no. 545 (2012) (62).

by day 5. SNP techniques may add to the amount of information gained, in the future. Also, in the armamentarium are first and second polar body studies for genetic information. Techniques used in these analyses are increasing: first with FISH and now with 24 chromosome SNP arrays, comparative hybridization- and PCR-based methods. A list of monogenic diseases detected by preimplantation genetic diagnosis may be found at http://web.mit.edu/7.72/restricted/readings/PGDreview.pdf (65).

OTHER TOPICS OF IMPORTANCE

Several important topics are beyond the scope of this chapter:
• Ethics of genetic counseling and testing (66,67)
• Dysmorphology: the study of abnormal human form and appearance (67)
• Genetic risks in medically assisted reproduction (68,69)
• Genetics and the law (70,71)
• Sonographic prenatal diagnosis
• Population genetics (37)
• Genetic anthropology (72)
• Genomics: the study of the human genome and its interaction in the human environment (73,74)

PATIENT EDUCATION

• All pregnant women should receive information about genetic risks and genetic screening early in the course of their prenatal care, including fetal aneuploidy (9,83–85).
• All pregnant women should be counseled on the risks of fetal aneuploidy and consented for accepting or declining screening.
• Using an interactive prenatal testing decision tool may provide a better understanding for women than health care provider counseling or reading materials (75).
• Women whose screening results indicate an increased aneuploidy risk should receive specific, nondirectional counseling to explain (76–78)
  • Results and their limitations
  • Risks and benefits of follow-up testing
  • Genetic testing procedure options
  • Implications of fetal karyotype results, both normal and abnormal (80–82)

- Women with inherited genetic abnormalities or diseases should receive specific, nondirectional counseling on the possible outcomes for the mother and fetus, fetal testing options, and management options for the pregnancy and newborn infant.
- Direct-to-consumer whole genome testing should be discouraged as it does not alter behavior after disease risk is identified and long-term outcomes of testing in the general population are unknown (76,77).

REFERENCES

1. Electronic Scholarly Publishing. Genetics in context. Available at http://www.esp.org/timeline/. Accessed March 6, 2013.
2. Oxford University Press. Genetic, genetics, heredity, counsel, counseling, risk. Available at http://www.askoxford.com. Accessed March 6, 2013.
3. Genetics. In: Cunningham FG, et al. *Williams obstetrics*. 23rd ed. New York: McGraw Hill, 2010:266–286.
4. Oxbridge Solutions. GP Notebook. Autosomal dominant inheritance. Available at http://www.gpnotebook.co.uk/Samplepage.cfm?ID = 1248526374. Accessed March 29, 2013.
5. Lee, J. Regulation of X-chromosome counting by Tsix and Xite sequences. *Science*. 2005;309:768–771.
6. Passare E, Wirth J, eds. *Color atlas of genetics*. 2nd ed. New York: Thieme, 2001.
7. National Center for Biotechnology Information. http://www.ncbi.nlm.nih.gov/entrez/query.fcgi?db = OMIM. Accessed March 8, 2013.
8. Kansagra S, List J. STUDENTJAMA. The clinical relevance of genomic variation. *JAMA*. 2004;291:1641.
9. Access excellence. Crossing-over and recombination during meiosis. Available at http://www.accessexcellence.org/RC/VL/GG/comeiosis.html. Accessed March 29, 2013.
10. The polymerase chain reaction. Available at http://dnalc.org/resources/animations/pcr.html. Accessed March 29, 2013.
11. Feuk L, Carson AR, Scherer SW. Structure variation I the human genome. *Nat Rev Genet* 2006;7:85.
12. Colorado State University. Mosaicism and chimerism from general and medical genetics. Available at, http://arbl.cvmbs.colostate.edu/hbooks/genetics/medgen/chromo/mosaics.html. Accessed March 29, 2013.
13. DeGroot N, Hochberg A. Gene imprinting during placental and embryonic development. *Mol Reprod Dev*. 1993;36:390–406.
14. Kimball JW. Restriction enzymes. Available at http://users.rcn.com/jkimball.ma.ultranet/BiologyPages/R/RestrictionEnzymes.html. Accessed March 29, 2013.
15. American College of Obstetricians and Gynecologists Committee on Genetics. ACOG committee Opinion 469. Carrier Screening for Fragile X Syndrome. *Obstet and Gynecol* 2010;116(4):1008–1010.
16. Thompson MW, McInnes RR, Willard HF. *Thompson & Thompson genetics in medicine*. 5th ed. Philadelphia: W.B. Saunders, 1991:352–363.
17. Nitromed. BiDil for treatment of heart failure in African Americans. Available at http://www.nitromed.com. Accessed March 29, 2013.
18. American College of Obstetricians and Gynecologists. ACOG Technology Assessment in Obstetrics and Gynecology. *Genetics and molecular diagnostic testing*. 2002;1:1–18.
19. National Center for Biotechnology Information. A new gene map of the human genome, the international RH mapping consortium. Available at http://www.ncbi.nlm.nih.gov/projects/genome/genemap99/. Accessed March 29, 2013.
20. The code of Life: the Genetic code. http://hyperphysics.phy-astr.gsu.edu/Nave-html/Faithpathh/codelife2.html. Accessed March 14, 2014.
21. Eukaryotic promoters. http://www.patentlens.net/daisy/promoters/239/g1/240.html. Accessed March 14, 2014.
22. Dolgin E. Human genomics: the genome finishers. *Nature* 2009;462:843.
23. Access Excellence. Southern Blotting gel transfer. Available at http://www.accessexcellence.orgRC/VL/GG/southBlotg.html. Accessed September 26, 2005.

24. Welt SI, Graham JB, Kosove DH, et al. Vitamin D-resistant rickets and hemophilia-A lack of close linkage on the X-chromosome. *Am J Hum Genet.* 1973;25:105–107.
25. Gill P. DNA as evidence—the technology of identification. *N Engl J Med.* 2005;352: 2067–2071.
26. Riley DE. DNA testing: an introduction for non-scientists. Scientific Testimony, an online journal. Available at http://www.scientific.org/tutorials/articles/riley/riley.html. Accessed April 24, 2013.
27. Feero WG, Guttmacher AE, Collins FS. Genomic Medicine–An updated primer. *N Engl J Med.* 2010;362:2001–2011.
28. ACOG Committee Opinion no. 446: array comparative genomic hybridization in prenatal diagnosis. *Obstet Gynecol* 2009;114:1161–1163.
29. Peng HH, VandenVeyer IB. Clinical application of Microarray-based Comparative Genomic Hybridization in prenatal diagnosis. http://cme.medscape.com/viewprogram/18786. Accessed March 17, 2013.
30. Hillman SC, Pretlove S, Coomarasamy A, et al. Additional information from array comparative genomic hybridization technology over conventional karyotyping in prenatal diagnosis a systemic review and meta-analysis. *Ultrasound Obstet Gynecol.* 2011;37:6–14.
31. Simpson JL. Genetic counseling and prenatal diagnosis. In: Gabbe S, et al., eds. *Obstetrics: Normal and problem pregnancies.* New York: Churchill Livingstone, 2002:187–219.
32. Maternal and Child Health Bureau. Advisory Committee on Heritable Disorders and Genetic Disease in Newborns and Children. Available at http://www.aphl.org/conferences/proceedings/Documents/2007_NBS_and_Genetic_Testing_Symposium/Follow-Up_of_Heritable_Disorders_and_Genetic_Diseases.pdf. Accessed March 30, 2013.
33. Institute for Medical Genetics. The frequency of inherited disorders database. Available at http://medicine.cf.ac.uk/cancer-genetics/medical-genetics/. Accessed March 30, 2013.
34. Ogino S, Wilson R. Bayesian analysis and risk assessment in genetic counseling and testing. *J Mol Diagn.* 2004;6:1–9.
35. Perinatology.com. Recurrence risks for multifactorial conditions. Available at http://www.perinatology.com/genetics/tools.htm#RECURRENCE. Accessed March 30, 2013.
36. Genetics Education Center, University of Kansas. Prevalence of genetic conditions/birth defects. Available at, http://www.kumc.edu/gec/prof/prevalnc.html. Accessed March 30, 2013.
37. Thompson MW, McInnes RR, Willard H. *Thompson and Thompson genetics in medicine.* 5th ed. Philadelphia: W.B. Saunders, 1991:150–164.
38. Kimball JW. The Hardy-Weinberg equilibrium. Available at http://users.rcn.com/jkimball.ma.ultranet/BiologyPages/H/Hardy_Weinberg.html. Accessed March 30, 2013.
39. Perinatology.com. Midtrimester risk of chromosome abnormalities. Available at http://www.perinatology.com/calculators/ama.htm. Accessed March 30, 2013.
40. Jones KI, Smith DW, Harvey MA, et al. Older paternal age and fresh gene mutation: data on additional disorders. *J Pediatr.* 1975;86:84–88.
41. American College of Obstetricians and Gynecologists. *Advanced paternal age: risk to the fetus. ACOG Committee Opinion no 30. 1997,* Washington: American College of Obstetricians and Gynecologists, 2002:19–20.
42. Rochebrochard E, Thomas P. Paternal age and maternal age are risk factors for miscarriage; results of a multicentre European study. *Hum Reprod.* 2002:17 1649–1656.
43. American College of Obstetricians and Gynecologists. *Genetic screening for hemoglobinopathies. ACOG Committee Opinion no. 238.* Washington: American College of Obstetricians and Gynecologists, 2002:30–32.
44. American College of Obstetricians and Gynecologists. *Screening for Tay-Sachs disease. ACOG Committee Opinion no. 162.* Washington: American College of Obstetricians and Gynecologists, 2002:42–43.
45. American College of Obstetricians and Gynecologists. *Screening for Canavan disease. ACOG Committee Opinion no. 212.* Washington: American College of Obstetricians and Gynecologists, 2002:40–41.
46. American College of Obstetricians and Gynecologists. *Maternal phenylketonuria. ACOG Committee Opinion no. 230.* Washington: American College of Obstetricians and Gynecologists, 2002:35–36.

47. Analytes. http://www.science direct.com/science/article/pii/50889854505702886. Accessed March 14, 2014..

48. Nicoaides KH, Sebire NJ, Snijders RJM. *The 11 to 14 weeks scan, the diagnosis of fetal abnormalities.* London: Parthenon Publishing Group, 1999.

49. Reddy UM, Mennuti MT, eds. Prenatal screening incorporating the first trimester studies. *Semin Perinatol.* 2005;29(4):189–279.

50. Prenatal diagnosis and fetal therapy. In: Cunningham FG, et al., eds. *Williams obstetrics.* 21st ed. New York: McGraw Hill, 2001:973–1004.

51. Franssen MTM, Korevaar JC, et al. Selective chromosome analysis in couples with two or more miscarriages: case–control study. *BMJ.* 2005;331:137–141.

52. Donnenfeld AE, Panke ES. What to do when your patient wants prenatal paternity testing. *Contemp OB GYN.* 2004;49:64–51.

53. Philip J, Silver RK, Wilson RD, et al. Late first-trimester invasive prenatal diagnosis: results of an international randomized trial. *Obstet Gynecol* 2004;103:1164–1173.

54. Eddleman KA, Malone FD, Sullivan L, et al. Pregnancy loss rate after midtrimester amniocentesis. *Obstet Gynecol.* 2006;108:1067

55. Ko TM, Tseng LH, Chaung MH, et al. Amniocentesis in mothers who are hepatitis B virus carriers does not expose the infant to an increased risk of hepatitis B virus infection, *Arch Gynecol Obstet* 1994; 255:25–30.

56. Simonazzi G, Curti A, Farina A, et al. Amniocentesis and chorionic villus sampling in twin pregnancies which is the best sampling technique? *Am J Obstet Gynecol.* 2010;202:365ei.

57. D'Alton M. Prenatal diagnostic procedure. *Semin Perinatol.* 1994;18:140–162.

58. Rodeck CH, Nicolaides KH. Fetal tissue biopsy: techniques and indications. *Fetal Therapy.* 1986;1:46–58.

59. Simpson JL. Noninvasive fetal diagnosis. Promise versus Practicality. *Contemp Ob Gyn* 2013:26–33.

60. Sehnert AJ, Rhees B, Comstock D, et al. Optimal detection of fetal chromosomal abnormalities by massively parallel DNA sequencing of cell-free fetal DNA from maternal blood. *Clin Chem.* 2011;57(7):1042–1049.

61. Sparks AB, Struble CA, Wang ET, et al. Noninvasive prenatal detection and selective analysis of cell-free DNA obtained from maternal blood: evaluation for trisomy 21 and trisomy 18. *Am J Obstet Gynecol.* 2012;206:319:e1–e9.

62. ACOG Committee no.545 noninvasive prenatal testing for fetal aneuploidy. *Obstet Gynecol.* 2012;120(6):1532–1534.

63. Bianchi DW, Platt LD, Goldberg JD, et al. Genome-wide fetal aneuploidy detection by maternal plasma DNA sequencing. *Obstet Gynecol.* 2012;119:890–901.

64. Ashoor G, Syngelaki A, Wagner M, et al. Chromosome-selective sequencing of maternal plasma cell-free DNA for first-trimester detection of Trisomy 21 and trisomy 18. *Am J Obstet Gynecol.* 2012;206:322.e1–322.e5

65. Massachusetts Institute of Technology. http://web.mit.edu/7.72/restricted/readings/PGDreview.pdf. Accessed March 17, 2013.

66. Church of Scotland. Society, religion, and technology project of the Church of Scotland. Available at http://www.churchofscotland.org.uk/speak_out/science_and_technology/articles/society_religion_and_technology_project. Accessed March 30, 2013.

67. Halsey D, Williams J, Donahue P. Ethical issues in genetic testing. *J Midwifery Womens Health.* 2005;50:234–240.

68. Koulischer L, Verloes A, et al. Genetic risk in natural and medically assisted procreation. *Early Pregnancy Biol Med.* 1997;3:164–171.

69. Schieve LA, Rasmussen SA, et al. Are children born after assisted reproductive technology at increased risk for adverse health outcomes? *Obstet Gynecol.* 2004;103:1154–1163.

70. Greely HT. Banning genetic discrimination. *N Engl J Med.* 2005;353:865–867.

71. Annas GJ, Elias S. Legal and ethical issues in obstetric practice. In: Gabbe S, et al., eds. *Obstetrics: normal and problem pregnancies.* New York: Churchill Livingstone, 2002:1349–1360.

72. National Geographic Society. A landmark study of the human journey, the Genographic Project. Available at https://genographic.nationalgeographic.com. Accessed March 30, 2013.

73. Centers for Disease Control and Prevention. Genomics and disease prevention. Available at http://www.cdc.gov/genomics/default.htm. Accessed March 30, 2013.
74. The American Society of Gene Therapy. Home page. Available at http://www.asgt.org/. Accessed March 30, 2013.
75. Kupperman M, Norton ME, Gates E. Computerized prenatal genetic testing decision-assisting tool a randomized controlled trial. *Obstet Gynecol.* 2009;113(1):53–63.
76. Bloss CS, Schork NJ, Topol EJ. Effect of direct-to-consumer genomewide profiling to assess disease risk. *N Engl J Med.* 2011;364:524–534.
77. Borry P, Henneman L, Lakeman PH, et al. Preconception genetic carrier testing and the commercial offer directly-to-consumers. *Human Reproduction* 2011;26(5):972–977.
78. Wikipedia. Intersexuality. Available at http://en.wikipedia.org/wiki/Intersexual. Accessed March 29, 2013.
79. Rauch A, Ruschendorf F, Huang J, et al. Molecular karyotyping using an SNP array for genome wide genotyping. *J Med Genet.* 2004;41:916.
80. Shaffer LG, Rosenfeld JA, Dabell MP, et al. Detection rates of clinically significant genomic alterations by microarray analysis for specific anomalies detected by ultrasound. *Prenat Diag.* 2012;32:986.
81. Wharton D.De Novo balanced chromosome rearrangements and extra marker chromosomes identified at prenatal diagnosis: clinical significance and distribution of break points. *Am J Hum Genet.* 1991;49:995.
82. Jones KL, ed. *Smith's recognizable patterns of human malformation.* 5th ed. Philadelphia: W.B. Saunders, 1997.
83. Carter CO. Genetics of common disorders. *Br Med Bull.* 1969;25:52–57.
84. Bonaiti-Pelle C, Smith C. Risk tables for genetic counseling in some common congenital malformations. *J Med Genet.* 1974;11:374–377.
85. Nora JJ, Nora AH. Updates on counseling the family with a first-degree relative with a congenital heart defect. *Am J Med Genet.* 1988;29:137.

30 Teratogens and Birth Defects

Bill Atkinson

KEY POINTS

- Teratogens are substances, organisms, or physical agents capable of causing abnormal fetal structural development, growth restriction, or death.
- Major defects are apparent at birth in about 3% of the general population.
- Many defects arise from multifactorial patterns of inheritance.
- The most common organ system for congenital abnormalities is the cardiovascular system.
- The incidence of neural tube defects (NTDs) and possibly other anomalies (particularly those associated with taking antiepileptic medications) may be significantly decreased by taking folic acid before conception.

BACKGROUND

Definitions

- A teratogen is a substance, an organism, or a physical agent capable of causing abnormal development. A teratogen can cause abnormalities of structure or function, intrauterine growth restriction, and death.
- Teratogenesis is a medical term from the Greek literally meaning "monster making." The term has gained a more specific usage for the development of abnormal cells causing physical defects in the fetus.
- Teratology is the study of the frequency, causation, and development of congenital malformations.
- *Congenital malformations* and *birth defects* are terms that are often used interchangeably. Congenital malformations are fetal physical defects. Birth defects have evolved beyond the original emphasis on congenital malformations to denote a broader category of developmental abnormalities that includes physical defects.

Pathophysiology

- It was once believed that the mammalian embryo developed in an impervious uterus, protected from extrinsic factors. The thalidomide disaster of the 1960s made it apparent that the developing embryo is highly vulnerable to extrinsic agents that may have a negligible effect on maternal well-being.
- Teratogens come from many sources. Research is focusing on the possible causative actions of teratogenic agents to determine their mechanism, as well as the site of action.
- James G. Wilson (1) developed the six principles of teratology for the development in the refinement of the mammalian embryo. These principles are
  - Susceptibility: Susceptibility to teratogenesis seems to depend on the genotype and the manner in which it interacts with environmental factors.
  - Timing of exposure: Susceptibility to teratogenic agents varies with the developmental stage at the time of exposure.
  - Mechanisms: Teratogenic agents act in specific ways on developing cells to initiate abnormal development in embryogenesis.
  - Manifestations: The final manifestation of abnormal development may be malformation, intrauterine growth restriction, functional disorders, or death.

- Access of adverse environmental influences to developing tissue depends on the nature of the agent (route and degree of maternal teratogen exposure, rate of placental transfer, and systemic absorption).
- Dose effect: Manifestations of abnormal development increase as the dosage increases from no effect to lethal levels.

Etiology
Known causes of developmental malformations include (2)
- Genetic transmissions (Mendelian disorders, single gene): 15% to 20%
- Chromosomal abnormalities: 5% to 10%
  - Aneuploidy (i.e., Down syndrome and Turner syndrome)
- Environmental causes
  - Maternal infections: 1% to 3%
  - Maternal conditions, including illicit substance abuse: 1% to 4%
  - Deformations: 1% to 2%
  - Drugs, chemicals, radiation, and hyperthermia: 1% to 2%
- Unknown: 65% (Table 30-1)

TERATOGENS
Background
Definitions
- The U.S. Food and Drug Administration (FDA) oversees the safety of drugs and provides the most widely used system to grade the teratogenic effects of medications.
- The FDA assigns a safety category for the use of medications during pregnancy using a five-letter system, A, B, C, D, and X (3,4):
  - Category A: Adequate and well-controlled studies in pregnant women have not shown an increased risk of fetal abnormalities.
  - Category B: Animal studies have revealed no evidence of harm to the fetus; however, there are no adequate and well-controlled studies in pregnant women, or animal studies have shown an adverse effect, but adequate and well-controlled studies in pregnant women have failed to demonstrate a risk to the fetus.
  - Category C: Animal studies have shown an adverse effect, and there are no adequate, well-controlled studies in pregnant women, or no animal studies have been conducted, and there are no adequate and well-controlled studies in pregnant women.
  - Category D: Adequate, well-controlled or observational studies in pregnant women have demonstrated a risk to the fetus; however, the benefits of the therapy may outweigh the potential risks.

Table 30-1	Estimated Incidents of the Leading Categories of Birth Defects
Birth defects	**Estimated incidence**
Heart and circulation	1 in 115 births
Musculoskeletal	1 in 130 births
Clubbed foot	1 in 735 births
Cleft lip and palate	1 in 930 births
Genitourinary	1 in 135 births
Anencephaly	1 in 8000 births
Spina bifida	1 in 2000 births
Respiratory tract	1 in 900 births

Data for this table are found in references 5 to 14.

- Category X: Adequate, well-controlled, or observational studies in animals or pregnant women have demonstrated positive evidence of fetal abnormalities. The use of the product is contraindicated in women who are or who may become pregnant.
- The safety category must be displayed on the labels of all drugs.

Etiology
- Major defects are apparent at birth in about 3% of the general population and in about 4.5% by 5 years of age. A cause or mechanism for the defect is typically determined in less than 50% of the cases (5,6).
- Health care providers and obstetricians are often asked about the potential teratogenic effect of various agents.
  - Some medications rarely cause birth defects, and others commonly cause them.
  - Some agents cause major defects if fetal exposure occurs during a specific critical period but cause no harmful effect at another time in gestation. After organogenesis has been completed (13 weeks of gestation), the observable effect of extrinsic agents may be limited to growth restriction rather than manifest as a defined structural abnormality.
  - Individual differences exist in susceptibility to teratogenic effects from the same agent. Unfortunately, when counseling patients, it is impossible at the present time to know the individual's genotypic sensitivity or resistance to a given agent. So the potential for abnormalities exists for each individual, although a wide spectrum of different outcomes can be anticipated.
- Animal studies have been used extensively to determine possible teratogenic effects, and the results have been used in counseling individuals and couples at risk. Although animal studies may be helpful in counseling, they do not reliably predict human effects. Specific teratogenic effects may be species specific. This was the case with thalidomide, where the teratogenic effect was not seen in animals (6,7).

Evaluation
- Prenatal testing should be provided when indicated by risk assessment or other findings.
- Some patients, once they are fully informed of the risk, may request pregnancy termination.
- Follow-up counseling is needed to provide emotional support, as well as education, regardless of whether the patient/couple chooses termination or continuation of the pregnancy.
- Multispecialty support for an abnormal infant is essential.

Diagnosis
- Prenatal diagnosis is available for many diseases and possible for many congenital anomalies that are linked to teratogenic agents. Unfortunately, not all abnormalities can be anticipated or detected, particularly those defects caused by environmental agents.
- Targeted ultrasound can be used to diagnose many structural and developmental abnormalities.
- Genetic amniocentesis provides access to amniotic fluid for karyotype determination, polymerase chain reaction for viral exposures, and assessment of specific markers such as α-fetoprotein (AFP).
- Chorionic villus sampling (CVS) and fetal blood sampling assist with prenatal diagnosis in specific situations.
- Confirmed or suspected agents are typically placed in one of three categories (4–13) (Table 30-2):
  - Infectious agents
  - Drugs and chemicals
  - Physical agents

| Table 30-2 | Suspected Human Teratogens |

Infectious agents	Drugs and chemicals	Physical agents
Cytomegalovirus	Alcohol	Hyperthermia
Herpes hominis type II virus	Folate antagonist	High-dose ionizing radiation
Parvovirus B19	Androgen hormones	
Rubella virus	Busulfan alkylating agents	
Toxoplasma gondii	Coumadin anticoagulants	
Treponema pallidum	Diethylstilbestrol	
Varicella virus	Vitamin A excess (isotretinoin)	
	Lead	
	Organic mercury compounds	
	Phenytoin	
	Polybrominated biphenyls	
	Polychlorinated biphenyls	
	Tetracyclines	
	Thalidomide	
	Trimethadione	
	Valproic acid	

From Shepherd TH. *Catalog of teratogenic agents.* 7th ed. Baltimore: Johns Hopkins University Press, 1992. (See also Beckman and Brent (2).)

INFECTIOUS AGENTS

Cytomegalovirus
Diagnosis
Clinical Manifestations
- Hydrocephaly, microcephaly with cerebral calcifications
- Chorioretinitis
- Intrauterine growth restriction, typically early onset or symmetric
- Microphthalmia and hearing loss
- Severe mental retardation, developmental delay

Characteristics
- Cytomegalovirus is one of the most common congenital infections.
- The congenital infection rate is 40% after primary infections during pregnancy and possibly only 15% after recurrent infections.
- Of the infected infants, physical effects may only be present in 20% after a primary infection and 8% after a secondary infection.
- No apparent effective therapy exists (4,8).

Herpes
Diagnosis
Clinical Manifestations
- Intrauterine growth restriction
- Microcephaly with cerebellar necrosis
- Chorioretinitis, cataract, microphthalmia
- Hepatosplenomegaly

Characteristics
- Passage of virus can be transplacental or transcervical.
- Majority of newborn infections occur by contact with infected genital secretions.

- With primary infection near the time of delivery, there is a 33% to 50% risk of transmitting the virus to neonate with vaginal delivery.
- With recurrent disease, the risk of transmission may be 2% to 5%.
- Prevention of transmission is primarily by cesarean delivery for those at risk at delivery (8).

Parvovirus
Diagnosis
Clinical Manifestations
- Hydrops
- Ascites
- Placentomegaly
- Hypertrophic myocardiopathy
- Ventriculomegaly

Characteristics
- Transplacental transmission.
- Parvovirus B19 leads to fetal anemia by affecting the erythroid precursor cells. It also has an affinity for cardiac myocytes, resulting in fetal myocarditis.
- Risk of congenital infection from an infected mother is 10% to 20%.
- Management is by in utero transfusion. Fetal anemia can be predicted with Doppler sonography of the middle cerebral artery peak systolic velocity (8).

Rubella
Diagnosis
Clinical Manifestations
- Microcephaly
- Mental retardation
- Cataracts and deafness
- Congenital heart defects (8)

Characteristics
- Malformation rate may exceed 50% if the infection occurs during the first trimester.
- The rate of severe malformations decreases to less than 10% by midpregnancy.
- Immunization of children and nonpregnant adults is necessary for prevention.
- Immunization is not recommended during pregnancy.
- The live, attenuated vaccine virus has not been shown to cause congenital rubella malformations (8).

Toxoplasmosis
Diagnosis
Clinical Manifestations
- Microcephaly, hydrocephalus, and cerebral calcifications.
- Chorioretinitis.
- Severity of malformations apparently depends on the duration of the disease.

Clinical Characteristics
- Overall, in the United States, infection during pregnancy is rare, occurring in less than 0.5% of pregnant women.
- For the fetus to be at risk, the primary infection has to occur during pregnancy.
- Transmission is by raw meat or exposure to cat feces that are infected.
- In the first trimester, with maternal infection, the incidence of fetal infection is less than 10%, but this increases to greater than 50% in the third trimester.
- The incidence and severity of congenital infections or malformations are greatest with first-trimester fetal infection.
- Pyrimethamine sulfadiazine and spiramycin are the antibiotic treatments of choice (8).

Syphilis
Diagnosis
Clinical Manifestations
- Congenital syphilis confers a 50% risk of intrauterine fetal death or neonatal death.
- An infant's symptoms may not be apparent until weeks or even years after birth.
- Early congenital syphilis is characterized by rhinitis, fever, pneumonia, skin problems, low birth weight, irritability, and hepatosplenomegaly.
- Skin rash is an early sign in the infant with congenital infection.
- Findings consistent with late congenital syphilis:
  - Dentition: Hutchinson teeth
  - Eye: Corneal scarring, chorioretinitis
  - Ear: Eighth nerve deafness
  - Nose: "Saddle nose"
  - Central nervous system: Mental retardation, palsies/paresis
  - Bones: Saber shins, Clutton joints
  - Late maculopapular rash on face and palms

Characteristics
- Congenital syphilis is potentially a preventable disease.
- Maternal serologic testing early in pregnancy is the key to prevention.
- Antibiotic treatment is effective for maternal infection but may not correct established fetal infection (8).

Varicella
Diagnosis
Clinical Manifestations
- Potentially, all organs can be affected by varicella, though skin scarring is a characteristic abnormality. Extremity and limb abnormalities with muscle atrophy and hypoplasia of the hands and feet are common.
- Chorioretinitis and cataracts are characteristic in the newborn infant.
- Microcephaly may be present.

Characteristics
- The risk of congenital varicella appears to be linked to maternal infection between 7 and 21 weeks of gestation.
- A separate syndrome of potentially fatal neonatal infection can occur with maternal varicella infection within 5 to 7 days of delivery. Zoster immunoglobulin is available for newborns delivered under this circumstance.
- Varicella vaccine is available for nonimmune women before conception (8).

DRUGS AND CHEMICALS
Folic Acid Antagonist and Disruption of Folic Acid Metabolism
Diagnosis
Clinical Manifestations
- Increased risk of spontaneous abortions
- Multiple anomalies

Characteristics
- Exposure to folic acid antagonists during the first trimester carries a malformation incidence of more than 30%.
- Preconception identification and counseling of women on folic acid antagonists is the important step in preventing these malformations.
  - Several congenital anomalies with examples of NTDs and cardiac defects may have an origin from disruption of folic acid metabolic pathways (9,10).

Genetic. Multifactorial anomalies are caused by interactions of environmental exposures by certain altered genes. An example is mutation of the gene for methylene tetrahydrofolate reductase. This genetic abnormality is associated with several malformations including the example of NTDs in women who have inadequate folic acid intakes.

Homeobox G. An example of homeobox gene creating teratogenicity is with retinoic acid. Retinoids such as vitamin A activate genes essential for normal growth and tissue development. Retinoic acid is a teratogen that can activate these genes prematurely. This mechanism has been linked to abnormalities in central nervous system development.

Anticonvulsant Medications
Background
A history of epilepsy presents an increased risk of fetal anomalies. It has been uncertain whether the risk is secondary to the underlying seizure disorder or to medication exposure (10). A meta-analysis of congenital malformation in women with epilepsy found an overall rate of 7.1% in pregnancies with epilepsy versus 2.2% in controls. Additionally, there are limited data available for the newer anticonvulsants:
- If possible, valproate and polytherapy should be avoided during pregnancy, particularly in the first trimester.
- With monotherapy, the malformation rates were
  - Valproate 10.7%
  - Phenytoin 7.3%
  - Carbamazepine 4.6%
  - Phenobarbital 4.9%
  - Lamotrigine 2.9%
- With polytherapy, overall the rate was 16.8% as compared to polytherapy with valproate that demonstrated a rate of 25.0%.
- Choice of antiepilepsy drug preconception should be
  - Most effective for seizure control
  - Monotherapy if possible
  - Least teratogenic
  - Lowest dose

Phenytoin
Diagnosis
Clinical Manifestations
- Microcephaly with mental retardation
- Craniofacial features with dysmorphism
- Intrauterine growth restriction
- Cardiac defects
- Hypoplasia of the distal phalanges and nail beds

Characteristics
- The full syndrome is seen in less than 10% of offspring exposed in utero.
- Some clinical manifestations are seen in up to 30% of exposed fetuses/infants.
- Mild to moderate mental retardation is noted frequently. The effects may depend on whether the fetus inherits a mutant gene that decreases the production of epoxide hydrolase, the enzyme necessary to decrease this production.
- Some studies suggest the possibility that folic acid supplementation could decrease the incidence of some of these anomalies. The dosage of folic acid necessary to achieve this may be 4 mg daily, as compared to the 0.4 mg/d normally used for pregnancy supplementation (11,12).

Valproic Acid (Depakote)
Diagnosis
Clinical Manifestations
- NTDs, particularly open spina bifida
- Increased risk for heart defects and skeletal abnormalities
- Minor facial defects, including cleft lip and palate

Characteristics
- Valproic acid exposure before closure of the neural tube between the third and fifth weeks of gestation results in a 1% incidence of NTDs.
- There is evidence that high-dose folic acid supplementation during the critical exposure period decreases the risk of NTDs. The recommended supplementation dose is 4 mg daily, which is significantly greater than the FDA-recommended dose of 0.4 mg daily during pregnancy (11,12).

Carbamazepine (Tegretol)
Diagnosis
Clinical Manifestations
- Neural tube defects
- Craniofacial defects
- Microcephaly with developmental delay
- Fingernail hypoplasia
- Intrauterine growth restriction

Characteristics
- Risk of NTDs is 1% to 2% and requires exposure before neural tube closure at the third to fifth weeks of gestation. Concurrent use with other antiepileptic agents may increase the risk.
- As with other anticonvulsant drugs, high-dose folic acid supplementation may decrease the incidence of NTDs. The recommended dose is 4 mg daily before conception and during early pregnancy (11,12).

Trimethadione
Diagnosis
Clinical Manifestations
- Characteristic facial appearance with cleft lip/cleft palate and ophthalmologic abnormalities
- Cardiac defects
- Microcephaly with mental retardation
- Intrauterine growth restriction
- Limb defects
- Genitourinary abnormalities

Characteristics
- The risk for defects or fetal loss exceeds 60% with first-trimester exposure.
- A syndrome characteristic for exposure includes V-shaped eye brows, low-set ears, and high, arched palate (11,12).

Lamotrigine (Lamictal)
- Registries report 2.7% to 3.2% risk of major malformation, similar to controls.
- Early studies noted a higher than expected rate of facial clefts 8.9/1000 compared with 1–2/1000.
- Drug level markedly increased with valproate and decreased with hormonal contraceptives and pregnancy (65% increased clearance).
- Lamotrigine Pregnancy Registry: 800-336-2176 (11,12).

Levetiracetam (Keppra)

- Mechanism of action unknown
- No adequate, well-controlled studies in pregnant women
- Two registries are available:
  - Antiepileptic Drug Pregnancy Registry 888-233-2334 www.mgh.harvard.edu/aed/
  - UCB AED Pregnancy Registry 888-837-7734 (11,12)

Phenobarbital

- One of the oldest anticonvulsant medications still in use.
- Phenobarbital is a folic acid agonist.
- Major cardiac, craniofacial, genitourinary abnormality rates similar to other therapy (e.g., Tegretol, Dilantin).
- Risk of congenital anomalies appears greater among infants whose mothers required phenobarbital and phenytoin during pregnancy compared to infants of mothers treated with phenobarbital alone.
- Associated with sedation in mother and nursing infants.
- Phenobarbital-exposed newborns may exhibit a withdrawal syndrome characterized by hyperactivity and tremors.
- Chronic maternal phenobarbital therapy may induce a vitamin K responsive bleeding abnormality in the neonate.

Choice of Antiepileptic Drugs (AEDs) (11,12)

First generation	Pregnancy category
Valproate (Depakote)	D
Carbamazepine (Tegretol)	D
Phenytoin (Dilantin)	D
Phenobarbital	D

Second generation	Pregnancy category
Lamotrigine (Lamictal)	C
Levetiracetam (Keppra)	C
Topiramate (Topamax)	C
Zonisamide (Zonegran)	C
Oxcarbazepine (Trileptal)	C

Antimicrobials

Penicillin, ampicillin, and amoxicillin appear to be safe in pregnancy. Collaborative perinatal project did not show an increased risk of anomalies. It has been suggested that amoxicillin and clavulanate may lead to abnormal microbial colonization of the gastrointestinal tract leading to a potentially increased risk of necrotizing colitis. It is recommended that amoxicillin and clavulanate be avoided in women at risk for preterm delivery.

Aminoglycosides

- Both nephrotoxicity and ototoxicity have been reported in preterm newborns treated with gentamicin.
- Congenital defects from prenatal exposure have not been documented.

Cephalosporins
- There is no consensus of teratogenicity.

Sulfonamides
No teratogenic effects have been noted. Sulfonamides can compete with bilirubin for binding sites on albumin. This can raise free bilirubin in the serum increasing the risk of hyperbilirubinemia in the neonate (13).

Trimethoprim
There are no studies that substantiate teratogenicity.

Nitrofurantoin (Macrodantin) is capable of inducing hemolytic anemia in patients deficient in G-6-PD deficiency. However, no studies have shown an increase in hemolytic anemia in newborns as a result of intrauterine exposure (13).

Fluoroquinolones
• **Quinolones (ciprofloxacin)** may cause cartilage damage and arthropathies in children. Its use has been discouraged during pregnancy.
Metronidazole (Flagyl) studies have failed to show any increased incidence of congenital defects.

Topical Antifungal Agents
• Mycostatin (nystatin), clotrimazole (Lotrimin), or miconazole (Monistat)
• Not known to be associated with any congenital malformations

Antivirals
• Amantadine may be used in treatment or preventive measures for influenza. At very high doses in animal studies, it has been reported to be teratogenic. Several case studies suggest that when the medication has been given in the first trimester, it may have a possible increased risk of congenital heart defects, but this information is very limited.
• Ribavirin is used to treat respiratory infections as an aerosol inhalation agent. This drug appears to be highly teratogenic in all animal studies. Human exposure is rare, but it is listed as a category X and is contraindicated in pregnancy.
• Antiviral medications used for human immunodeficiency virus (HIV) inhibit the host intercellular viral replication. There is a large registry established by several manufacturers. No significant increase in birth defects has been noted following the exposure to the most common agents used (7,11).

Tetracyclines
Diagnosis
Clinical Manifestations
• Hypoplasia of tooth enamel
• Permanent yellow-brown discoloration of deciduous teeth

Characteristics
• The effect appears to occur with exposure in the second and third trimesters.
• Tetracyclines should be considered contraindicated during pregnancy (11).

Streptomycin/Kanamycin
Diagnosis
Clinical Manifestations
• Ototoxicity with hearing loss
• Eighth nerve damage

Characteristics
• Theoretically, the fetus may be at risk from other mycin antibiotics.
• There are no definitive studies that have reported ototoxicity with gentamicin or vancomycin (11).

Hormones and Vitamins
Androgens
Clinical Manifestations
• Androgen hormones lead to various degrees of virilization of female fetuses.

Characteristics
• The effect appears to be dose dependent and related to exposure at a critical time during embryonic development.

- If exposure is before 9 to 10 weeks, labial/scrotal fusion may occur. Clitoromegaly may occur with exposure at any gestational age.
- The risks from brief androgenic exposure for a female fetus appear to be minimal (11).

Oral Contraceptives/Progestins
- Studies have not confirmed any teratogen risk.

Corticosteroids
- Although some animal studies have suggested a possible increased risk of midfacial anomalies, hydrocortisone and prednisone have been extensively used in human pregnancies without association with such anomalies.
- Corticosteroids are not considered to represent a major teratogenic risk, though systemic corticosteroids if used in the first trimester are category D (11).

Diethylstilbestrol
Diagnosis
Clinical Manifestations
- Clear cell adenocarcinoma of the vagina or cervix
- Vaginal adenosis
- Abnormalities of the cervix and uterus in the female. Abnormalities of the testes in the male
- Infertility
- Incompetent cervix and preterm delivery

Characteristics
- Vaginal adenosis is detected in more than 50% of women whose mothers were exposed to diethylstilbestrol (DES) before the ninth week of gestation.
- The risk of vaginal adenocarcinoma is relatively low.
- Males exposed in utero have a 25% incidence of hypertrophic testes and epididymal cysts.
- Note that the women who were born during the era of DES use during pregnancy have just about completed their own reproductive years (7).

Vitamin A Isotretinoin (Accutane)
Diagnosis
Clinical Manifestations
- Increased rate of fetal loss
- Central nervous system defects with sequelae of mental retardation
- Microphthalmia
- Thymic agenesis
- Cardiovascular defects
- Craniofacial dysmorphism including cleft lip and palate

Characteristics
- Vitamin A intake greater than 15,000 IU/d is associated with an increased risk of fetal malformation.
- The risk of malformation associated with Accutane may exceed 28%.
- Accutane has a relatively short half-life (96 hours). If the medication is discontinued within days of conception, the risk may not be increased (11).
- Tretinoin (Retin-A) topical application does not have a known risk. However, its use is still not recommended during pregnancy.

Thyroid and Antithyroid Medications
- The antithyroid medications propylthiouracil (PTU) and methimazole (Tapazole) both cross the placenta and can potentially cause fetal goiter. Methimazole has been associated with scalp defects and esophageal atresia. In 2009, the FDA released a black box warning highlighting serious liver injuries with PTU treatment, so some have suggested

PTU during the first trimester and then switching to methimazole for the remainder of the pregnancy.
- Thyroid hormones cross the placenta poorly, so fetal hypothyroidism produced by antithyroid drugs cannot be corrected.
- Radioactive iodine for thyroid ablation or diagnostic studies is not concentrated by the fetal thyroid until after 12 weeks of pregnancy; thus, inadvertent exposure before 12 weeks does not identify a specific risk to the thyroid. After 12 weeks of pregnancy, radioactive iodine can be destructive (11).

Psychiatric Medications
Selective Serotonin Reuptake Inhibitors
- Paroxetine exposure appears to have potentially twofold increased risk of congenital heart malformations. The manufacturer has changed the pregnancy category of paroxetine from a C to a D. The American College of Obstetrics and Gynecology recommend that paroxetine be avoided in women either pregnant or planning to be pregnant. Overall, the use of selective serotonin reuptake inhibitors (SSRIs) does not appear to cause major teratogenic effects. Neonatal effects have been evaluated from maternal exposure of SSRI. Features have been described as jitteriness, irritability, and increased muscle tone. Generally, these characteristics are considered to be mild and only last 2 days. The second neonatal syndrome though rare associated with SSRI exposures includes high pulmonary vascular resistance. The American College of Obstetricians and Gynecologists stresses that the potential risk of SSRI use in pregnancy must be considered in comparison of the risk of recurrent depression if the medication was discontinued. Treatments of these medications should be individualized. Persistent pulmonary hypertension in a newborn (PPHN) has been from case–control studies and appears to be associated with fetuses exposed after 20 weeks' gestation. The risk appears to be approximately 1% (12).

Lithium
Diagnosis
Clinical Manifestations
- Congenital cardiac defects, particularly Ebstein anomalies
- Renal, thyroid, and neuromuscular toxicity

Characteristics
- Lithium exposure in the first trimester may cause cardiac malformation. The effect though may not be severe as earlier studies reported.
- Late third-trimester exposure may produce toxic effects on the renal, neuromuscular, and thyroid systems.

Benzodiazepines
- Benzodiazepines have been associated with a possible increase in the incidence of cleft lip or palate.
- Benzodiazepine withdrawal syndrome is most significant in neonates (12).

Recreational Drugs/Dietary and Social Exposures
Alcohol
Diagnosis
Clinical Manifestations
- Fetal alcohol syndrome (FAS) has a variable clinical presentation.
- Intrauterine growth restriction (IUGR) is a characteristic manifestation of FAS.
- Microcephaly and subsequent mental retardation may be present.
- The infant may have midfacial hypoplasia with atypical facial appearance.
- Renal/cardiac abnormalities may be present (14).

Characteristics
- The threshold amount of alcohol ingestion required to produce FAS has not been determined, but any level of consumption during pregnancy appears to have some risk of sequelae. As few as one to two drinks per day can result in intrauterine growth restriction.
- Women who ingest more than the equivalent of six drinks per day have a greater than 50% risk of developing a fetus with FAS.

Amphetamines
- Various amphetamines may be teratogenic at high doses in animal studies. They have been associated with symmetric IUGR. There does not appear to be an association with defined congenital anomalies in human studies.

Cocaine
Diagnosis
Clinical Manifestations
- Genitourinary tract malformations
- Bowel atresia
- Microcephaly and cerebral infarcts
- Facial, cardiac, and limb defects
- Intrauterine growth restriction

Characteristics
- Risk is most likely confounded by other factors, including environmental factors and concurrent use of other substances.
- Increased risk of placental abruption with subsequent risk for hemorrhage, hypoxic fetal distress, preterm delivery, and perinatal death (14,15).

Opiates: Narcotics
- Heroin. Antenatal effects of fetal growth restriction and fetal demise have been associated with narcotic-addicted mothers. Concerns also exist for withdrawal symptoms, which may occur in 40% to 80% of newborns delivered from heroin-addicted mothers. Some symptoms of neonatal withdrawal may persist for 10 days.
- Methadone. Methadone has not been shown to be teratogenic, but the primary concern is withdrawal symptoms. Withdrawal from methadone may be more severe than from heroin and may have a duration of 3 weeks secondary to methadone's longer half-life.
- Marijuana. There is no evidence that it is associated with human abnormalities. There may be association with SGA and fetal growth restriction (14,15).

Caffeine
- There is no evidence of teratogenic effects from caffeine in humans. One study suggests that if women consumed greater than 300 mg of caffeine per day, it may increase risk of low birth weight. The American Congress of Obstetrics Gynecologist (ACOG) states that moderate caffeine consumption (less than 200 mg/d) does not appear to be a major contributing factor in fetal loss or preterm delivery (15).

Smoking
- Smoking appears to be associated with increased risk of small for gestational age as well as potential for increased prematurity rate. This appears to be attributable to an increased risk of abruption, premature and prolonged abruption of membranes, and intrauterine growth restriction. There is also an association between smoking and sudden infant death syndrome as well as increased respiratory illnesses in children (17).

Smoking Cessation During Pregnancy
- Typically, it is recommended that nicotine is the agent to be avoided in pregnancy. Carbon monoxide decreases oxygen delivery to the fetus where nicotine decreases uterine blood flow. Tobacco contains nicotine and carbon monoxide. Nicotine medications are indicated for patients with nicotine dependence, but the studies regarding safety are limited using these agents. They are available in patches, gum, or inhalers (17).

Marijuana
- No significant teratogenic effect of marijuana has been documented.

Aspartame Nutricillin
- A medical review in 2007 concluded that existing scientific evidence indicated that aspartame at current levels of consumption was safe. The possibility of relative high doses being teratogenic has been suggested in animal studies.
- The breakdown products of aspartame include phenylalanine, which must be avoided by those with the genetic condition phenylketonuria (PKU) (18).
- Aspartame (Equal, NutraSweet).
- Saccharin (SugarTwin, Sweet'N Low).
- Acesulfame potassium (Sunnet, Sweet One).
- Artificial sweeteners.

Herbal Remedies
- Herbal remedies are not regulated by the FDA, and very few human/animal studies have been reported as far as causing teratogenicity because it is not possible to assess the effects of herbal remedies on fetal development. It is recommended that pregnant women be counseled to avoid exposure or continuation of these substances (11).

Thalidomide
Diagnosis
Clinical Manifestations
- Bilateral limb deficiencies and anotia and microtia
- Cardiac and gastrointestinal anomalies

Characteristics
- The clinical manifestations are specific to humans.
- The critical time of exposure appears to be between 35 and 50 days of gestation.
- Twenty percent of exposed fetuses will develop clinical manifestations (11).

Cardiovascular/Antithrombotic Agents
Coumadin Derivatives
Diagnosis
Clinical Manifestations
- Nasal hypoplasia
- Stippled bone epiphysis
- Abnormal hands that are broad and short with shortened phalanges
- Ophthalmologic abnormalities
- Intrauterine growth restriction
- Developmental delay (11)

Characteristics
- The risk of having an affected child may exceed 15% to 25% with first-trimester exposure.
- Later exposure may result in spontaneous abortions, intrauterine fetal death, and central nervous system abnormalities.
- There is an increased risk of vaginal bleeding, placental abruption, and fetal or neonatal hemorrhage.

Angiotensin-Converting Enzyme Inhibitors
Diagnosis
Clinical Manifestations
- Renal tubular dysplasia with oligohydramnios
- Neonatal renal failure
- Possible lack of cranial ossification
- Intrauterine growth restriction (11)

Characteristics
- Fetal/neonatal morbidity may exceed 30%.
- Risk is greatest with second- and third-trimester exposure.
- Risk of fetal hypotension with decreased renal blood flow and subsequent renal failure.

Antihypertension Medications
- Methyldopa (Aldomet) has been widely used for the treatment of chronic hypertension in pregnancy. No unusual fetal effects have been identified.
- Hydralazine (Apresoline) has not shown any deferred teratogenic effects.
- Beta-blocking agents. No evidence of teratogenicity has been found. Several studies have suggested increased risk of intrauterine growth restriction.
- Calcium channel blockers have been widely used without teratogenicity (11).

Heparin
- Unfractionated heparin (UFH) and low molecular weight heparin (LMWH) do not cross the placenta and would not be expected to produce fetal complications. It is recommended that women with mechanical heart valves require warfarin anticoagulation because heparin is not effective.
- Lovenox and enoxaparin are cleared more rapidly during pregnancy (11).

Aspirin/Nonsteroidal Agents
- There is no clear evidence of teratogenic effect though it may increase perinatal risk by inhibiting prostaglandin synthesis. It may also have antiplatelet aggregation effect with decreased platelet aggregation increasing the risk of bleeding.
- Nonsteroidal anti-inflammatory drugs (NSAIDS) given to pregnant women cross the placenta and may cause embryo, fetal, and neonatal adverse effects, depending on the type of agent and the dose and duration of therapy.
- Increased risk of miscarriage and malformation is associated with NSAID use in early pregnancy, and conversely, exposure after 30 weeks is associated with an increased risk of premature closure of the fetal ductus arteriosus and oligohydramnios (11).

PHYSICAL AGENTS
High Temperature
Hyperthermia
- When body temperature reaches 102°F (38.9°C) or higher during pregnancy, a concern exists. Hyperthermia can be from fever, hot tubs, baths, or saunas.
- Animal studies show that the central nervous system appears to be at the greatest risk. Also, abnormalities include microcephaly, defects of eyes and palate, maxillary hypoplasia, limb reduction, renal agenesis, and hearing impairments.
- Bathing in hot tubs can elevate core body temperature much greater than saunas. The suggestion has been made that pregnant women limit exposure to 15 minutes in 39°C (102°F) or 10 minutes in 40°C to 41°C (104°F to 106°F) (11,19,20).

Radiation
Diagnosis
Clinical Manifestations
- Acute high dose
  - Microcephaly
  - Mental retardation
  - Intrauterine growth restriction

Characteristics
- Medical/diagnostic radiation delivering less than 0.05 Gy or 5 rad (1 Gy = 100 rad) to the fetus does not appear to have a teratogenic effect.
- Estimated fetal exposure of common radiologic procedures is 0.01 Gy or less.
- Chronic low-dose radiation exposure of the fetus has no defined sequelae, but there has been a suggestion of an increased rate of Down syndrome (21).

Methyl Mercury
Diagnosis
Clinical Manifestations
- Abnormal neuronal migration
- Mental retardation, cerebral palsy
- Increased risk of deafness, blindness, or seizures

Characteristics
- Methyl mercury was widely used as a fungicide until the 1960s. Today, exposure mainly occurs through consumption of contaminated fish.
- Accumulation of methyl mercury in the hair makes it possible to reconstruct prenatal exposure.
- Methyl mercury crosses the placenta and easily accumulates in embryonic and fetal tissues, particularly brain tissues, at concentrations exceeding those in the mother.
- The most devastating effects may not be apparent at birth but are manifested later in childhood.
- Cerebral palsy can occur even with exposures in the third trimester to fish contaminated with methyl mercury (11).

Lead
Diagnosis
Clinical Manifestations
- Increased rate of fetal loss.
- Intrauterine growth restriction.
- Associated with psychomotor retardation and seizures.
- Increased risk for intrauterine fetal death.
- Chronic low-dose exposure may impair central nervous system function with abnormal cognitive development, lower intelligence quotients, and potential for attention deficit problems.

Characteristics
- Assessment of environmental lead exposure risk before pregnancy is helpful.
- For women at risk for excessive lead exposure, determining preconception lead levels may be beneficial for counseling and pregnancy planning (23).

Polychlorinated Biphenyls
Diagnosis
Clinical Manifestations
- Increased rate of fetal loss.
- Intrauterine growth restriction.
- Neural epidermal dysplasia may develop with skin staining, as well as dysplastic nails, skin hyperpigmentation, and skull calcifications.
- Developmental and psychological deficits.
- Abnormal bone calcification.

Characteristics
- Polychlorinated biphenyls (PCBs) are highly lipid soluble. They accumulate in fat and can be found in high concentrations in the breast milk.
- Although transplacental transfer of PCBs occurs, the largest dose is delivered from nursing, via breast milk.
- PCBs are no longer produced in the United States but are still found in the environment in items such as transformers, older fluorescent lighting fixtures, and refrigerators.
- Exposure also occurs from contaminated food, such as fish from contaminated lakes or rivers (11,19).

Polybrominated Biphenyls
Diagnosis
Clinical Manifestations
• Intrauterine growth restriction
• Microcephaly and cognitive impairment (11,19)

Characteristics
• Polybrominated biphenyl (PBB) compounds are similar to PCBs. Both are highly lipid soluble.
• PBB exposure is primarily by ingesting contaminated foods, mainly fish, meat, and dairy products.
• The greatest exposure occurred in Michigan in the early 1970s when animal feed was accidentally contaminated with PBBs. The risk may still exist if contaminated fish, dairy products, and meat are consumed.
• Exposure can also come from PBBs in the air if one lives near a waste site containing PBBs.

Organic Solvents
Diagnosis
Clinical Manifestations
• Developmental impairment from chronic, high-dose exposure
• Facial dysmorphism
• Intrauterine growth restriction

Characteristics
• Abnormalities appear to be similar to those found in fetal alcohol embryopathy.
• Exposure occurs through the use of household products, as well as drinking water contamination.
• Chronic, low-dose exposure carries an increased risk of fetal loss and a potential increased risk of central nervous system malformations and facial clefts.
• High-dose exposures frequently result from sniffing solvents as a type of recreational drug use. Lower-level exposures are usually occupational, and the risk may be lower, although some reports suggest an increased risk of first-trimester losses (11,19).

NEURAL TUBE DEFECTS
Background
Definition
• NTDs are frequently defined as a midline defect resulting in the exposure of contents of the neural tube.

Etiology
• Most commonly inherited in a multifactorial pattern.
• Genetic factors play a role because there are ethnic differences in NTD risk. This may be part of a Mendelian syndrome or a chromosomal anomaly.
• Environmental factors or teratogens may play a role.
• Maternal diabetes is recognized as a predisposing factor.
• There is evidence for a direct association of NTDs with folic acid deficiency in early pregnancy. Therefore, specific recommendations have been developed for women at risk.
  • The recommended folic acid supplementation during normal pregnancy is 0.4 g/d.
  • Women at high risk for NTDs should take 4 mg of folic acid per day, starting well before conception (21).

Diagnoses
• Maternal serum AFP screening has been available for a number of years. It relies on an increase in AFP in the amniotic fluid because of the fetal defect. The AFP crosses the placenta and is measurable in the maternal serum (21).

- Ultrasound evaluation of the fetal central nervous system is used to diagnose an NTD. Ultrasound detection of NTDs is reported to be 95% to 99%.
- In almost all cases of spina bifida, an abnormality of the posterior fossa is found.
  - This is described as an Arnold-Chiari malformation type II, characterized by herniation of the cerebellar vermis through the foramen magnum.
  - Arnold-Chiari malformations are almost invariably associated with obstructive hydrocephalus due to the NTD causing "tenting" of the spinal cord and obstruction of the foramen magnum.

Treatment
Prognosis
- NTDs carry significant neonatal morbidity/mortality.
- The degree of paralysis is influenced by location of the lesion, as well as size. Various studies have examined whether an association can be made with in utero antenatal assessment and neonatal outcome. The presence of severe hydrocephaly may be a poor prognostic sign.
- There appears to be an association of decreased intelligence with those requiring shunting with hydrocephalus.

Obstetrical Management
- If the abnormality is diagnosed before the fetus is viable, the patient should receive detailed counseling and be offered the option of pregnancy termination.
- If the patient decides to continue the pregnancy, then expectant management is followed with serial ultrasound assessments. Fetal surgical repair may be an option in select cases.
- Data regarding the appropriate mode of delivery are inadequate. Theoretically, the concern for vaginal delivery traumatizing the defect and exposing the open neural tube to bacteria has been raised. Data from clinical studies on this issue are conflicting, with no clear agreement on vaginal versus cesarean delivery (21).

CONGENITAL HEART DEFECTS
Background
Etiology
- Most congenital heart defects arise from multifactorial disorders.
- The overall incidence may approach 1 in 100 of all liveborn infants.
- The recurrence risk after the birth of one affected child is 2% to 5%.
- An association exists for a high frequency of congenital heart defects with various medical conditions and environmental exposures (Table 30-3).

Treatment
Obstetrical Management
- Fetal echocardiogram is recommended for those at risk based on history or if a screening ultrasound examination suggests the possibility of an abnormality.
- Consultation with pediatric cardiology should be sought for abnormal ultrasound findings.
- Amniocentesis for fetal karyotype should be offered because of the increased risk of aneuploidy.
- Appropriate counseling should be provided to the couple to give them a thorough and realistic understanding of the suspected cardiac defect, its implications, and potential therapy after delivery.
- Delivery should be coordinated with neonatology and pediatric cardiology, particularly if the anomaly will warrant dependency on a patent ductus and the need for immediate therapy.
- Referral to a tertiary care center that performs the corrective procedures is recommended. Ideally, maternal rather than neonatal transport should be performed, so that delivery can occur at the tertiary center that will perform the neonatal surgery (21).

Table 30-3	Conditions Associated with Congenital Heart Defects
Condition	**Frequency of heart defects**
Drugs (e.g., hydantoin)	2%–3%
Trimethadione	15%–30%
Lithium	10%
Infections (e.g., rubella)	35%
Maternal conditions (e.g., diabetes)	3%–5%
Environmental exposure (e.g., alcoholism)	20%–30%

ABDOMINAL WALL DEFECTS
Background
Definition
- Gastroschisis and omphalocele are both abdominal wall defects, but otherwise, they are unique conditions. Accurate antenatal diagnosis is important for overall prognosis and evaluation of association with other abnormalities (21).
- Omphalocele is ventral wall defect with herniation of intraabdominal contents into the base of the umbilical cord. It is covered by fetal peritoneum.
- Gastroschisis is a ventral wall periumbilical defect with evisceration of abdominal organs (21). There is no membrane covering the eviscerated bowel.

Omphalocele
Background
Etiology
- Typically, cases are sporadic, though omphalocele can be associated with chromosomal abnormalities and with Beckwith-Wiedemann syndrome, as well as pentalogy of Cantrell.

Associated Anomalies
- The frequency of chromosomal trisomies with omphalocele is 35% to 58%.
- Cardiac anomalies are present in up to 47% of patients.
- IUGR may exceed 20%.

Diagnosis
- The diagnosis relies on demonstrating a mass protruding from the ventral wall representing herniated visceral organs. Gastroschisis is part of the differential.

Treatment
Prognosis
- The prognosis is largely dependent on the presence or absence of associated anomalies.

Obstetrical Management
- Evaluation for associated anomalies is indicated.
- Amniocentesis to evaluate karyotype should be offered.
- Fetal echocardiogram to evaluate for cardiac defects is warranted.
- The mode of delivery for fetuses with omphalocele is frequently controversial. There are no studies that demonstrate a benefit of cesarean over vaginal delivery. The size of the omphalocele may create a dystocia; a large omphalocele with external protrusion of the liver may warrant cesarean delivery.

Gastroschisis
Background
Etiology
- Gastroschisis is sporadic, though familial transmission may occur. Gastroschisis is a defect that results from vascular compromise of either the umbilical vein or the omphalomesenteric artery.

Associated Anomalies
- Gastroschisis does not appear to be associated with an increased incidence of other anomalies.
- IUGR is commonly associated with gastroschisis, with the incidence possibly exceeding 75%.

Diagnosis
- Ultrasound is an effective method for identifying the ventral wall defect and then differentiating omphalocele from gastroschisis.

Treatment
Prognosis
- Morbidity may be associated with antenatal events, but, more commonly, neonatal intraoperative complications and herniation of the liver are the cause of the higher neonatal mortality rate.

Obstetrical Management
- If IUGR is present, then fetal surveillance is warranted. Ultrasound has been used to evaluate the herniated bowel for compromise and obstruction in order to inform management decisions. There are few studies to support the benefit and the outcomes from this approach.
- The optimal mode of delivery remains uncertain, with vaginal delivery still the most common. Studies have not demonstrated a benefit of a cesarean delivery to avoid birth injury.
- It is recommended that delivery be in a tertiary care center with access to pediatric surgery.

CONGENITAL CLUBBED FEET
Background
Epidemiology
- The incidence is 1 to 4 per 1000.
- An association exists with other abnormalities, including neuromuscular disease, intrauterine confinement, or constraints.
- There is an increased risk for clubbed feet with NTDs (21).

Diagnosis
- Ultrasound is the method of diagnosis.
- If other malformations are identified, then the feet should be carefully examined for evidence of clubbing.
- The presence of clubbed feet on ultrasound exam should trigger a careful examination of the rest of the fetal anatomy to exclude the possibility of other malformations.

Treatment
Obstetrical Management
- The presence of clubbed feet, in the absence of any other malformations, does not alter normal obstetric management.

DIAPHRAGMATIC HERNIA
Background
Definition
- A protrusion of abdominal organs into the thoracic cavity through a defect in the diaphragm.
Etiology
- Sporadic or familial.
- A multifactorial type of inheritance has been suggested.
- Recurrence risk may exceed 2%.

Embryology

The hernia is classified according to its location:

- Bochdalek hernia: Posterolateral defect
- Morgagni foramen hernia: Parasternal defect located in the anterior portion of the diaphragm
- Septum transversum defects
- Hiatal hernia (21)

Treatment

Prognosis

- Aside from the diaphragmatic defect, the obstruction to physical development of the fetal lung results in varying degrees of pulmonary hypoplasia with a high risk of neonatal mortality.
- Historically, patients were given a relative rather poor prognosis.
- Neonatal management has improved outcomes with the benefit of various ventilatory support techniques and the availability of extracorporeal membrane oxygenation.
- Suggestions have been made that abnormally low lecithin/sphingomyelin (L/S) ratios, as markers of fetal pulmonary maturity, may be associated with decreased surfactant production in hypoplastic lungs. It has not been determined if one can use L/S ratios as a prognostic value.
- Outcome is directly associated with the degree of hypoplastic lungs. Postnatal survival also may depend on other factors, including the presence or absence of polyhydramnios; the degree of mediastinal shift, whether the liver has been displaced into the thoracic cavity; and most likely, the degree of pulmonary compromise or response immediately after delivery.

Obstetrical Management

- If diagnosed before the fetus is viable, the option of termination should be offered.
- Thorough evaluation is indicated with amniocentesis for karyotype and fetal echocardiogram.
- A number of intrauterine surgical approaches have been considered but have not been demonstrated an improvement in the outcome (21).

GASTROINTESTINAL MALFORMATIONS

Atresia of the Small Bowel

Background

Etiology

- Generally associated with vascular accident, intussusception, or volvulus. Occurrence is approximately 1 in 5000 live births.

Diagnosis

- Ultrasound typically will demonstrate multiple distended bowel loops. Polyhydramnios is a frequent feature, particularly in upper gastrointestinal obstruction, but is rare in distal obstruction (21).

Treatment

Prognosis

- Prognosis depends on the site of obstruction, the length of remaining bowel, as well as on the association of other congenital anomalies.
- If there is bowel perforation and meconium peritonitis, the prognosis will be worse.
- In general, the lower the obstruction, the better the outcome.

Obstetrical Management

- The recognition of intestinal obstruction typically does not change obstetrical management.

- Primary concerns may be associated with polyhydramnios with increased risk of preterm labor and delivery and potential for fetal compromise.
- Delivery in a tertiary care center is recommended for accessibility to pediatric surgery.

Duodenal Atresia
Background
Etiology
- Most cases are sporadic, but a genetic component has been suggested.

Associated Anomalies
- Duodenal atresia may be an isolated abnormality in 30% to 50% of patients.
- Up to one-third of cases are associated with trisomy 21.
- Other gastrointestinal anomalies occur in more than 25% of patients.
- Cardiac defects occur in 8% to 20% of fetuses.
- Renal anomalies have been reported to be as high as 8%.
- Vertebral anomalies may be found in greater than one-third of patients (21).

Diagnosis
- The typical double bubble sign is demonstrated on ultrasound. This is secondary to the simultaneous distension of the stomach and the first portion of the duodenum.
- The gestational age at which the diagnosis can be reliably established remains an issue. Some have reported that the diagnosis may not be possible until the third trimester (21).

Prognosis
- Prognosis is primarily determined by associated anomalies, as well as the association of polyhydramnios with preterm labor and delivery.

Obstetrical Management
- The critical issue is the association of other anomalies.
- Amniocentesis with karyotype and fetal echocardiogram are warranted.
- Serial amnioreduction may prove beneficial in decreasing the risk of preterm labor and fetal compromise.

Tracheal Esophageal Fistula
Background
Definition
- Esophageal atresia is the presence or absence of a segment of esophagus where the fistula creates a communication between the esophagus and respiratory tracts.

Etiology
- The etiology is unknown. There does not appear to be a genetic predisposition (21).

Pathophysiology
- The most common is esophageal atresia with a fistula connecting the distal portion of the esophagus with the trachea, which accounts for 90% of cases. Five major varieties of tracheal esophageal abnormalities have been reported:
  - Isolated esophageal atresia
  - Esophageal atresia with fistula connecting the proximal portion of the esophagus and trachea
  - Esophageal atresia with a fistula connecting the distal portion of the esophagus and trachea
  - Esophageal atresia with double fistula
  - Tracheal esophageal fistula without esophageal atresia
- Associated anomalies.
  - Greater than 50% have an associated chromosome abnormality or cardiac, genitourinary, or gastrointestinal anomalies.
  - Congenital heart defects may be present in more than one-third of patients.

Diagnoses
- Esophageal atresia or tracheoesophageal fistula is suspected in the presence of polyhydramnios. Increased amniotic fluid is related to a decreased turnover secondary to esophageal obstruction.
- Failure to visualize the stomach on serial ultrasounds raises a suspicion of the diagnosis, particularly if esophageal atresia is present.

Treatment
Prognosis
- Associated congenital anomalies affect the outcome.
- The risk of preterm labor and delivery is increased by polyhydramnios.
- The risk of respiratory complications is increased with this anomaly.

Obstetrical Management
- Amniocentesis with karyotype and fetal echocardiogram are warranted with severe polyhydramnios.
- Serial amniotic reductions may be beneficial to decrease the risk of preterm labor and delivery and fetal compromise (21).

Facial Clefts, Including Cleft Lip and Palate
Background
Etiology
- Causes appear to be multifactorial, with both genetic and environmental factors. Inherited patterns of transmission may also be present. There has been an increased incidence of clefts with medical therapy, including phenytoin (Dilantin) (21).
- The incidence is 1 in 1000 live births.
- Facial clefts are the second most common congenital malformation, accounting for 13% of all anomalies.
- The male/female ratio is 2 to 1.
- The left side is involved twice as often as the right side.

Diagnosis
- Ultrasound, particularly in three-dimensional mode, can reliably detect cleft lip with the appropriate views. Conversely, the ultrasound diagnosis of an isolated cleft palate remains difficult.

Treatment
Prognosis
- Minimal defects are readily correctable with surgery. Large defects may cause cosmetic, swallowing, or respiratory problems; however, recent advances in surgical technique have produced excellent cosmetic and functional results.

Obstetrical Management
- Careful evaluation for associated anomalies is indicated. Amniocentesis for karyotype is controversial. In the absence of other anomalies, amniocentesis may not be necessary.
- Referral for consultation by pediatrics and pediatric surgery is beneficial for educating and lessening the anxiety of the parents (21).

RENAL MALFORMATIONS
Bilateral Renal Agenesis
Background
Etiology
- Renal agenesis can be an isolated finding or can be part of a syndrome including
  - Chromosomal disorders
  - Autosomal recessive or dominant disorders

- Nonmendelian disorders, including association with VATER (vertebral defects, imperforate anus, tracheoesophageal atresia, and radial and renal dysplasia)

Diagnosis by Ultrasound
- Absence of a fetal bladder can typically be confirmed after 12 to 13 weeks.
- The definitive diagnosis is made by ultrasound with the absence of bilateral fetal kidneys. Fetal kidneys can typically be visualized by the 12th week. Kidneys may be confused with the adrenal glands, which are often enlarged during the second trimester.
- Severe oligohydramnios or anhydramnios will be present typically by the middle of the second trimester, when the amniotic fluid originates only from the fetal kidneys (21).

Treatment
Prognosis
- Bilateral renal agenesis is invariably fatal.

Obstetrical Management
- The option of pregnancy termination should be offered before the fetus is viable.
- If the patient decides to continue the pregnancy, it should be made clear that this is a uniformly lethal abnormality and that intervention by cesarean delivery is not recommended (21).

Infantile Polycystic Kidney Disease
Background
Etiology
- The disease is an inherited autosomal recessive disorder.
- The recurrence risk is 25% (21).

Diagnosis
- Criteria for diagnosis are bilaterally enlarged kidneys with oligohydramnios and absence of fetal bladder.

Treatment
Prognosis
- Severe renal involvement typically leads to intrauterine fetal death or neonatal death secondary to pulmonary hypoplasia (21).

Adult Polycystic Kidney Disease
Background
Etiology
- This is an autosomal dominant disorder in which cystic structures replace normal renal parenchyma.

Associated Anomalies
- Polycystic kidney disease is associated with cystic lesions in other organs, including liver, pancreas, spleen, lungs (21).

Treatment
Prognosis
- This disease has variable expression. It can be a chronic disease, becoming symptomatic over a wide range of ages from newborn to adulthood. It can also be completely asymptomatic.
- Hypertension is present in greater than 50% of patients at some point in their life (21).

OBSTETRICAL MANAGEMENT
- The diagnosis of adult polycystic kidney disease typically does not alter standard obstetrical management.
- Enlarged hyperechoic kidneys on ultrasound examination warrant screening of other family members, particularly using renal ultrasound (22).

Multicystic Kidney Disease

Background

Definition

- Multicystic kidney disease (MKD) is a renal disorder characterized by cystic lesions. MKD may be bilateral, unilateral, or segmental.

Etiology

- MKD is generally sporadic but can be a familial occurrence with an association of autosomal recessive, autosomal dominant syndromes, or chromosomal defects.
- The pathogenesis suggests a complex abnormality that may result from two types of insults, developmental failure or early obstructive uropathy (21).

Diagnosis

- Ultrasound is the appropriate modality.
- Multicystic kidneys have a typical appearance on ultrasound, and antenatal diagnosis can be made.
- There may be failure to visualize the fetal bladder. Oligohydramnios is usually present.
- The differential diagnosis includes ureteropelvic junction obstruction.

Treatment

Prognosis

- Bilateral MKD is typically fatal.

Obstetrical Management

- Unilateral MKD without associated abnormalities may not influence obstetrical management. If an obstructive uropathy is suspected, delivery should be performed when pulmonary maturity is demonstrated.
- Amniocentesis may be warranted to assess for karyotype abnormalities.
- If diagnosis of bilateral MKD is made before the fetus is viable, then termination of the pregnancy should be offered.
- Delivery in a tertiary care center for neonatal evaluation may be warranted (21).

Ureteropelvic Junction Obstruction

Background

Incidence

- The diagnosis appears more commonly in males, with a 5:1 male-to-female ratio.

Etiology

- Typically ureteropelvic junction obstruction is sporadic, although familial cases have been reported.

Diagnosis

- Ultrasound will demonstrate a dilated renal pelvis. Several definitions of a dilated renal pelvis exist. Most commonly, a renal pelvis of less than 5 mm is normal. Those between 5 and 10 mm may require follow-up. If greater than 10 mm, an anatomic abnormality is frequently confirmed postnatally (22).

Treatment

Prognosis

- The overall prognosis overall is good in unilateral ureteropelvic junction obstruction, and intervention is usually not necessary. If bilateral involvement is present, there may be an increased risk of renal compromise with a poorer prognosis and indication for earlier delivery.

Obstetrical Management

- A unilateral ureteropelvic junction obstruction typically does not alter obstetrical management.
- Bilateral ureteropelvic junction obstruction may affect management based on gestational age and the degree of obstruction (21).

- A thorough evaluation for associated anomalies, including possible abnormal karyotype, should be considered.

Posterior Urethral Valve Syndrome
Background
Definition
- Obstruction of the lower urinary tract.
- Affects male fetuses almost exclusively.
- Etiology is typically sporadic.

Associated Anomalies
- Associated anomalies are unusual and appear to be confined to the urinary tract.

Diagnosis
- The diagnosis is typically suspected in the presence of a large, dilated bladder with hydro-ureter and hydronephrosis in a male fetus. The ureters are characteristically dilated. The degree of dilatation in the renal pelvis is variable.
- Diagnostic indices to evaluate renal function had been described. Sampling of fetal urine from the dilated bladder can be used to assess fetal renal function by evaluation of urinary sodium chloride and osmolarity, as well as the degree of oligohydramnios.

Treatment
Obstetrical Management
- A search for associated anomalies is indicated because they will impact management, as well as prognosis.
- If a bladder sample is obtained, the option of intrauterine management is available. Suprapubic vesicostomies have been performed.
- Procedures of catheter placement to drain the bladder have shown potential for intrauterine management (21).

Fetal Surgery
- Surgical repair of specific fetal anatomic defects is currently available in a few centers in the United States and Europe.
- This is a rapidly evolving field that can be associated with substantial fetal and maternal risk. These types of procedures are only considered when they might be able to improve fetal outcome.
- The reader is referred to Chapter 37, Fetal Surgery, for a more comprehensive review of this topic.

PATIENT EDUCATION
- All pregnant women should receive screening when prenatal care is initiated for teratogen exposures and birth defect risks.
- Women with known teratogenic risks, such as medical problems, family history, medication, or environmental exposure, should receive counseling before conception about their risk for birth defects with a future pregnancy.
- When explaining the diagnostic methods available for evaluation of fetal malformations, it is important that the couple understand the diagnostic limitations of each method and of the overall process.
- Nondirectional, full disclosure counseling is necessary for couples with fetuses that have lethal or severely compromising malformations so that they can fully participate in the decision-making process.
- Every woman who has had a pregnancy complicated by an NTD should receive counseling before conception about the importance of taking high doses of folic acid before becoming pregnant again and maintaining this dose during the first trimester of pregnancy.

REFERENCES

1. Wilson JG. Current status of teratology–general principles and mechanisms derived from animal studies. In: Wilson JG, Fraser FC, eds. *Handbook of teratology.* Vol 1. New York: Plenum, 1977.
2. Beckman DA, Brent RL. Mechanisms of teratogenesis. *Annu Rev Pharmacol Toxicol.* 1992;24:483–500.
3. U.S. Food and Drug Administration. Pregnancy labeling. *FDA Drug Bull.* 1979;9:23–24.
4. Shepard TH. *Catalog of teratogenic agents.* 7th ed. Baltimore: Johns Hopkins University Press, 1992.
5. March of Dimes Birth Defect Foundation. Pregnancy and Newborn Health Education Center. In: *Birth defects and genetic conditions.* White Plains: March of Dimes Birth Defect Foundation.
6. Centers for Disease Control and Prevention. Congenital malformations surveillance. *Teratology.* 1993;48:545.
7. Friedman JM, Polifka JE. *Teratogenic effects of drugs.* Baltimore: Johns Hopkins University Press, 1994.
8. American College of Obstetricians and Gynecologists. ACOG Practice Bulletin No 20: Perinatal viral and parasitic infections. *Obstet Gynecol.* 2000;96(3).
9. Centers for Disease Control and Prevention. National Center of Birth Defects and Developmental Disabilities Division of Birth Defects and Developmental Disabilities.
10. Centers for Disease Control and Prevention. Recommendations for the use of folic acid to reduce the number of cases of spina bifida and other neural tube defects. *Morbid Mortal Wkly Rep.* 1992;41:1.
11. The Reproductive Toxicology Center. *ReproTox database.* Washington: The Reproductive Toxicology Center.
12. American College of Obstetricians and Gynecologists. ACOG Practice Bulletin No 92: Use of psychiatric medications during pregnancy and lactation. *Obstet Gynecol.* 2012
13. American College of Obstetricians and Gynecologists. ACOG Committee Opinion No 494: Sulfonamides, nitrofurantoin, and risk of birth defects. *Obstet Gynecol.* 2011;117(6):1484–1485.
14. American College of Obstetricians and Gynecologists. ACOG Educational Bulletin No 524: Opioid abuse, dependence and addiction in pregnancy. *Obstet Gynecol.* 2012;119(5):1070–1076.
15. American College of Obstetricians and Gynecologists. ACOG Educational Bulletin No 473: Substance abuse reporting and pregnancy: the role of the obstetrician gynecologist. *Obstet Gynecol.* 2011;117(1):200–201.
16. American College of Obstetricians and Gynecologists. ACOG Educational Bulletin No. 462: Moderate caffeine consumption during pregnancy. *Obstet Gynecol.* 2010;116(2 pt 1):461–468.
17. American College of Obstetricians and Gynecologists. ACOG Educational Bulletin No 471: Smoking cessation during pregnancy. *Obstet Gynecol.* 2010;116(5):1241–1244.
18. Halldorsson T, Strom, M, Petersen S, et al. Intake of artificially sweetened soft drinks and risk of preterm delivery: a prospective cohort study in 59,334 Danish pregnant women. *Am J Clin Nutr.* 2010;92(3):626–633.
19. American College of Obstetricians and Gynecologists. ACOG Educational Bulletin No 575: Exposure to toxic environmental agents. *Obstet Gynecol.* 2013;122(4):931–935.
20. American College of Obstetricians and Gynecologists. ACOG Educational Bulletin No 267: Exercise during pregnancy and the postpartum period. *Obstet Gynecol.* 2002;99(1):171–173.
21. Romero R, Pilu G, Jeanty P, et al. *Prenatal diagnosis of congenital anomalies.* Norwalk: Appleton & Lange, 1988.
22. American College of Obstetricians and Gynecologists. ACOG Educational Bulletin No. 299: Guidelines for diagnostic imaging during pregnancy. *Obstet Gynecol.* 2004;104(3):641–651.
23. American College of Obstetricians and Gynecologists. ACOG Educational Bulletin No 533: Lead screening during pregnancy and lactation. *Obstet Gynecol.* 2012;120(2 Pt 1):416–420.

Obstetric Ultrasound

Eliza M. Berkley and Alfred Z. Abuhamad

KEY POINTS

- Since its introduction into clinical obstetrics, obstetric ultrasound imaging (OUI) has become an essential component of prenatal care.
- OUI requires careful documentation of findings, particularly in regard to confirmation of dates and fetal anatomy.
- While OUI has assumed important social significance to mothers and their families, it is important patients understand that it is a medical examination with certain limitations.

BACKGROUND

Applications

- Biometry
  - Biometry is direct ultrasonic measurements of the fetus.
  - Biometric information is used to estimate gestational age and fetal weight.
  - When combined with appropriate clinical information, biometry is used to document normal or altered growth patterns of the fetus and fetal organ systems.
- Structural assessment
  - High-resolution ultrasound images can detect
    - Structural abnormalities of the fetal gastrointestinal, skeletal, genitourinary, cardiac, and central nervous systems
    - Multiple gestations
    - Placental abnormalities
- Assessment of fetal well-being
  - Real-time ultrasound is used to obtain biophysical profiles (BPPs), amniotic fluid volume assessments, and Doppler studies of the fetal vasculature in the antepartum period.
  - These tests provide information on the well-being of the fetus and have helped reduce perinatal mortality.
- Screening for chromosomal abnormalities
  - Ultrasound can be used in the first and second trimester to screen for chromosomal abnormalities, such as Down syndrome.
    - A first-trimester screen involves measuring fetal nuchal translucency between 10 and 14 weeks' gestation.
    - A second-trimester screening involves multiple serum analyte and ultrasound markers that correlate with chromosomal abnormalities.
- Guidance for invasive procedures
  - Real-time ultrasonography is used to guide needle placement during invasive procedures such as amniocentesis, chorionic villus sampling (CVS), and cordocentesis.
- Early pregnancy assessment
  - Ultrasonography is useful for evaluating early pregnancy issues, such as
    - Verifying the presence (or absence) of a viable intrauterine gestation when bleeding occurs
    - Excluding ectopic pregnancy when pain is present
    - Assigning accurate dates

EVALUATION
General Principles
- Safety concerns.
  - As a general principle, obstetrical ultrasound studies should be performed only for specific clinical indications.
  - Ultrasound imaging uses focused, high-frequency sound waves to generate images.
  - Ultrasound waves transmit energy and can theoretically cause damage to the fetus through the mechanisms of heat and cavitation (the production and collapse of bubbles).
  - At much higher intensities than are in current clinical use, ultrasound waves have been shown to disrupt biologic systems.
  - The relative susceptibility of a given organ system to ultrasound damage is related to the intensity and duration of ultrasound exposure, its distance from the sound source, and the thermal dissipation characteristics of the organ system (related to blood flow through the organ).
- In a review of the safety of ultrasonography in obstetrics, the U.S. Food and Drug Administration (FDA) stated that, although no definite effects could as yet be documented for current exposure levels, the possibility of long-term side effects could not be excluded. Further, the report warned that such effects might be subtle in nature and not easily detected.
- A long-term follow-up study (8 to 9 years) of children exposed to routine ultrasonography in utero showed that the risk of having poor skills in reading and writing was no greater for children whose mothers had routine ultrasonography than for those whose mothers had not had the procedure (1).

Principles of Ultrasound Image Generation
- Ultrasound images are generated by coordinating a transducer, which is a combined sound generator and receiver, with an electronic processor.
- Timed high-frequency pulses of sound (usually in the range 2 to 8 MHz) are sent out and then reflected back to the transducer by objects in the field.
- The time delay between signal generation and return is calculated by the electronic processor, and because the average speed of sound waves in human tissues is known (1540 m per second), this delay in signal return can be displayed as depth.
- By simultaneously obtaining images from adjacent points, the electronic processor can assemble a real-time cross-sectional image of structures within the sound field. This image can be oriented in a linear, curvilinear, or radial manner, depending on the shape of the transducer apparatus.
- Transabdominal and transvaginal transducers rely on the same technology and are commonly used in obstetric and gynecologic ultrasound:
  - Imaging energy frequencies
    - Multiple-energy frequencies are available; however, the range that is used for obstetrical imaging is typically between 2 and 9 MHz.
    - The exact frequency used for imaging depends on the clinical setting and variables such as tissue density and required depth of penetration. Although fixed frequency transducers can be used, the transducers that are currently in use are variable over a preset energy range with continuous adjustment provided by the electronic processor. Typical energy ranges are
      - Abdominal curvilinear probe: 2 to 7 MHz
      - Vaginal probe: 5 to 9 MHz
      - 3D/4D probe: 4 to 8 MHz
    - Generally, 5 or 6 MHz provides the best resolution. However, these high-frequency sound waves are easily attenuated by bodily tissues and do not adequately image fetuses more than 6 to 8 cm from the transducer. When this is a problem, lower frequencies of 3 to 4 MHz are used.

- Tissue interfaces
  - Highly dense structures such as bones are hyperechoic, meaning they reflect a large portion of an incident sound signal, sometimes resulting in a shadowing of structures lying behind them.
  - Fluid-filled structures are hypoechoic, meaning they generate few return images and appear empty on the display.
  - Interfaces between areas of differing tissue densities (e.g., fluid–tissue, tissue–bone) are the most easily visualized.
  - Fetal imaging is more difficult if little difference exists between the structure of interest and surrounding tissues (e.g., distinguishing fetal abdominal circumference (AC) from the uterus if oligohydramnios is present, distinguishing renal parenchyma from surrounding retroperitoneal structures if calyceal structures are not well developed).
- Doppler ultrasound
  - Ultrasound can be used to measure the direction and velocity of fluid flow by means of the Doppler principle.
  - The Doppler effect, which is a change in frequency of sound with motion, means that predictable changes in the frequency of a sound wave occur when it is reflected by moving red cells. Cells moving toward a sound wave source will reflect sound waves back at a higher frequency; cells traveling away from a source will reflect sound at a diminished frequency. Furthermore, blood cells moving with a higher velocity reflect sound waves back at a higher frequency than cells moving with a slower velocity. By comparing initial and returning sound frequencies, a Doppler shift is calculated. This information can then be combined ("duplexed") with simultaneous standard ultrasound images to provide information regarding blood flow in a given area.
  - Blood flow direction.
    - In color Doppler imaging, color converters are added to assign color codes to the directions of blood flow.
    - By convention, flow toward the transducer is colored red, and flow away from the transducer is colored blue. Such information is superimposed on a standard sonographic image.
    - Color flow Doppler ultrasound is particularly useful for evaluating the fetal cardiovascular system and for improving the efficiency of pulsed Doppler measurements.
    - Color Doppler ultrasound is pulsed energy transmission. A relatively large amount of sound energy is required to generate these images. The FDA has approved these energy levels for use in pregnancy. But pulsed Doppler ultrasound should not be used continuously in first-trimester scanning due to the total amount of energy to which the fetus could be exposed.
  - Blood flow velocity.
    - Doppler ultrasound can also be used to calculate blood flow velocity either
      (a) In direct terms as centimeters per second or
      (b) As the Pourcelot index (RI) or pulsatility index (PI), which are modified ratios of frequency shifts during systole and diastole
    - These measurements have been performed for various fetal vessels, including the umbilical artery, the aorta, the carotids, the renals, the splenic, the uterine, the middle cerebral artery, and the ductus venosus in an attempt to facilitate diagnosis of fetal disease states (2).

Types of Ultrasonographic Studies

The American College of Obstetricians and Gynecologists (ACOG), in its technical bulletin on ultrasonography in pregnancy (number 101, December 2011), divided obstetric ultrasound examinations into three types in the second and third trimesters: standard, limited, and specialized. The first-trimester ultrasound is distinct and discussed separately.

Table 31-1	Essential Elements of Fetal Anatomic Ultrasound Survey

Head, face, and neck
- Cerebellum
- Choroid plexus
- Cisterna magna
- Lateral cerebral ventricles
- Midline flax
- Cavum septi pellucidi
- Upper lip

Chest
- The basic cardiac examination includes a four-chamber view of the fetal heart. If technically feasible, an extended basic cardiac examination also can be attempted to evaluate both outflow tracts.

Abdomen
- Stomach (presence, size, and situs)
- Kidneys
- Bladder
- Umbilical cord insertion site into the fetal abdomen
- Umbilical cord vessel number

Spine
- Cervical, thoracic, lumbar, and sacral spine

Extremities
- Legs and arms (presence or absence)

Sex
- For evaluation of multiple gestations

From American College of Obstetricians and Gynecologists. *ACOG Tech Bull.* 2009;101; and American College of Radiology. ACR practice guideline for the performance of antepartum obstetrical ultrasound. In: *ACR practice guidelines and technical standards.* Philadelphia: American College of Radiology, 2007:1025–1033.

- Standard examination: The standard examination is performed during the second and/ or third trimesters of pregnancy.
  - It includes an evaluation of fetal presentation, amniotic fluid volume, cardiac activity, placental position, fetal biometry, fetal number, and an anatomic survey of the fetus. If technically feasible, the uterus and the adnexa should be evaluated.
  - The essential elements of the standard ultrasound examination fetal anatomic survey, as defined by the ACOG, are listed in Table 31-1.
  - Details of the standard examination include
    - ○ A general description of the intrauterine contents, including the number and orientation of fetuses, the placement of the placenta with relation to the uterine cavity and the cervix, and the estimation of the amniotic fluid volume (individual estimations for all fetuses in multiple gestations)
    - ○ Measurement of the following fetal features:
      - – Biparietal diameter (BPD)
      - – Head circumference (HC)
      - – Abdominal circumference (AC)
      - – Femur length (FL)
    - ○ For all fetuses beyond 22 weeks of gestation, an estimated fetal weight (EFW) should be calculated from proved regression equations or by using suitable fetal weight nomograms. This estimated weight should then be interpreted as a percentile for

gestational age (e.g., "The EFW based on a BPD-AC table was 1720 g, placing the fetus at the 25th percentile for gestational age").
- A survey of the fetal anatomy (Table 31-1).
- Comment about the fetal heart rate and rhythm.
- A cursory evaluation should be carried out for other problems such as an abnormally thickened (hydropic) placenta, an overly distended fetal bladder, cystic dilation of a renal pelvis, evidence of fetal ascites or other effusions, or uterine abnormalities (such as leiomyomas); a survey of the maternal pelvic organs should also be performed.
- In multifetal gestations, the presence of a dividing membrane should always be sought (because this effectively excludes the possibility of monochorionic/monoamniotic twins). Multifetal gestations beyond 24 weeks of gestation should be evaluated for growth restriction and discordance. Discordance in twins has been defined as a difference in EFWs of more than 20% (3,4).

- Limited examination
  - When a specific question requires investigation, a limited ultrasound examination may be performed.
  - Limited examinations focus on a specific ultrasonic finding that is usually being surveyed serially, such as the assessment of amniotic fluid volume, confirmation of fetal viability, localization of placenta, evaluation of the cervix, and confirmation of fetal presentation.
  - If a limited study is selected, a previous standard examination should have been performed and the determination made that a repeat standard examination is not warranted (3).

- Specialized examination
  - A specialized examination (detailed or targeted) is a more extensive examination of the entire fetus, often with special attention on a specific fetal organ system. It may be indicated for a fetus with a suspected congenital anomaly or in pregnancies with severe growth abnormalities.
  - It must be emphasized that the accuracy of ultrasonography, even in the most expert hands, does not approach 100%. Patients should be informed of this limitation.
  - The specialized study is best performed under the direct supervision of an experienced sonographer as a real-time examination (3).

- Biophysical profile
  - The BPP is a specialized type of ultrasound examination that was originally described by Manning and colleagues (5).
  - The BPP is a scoring system that has proved to be a valuable method of fetal antepartum assessment. Its principal advantage over other methods of fetal evaluation is that it retains sensitivity (i.e., the ability to diagnose impending fetal compromise) but offers improved specificity (fewer false-positives or abnormal findings).
  - There are four sonographic criteria for the BPP (fetal breathing movements, gross body–limb movements, general body tone, and amniotic fluid volume) and a fetal heart rate nonstress test (NST) component. Each is scored as either normal or abnormal. Two points are assigned for normal findings and no points if a category is judged abnormal. (Note that there are no 1-point scores.)
  - These points are added to give the total score:
    - 8 or 10 is normal.
    - 6 is equivocal.
    - 4 or less is abnormal.
    - 0 or 2 is ominous.
  - The BPP and other similar tests are clinical applications of available technology. They must be interpreted in light of all relevant clinical data pertaining to a given patient. Caution should be used in inferring a particular prognosis from an individual test result viewed outside the clinical context.

- First-trimester examination. The first-trimester examination is performed prior to 14 weeks' gestation.
  - It may be performed transabdominally or transvaginally. A transvaginal exam should be performed if the transabdominal exam is not definitive.
  - It includes an evaluation of the uterus including the cervix and adnexa, the description of the gestational sac including its location and the presence or absence of a yolk sac or embryo, measurement of the crown–rump length (CRL), and documentation of cardiac activity, fetal number, chorionicity, and amnionicity.
  - If ultrasound screening for aneuploidy is desired, a nuchal translucency should be measured (3).

Overview of Technique for Various Fetal Measurements

- Four fetal measurements are essential to every fetal ultrasound examination.
- Biparietal diameter
  - The fetal BPD is measured in a plane transverse to the long axis of the head, which allows visualization of the midline falx cerebri, the cavum septum pellucidum, and the thalamus (which can be seen straddling the midline centrally) (Fig. 31-1). If structures such as the cerebellum, orbits, or basal skull (the petrous ridges and wings of the sphenoid give an X-shaped appearance) are seen, a more accurate plane should be sought before measurements of the head are taken.
  - Technically difficult studies: When the fetal head is low and engaged in the maternal pelvis, it will occasionally be impossible to obtain an accurate BPD. In such circumstances, it is usually best to report that the measurement was "not technically possible" rather than reporting and according clinical significance to a suspect measurement that may be erroneous.
  - Imaging landmarks: The BPD is traditionally measured from the external surface of the cranium anteriorly to the internal surface of the cranium posteriorly. The cranium is most often found to be slightly elliptic in shape. Some fetuses will present with cranial shapes that are either overly rounded (brachycephalic) or an exaggerated narrowed, longitudinally lengthened, elliptical shape (dolichocephaly).
  - The *cephalic index* has been developed to assess the degree of alteration in fetal head shape. It is obtained by dividing the transverse cranial diameter by the occipitofrontal diameter. Cephalic indices of 0.74 to 0.83 are within one standard deviation of the mean.
  - Brachycephaly and dolichocephaly are not intrinsically abnormal but can result in false estimates of gestational age (EGA) or EFW. Infants with brachycephaly will

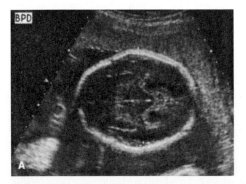
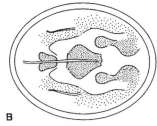

Figure 31-1. Intracranial anatomy for the BPD. **A:** ultrasound picture. CSP, cavum septum pellucidum; 3 V, third ventricle. **B:** diagram of the ultrasound picture.

tend to have overestimated EFW and EGA determinations because of the exaggerated width of the BPD measurement relative to the overall fetal size. The converse is true for dolichocephalic infants. This problem can be overcome by using other parameters to assess gestational age (such as FL and HC) and by using EFW nomograms based on HC or FL, or both, in combination with AC.

- Head circumference
  - The HC is measured in the same plane as the BPD. It can be measured directly with the ultrasound computer's calipers, or its length can be accurately estimated by measuring the diameter of the head in the occipitofrontal dimension and in the transverse dimension. All measures can be obtained from the external surface of the relevant portions of the cranium or at a midpoint within the cranial bones:
    - If the occipitofrontal dimension and transverse dimension are used to estimate the HC, the following formula can be used: $HC = 1/2 \times (OFD + TD) \times 3.1416$. This formula is modeled for a circle, but it closely approximates the results obtained if formulas for elliptic circumference are used.
  - The HC has the advantage of being unaffected by alterations in the shape of the fetal head. Thus, it is an ideal parameter for estimating fetal weight. Unfortunately, HC offers a much wider range of possible values than BPD, and nomograms relating HC to EFW are less often used clinically. If computers or hand calculators are used to directly compute EFW, regression equations using HC are good options.
  - HC is also used in diagnosing microcephaly. Typically, measurements below two standard deviations for a corresponding gestational age are required for a diagnosis of microcephaly.
- Abdominal circumference
  - The fetal AC is measured in a plane perpendicular to the long axis of the torso. The image at the level of AC measurement should contain the stomach bubble and the midportion (not umbilical insertion) of the umbilical vein (Fig. 31-2). The superior poles of the kidneys usually lie slightly caudal to this plane.
  - To obtain this cross-section image, it is usually best to orient the transducer parallel to the spine and slightly caudal to the heart. The transducer should then be rotated 90°, taking care to avoid the oblique transabdominal planes. A full fetal rib should be visible on either side when an accurate transverse plane of the abdomen is obtained. The AC should then be measured several times until two or three consistent values have been obtained. Care should be taken to include the skin in these measurements. As with the HC, if computed planimetry is unavailable, two

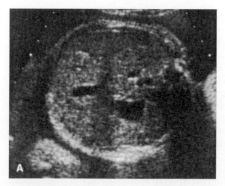
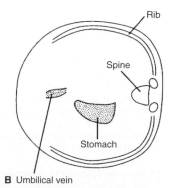

Figure 31-2. Anatomic landmarks of the AC. **A:** ultrasound picture. **B:** diagram of the ultrasound picture.

diameters can be obtained and an estimated AC calculated with the following formula: $AC = 1/2 \times (D_1 + D_2) \times 3.1416$.
- The AC measurement is very sensitive to fetal intrauterine growth restriction (IUGR), as evidenced by the use of FL/AC and HC/AC ratios in screening for IUGR.
- The AC measurement is also the first biometric measurement in the fetus to be affected by growth abnormalities.
- Femur length
  - The part of the femur measured by ultrasound is the ossified portion of the diaphysis. The epiphyseal cartilages are hypoechoic and not easily visualized by ultrasound because they are not well calcified in utero. The femur itself is somewhat bowed, but the proper FL should be the linear distance between the proximal and distal diaphyses.
  - Embryologically, the distal femoral epiphysis becomes ossified at 28 to 35 weeks of gestation. At times, this observation can be used to help assess fetal gestational age (6,7).
- Other fetal measures
  - For a more complete discussion of fetal biometry, see the references and "Selected Readings" at the end of this chapter. These publications provide appropriate nomograms for estimation of fetal weight and gestational age–specific tables of fetal measurements.

Indications for Obstetric Ultrasound Imaging Evaluation
- The ACOG and the National Institutes of Health special study groups now consider routine second-trimester OUI to be standard care in the United States.
- As experience with OUI has accumulated, the indications for such imaging have expanded broadly.
- Routine performance of ultrasound examinations around 18 to 20 weeks of gestation is widely practiced. Ultrasound examination provides important information regarding confirmation of gestational age and fetal anatomic survey. The value of this routine ultrasound examination, although not clearly demonstrated in the United States, is directly related to the expertise of the operator. We recommend routine ultrasound examinations around 18 to 20 weeks of fetal gestation if expertise in performing and interpreting this examination is available.
- The National Institutes of Health's 1984 *Consensus Report on Safety of Ultrasound* reported a number of indications for OUI:
  - Estimation of gestational age for confirming clinical dating among patients who are to undergo elective repeat cesarean delivery, induction of labor, or elective pregnancy termination.
  - Evaluation of fetal growth among patients with suspected or known medical complications associated with either IUGR or macrosomia; these conditions include severe preeclampsia, chronic hypertension, chronic renal disease, and diabetes mellitus.
  - Vaginal bleeding of undetermined cause in pregnancy.
  - Determination of fetal presentation when the fetal presentation cannot be adequately assessed in labor or when the fetal presentation is variable in late pregnancy.
  - Suspected multiple gestation if multiple fetal heart rate patterns are auscultated, if the fundal height is larger than expected for gestational age, or if fertility-enhancing medications have been taken.
  - Ultrasound guidance during invasive procedures, such as amniocentesis, assists the operator to avoid the fetus and placenta during the procedure, thus decreasing the risk to the fetus.
  - For uterine size–dates discrepancy, OUI facilitates accurate assessment of gestational age, potential growth abnormalities, and detection of conditions such as oligohydramnios and polyhydramnios.
  - Evaluation of pelvic mass noted on the clinical examination.

- Suspected hydatidiform mole based on symptoms such as hypertension, proteinuria, or ovarian cysts, uterine size greater than dates, or a combination, or the absence of fetal heart tones by Doppler ultrasound after 12 weeks of gestation.
- As an adjunct to timing of cervical cerclage and placement of the cerclage suture.
- Suspected ectopic pregnancy or pregnancy in a patient at high risk for ectopic pregnancy.
- Suspected intrauterine fetal death.
- As an adjunct to special procedures such as fetoscopy, intrauterine transfusion, percutaneous fetal blood sampling, shunt catheter placement, or CVS.
- Suspected uterine anomaly such as clinically significant leiomyomas, didelphic uterus, or bicornuate uterus.
- Localization of intrauterine contraceptive device.
- Surveillance of ovarian follicle development.
- BPP to assess fetal well-being after 28 weeks of gestation.
- Observation of intrapartum events such as the version or extraction of the second twin.
- Suspected polyhydramnios or oligohydramnios.
- Suspected abruptio placentae.
- As an adjunct to external cephalic version.
- Estimation of fetal weight and presentation in premature rupture of membranes and preterm labor.
- Abnormal maternal serum α-fetoprotein (AFP) value for clinical gestational age when drawn. OUI provides an accurate assessment of gestational age and detects several conditions that may cause elevations of maternal serum AFP, such as multiple gestations, anencephaly, and neural tube defects.
- Serial evaluation of identified fetal anomaly.
- Family history of congenital anomaly.
- Serial evaluation of fetal growth in multiple gestations.
- Estimation of gestational age in patients presenting late for prenatal care.

APPLICATION OF OBSTETRIC ULTRASOUND IMAGING TO COMMON CLINICAL PROBLEMS

Discordant Uterine Size for Gestational Age

- Uterine fundal height inappropriate for expected dates
  - If gestational age is well established, the fundal height approximately equals the gestational age in weeks.
  - A fundal height measurement that is 2 to 3 cm more or less than expected for gestational age is considered abnormal and should be evaluated by OUI to determine fetal biometry with EFW and amniotic fluid volume assessment.
- Uncertain pregnancy dating
  - In pregnancies with poor or uncertain dates, fetal measures of BPD, HC, and FL can be used to estimate gestational age and, in combination with the fetal AC, can be used to estimate fetal weight and serially evaluate fetal growth.
- Good pregnancy dating with fundal height less than expected
  - If the gestational age is known with reasonable certainty, the EFW can be compared to the expected EFW for gestational age.
  - Fetuses below the 10th percentile for gestational age are considered small for gestational age, possibly due to fetal growth restriction.
  - Ratios of HC/AC and FL/AC can also be used to assess possible IUGR. Interpretation of the HC/AC ratio depends somewhat on fetal gestational age (1.12 at 24.0 weeks, 1.05 at 32 weeks, and 0.98 at 40 weeks); the FL/AC ratio (normally ~0.20 to 0.22) does not vary during pregnancy. Together, these measures and ratios provide a relatively sensitive and specific means of assessing gestational age and fetal growth.

- The two general categories of IUGR are asymmetric growth restriction and symmetric growth restriction.
- Asymmetric IUGR is most common and results in "sparing" of fetal brain growth with consequently normal BPD and HC with small AC and EFW estimates.
- Symmetric IUGR is characterized by abnormally decreased EFW with paradoxically normal FL/AC and HC/AC ratios. Symmetric IUGR can also be falsely diagnosed in infants who are growing at rates that are individually normal but below the 10th percentile for the general population.
- Although a distinction has been made between symmetrical and asymmetrical IUGR with regard to the timing of the insult and the pathogenesis of the disease, in clinical practice, the distinction is not that evident; ultrasound may not be specific, and management is uniform for both types.
- Good pregnancy dating with fundal height greater than expected
  - A fundal height of ≥3 cm more than expected for gestational age is considered large for dates. Potential causes of a fundal height greater than expected for age include
    - Incorrect pregnancy dating. If no prior ultrasonic evaluations have been performed to establish pregnancy dating, the possibility of incorrect pregnancy dates should be considered.
    - Large for gestational age fetus.
    - Multiple gestations.
    - Polyhydramnios.
    - Uterine leiomyomas.
- Repeat evaluation should be considered near term to assess interval growth and evaluate for possible fetal macrosomia.

HIGH-RISK PREGNANCY EVALUATION

- Serial evaluations of fetal growth in most cases are best initiated at 24 to 26 weeks of gestation and then repeated at monthly intervals.
- Fetuses not growing normally for gestational age (using population-specific percentile growth tables) should be monitored with other methods of antepartum assessment (such as contraction stress tests, nonstress tests, Doppler velocimetry, or BPPs).
- Patients at high-risk for preterm labor may benefit from early ultrasonic confirmation of pregnancy dating because accurate pregnancy dating helps in the management of preterm labor. These patients do not require serial sonographic evaluation unless clinical suspicion of fetal growth abnormality is noted.

Complications

- OUI facilitates the management of pregnancies at risk for complications. Accurate pregnancy dating allows more precise evaluation of fetal growth. Precise knowledge of obstetric dating may also affect decisions regarding certain therapeutic interventions (choice of tocolytic agents, use of fetal lung-maturing agents) or timing of delivery in complicated pregnancies.
- The following pregnancy complications are best managed by an ultrasound evaluation obtained in the first trimester to confirm pregnancy dating, followed by a fetal anatomic evaluation at 18 to 20 weeks' gestation and then serial sonographic evaluation of fetal growth and EFW:
  - Chronic renal disease
  - Collagen vascular disease
  - Diabetes or prior gestational diabetes
  - Hypertension or prior preeclampsia
  - Isoimmunization (rhesus or other)
  - Lupus or antiphospholipid antibody syndrome
  - Maternal malignancy
  - Multiple gestation

MULTIPLE GESTATION

Background

- Multiple gestations are at increased risk for preterm labor, growth discordance, and fetal demise.
- Monoamniotic gestations have complications secondary to cord entanglement, which may lead to fetal demise of one and often both fetuses.
- Monochorionic gestations are at increased risk of developing specific complications related to vascular communications in a single placenta including twin–twin transfusion syndrome (TTTS), selective intrauterine growth restriction (sIUGR), and twin anemia polycythemia sequence (TAPS). They are also at greater risk of fetal death, preterm delivery, and perinatal death compared to dichorionic twin gestations.
- In multifetal gestations, normal growth references are not well established because a population of "normal" twin gestations has not been clearly defined. In general, twin gestations at term yield fetuses weighing approximately 10% less than matched singleton fetuses.

Evaluation

- Amnionicity and chorionicity should ideally be established in the first trimester by documentation of the number of gestational sacs, placental number, and presence of a dividing membrane.
- The thickness and shape of the membrane should be documented, and the presence of a thick dividing membrane and "lambda" sign if dichorionic or thin dividing membrane and "T" sign if monochorionic should be reported.
- Monochorionic gestations are best managed by an ultrasound evaluation at 16 and 18 weeks to confirm growth concordance with biometric measures and single deepest amniotic pockets as well as assessing for the presence of fetal bladders to screen for evidence of TTTS. Ultrasound screening for TTTS may then be considered every 2 weeks thereafter.
- After completion of a morphology ultrasound of twins, serial assessments of EFW should be evaluated for discordant growth. Fetuses with differences of more than 20% in EFW or with BPDs varying by more than 4 mm exhibit abnormal discordance and should be placed into an antepartum assessment protocol as described before (4).

SUSPECTED FETAL ANOMALY

Background

OUI is a useful method for detecting major fetal anomalies, with a sensitivity of approximately 50% and close to 100% specificity for major anomalies.

Evaluation

History

- Patients with family or obstetric histories suggestive of fetal anomalies should undergo a thorough ultrasound evaluation to screen for fetal anomalies. This evaluation should initially survey all fetal organ systems and then focus on the index organ system (i.e., the system with a history of prior anomaly).
- The optimal timing of this study has not been clearly elucidated because major central nervous system abnormalities (such as anencephaly) can often be detected by 15 weeks of gestation, whereas cardiac structure is much more easily assessed at 22 weeks of gestation.
- Maternal serum AFP abnormalities.
  - OUI is a valuable adjunct for evaluating fetal anatomy and potential viability when abnormal maternal serum AFP values are present on quadruple screen results (see below).
  - Elevated maternal serum AFP values may be an indication of open neural tube defects as well as ventral abdominal wall defects, multiple gestations, fetal death (in multifetal gestations), and other less common conditions.

- An ultrasound evaluation should always be performed to establish the correct gestational age:
  - If the confirmed or corrected gestational age places the maternal serum AFP in the normal range, no further evaluation is necessary. Otherwise, a thorough fetal ultrasonic evaluation is required, with emphasis on visualizing intracranial structure and the entire neural axis.
  - A negative ultrasonic evaluation does not negate the significance of an elevated maternal serum AFP. Small neural tube defects can potentially be missed despite a thorough ultrasound evaluation.
- If the cause for elevated maternal serum AFP is not obvious, ultrasound-guided amniocentesis may be performed to directly measure the amniotic fluid AFP, to measure the amniotic fluid acetylcholinesterase, and to perform a fetal karyotype.
  - Acetylcholinesterase is found in high concentrations within the central nervous system and is present in the amniotic fluid very early in pregnancy.
  - If present after 14 weeks of gestation, amniotic fluid acetylcholinesterase is considered direct evidence of an open neural tube defect. Contamination of amniotic fluid with fetal blood can raise the level of amniotic fluid AFP but does not affect the level of amniotic fluid acetylcholinesterase.
  - However, many patients decline amniocentesis when the targeted ultrasound is normal in association with an elevated maternal serum AFP.
- Abnormal quadruple screen. The quadruple ("quad") screen is a biochemical test performed on maternal blood between 14 and 22 weeks. It is performed for the detection of fetal chromosomal abnormalities, the most common of which is Down syndrome, and includes maternal serum AFP to screen for risk of open neural tube and other defects as discussed above.
  - Patients with an abnormal quad screen are at increased risk for having infants with chromosomal abnormalities such as trisomies 21 and 18. Such syndromes cannot be reliably excluded by ultrasound evaluation. Thus, amniocentesis for fetal karyotype should be offered in these circumstances and/or targeted fetal DNA screening from maternal blood.
  - A modification of a patient's risk for Down syndrome can be accomplished by a quad screen in combination with a comprehensive ultrasound examination between 18 and 22 weeks of gestation.
  - Markers of Down syndrome on ultrasound include thickened nuchal fold, short femurs and humerii, echogenic intracardiac foci, fetal pyelectasis, and echogenic fetal bowel. The absence of these markers may reduce the patient's risk profile significantly.
  - Several prenatal diagnosis and ultrasound centers are combining the quad screen with the ultrasound findings in modifying a patient's risk for Down syndrome.
- Abnormalities of amniotic fluid volume.
  - Measurement of amniotic fluid volumes
    - Abnormalities of amniotic fluid volume may be indicators of functional abnormalities within the renal, gastrointestinal, or central nervous systems.
    - Amniotic fluid index (AFI) is a measure of amniotic fluid volume. Derivation of the index involves measuring, in a longitudinal plane, the largest fluid pocket in each of the four quadrants of the uterus and adding the four measurements. The pockets are measured when no fetal parts or umbilical cord is visualized within the measured pocket.
    - Normal AFI values are between 10 and 24 cm (6,9).
    - Alternatively, the single deepest pocket of amniotic fluid can be used to assess for oligohydramnios and polyhydramnios. This method is helpful in multiple gestations.
    - When using a single deepest pocket, a maximum vertical pocket value of less than 2 cm defines oligohydramnios, and a maximum vertical pocket value greater than 8 defines polyhydramnios (10).

POLYHYDRAMNIOS

Background
- No exact definition for polyhydramnios exists, but two suggested definitions are as follows:
  - Subjectively increased amniotic fluid volume and a maximum vertical pocket ≥8 cm (3)
  - AFI (the sum of largest vertical amniotic fluid pocket depths from the four uterine quadrants) of 24 or greater (3)

Evaluation
- Polyhydramnios may be seen in association with diabetic pregnancies, isoimmunization syndromes, open neural tube defects, fetal anomalies affecting the fetal swallowing mechanism (esophageal atresia, tracheoesophageal fistula) or the gastrointestinal tract (duodenal atresia), or other rare metabolic or genetic syndromes. However, polyhydramnios is often idiopathic with no identifiable underlying pathophysiologic process.
- If polyhydramnios is judged to be severe, fetal chromosomal evaluation should be considered.

OLIGOHYDRAMNIOS

Background
- Oligohydramnios is defined as an amniotic fluid volume less than expected for gestational age.
- Oligohydramnios is of great clinical significance because severe prolonged reductions in amniotic fluid volume, especially when present at early gestational ages, may alter fetal mobility and predispose to abnormal facies, limb contractures, and pulmonary hypoplasia.
- In the term pregnancy, oligohydramnios (with intact membranes) is associated with increased risk of adverse fetal outcomes and requires close surveillance.
- Oligohydramnios can be caused by rupture of membranes or decreased production of amniotic fluid. After 18 weeks of gestation, the fetal kidneys produce most amniotic fluid. Renal agenesis, dysplasia, or obstruction of the urinary system may cause oligohydramnios.

Evaluation
- Two commonly used methods of quantifying oligohydramnios are the AFI (9,13) and the deepest vertical pocket (DVP) method.
- The AFI (9,13) was described above. A four-quadrant total of 5 cm or less is defined as oligohydramnios; values greater than 10 cm are normal, while values between 5 and 10 mm are considered to be decreased amniotic fluid volume.
- The DVP method defines oligohydramnios as a single DVP less than 2 cm.
- Patients with diminished amniotic fluid volumes should be carefully monitored with antenatal tests of fetal well-being and with serial sonographic evaluation of amniotic fluid volume.

SHORT CERVICAL LENGTH

Background
- A short cervical length is commonly defined as less than 25 mm on transvaginal ultrasound in the midtrimester of pregnancy (18 to 24 weeks of gestation).
- A short cervical length is associated with an increased risk of preterm birth, which is the leading cause of neonatal mortality.
- The shorter the cervical length, the higher the risk of preterm birth.
- Patients with a prior history of preterm birth are at risk for a short cervical length and subsequent preterm birth.

Evaluation

- Transvaginal ultrasound assessment of cervical length can be performed easily and quickly and has been shown to be reproducible.
- The distance between the internal and external os should be measured and the shortest of three measurements used.
- Knowledge of a short cervical length may allow providers to offer therapeutic interventions such as cerclage placement or vaginal progesterone in efforts to prevent preterm birth.

SINGLE UMBILICAL ARTERY

- In a normal pregnancy, three umbilical blood vessels (two arteries and one vein) are present. This should be confirmed by OUI.
- Two-vessel umbilical cords (single umbilical artery) occur in up to 1% of pregnancies.
- Two-vessel cords are commonly associated with other fetal abnormalities.
- There is some controversy as to whether fetuses with two-vessel umbilical cords are at risk for intrauterine growth restriction.
- Some studies have also reported an increased incidence of congenital heart defects in fetuses with a single umbilical artery (14). Therefore, a detailed fetal anatomic cardiac examination with consideration of fetal echocardiogram is indicated in the pregnancy with a single umbilical artery.
- If fetal anomalies are identified by OUI, prenatal genetic screening and diagnostic testing options should be offered to the patient. The incidence of karyotypic abnormalities increases if one anomaly is present. The presence of two or more anomalies is much more strongly associated with fetal karyotypic abnormalities.

UNCERTAIN DATING OF PREGNANCY
Background

- Patients who do not have well-established menstrual dating (i.e., history confirmed by early physical examination) should have an ultrasound evaluation to confirm or establish the gestational age and estimated date of confinement.

Evaluation
History

- The earliest available sonographic study is generally used to establish obstetric dates, provided it was performed before 24 weeks of gestation.
- Patients should be questioned as to prior ultrasound evaluations at other facilities, and every effort should be made to obtain existing information. If the examination was performed by suitably experienced practitioners, it should be used as the basis for establishing the pregnancy dates.
- Estimated gestational age.
  - The margin of error associated with ultrasonic determination of EGA is approximately 10% of the determined gestational age (±1-week margin of error before 12 weeks of gestation, ±1 to ±2 weeks error from 12 to 20 weeks of gestation, and ±2 to ±3 weeks error after 20 weeks of gestation).
  - If OUI is performed between 7 and 10 weeks of gestation, the fetal CRL should be used to determine the EGA.
  - For OUIs obtained later in pregnancy, the EGAs associated with the fetal biometric measures of the BPD, HC, and FL should be obtained and (as available) averaged.
  - If OUI is obtained before 6 weeks of gestation and no fetal pole is clearly visible, the gestational sac measure should not be used to establish the EGA. The ultrasound should be repeated several weeks later to measure the CRL and to document fetal cardiac activity within the uterus (excluding the possibility of ectopic gestation). The pregnancy is then dated using the CRL from the later exam.

- If the ultrasound estimates an EGA that agrees with the menstrual dates (within the procedural error limits), the menstrual dates are considered confirmed.
- For pregnancies that are less than 24 weeks of gestation by ultrasound with discrepancies between the menstrual dates and ultrasound measurements of more than 2 to 3 weeks, it is generally safe to accept the ultrasound EGA as the correct obstetric EGA.

Fetal Growth Restriction
- In pregnancies of more than 24 weeks' gestation as estimated by ultrasound with reported menstrual date–derived EGAs that are 3 weeks or more ahead of the ultrasound measurements, the possibility of intrauterine growth restriction should be considered. If underlying maternal disease is present, this diagnosis is more likely.
- If the AC is disproportionately decreased relative to the ultrasound composite gestational age, then asymmetric IUGR may be present. Conversely, if FL/AC and HC/AC ratios are within normal limits (i.e., if all fetal measures are symmetric), then the possibility of symmetric IUGR should be considered.
- When growth restriction is believed to be a reasonable possibility, the fetus should be evaluated with ongoing antepartum testing, and a repeat sonogram for growth should be conducted in approximately 3 to 4 weeks:
  - If the repeat examination shows normal growth for assigned ultrasonic gestational age, the obstetric EGA should be accepted, and antepartum testing can be discontinued.
  - If little or no growth occurs, the fetus should be managed as a high-risk pregnancy (see Chapter 33).

Changing the Estimated Date of Delivery
- Once properly established, the gestational age and estimated date of delivery should be strictly adhered to.
- If better information becomes available and it is judged necessary to change the estimated date of delivery, this information should be carefully documented in the patient's chart.

Serial Obstetric Ultrasound Exams
- OUI allows accurate interval assessment of fetal growth throughout pregnancy. Pregnancies at risk for IUGR (maternal disease states, multiple gestations) should have initial ultrasound exam performed early in pregnancy and then repeated at established intervals throughout pregnancy.
- A commonly used scheme is for pregnancies at risk of fetal growth restriction:
  - Twelve-week ultrasound to confirm gestational age
  - Eighteen- to twenty-week detailed ultrasound for fetal anatomy and confirmation of appropriate growth
  - Repeat ultrasound exams at 4- to 6-week intervals
- The fetus can also be surveyed at other intervals if findings necessitate therapeutic intervention or early delivery. Anomalies such as hydrocephalus or hydronephrosis or fetal risk for hydrops or cardiac compromise may require individualized schedules for serial ultrasound exams.

UNEXPLAINED ABDOMINAL PAIN OR VAGINAL BLEEDING
Failed Pregnancy
- A failed pregnancy may be diagnosed when a gestational sac greater than 25 mm in mean diameter does not contain a yolk sac or embryo or when an embryo measuring ≥7 mm does not have cardiac activity (ACR Appropriateness Criteria 2012).

Ectopic Pregnancy
- The management of unexplained abdominal pain and vaginal bleeding in pregnancy has been greatly aided by abdominal and vaginal ultrasonography.
- If an ectopic pregnancy is suspected, ultrasonic evaluation of the uterine cavity should be performed, and a serum β-human chorionic gonadotropin (β-hCG) titer obtained.
- If the β-hCG titer is greater than 1500 IU, an intrauterine gestation should be seen by endovaginal ultrasound examination, and if not, an ectopic gestation is likely (15,16).

Abnormalities of Placentation

- Abnormal placentation is strongly associated with bleeding complications in all stages of pregnancy.
- Ultrasonic studies allow relatively precise delineation of the site of placentation. Of greatest concern is establishing or excluding the diagnosis of placenta previa, although there are numerous other placental abnormalities that can be identified by ultrasound.
- Before 20 weeks of gestation, the placenta is frequently seen to be low lying in relation to the cervix. In 60% to 90% of second-trimester marginal placenta previae, normal placentation will be noted at term.
- Placentas found to be implanted both anteriorly and posteriorly over the internal cervical os (e.g., central placenta previa) most commonly do not resolve as pregnancy progresses).

PATIENT EDUCATION

- For more information to provide to patients about ultrasound, please refer to the American Institute of Ultrasound in Medicine Web site at www.AIUM.org.

REFERENCES

1. Salvesen KA, Bakketeig LS, Eik-Nes SH, et al. Routine ultrasonography *in utero* and school performance at age 8–9 years. *Lancet.* 1992;339:85–89.
2. Zacko A, Neilson JP. Doppler ultrasonography in high-risk pregnancies: systematic review with meta-analysis. *Am J Obstet Gynecol.* 1995;172:1379–1387.
3. American College of Obstetricians and Gynecologists. ACOG Tech Bull No. 101: ultrasonography in pregnancy. *Obstet Gynecol.* 2011;113(2 Pt 1):451–461.
4. Simpson LL. Twin-Twin transfusion syndrome. SMFM Clinical Guideline. *Am J Obstet Gynecol.* 2013;208(1):3–19.
5. Manning FA, Baskett TF, Morrison I, et al. Fetal biophysical profile scoring: a prospective study of 1,184 high risk patients. *Am J Obstet Gynecol.* 1981;140: 289–294.
6. Mahony BS, Bowie JD, Killam AP, et al. Epiphyseal ossification centers in the assessment of fetal lung maturity: sonographic correlations with the amniocentesis lung profile. *Radiology.* 1986;159:521–524.
7. McLeary RD, Kuhns LR. Sonographic evaluation of the distal femoral epiphyseal ossification center. *J Ultrasound Med.* 1983;2:437–438.
8. Wald NJ, Kennard A, Hackshaw A, McGuire A. Antenatal screening for down's syndrome. *J Med Screen.* 1997;4(4):181–246.
9. Phelan JP, Ahn MO, Smith CV, et al. Amniotic fluid index measurements during pregnancy. *J Reprod Med.* 1987;32:601–604.
10. Chauhan SP, Doherty DD, Magann EF, et al. Amniotic fluid index vs single deepest pocket technique during modified biophysical profile: a randomized clinical trial. *Am J Obstet Gynecol.* 2004;191:661–667; discussion 667–668.
11. Iams JD, Goldenberg RL, Meis PJ, et al. The length of the cervix and the risk of spontaneous premature delivery. National Institute of Child Health and Human Development Maternal Fetal Medicine Unit Network. *N Engl J Med.* 1996;334:567–572.
12. Owen J, Iams JD. What we have learned about cervical ultrasound. National Institute of Child Health and Human Development Maternal-Fetal Medicine Units Network. *Semin Perinatol.* 2003;27:194–203.
13. Phelan JP, Smith CV, Broussard P, et al. Amniotic fluid volume assessment with the four-quadrant technique at 36–42 weeks' gestation. *J Reprod Med.* 1987;32:540–542.
14. Abuhamad AZ, Shaffer W, Mari G, et al. Single umbilical artery: does it matter which artery is missing? *Am J Obstet Gynecol.* 1995;173:728–732.
15. Nyberg DA, Filly RA, Filho DL, et al. Abnormal pregnancy: early diagnosis by ultrasound and serum chorionic gonadotropin levels. *Radiology.* 1986;158:393–396.
16. Nyberg DA, Filly RA, Laing FC, et al. Ectopic pregnancy: diagnosis by sonography correlated with quantitative HCG levels. *J Ultrasound Med.* 1987;6:145–150.

32 Fetal Monitoring and Testing

Kathleen M. Berkowitz and Michael P. Nageotte

FETAL HEART RATE MONITORING

Key Points

The goals for performance of fetal monitoring are to
- Decrease risk for stillbirth in the antepartum population
- Assess the physiologic stresses of labor on the metabolic status of the fetus
- Identify at-risk fetuses before permanent damage occurs, so that therapeutic interventions can be used to decrease complication rates

Background

The idea that abnormal fetal heart rates correlate with fetal distress was initially proposed by Kilian in 1848 (1). Since its inception, the goal of fetal heart rate monitoring (FHRM) has been early identification of fetuses at risk for hypoxic insult. FHRM now occurs nearly universally during the intrapartum period and in selected patients at high risk for stillbirth in the antepartum population.
- Retrospective studies have confirmed the safety of FHRM.
- Prospective trials have shown a decreased perinatal mortality rate associated with electronic FHRM (2–4).
- Despite improved perinatal mortality, the goal of reducing fetal asphyxia and brain damage remains elusive.
- The benefit of electronic FHRM is that it is very reliable in prediction of normal fetal acid–base status (it has a high specificity) when the pattern is normal or indeterminate:
  - Normal FHRM patterns have a positive predictive value of approximately 99% for the absence of fetal acidosis.
- Electronic FHRM is of limited utility in that its sensitivity (the ability to identify abnormal fetuses) is poor when there is an abnormal pattern. Abnormal FHRM monitoring patterns have poor positive predictive value for the presence of significant fetal acidosis (5). Standardized guidelines for interpretation of fetal heart rate patterns and estimation of the risk for acidosis have been adopted by the National Institute of Child Health and Human Development to help identify the subset of patients at highest risk for the development of metabolic acidosis (6).

Epidemiology
- Electronic fetal monitoring is used in two settings:
  - Intrapartum monitoring for the development of clinically significant fetal hypoxia/acidosis during labor
  - Antepartum monitoring for pregnancies deemed high risk because of maternal or fetal complications
- When intrapartum electronic fetal monitoring is used, the perinatal death rate decreases (7).
- Antepartum use of FHRM combined with evaluation of amniotic fluid volume decreases the stillbirth rate in populations at higher than average risk for stillbirth (women with chronic medical conditions, presence of intraamniotic infection, fetal congenital anomalies, and fetal intrauterine growth retardation) (8).

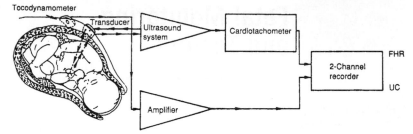

Figure 32-1. Schematic diagram of an indirect fetal monitoring system. The fetal heart rate (FHR) is obtained using Doppler techniques and then counted by a cardiotachometer. Uterine activity is measured by tocodynamometry. (UC, uterine contraction.) (Reproduced with permission from Berkowitz KM, Nageotte M. Intrapartum fetal monitoring. In: Moore T, et al., eds. *Gynecology and obstetrics: a longitudinal approach.* New York: Churchill-Livingstone, 1993:568.)

- Several retrospective studies published during the 1970s associated the use of electronic FHRM with an observed decrease in the fetal death rate (9–12). Other randomized controlled trials during the same era did not show similar benefit (13,14). In previously unmonitored populations with high perinatal mortality rates, randomized studies of electronic fetal monitoring confirmed a decrease in perinatal mortality (2). Using data from 1,732,211 pregnancies recorded in the US 2004 birth cohort–linked birth/infant death data set, the use of EFM was associated with a significant decrease in the risk for perinatal mortality (3). However, it should also be noted that electronic fetal monitoring has a high false-positive rate for identification of clinically significant fetal stress, which increases the incidence of interventions such as cesarean delivery or operative vaginal delivery (15). The percentage of these operative interventions that actually improve neonatal outcome is uncertain.

Physiologic Basis of Fetal Heart Rate Monitoring
- External monitoring
  - The external fetal monitoring system consists of a transmitter that emits ultrasound waves that penetrate the uterine cavity and encounter interfaces of differing density.
  - When the interfaces are moving, as the fetal heart chambers do with each cardiac cycle, the reflected signals undergo a Doppler shift, which is measured by the receiving device. The highest Doppler shift of the returning waveform passes to a cardiotachometer (Fig. 32-1).
  - Fetal movement can also cause Doppler shifts and must be filtered out of external monitoring.
- Internal monitoring
  - Internal FHRM is accomplished by attaching an electrode to the fetal scalp.
  - The signal generated by electrical activity of the heart is acquired by the electrode, amplified, and transmitted to a cardiotachometer (Fig. 32-2).
  - The cardiotachometer counts the interval between the R waves of the fetal electrocardiogram (ECG) and displays fetal heart rate as the reciprocal of this interval. A new rate is set with the transmission of each R wave, and the tiny differences in arrival intervals between R waves are recorded. These small, instantaneous differences are known as beat-to-beat variability and can be measured accurately only by internal monitoring systems.
  - If the fetal R–R interval is shorter than 250 milliseconds (i.e., the heart rate exceeds 240 beats per minute [bpm]), the cardiotachometer cannot differentiate between arriving signals and will either divide the true rate in half or not register it at all.
  - Fetal movement does not affect internal FHRM.

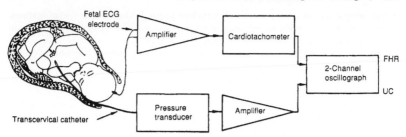

Figure 32-2. Schematic diagram of a direct fetal monitoring system depicting internal fetal scalp electrode and intrauterine pressure catheter. (FHR, fetal heart rate; UC, uterine contraction.) (Reproduced with permission from Berkowitz KM, Nageotte M. Intrapartum fetal monitoring. In: Moore T, et al., eds. *Gynecology and obstetrics: a longitudinal approach* New York: Churchill-Livingstone, 1993:569.)

- Uterine contractions
  - Assessment of uterine contraction patterns is necessary to determine the pattern of any accelerations and decelerations in the fetal heart rate.
  - *External* acquisition of uterine contractile activity is obtained using a transducer, which acts as a strain gauge and senses changes in uterine shape and rigidity. When the transducer's plunger is depressed, an electrical signal is emitted and recorded on the tracing paper as an upward deflection, indicating a uterine contraction. The external transducer does not sense true intrauterine pressure, and the early stages of a contraction may not depress the plunger enough to record small changes in uterine pressure.
  - *Internal* intrauterine catheters are open-ended, fluid-filled catheters that measure the intrauterine pressure as the difference in hydrostatic pressure present between the closed intrauterine space and the external environment.
- Maternal–fetal nutrient exchange
  - Eighty-five percent of the uterine blood flow supplies the fetoplacental circulation, while the remaining 15% nourishes the myometrial wall.
  - Oxygen crosses the placental barrier by simple diffusion and is more avidly bound to fetal hemoglobin than to maternal hemoglobin.
  - During a normal uterine contraction, there is a short interruption of blood flow through the intervillous space when the pressure generated by the myometrial contraction exceeds the blood pressure in the spiral arterioles and the intervillous space adjacent to the placenta. If the contractions are prolonged or tetanic (16), the interruption of placental perfusion may be prolonged and fetal oxygen reserves may be exceeded, leading to fetal hypoxia.
  - Any factor that decreases uterine blood flow or that affects oxygen diffusion may decrease the amount of oxygen delivered to the fetus.
    - Maternal position (17), exercise, hypotension, or chronic maternal medical conditions such as hypertension and diabetes may be associated with decreased placental blood flow.
    - Placental infarcts or premature placental separation may impair oxygen delivery to the fetus.
- Neurologic control of fetal heart rate
  - The average baseline fetal heart rate is about 160 bpm in the early second trimester. An atrial pacemaker determines the baseline fetal heart rate.
  - Opposing effects of parasympathetic and sympathetic innervation of the heart modulate variations in this rate. Initially, the fetal heart rate is predominantly regulated by

the sympathetic nervous system and chemoreceptors. As the nervous system matures, parasympathetic regulation becomes more pronounced. This results in a decrease in average baseline heart rate and an increase in its variability.

- o Parasympathetic nerve impulses arise in the brainstem and reach the heart via the vagus nerve.
- o Sympathetic stimuli are carried from the brainstem to the heart via cervical sympathetic nerve fibers.
- o Parasympathetic tone primarily affects the short-term beat-to-beat variability, whereas sympathetic stimulation is the strongest determinant of long-term variability and accelerations in heart rate (18).
- o Even combination autonomic blockade may not abolish all variability, which suggests that unknown, nonautonomic neural factors may play a role in fetal heart rate variability (19).

- Parasympathetic tone increases as gestation advances, which gradually decreases the baseline fetal heart rate.
- Transient loss of variability may result from infection, drugs, hypoxia, or sleep cycles.
- Prematurity is also associated with decreased variability, but by 28 weeks of gestation, the neurologic pathways stimulating variability are functional. Consequently, it should be kept in mind that a persistent absence of variability beyond 28 weeks of gestation occurs less than 15% of the time. Such a finding may indicate the occurrence of a significant insult to the fetal central nervous system.

Definitions of Terms

The process of fetal assessment requires definition of fetal heart rate baseline, reactivity, variability, and the presence and patterns of accelerations and decelerations. The analysis of these characteristics is then interpreted in the context of the setting in which the testing is occurring. In antepartum testing situations, the FHR pattern is assessed for a fixed time interval and interpreted as normal or abnormal assessment of fetal acid–base and oxygenation status. In the case of intrapartum FHR monitoring, the FHR pattern is evaluated continuously and categorized as normal (Category 1, Fig. 32-3), indeterminate (Category 2, Fig. 32-4), or abnormal (Category 3, Fig. 32-5) (6). Several factors must be considered in order to properly characterize an FHR pattern.

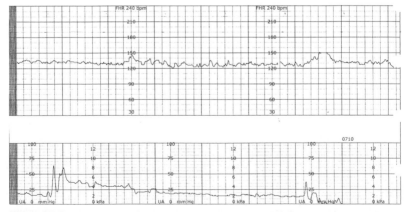

Figure 32-3. The presence of a normal baseline, normal variability, and accelerations. This is a Category 1 FHR tracing.

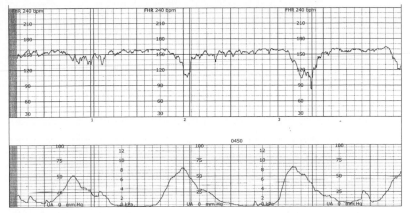

Figure 32-4. Variable decelerations. Baseline heart rate and variability are normal. This is a Category 2 FHR pattern.

- Fetal heart rate baseline.
  - The National Institute for Child Health and Human Development defines baseline fetal heart rate as "the approximated mean fetal heart rate, rounded to increments of 5 bpm during a 10-minute window, excluding periodic or episodic changes, periods of marked fetal heart rate variability, or segments of the baseline that differ by greater than 25 bpm" (20). A normal fetal heart rate baseline is 110 to 160 bpm.
- Fetal heart rate reactivity.
  - Fetal heart rate reactivity is two or more accelerations in a 20-minute period (21).
  - The presence of accelerations and reactivity indicates the presence of an intact and functioning fetal central nervous system and the existence of normal intrauterine acid–base and oxygenation conditions.

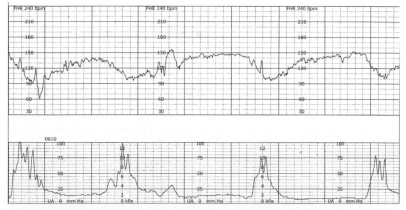

Figure 32-5. Severe variable decelerations with decreased variability and "overshoot." This is a Category 3 FHR pattern.

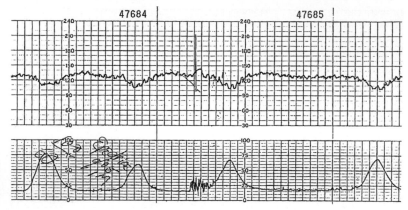

Figure 32-6. Early decelerations during FHRM. (Reproduced with permission from Parer JT. *Handbook of fetal heart rate monitoring.* 2nd ed. Philadelphia: WB Saunders, 1997:162.)

- Variability.
  - Baseline variability is defined as fluctuations from baseline fetal heart rate of two cycles or more per minute (22).
  - Beat-to-beat variability is the small, instantaneous differences in the R–R interval:
    o It is literally the difference in the FHR baseline from one beat to the next beat.
    o Beat-to-beat variability can only be measured accurately by internal monitoring systems.
  - Long-term variability refers to state changes induced by alternating periods of fetal sleep and activity.
  - Gradations of variability include undetectable, minimal, moderate, marked, and sinusoidal.
- Accelerations (see Fig. 32-3).
  - Accelerations are elevations of fetal heart rate at least 15 bpm above baseline, lasting at least 15 seconds.
  - Accelerations are typically abrupt in onset and are associated with fetal movements.
  - Any factor that suppresses central nervous system activity (sleep, drugs, acidosis, etc.) can also suppress accelerations and reactivity.
- Decelerations: Episodic patterns of decelerations are not associated with uterine contractions. Periodic patterns of deceleration occur in association with uterine contractile activity.
  - Early decelerations (Fig. 32-6)
    o Early decelerations are secondary to fetal head compression and are benign. They can be seen during labor in Category 1 FHR patterns.
    o Early decelerations are uniformly shaped decelerations of minimal amplitude, have a slow onset and slow return to baseline, and are in phase with the uterine contraction cycle. The time from onset of deceleration to nadir is typically greater than 30 seconds.
    o An early deceleration begins early in the contraction cycle, drops to its lowest point with the peak of the contraction force, and returns to baseline before the contraction ceases.
    o The amplitude of the deceleration roughly parallels the strength of the contraction but rarely exceeds 30 bpm below the baseline. The nadir of the contraction occurs with the peak of the contraction.

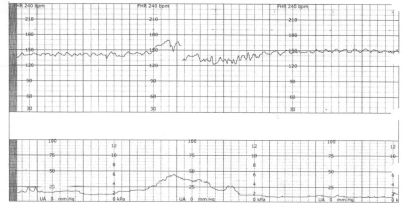

Figure 32-7. Late decelerations during external monitoring. Note the latency period in contrast to the similarly shaped early decelerations in Figure 32-6.

- Variable decelerations (Figs. 32-4 and 32-5)
  - Variable decelerations are V-shaped decelerations associated with umbilical cord compression and reduction in blood flow through the umbilical vein. During labor, variable decelerations are features of Category 2 or Category 3 FHR patterns.
  - Variable decelerations have an abrupt onset and quick return to baseline. The duration, intensity, and timing of each variable deceleration relative to its contraction may differ markedly. The onset of the deceleration to the nadir occurs within 30 seconds. The deceleration itself lasts more than 15 seconds but less than 2 full minutes. Accelerations occurring just prior to the onset of the decelerations are commonly referred to as "shoulders" and are not part of the variable deceleration.
- Late decelerations (Fig. 32-7)
  - Late decelerations are named for the timing of their onset and cessations. The decrease in fetal heart rate occurs after the start of a uterine contraction, and the return to baseline is delayed until after the end of the contraction.
  - The onset of a late deceleration occurs up to 30 seconds after the start of a contraction, and its nadir occurs well after peak contraction strength has been reached.
  - The decreased fetal heart rate continues after the contraction has ended, with return to baseline delayed for up to 30 seconds.
- Normal, indeterminate, and abnormal fetal heart rate patterns.
  - The FHR pattern is categorized by assessment of the following four variables:
    - Baseline fetal heart rate
    - Presence of accelerations or decelerations
    - Frequency, type, and severity of decelerations
    - Presence or absence of variability
- In the setting of antepartum testing, the pattern is described as normal, equivocal, or abnormal. A normal antepartum tracing is present when
  - The baseline fetal heart rate is between 110 and 160 bpm.
  - There is moderate variability.
  - At least two accelerations are present in a 20-minute time interval.
  - There are no significant decelerations.
- When features such as abnormal FHR baseline, the absence of reactivity, and the presence of decelerations are noted during antepartum testing, the test is read as equivocal

or abnormal. Further evaluation or treatment of the fetal condition is indicated when an equivocal or abnormal FHR pattern is present.

- In the setting of continuous intrapartum monitoring, the same process is used to determine if the FHR is normal (Category 1), indeterminate (Category 2), or abnormal (Category 3).
  - ○ Category 1 (normal) FHR patterns are highly predictive of normal fetal acid–base status and have the following four characteristics:
    - − The baseline fetal heart rate is between 110 and 160 bpm.
    - − There is moderate variability (6 to 25 bpm).
    - − Accelerations can be present or absent.
    - − Absence of late or variable decelerations. Early decelerations may be present.
  - ○ Category 2 (indeterminate) FHR patterns comprise any pattern that does not meet criteria for Category 1 or Category 3. They are not predictive of abnormal fetal acid–base status. Any of the following features may be observed:
    - − Tachycardia, bradycardia without absent variability, minimal variability, absent variability without recurrent decelerations, marked variability, recurrent variable decelerations with minimal or moderate variability, prolonged deceleration ≥2 minutes but less than 10 minutes, recurrent late decelerations with moderate variability, and variable decelerations with other characteristics such as slow return to baseline or the presence of "shoulders"
  - ○ Category 3 (abnormal) FHR patterns are the only patterns that suggest a likelihood of abnormal fetal acid–base status. There are four types of abnormal fetal heart rate patterns. They are predictive of abnormal fetal acid–base status and suggest that a concerted effort should be made to alleviate the conditions leading to the development of these patterns.
    - − Sinusoidal heart rate: a pattern of regular variability resembling a sine wave, with an amplitude of 5 to 40 bpm occurring at a rate of three to five cycles per minute. The pattern is classically associated with fetal anemia.
    - − Absent variability and recurrent late decelerations.
    - − Absent variability and recurrent variable decelerations.
    - − Bradycardia.
- Uncommon patterns of fetal heart rate (Fig. 32-8) include
  - Prolonged decelerations (isolated decelerations longer than 60 to 90 seconds)
  - Saltatory patterns (characterized by frequent high-amplitude accelerations greater than 25 bpm)
  - Bradyarrhythmias (slow fetal heart rate baseline below 90 bpm)
  - Tachyarrhythmias (sustained fetal heart rate in excess of 200 bpm)
  - Sinusoidal heart rate pattern

Pathophysiology of Fetal Heart Rate Monitoring

- The presence of a normal or indeterminate fetal heart rate pattern indicates an intact, functioning fetal central nervous system. It also indicates that the intrauterine environment is capable of sustaining continued fetal oxygenation.
- The presence of an abnormal fetal heart rate pattern indicates some degree of fetal compromise, ranging from intermittent hypoxia to metabolic acidosis, and even, rarely, intrapartum stillbirth.
- Indeterminate or abnormal fetal heart rate patterns may occur transiently as result of reversible conditions (Table 32-1) or as a result of long-standing fetal compromise.

Etiology of Late Decelerations

- Regardless of the underlying etiology (transient or long standing), the uteroplacental–fetal events that cause indeterminate or abnormal FHR patterns with late decelerations are as follows:
  - A contraction begins in a woman with uteroplacental insufficiency, and the intervillous oxygen content drops significantly, lowering the fetal PO_2 below 15 to 20 mm Hg.

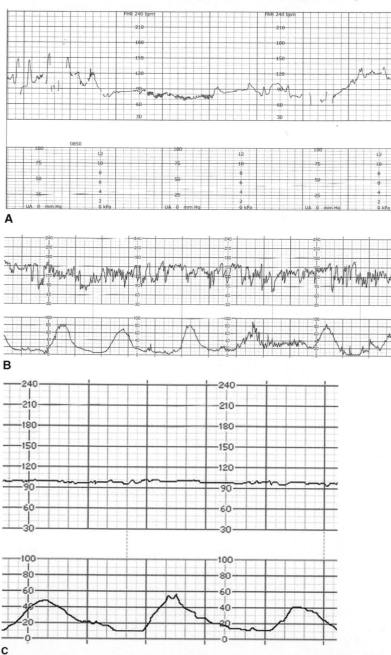

Figure 32-8. Other types of fetal heart rate abnormalities. **A:** Prolonged deceleration. **B:** Saltatory pattern. **C:** Bradyarrhythmia.

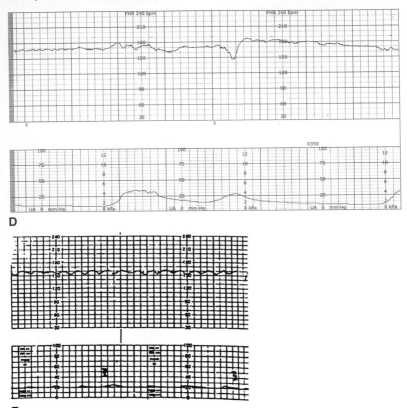

Figure 32-8 (Continued). D: Tachyarrhythmia. **E:** Sinusoidal pattern. (Reproduced with permission from Berkowitz KM, Nageotte M. Intrapartum fetal monitoring. In: Moore T, et al., eds. *Gynecology and obstetrics: a longitudinal approach*. New York: Churchill-Livingstone, 1993:566.)

Table 32-1	Reversible Conditions Leading to Abnormal Fetal Heart Rate Patterns

Excessive uterine activity
Maternal hypotension
Bronchospasm
Maternal fever
Diabetic ketoacidosis
Thyrotoxic crisis
Hypertensive disorder
Status epilepticus
Maternal or fetal anemia
Alcohol or drug intoxication
Acute renal failure
Fetal supraventricular tachycardia

- Fetal chemoreceptors are activated, and α-sympathetic stimulation occurs.
- The α-stimulation increases fetal blood pressure, which in turn activates the baroreceptors.
- Baroreceptor impulses are transmitted back to the brainstem, increasing vagal tone and decreasing fetal heart rate.
- The onset of the late deceleration is delayed (or "late") in relation to the pattern of uterine contraction because of the complexity of the feedback mechanism that produces it.
- When uteroplacental insufficiency is severe enough to generate an intervillous partial pressure of oxygen less than 18 mm Hg, chronic metabolic acidosis can evolve and directly depress fetal myocardial performance.
- Isolated or intermittent late decelerations are common and are not worrisome.
- Persistent late decelerations over a period of time are cause for concern because they carry a risk of progression to persistent hypoxia, acidosis, and asphyxia.
- Late decelerations due to myocardial depression are usually of low amplitude, resulting in the appearance of shallow decelerations.

Etiology of Variable Decelerations
- The critical event that leads to variable decelerations is reduction in blood flow through the umbilical vein.
- Blood pressure in the umbilical vein is lower than in the umbilical arteries, so cord compression produces earlier and relatively greater occlusion of the vein than the arteries.
- When cord compression decreases the return of oxygenated blood from the placenta through the umbilical vein and occludes flow of deoxygenated blood to the placenta through the umbilical arteries, the fetal baroreceptors initiate a parasympathetic response that lowers fetal heart rate via the vagus nerve.
- Variable decelerations will occur when umbilical cord blood flow is reduced by 10% or more.
- Because the degree of umbilical cord compression is not consistent and varies throughout a contraction, the shape of these decelerations is variable and not directly related to fetal hypoxia.
- Although variable decelerations are not directly due to fetal hypoxia, the fetus will eventually develop hypoxia if these decelerations persist for a long enough time.
- Although mild variable decelerations are often observed in normal and indeterminate FHR patterns (Fig. 32-9), severe variable decelerations are more ominous. The presence of severe variable decelerations requires careful observation and the ability to intervene rapidly if they persist or become associated with more worrisome features.

Prolonged Decelerations/Bradycardias
- Prolonged decelerations are ominous patterns associated with poor fetal outcomes if they are not quickly resolved. Prolonged decelerations derive from a variety of causes, all of which work through the common pathway of severe, sustained interruption of the fetal supply of oxygenated blood.
- Prolonged decelerations last at least 60 to 90 seconds and may be longer in duration. The longer the deceleration lasts, the greater the risk of fetal acidosis and compromise.
- Decelerations that last longer than 3 to 4 minutes require preparation for immediate delivery due to the risk to the fetus of sustained reduced perfusion.

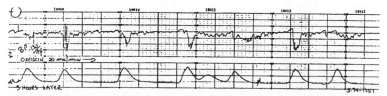

Figure 32-9. Variable decelerations. (Reproduced with permission from Freeman RK, Garite TJ. *Fetal heart rate monitoring.* Baltimore: Williams & Wilkins 1981:71.)

Sinusoidal Patterns
- Sinusoidal patterns are rare, ominous patterns that occur with severe fetal anemia and associated hypoxia.
- Sinusoidal patterns are classically associated with fetal anemia due to Rh isoimmunization or fetal–maternal hemorrhage.
- Management requires either correction of the fetal anemia or delivery.

Saltatory Patterns
- Saltatory patterns are considered indicative of early, intermittent hypoxia without acidosis.
- The exaggerated accelerations characteristic of a salutatory pattern are a response generated by the central nervous system in an attempt to correct intermittent hypoxia. The fetal heart rate increases in order to increase cardiac output and thereby improve return of oxygenated blood from the placenta to the fetus.

ANTEPARTUM FETAL MONITORING

Background
- Patient identification
  - If clinical evaluation of an antepartum patient indicates a fetal or maternal condition associated with an increased risk for perinatal complications, antepartum FHRM should be initiated (Table 32-2).
  - Common indications include postdate pregnancy, diabetes, hypertensive disorders, growth restriction, and multiple gestation with discordant growth.

Table 32-2	Maternal and Fetal Conditions Associated with an Increased Risk for Uteroplacental Insufficiency
Indication	**When to start testing**
Preeclampsia/eclampsia	At diagnosis
Chronic hypertension	34 wk
Collagen vascular disease	34 wk
Diabetes mellitus	
Class A1 (uncomplicated)	40 wk
Class A (A2 or complicated A1)	34 wk
Class B, C, D	32–34 wk
Class R, F, H	26–28 wk
Anemia, hemoglobinopathy	32–34 wk
Rh isoimmunization	26–34 wk (consider using weekly peak evaluation of peak systolic velocity of middle cerebral artery)
Hyperthyroidism	34 wk
Maternal cyanotic heart disease	34 wk
Prolonged pregnancy	41 wk
Previous stillbirth	28–34 wk
Fetal growth retardation	At diagnosis
Advanced maternal age	34–40 wk
Decreased fetal movement	At diagnosis
Discordant twin growth (>25% discordance or IUGR <10th percentile)	At diagnosis

IUGR, intrauterine growth retardation.

Evaluation
Testing Protocols
- Low-risk populations are best evaluated using noninvasive protocols such as fetal movement counting.
- In higher-risk populations, typical testing protocols combine short-term indicators of fetal well-being (FHRM) with long-term indicators such as amniotic fluid volume. A popular and easily implemented protocol is the nonstress test (NST) and assessment of amniotic fluid volume. If the NST reveals a reactive tracing without decelerations and if the amniotic fluid volume is normal (greater than 5 cm is the usual criteria), testing continues on a twice-weekly basis. If features such as decelerations or abnormal fetal heart rate are present, further evaluation can include a biophysical profile (BPP), contraction stress testing (CST), or admission for intensive evaluation of the fetal condition.
- Fetal movement counting.
  - Low-risk populations can be asked to count fetal movements at term daily for 1 hour. If fewer than ten movements are felt, or if it takes progressively longer to feel ten movements, the patient should call her physician immediately (23).
  - High-risk populations should receive more sensitive testing protocols.
- NST.
  - The patient is placed in a lateral recumbent position for assessment of fetal heart rate patterns and uterine contractility. After approximately 30 minutes, fetal heart rate baseline, accelerations, and decelerations are evaluated.
- Amniotic fluid assessment.
  - The uterine corpus is divided into quadrants, and the deepest vertical pocket of amniotic fluid is measured in each quadrant. Adding the amount of fluid in the quadrants in a singleton, term patient should yield a value generally between 5 and 22 cm (24). The fluid pocket should be measured while the ultrasound transducer is held parallel to the patient's long axis and perpendicular to the floor. The pocket must be free of umbilical cord loops or fetal parts.
- BPP.
  - The BPP evaluates the combined effects of acute and chronic factors upon the metabolic status of the fetus and uteroplacental blood flow. Acute markers include presence or absence of fetal breathing, movement, tone, and FHR reactivity. Amniotic fluid volume is considered a marker for chronic conditions. Each of the five markers is scored as present (2 points) or absent (0 points). The presence of an AFI of at least 50 cm scores 2 points. The presence of sustained fetal breathing for 30 seconds scores 2 points. The observation of two or more gross body movements scores 2 points. The presence of fetal tone is confirmed by observation of flexion and/or extension of fetal extremities and scores 2 points. If tone, movement, or breathing is not seen during a 30-minute period of observation, the score for each factor not seen is 0.
- CST.
  - The CST evaluates fetal heart rate in response to uterine contractions induced by breast stimulation or oxytocin infusion. Once three contractions occur in a 10-minute period, the fetal heart rate is observed for reactivity and the occurrence of late or variable decelerations.
  - A negative test indicates the absence of decelerations.
  - Equivocal tests occur when fewer than 50% of the contractions are associated with decelerations.
  - A positive test indicates that more than 50% of the contractions are associated with decelerations.
- BPP.
  - The BPP combines the NST with assessment of fetal breathing, tone, gross body movements, and amniotic fluid volume.

Table 32-3	Scoring of the BPP	
	Score	
Parameter	**2**	**0**
Fetal heart rate	Presence of reactivity, without or without presence of decelerations	Absence of reactivity
Fetal tone	At least one episode of fetal extremity extension and flexion within 30 min	No episodes of fetal extremity extension/flexion
Fetal movement	At least three gross body movements observed within 30 min	Fewer than three gross body movements within 30 min
Fetal breathing	Sustained episode of breathing >30 s in duration, occurring at least once during a 30-min period	Absence of sustained episode of fetal breathing
AFI	At least one pocket of fluid >2.0 cm or an AFI >5.0 cm	Less fluid

- The advantage of the BPP is that it evaluates both acute and chronic markers for fetal compromise by combining the NST and amniotic fluid index (AFI), respectively. The BPP requires proficiency in ultrasonography and should be done twice weekly (25).
- Each of the five markers is scored as either 0 (absent) or 2 (present). Scores of 8 or 10 signify fetal well-being (Table 32-3).
- Primary surveillance and backup tests.
  - There is no one method of antepartum fetal surveillance that is superior to others. Selection of a method of primary surveillance is based on the cost and availability of services in a particular region.
  - The use of weekly CST, biweekly NST, biweekly BPP, or biweekly modified BPP should result in perinatal mortality rates of 0.4 to 3 per 1000 live births within 1 week of a normal test (26).
  - The most common method of primary surveillance currently in use is the modified BPP, which is actually an NST combined with amniotic fluid assessment by ultrasound. When this test is abnormal, a CST or BPP can be performed as a backup test (27). The need for subsequent interventions is determined by the test result, the patient-specific setting, and the clinical judgment of the assessor.

FETAL HYPOXIA/ACIDOSIS

Differentiating between a truly hypoxic, compromised fetus and a fetus with normal acid–base status that has some abnormal features of FHRM is difficult. The use of standardized guidelines can decrease intraobserver variability and identify a subset of patients in whom obstetric interventions are likely to alleviate fetal acidosis or clinically significant hypoxia.
- The principles of FHRM indicate that
  - The presence of a normal fetal heart rate baseline is a reassuring feature that persists until fetal compromise is firmly established
  - Loss of variability and presence of decelerations precede the loss of a normal fetal heart rate baseline. Persistently minimal or absent fetal heart rate variability is a strong indicator of fetal compromise (28)
- During the intrapartum period, additional information can be acquired with rupture of the membranes and with further tests to identify a truly compromised fetus.

- Fetal scalp and acoustic stimulation
  - Stimulation of the fetal scalp either digitally at the time of cervical examination or atraumatically with an Allis clamp is a valuable adjunct for intrapartum fetal assessment.
  - When accelerations occur following stimulation, fetal acidosis is not present (29).
  - In the absence of accelerations, at least 20% of the patients have a fetus with a pH less than 7.20 (30).
  - Vibroacoustic stimulation–induced fetal heart rate accelerations are also reassuring of normal fetal pH. Absence of an acceleration after acoustic stimulation is associated with fetal pH less than 7.20 in a significant percentage of cases (31).
  - STAN—ST segment waveform analysis. The placement of an internal fetal scalp electrode allows for direct assessment of the fetal cardiotocography (CTG) and changes in the ST segment (32). Changes are categorized as normal, intermediary, abnormal, or preterminal. Improvements in neonatal outcome with the STAN system appear modest at best (33).
- Acid–base determination
  - Fetal acid–base determination can be assessed from a fetal scalp blood sample obtained during labor or from cord blood at the time of delivery. It directly measures the type and degree of acidosis present. Due to risks for fetal infection and hemorrhage, fetal scalp sampling procedures are rarely indicated. Fluid obtained from the fetal scalp may not accurately reflect the true acid–base status of the fetus.
  - Fetal respiratory acidosis can be differentiated from metabolic or mixed acidosis by measuring the partial pressure of carbon dioxide (PCO_2) and base deficit present. The normal fetal PCO_2 is 40 to 50 mm Hg. Normal base deficit is approximately 7 mEq/L. Normal pH values decrease slightly as labor progresses. Fetal respiratory acidosis is associated with intermittent umbilical cord occlusion and increased PCO_2 levels. The pH is usually in the range of 7.20 to 7.25. A hypoxic fetus produces lactic acid, and the resulting metabolic acidosis is reflected in an increase of the base deficit.
  - The U.S. Food and Drug Administration approved fetal pulse oximetry for clinical use in 2000. Currently, the American College of Obstetricians and Gynecologists does not recommend adjunctive use of fetal pulse oximetry during labor (21). Two large randomized trials have been conducted (34,35). Neither was able to demonstrate a reduction in overall cesarean delivery rate, although one study (34) did show a decrease in rate of cesarean delivery for "non-reassuring" fetal status.

Treatment
Management
- When an indeterminate or abnormal fetal heart rate pattern is identified, management depends on
  - Setting (antepartum vs. intrapartum)
  - Gestational age
  - Clinical circumstances
- If a reversible condition is generating, the abnormal fetal heart rate pattern should be corrected. Reversible conditions (Table 32-1) can be treated with appropriate measures of intrauterine resuscitation.
- Irreversible conditions are best treated by expeditious delivery and extrauterine resuscitation by experienced neonatal personnel.
- When indeterminate or abnormal fetal heart rate patterns are encountered in the outpatient setting, backup testing should be performed promptly.
- When there are specific fetal concerns about gestational age and the possible need for neonatal intensive care unit services, hospitalization should be arranged at a facility where such services are available.

- Transfer of a patient in labor with an indeterminate or abnormal fetal heart rate pattern is difficult and should be approached with great caution, regardless of gestational age or complications. A diagnosis of abnormal fetal status with failure to respond to intrauterine resuscitative measures requires prompt delivery, with neonatal support provided until transport can be arranged.

Treatment of Maternal Conditions
- Reversal of an unstable maternal condition can convert an indeterminate or abnormal fetal heart rate pattern to one that is normal.
  - Uncontrolled diabetes should be treated with insulin, fluid support, and correction of electrolyte abnormalities.
  - Hypertension should be controlled with short-acting medications. Care should be taken not to overcorrect hypertension, as this can abruptly decrease intrauterine blood flow.
  - Maternal conditions that are not readily reversible, such as acute or severe abruption, should be treated by delivery.
- Correction of intrapartum complications will often improve indeterminate or abnormal fetal heart rate patterns.
  - Excessive uterine activity should be addressed by decreasing or discontinuing the use of Pitocin. If it is severe or persistent, the administration of a short-acting β-mimetic agent may also be indicated. Both of these actions decrease uterine activity, allowing the fetus to regain metabolic reserve.
  - Hypotension should be corrected with fluid and vasopressor support.
  - Fetal heart rate patterns indicative of cord compression can often be improved or alleviated by changing maternal position. The presence of recurrent variable decelerations should prompt consideration to treat with amnioinfusion (21).
  - Oxygen administration will improve the maternal–fetal oxygen gradient and allow for quicker fetal recovery from hypoxia. Oxygen should be administered at 100% concentration via face mask.
  - Correction of maternal fever using antipyretics will reverse fetal tachycardia.

Treatment of Fetal Conditions
- During labor, fetal conditions are generally treated via management of the mother. The primary decisions regard circumventing or intervening in the normal labor process through cesarean delivery for abnormal or ominous fetal heart rate patterns. The American College of Obstetrics and Gynecology considers the use of FHRM to be associated with a high false-positive rate and increased rate of obstetric interventions. The use of a three-tiered system of categorization of fetal heart rate is recommended to decrease interobserver variability and limit the scope of such intervention to the subset of patients most likely to benefit (21).
- Tachycardia.
  - Sinus tachycardia must be differentiated from supraventricular tachycardia.
  - Intermittent supraventricular tachycardia is usually of little clinical significance, but persistence of this rhythm is associated with high-output cardiac failure, fetal hydrops, and eventual death.
  - Digoxin is the most commonly used initial treatment; other available agents include quinidine, verapamil, and propranolol.
  - β-Mimetics, theophylline, caffeine, and some over-the-counter drugs may induce mild fetal tachycardia. Discontinuation of the drug and substitution of an appropriate alternative medication is indicated when the tachycardia is concerning or prolonged.
  - Fetal anemia may also cause tachycardia.
- Bradyarrhythmia.
  - Persistent antepartum fetal bradyarrhythmia is generally due to heart block. Sustained, prolonged bradyarrhythmia can lead to heart failure and death. Careful fetal surveillance is required to determine the proper timing of delivery.

- Intrapartum fetal bradycardia is indicative of fetal compromise, as discussed earlier in this chapter. Bradycardias that last longer than 3 to 4 minutes require immediate response and progression to delivery. Repetitive bradycardias of 2 to 4 minutes in length require delivery after three or four occurrences.

Risk Management

- The presumption that antepartum and intrapartum FHRM could prevent stillbirth and neonatal complications due to a compromised intrauterine environment preceded investigations designed to confirm the promise of these interventions.
- Ironically, the widespread use of intrapartum electronic FHRM led to an increase in cesarean deliveries, with little evidence to support a concomitant decrease in cerebral palsy or other neonatal complications. It has further led to a widespread popular assumption that we can prevent these complications and that failure to do so must be a result of inadequate implementation of infallible technology.
- The dichotomy between public expectation and the observed limitations of FHRM makes this an area of medicolegal risk. Risk management in this area revolves around expeditious response to perceived abnormalities noted in the testing protocols.
  - In the antepartum and outpatient setting, all fetal surveillance tests should be read the same day as performed. Indeterminate and abnormal results should be investigated promptly. The patient should be informed of the results and of any improvements resulting from further interventions. She should also be informed about how those results will affect her ongoing plan of care.
  - Intrapartum categorization of the fetal heart rate as Category 1, 2, or 3 should occur on an ongoing basis as labor progresses. The use of standardized definitions can limit the number of unindicated interventions and focus resources on the subset of patients most likely to benefit from those interventions. In cases where a Category 3 FHR pattern cannot be improved, prompt intervention and neonatal resuscitation should be implemented.
- The most common complication of fetal heart rate assessment is the overtreatment of a fetus not truly compromised. If appropriate clinical judgment is not employed, this may result in unnecessary interventions, higher cesarean delivery rates, or even premature delivery.

PATIENT EDUCATION

- Patients who have been identified as at high risk for antepartum or intrapartum complications should be informed of the specific risks involved.
- Patients should be informed of the benefits, limitations, and physiologic basis of FHRM.
- When antepartum testing is performed, the patient should be aware of the time needed for the test to be completed, the process by which the results are reviewed, and the frequency with which testing will occur. It is helpful to advise the patient that, although the diagnosis of a reassuring test truly is reassuring, the presence of some nonreassuring features does not necessarily indicate that a problem exists. This is particularly true when CSTs are used, as there is a high false-positive rate for this test compared to NST or BPP testing.
- Patients should be aware that the identification of indeterminate or abnormal features of the fetal heart rate will be fully and promptly investigated, whether she is in the antepartum or intrapartum setting.

REFERENCES

1. Goodlin RC. History of fetal monitoring. *Am J Obstet Gynecol.* 1979;133:323–352.
2. Vintzileos AM, Nochimson DJ, Antsaklis A, et al. Comparison of intrapartum electronic fetal heart rate monitoring versus intermittent auscultation in detecting fetal acidemia at birth. *Am J Obstet Gynecol.* 1995;173(4):1021–1024.
3. Ananth CV, Joseph KS, Oyelese Y, et al. Trends in preterm birth and perinatal mortality among singletons: United States, 1989 through 2000. *Obstet Gynecol.* 2005;105:1084–1091.

4. Chen HY, Chauhan SP, Ananth CV, et al. Electronic fetal monitoring and its relationship to neonatal and infant mortality in the United Sates. *Am J Obstet Gynecol.* 2011;204: 401.e1–401.e10.
5. Larma JD, Silva AM, Holcroft CJ, et al. Intrapartum electronic fetal heart rate monitoring and the identification of metabolic acidosis and hypoxic-ischemic encephalopathy. *Am J Obstet Gynecol.* 2007;197:301.31–38.
6. Macones GA, Hankins GDV, Spong CY, et al. The 2008 National Institute of Child Health and Human Development workshop report on electronic fetal monitoring: update on definitions, interpretation, and research guidelines. *Obstet Gynecol.* 2008;112:661–666.
7. Ananth CV, Chauhan SP, Chen HY, et al. Electronic Fetal Monitoring in the United States: Temporal trends and adverse perinatal outcomes. *Obstet Gynecol.* 2013;121:927–933.
8. Kontoupoulos EV, Vintzileos AM. Condition specific antepartum fetal testing. *Am J Obstet Gynecol.* 2004;191:1546–1551.
9. Nichols PL, Chen T-C. *Minimal brain dysfunction: a prospective study.* Hillsdale, NJ: Lawrence Erlbaum Associates, 1981.
10. Hobel CJ, Hyvarinen M, Oh W. Abnormal fetal heart rate patterns and fetal acid-base balance in low birth weight infants with respiratory distress syndrome. *Obstet Gynecol.* 1972;39:83.
11. Chan WH, Paul R, Toews J. Intrapartum fetal monitoring, maternal and fetal morbidity and perinatal mortality. *Obstet Gynecol.* 1973;41:7–13.
12. Tutera G, Newman RL. Fetal monitoring: its effect on the perinatal mortality and cesarean section rates and its complications. *Am J Obstet Gynecol.* 1975;122:750–754.
13. Paul RH, Huey JR, Yaeger CF. Clinical fetal heart rate monitoring—its effect on cesarean section rate and perinatal mortality: five year trends. *Postgrad Med.* 1977;61:160–166.
14. Lee WK, Baggish MS. The effect of unselected intrapartum fetal monitoring. *Obstet Gynecol.* 1976;47:516–520.
15. Alfirevic Z, Devane D, Gyte GM. Continuous cardiotocography (CTG) as a form of electronic fetal monitoring (EFM) during labour. *Cochrane Database Syst Rev.* 2006;(3):CD006066. DOI: 10.1002/14651858.CD006066.
16. Lees MH, Hill JD, Ochsner AJ III, et al. Maternal and placental myometrial blood flow of the rhesus monkey during uterine contractions. *Am J Obstet Gynecol.* 1971;110:68–81.
17. Poseiro JJ, Mendez-Bauer C, Pose SV, et al. Effect of uterine contractions on maternal blood flow through the placenta. In: *Perinatal factors affecting human development. Scientific Publication 185.* Washington: Pan American Health Organization, 1969:161.
18. Druzen M, Ikenoue T, Murata Y, et al. A possible mechanism for the increase in FHR variability following hypoxemia. Paper presented at: The 26th Annual Meeting of the Society for Gynecologic Investigation; March 23, 1979; San Diego, CA.
19. Hammacher K. In: Kaser O, Friedberg V, Oberk K, eds. *Gynakologie v Gerburtshilfe. Bd II.* Stuttgart: Georg Thieme Verlag, 1967.
20. Dalton KJ, Dawes GS, Patrick JE. The autonomic system and fetal heart rate variability. *Am J Obstet Gynecol.* 1983;146:456–462.
21. American College of Obstetricians and Gynecologists (ACOG). *Intrapartum fetal heart rate monitoring: nomenclature, interpretation, and general management principles.* Washington, DC: American College of Obstetricians and Gynecologists (ACOG), 2009 Jul. 11 p. (ACOG practice bulletin; no. 106).
22. Electronic fetal heart rate monitoring: research guidelines for interpretation. National Institute of Child and Human Development Research Planning Workshop. *Am J Obstet Gynecol.* 1997;177:1385–1390.
23. Piaquadio K, Moore TM. A prospective evaluation of fetal movement screening to decrease the incidence of antepartum fetal death. *Am J Obstet Gynecol.* 1989;160:1075.
24. Nwosu CE, Welch CR, Manasse PR, et al. Longitudinal assessment of amniotic fluid index. *Br J Obstet Gynecol.* 1993;100:816–819.
25. Miyazaki F, Nevarez F. Saline amnioinfusion for relief of repetitive variable decelerations: a prospective randomized study. *Am J Obstet Gynecol.* 1985;153:301–306.
26. Greiss FC Jr, Crandell DL. Therapy for hypotension induced by spinal anesthesia during pregnancy. *JAMA.* 1965;191:793–796.

27. Nageotte MP, Towers CV, Asrat T, et al. The value of a negative antepartum test: contraction stress test and modified biophysical profile. *Obstet Gynecol.* 1994;84:231–234.
28. Williams KP, Galerneau F. Intrapartum fetal heart rate patterns in the prediction of neonatal acidemia. *Am J Obstet Gynecol.* 2003;188(3):820–823.
29. McDonald D, Grant A, Sheridan-Pereira M, et al. The Dublin randomized control trial of intrapartum fetal heart rate monitoring. *Am J Obstet Gynecol.* 1985;152:524.
30. Haverkamp AD, Thompson HE, McFee JG, et al. The evaluation of continuous fetal heart rate monitoring in high risk pregnancy. *Am J Obstet Gynecol.* 1976;125:310.
31. Luttkus AK, Norén H, Stupin JH, et al. Fetal scalp pH and ST analysis of the fetal ECG as an adjunct to CTG. A multi-center, observational study. *J Perinat Med.* 2004;32:486–494.
32. Neilsen J. Fetal electrocardiogram (ECG) for fetal monitoring during labor. *Cochrane Database Sys Rev.* 2006(3).
33. Clark S, Gimovsky M, Miller F. Fetal heart rate response to fetal scalp blood sampling. *Am J Obstet Gynecol.* 1982;144:706.
34. Garite TJ, Dildy GA, McNamara H, et al. A multicenter controlled trial of fetal pulse oximetry in the intra-partum management of non-reassuring fetal heart rate patterns. *AJOG.* 2000;183(5):1049–1058.
35. Klauser CK, Christensen EE, Chauhan SP, et al. Use of fetal pulse oximetry among high-risk women in labor: a randomized clinical trial. *Am J Obstet Gynecol.* 2005;192:1810–1819.

PART V

Fetal Complications

33 Fetal Growth Abnormalities

Carri R. Warshak and Todd Fontenot

KEY POINTS

- Aberrations of fetal growth increase the risk of fetal and neonatal morbidity and mortality.
- Maternal comorbidities such as obesity, diabetes, hypertension, and other vascular diseases predispose to complications from fetal growth abnormalities. Comprehensive management of these conditions may prevent perinatal complications.
- Women at risk for growth abnormalities should be screened with sonographic evaluation of fetal growth and well-being and other fetal surveillance as appropriate. Delivery management may be dramatically influenced by fetal growth abnormalities.

INTRAUTERINE GROWTH RESTRICTION

Background

Definitions
- The most commonly used definition for intrauterine growth restriction (IUGR) in the United States is an estimated fetal weight less than the 10th percentile (1,2). Fetuses with lagging abdominal circumference are deemed "at risk" and should be followed closely for development of IUGR.
- Estimation of fetal weight is heavily influenced by parental race, fetal gender, genetic influences, maternal body mass index (BMI), and altitude (2,3).
- Many fetuses with estimated weights less than the 10th percentile, or with small abdominal circumferences, are constitutionally small, and it is often challenging to differentiate the growth-restricted fetus from the constitutionally small fetus that is meeting its growth potential.

Etiology and Pathophysiology

- Fetal life is a period characterized by phases of rapid cell proliferation and differentiation (1). IUGR is the result of disruption of this normally proliferative state. IUGR may be symmetrical if the disruption occurs early and globally within the fetus or asymmetrical when the insult occurs later in gestation and preferentially impairs growth of the fetal abdominal circumference. Different etiologic mechanisms lead to varying degrees and patterns of growth restriction.
- Pathologic findings on placental examination are the hallmark for the diagnosis of true IUGR versus a constitutionally small fetus. However, for obvious reasons, this

information is not available to the clinician to aid in the management of the pregnancy. Placental abnormalities associated with IUGR include decreased placental weight, decidual necrosis, and infarction. Histologic changes in placental villi including hypermaturity, villus edema, and infarction are characteristic of placental insufficiency and resultant fetal hypoxia. Massive intervillus fibrin deposition, or "maternal floor infarction," is a lesion of particular importance because it is associated with high rates of severe fetal compromise and stillbirth and tends to be recurrent with future pregnancies (3).

- Maternal, placental, and fetal factors may lead to the development of IUGR. Maternal factors are as follows:
  - Medical comorbidities: including chronic hypertension, pregestational diabetes, lupus, cardiovascular disease, thyroid dysfunction, nephrotic syndrome, hemoglobinopathies, antiphospholipid antibody syndrome, severe pulmonary conditions, and severe nutritional deficiencies.
  - Medications used to treat comorbidities may increase the risk of IUGR:
    - Antiepileptics
    - Warfarin
    - Folic acid antagonists
    - Possibly beta-blockers
  - High doses of radiation have been shown to cause symmetrical growth restriction.
  - Social habits:
    - Tobacco use
    - Excessive alcohol intake
  - Cocaine/amphetamine exposures and other drug exposures.
  - Severe maternal nutrition deficiencies.
    - In the adequately nourished woman, regardless of weight, minimal weight gain and even weight loss are unlikely to cause IUGR.
    - Women with severe nutritional deficiencies secondary to poor resources, extremely poor diet, or conditions such as severe hyperemesis gravidarum are at risk for IUGR.
- Obstetrical complications predispose a pregnancy to an increased risk of IUGR.
  - Preeclampsia
    - Both placental vascular changes and a contracted maternal intravascular volume contribute to restriction in fetal growth.
  - Multiple gestation
    - As many as 30% of twin pregnancies may have IUGR in one or both twins. This is especially true in monochorionic twins and specifically in the setting of twin–twin transfusion syndrome (4).
  - Recurrent bleeding
  - Preterm premature rupture of membranes
- Placental abnormalities that have been associated with an increased risk of IUGR:
  - Placenta previa
  - Subchorionic hemorrhage
  - Partial/chronic abruption
  - Aberrant cord insertions
- Fetal factors.
  - Fetal karyotype abnormalities, such as trisomy 21, trisomy 18, trisomy 13, and triploidy, commonly have significant IUGR.
  - Major fetal malformations are often associated with poor fetal growth.
    - Abdominal wall defects, skeletal dysplasias, and others interfere with the ability to accurately estimate fetal weight using ultrasound and may not be associated with true growth restriction.
    - Neural tube defects, heart defects, or fetal tumors may be associated with growth restriction both because of increased demand on the fetal cardiovascular system and because of association as part of a fetal syndrome associated with IUGR.

- Congenital infections are relatively uncommon causes of growth restriction but should be considered especially when other markers for congenital infection are present.
  - Viral infections such as cytomegalovirus, parvovirus, rubella, and HSV are associated with IUGR.
  - Protozoan parasites such as Toxoplasma gondii have also been shown to cause IUGR.

Fetal Adaptation
- The fetus with growth restriction secondary to uteroplacental insufficiency with hypoxia adapts to its environment by a variety of mechanisms.
- Fetal metabolism is shifted toward anaerobic metabolism, producing lactic acid and altering the acid–base status of the fetus.
- Compensatory polycythemia to improve oxygen delivery to tissues that when pronounced may paradoxically decrease tissue perfusion.
- Cardiovascular changes that redirect blood flow to vital organs such as the fetal brain, heart, and adrenal glands develop and offer an opportunity to quantitate the degree of fetal impairment.
- Decrease in fetal urine output as blood is shunted from the fetal kidneys, leading to a consequent decreased amniotic fluid volume.
- Ultimately, the fetus adapts to the hypoxic, hypoglycemic environment by conserving energy, and behavioral changes, as measured by the nonstress test and biophysical profile, become evident.

Evaluation
- **History**
  - A detailed history can help to identify patients at risk for IUGR such that more aggressive surveillance is undertaken. In addition, information gained from a detailed history can help direct the diagnostic evaluation when a fetus with IUGR is discovered.
- **Physical exam**
  - The fundal height measurement is considered the primary method of screening for IUGR in the general obstetric population. Although it is nonspecific and poorly sensitive, it remains the most common method for screening for IUGR in low-risk patients (2).
  - Assessing maternal weight gain is not a sensitive or specific method for the detection of IUGR.
  - When IUGR is identified, a detailed exam for signs of preeclampsia and other medical comorbidities is useful.
- **Ultrasound**
  - Ultrasound is the primary diagnostic tool for the evaluation of IUGR.
    - Equations that use abdominal circumference, biparietal diameter, and femur length have been shown to be the most accurate at estimating the fetal weight (4,5).
    - While both first-trimester biometry and second-trimester biometry have been used to predict subsequent small for gestational age (SGA) neonates, second-trimester biometry appears to be superior (6).
    - Accurate pregnancy dating is a prerequisite to the ability to accurately diagnose IUGR.
    - Customized growth curves may lower the false-positive rate of biometry for the prediction of true growth restriction, although such curves are variably used (7,8).
  - The finding of IUGR on ultrasound should prompt a detailed evaluation of fetal anatomy, quantification of the amniotic fluid volume, and performance of umbilical artery Doppler studies. In appropriately aged fetuses, additional measures of fetal well-being such as a biophysical profile or nonstress test can provide meaningful information regarding the overall status of the fetus.
  - In fetuses found to have IUGR who remain undelivered, serial ultrasounds at intervals of at least every 2–4 weeks should be considered. In the specific setting of preeclampsia, more regular measurements of the fetus may be indicated, but it is not generally

recommended to repeat biometry at intervals less than 2 weeks given the inherent error range of biometric measurements.

- **Laboratory**
  - When IUGR is diagnosed in the midtrimester, consideration for karyotype analysis should be undertaken, particularly if there are associated fetal malformations. Genetic amniocentesis has traditionally been recommended to evaluate for aneuploidy in high-risk patients. In patients at moderate or low risk who wish to avoid an invasive procedure, there may be a role for newer cell-free fetal DNA aneuploidy screening. Although ffDNA is useful for the detection of certain karyotype abnormalities, it is not able to detect a wide range of less common karyotype abnormalities, such as triploidy, trisomies of chromosomes other than 21,13, and 18 and partial deletions/duplications/inversions that would be diagnosable with traditional amniocentesis and karyotype analysis via cell culture.
  - Infectious causes for IUGR are relatively uncommon. Maternal serology and/or amniotic fluid evaluation with microbial culture and polymerase chain reaction (PCR) testing should be considered in cases of midtrimester onset IUGR or when ultrasound findings suggestive of congenital infection are present.
  - Thrombophilias.
    - Inherited thrombophilias do not appear to be associated with IUGR (9).
    - Acquired thrombophilia as part of the antiphospholipid syndrome does appear to be associated with IUGR, particularly when there is severe IUGR and/or preeclampsia occurring prior to 34 weeks. In this subset of patients testing for lupus anticoagulant, anticardiolipin antibodies and anti–β2-glycoprotein I should be considered (10).
  - Several biomarkers have been associated with IUGR such as maternal serum α-fetoprotein, endothelin 1, leptin, placental growth factor, urinary S100B, insulin-like growth factors, myoinositol, and D-chiro-inositol (1). At the current time, there are no markers available for diagnostic purposes in the clinical setting of suspected IUGR.

MANAGEMENT
Fetal Surveillance
- Fetal kick counting.
  - It is an important daily measure of fetal well-being and should be instituted both in the uncomplicated pregnancy and the pregnancy complicated by IUGR.
  - Various methods of measurement are available, and none are known to be superior.
- A variety of antenatal testing options are available to assist in the surveillance of the preterm fetus in pregnancies complicated by IUGR.
  - The fetal nonstress test, biophysical profile, amniotic fluid volume measurements, and Doppler velocimetry have all been found to be useful in this context.
  - In the setting of IUGR, decreased amniotic fluid volume (in particular, the absence of a 2-cm pocket of amniotic fluid) has been shown to be associated with significant increase in the risk of stillbirth.
  - Doppler velocimetry has been shown to be a useful adjunct in predicting perinatal outcomes. Normal results are associated with reduced perinatal mortality in this setting (11–13).
  - The optimal frequency of testing is unclear, although testing twice per week appears to lower the risk of stillbirth as compared to once per week (14).

Treatments
- Aspirin.
  - Aspirin may have a role in prevention of recurrent IUGR, especially in women with thrombophilia or in those that have pregnancies complicated by preeclampsia (15).
  - There is little support that aspirin started after the development of IUGR influences further growth or improves perinatal outcomes.
- Additional nutritional supplementation, high protein diets, zinc supplementation, calcium supplementation, heparin, maternal oxygen therapy, maternal bed rest, and plasma

volume expansion have been studied as potential therapies for IUGR; however, none has been conclusively shown to improve fetal growth or reduce perinatal morbidities or mortality and may come with considerable maternal risk. It is recommended these interventions be considered only in experimental protocols (2). In the setting of maternal hypertensive disease related to chronic hypertension or preeclampsia, bed rest may improve hypertension and prolong latency to delivery.

Delivery Management
- Preterm IUGR
  - When patients have significant IUGR and delivery is likely to be indicated prior to 34 weeks, consideration for a course of glucocorticoids is warranted (2). This is especially true when significant Doppler abnormalities, such as absent end-diastolic flow or reversal of end-diastolic flow, are present or, in the setting of preeclampsia, remote from term.
  - Timing of delivery in the preterm fetus found to have IUGR is a complex decision requiring consideration of both risks of prematurity and risks of pregnancy prolongation. The Growth Restriction Intervention Trial (GRIT) randomized women with IUGR to delivery versus expectant management (14,16). These investigators found similar perinatal mortality between groups, with higher stillbirth rate in the delayed delivery group as compared to higher neonatal mortality rate in the group immediately delivered. Two-year follow-up of development in survivors was also comparable (14). However, in the group immediately delivered prior to 31 weeks, a higher rate of morbidity and disability was seen (13% vs. 5% in those expectantly managed). Of note, the mean latency for the expectantly managed group was only 4.9 days and 3.2 days if IUGR was diagnosed at less than 32 weeks, which may explain their similar outcomes.
- Term IUGR
  - Management options for the IUGR fetus at term have also been studied. The DIGITAT Study Group randomized fetuses with IUGR beyond 36 0/7 weeks to induction versus expectant management (17). Fetuses expectantly managed were delivered an average 10 days later and were slightly larger; however, there was no difference in the composite adverse neonatal outcome. In addition, there was a similar rate of cesarean section in both groups. Thus, these authors concluded induction did not appear to increase maternal morbidity and cesarean rate; however, there were not significantly increased adverse fetal outcomes with expectant management, and induction may prevent possible neonatal morbidity and stillbirth.

Prognosis
- The fetuses with IUGR have higher rates of fetal and neonatal complications. Rates of stillbirth are significantly elevated and, in the setting of reversal of end-diastolic flow in umbilical artery Doppler, may be as high as 20%. Conversely, evidence of growth restriction is found in 23% to 65% of stillbirths (13,18). A recent cohort study of all births in the United States in 2005 demonstrated that the risk for IUFD was 58, 43.9, and 26.3 per 10,000 at-risk fetuses at the less than 3rd, less than 5th, and less than 10th percentiles, respectively (19). Other perinatal morbidities include hypoxia, acidemia, polycythemia, hyperbilirubinemia, hypoglycemia, seizures, sepsis, need for ventilation, and hypothermia (13,20,21). Ultimately, these complications lead to an increased risk of long-term neurologic sequelae and increased risk of developmental delay (20).
- Efforts to understand "perinatal programming" have greatly expanded (1). It is becoming increasingly clear that intrauterine environmental factors alter the development of organs and tissues in the fetus, leading to susceptibility to childhood and adult disease. Ischemic heart disease, hypertension, cardiovascular disease, obesity, and diabetes have all been demonstrated to be associated with a hypoxic, hypoglycemic intrauterine environment (20). No longer does the concept of "correction" by delivery or "catch-up" in neonatal life appear to be the resolution of IUGR, but in fact, there appear to be long-standing medical effects on the health of the child persistent even into adulthood.

Prevention

- When IUGR is caused by modifiable maternal risk factors such as tobacco use, alcohol intake, and potentially medication exposures, patients should be encouraged to reduce or eliminate these exposures to improve perinatal outcome. Smoking cessation programs are associated with a 6% increase in smoking cessation and a 19% reduction in low birth weight and perinatal morbidity and mortality (20).
- Optimization of maternal health when concurrent maternal medical comorbidities are thought to be the underlying etiology for the IUGR can reduce the risk for an SGA fetus. In particular, in patients with severe hypertension, SGA can be prevented with aggressive antihypertensive therapy (22). When IUGR occurs in the setting of preeclampsia and maternal obesity, interpregnancy weight loss has been demonstrated to reduce the recurrence risk of preeclampsia (23,24).
- Aspirin for the prevention of preeclampsia and IUGR is controversial. Despite dozens of trials, a conclusive improvement in outcomes eludes researchers. However, a Cochrane meta-analysis demonstrated a 10% reduction in SGA when aspirin is started early in pregnancy to prevent IUGR (15). Other studies have similarly demonstrated reduction in IUGR when aspirin is initiated early in pregnancy in women at risk for preeclampsia and IUGR (25). Finally, initiation of aspirin therapy when abnormal uterine artery Doppler studies early in pregnancy predict the likely development of IUGR and/or preeclampsia has shown a significant reduction in IUGR (20).
- Worldwide, malaria is a major causative factor for IUGR, and prevention of malaria could greatly impact the rate of this pregnancy complication (20).

MACROSOMIA

Background

Definitions

- Fetal macrosomia is a categorical definition used to describe fetuses with an estimated or actual weight above a predefined cutoff. Most consider a fetal weight above 4000 or 4500 g to be macrosomic, with weights above 4500 g being the most commonly used definition (26).
- A similar term, large for gestational age (LGA), is used to describe the fetal weight in relation to the gestational age of the fetus, and in general, weights above the 90th percentile are considered LGA (26).
- Macrosomia leads to maternal and fetal morbidity. Macrosomia is associated with a near doubling of the risk for cesarean section (27). In addition, maternal pelvic floor injury may be related to delivery of the macrosomic fetus (28). Fetal complications include neonatal intensive care unit (NICU) admission, hypoglycemia, shoulder dystocia, brachial plexus injury, and Erb palsy (27,29–31).

Etiology and Pathophysiology

- Incorrect dating can falsely identify a fetus as LGA. Therefore, when a fetus is found to be measuring ahead of the clinical dating, reexamination of the accuracy of gestational dating should be undertaken.
- Maternal comorbidities such as diabetes and obesity are the most commonly identified causes for fetal macrosomia. Maternal BMI greater than 30 has been found to double the rate of fetal macrosomia (27). Gestational diabetes not only increases the risk of fetal macrosomia but also increases the risk of morbidity in fetuses with macrosomia when compared to nondiabetics (29,32).
- Maternal and paternal genetic factors play a role in the predetermination of the fetal size, and therefore, the fetal size appears to be an interplay between genetic predetermination and intrauterine environmental influences.

- Fetal factors can also contribute to fetal size. Male gender has consistently been associated with increased fetal size. Fetal anomalies such as intra-abdominal masses, bladder outlet obstruction, severe ventriculomegaly, and hydrops can also lead to an increased fetal size. Rarely, genetic syndromes, such as Beckwith-Wiedemann or Pallister-Killian syndrome, cause a fetus to grow abnormally large. The prognosis for the fetus in these settings is determined by the underlying causative factor rather than the absolute fetal size.

Evaluation
Risk Factors
- Maternal diabetes.
  - Most important risk factor for the development of fetal macrosomia secondary to both its impact on the rate of fetal macrosomia and its influence on the occurrence of complications in the setting of fetal macrosomia.
  - Even in women who do not meet the classic criteria for gestational diabetes, increasing insulin resistance has been found to increase the rate of LGA (26,33).
- Nondiabetic patients may have additional risk factors for the development of macrosomia:
  - Prior history of macrosomia
  - High maternal prepregnancy weight
  - Male fetus
  - Gestational age greater than 40 weeks
  - Ethnicity
  - LGA maternal birth weight
  - Tall maternal stature
  - Maternal age younger than 17 years
  - Positive glucose screen with a negative glucose tolerance test (26,34)
- Excessive maternal weight gain has also been associated with the development of fetal macrosomia, especially in the obese pregnant woman (35,36).

Diagnosis
Physical Exam
- Fundal height measurement is used as a general screening tool for assessing fetal growth abnormalities. Near delivery, Leopold maneuvers can be used to roughly estimate the fetal size, but are imprecise. Obesity is a major hindrance to the performance of both of these measurements, in addition to being a major risk factor for the development of macrosomia. For these reasons, ultrasound estimation of fetal weight is performed in women at risk for macrosomia or with suspected macrosomia.

Ultrasound
- Ultrasound estimation of fetal weight using biometric measures such as the head circumference, biparietal diameter, abdominal circumference, and femur length is commonly used to evaluate for fetal macrosomia.
- Sonographic estimation of fetal weight has a considerable error range, which increases with fetal size. It is likely that high maternal BMI also influences the accuracy of ultrasound-obtained estimations of fetal weight.
- Measurements of subcutaneous fat in various fetal anatomical landmarks have been found to correlate with postnatal adiposity, but not necessarily with greater accuracy in the prediction of estimated fetal weight from standard ultrasound biometry (37).

Laboratory Testing
- Cord blood serum C-peptide is a biomarker that correlates with LGA; however, it has limited clinical utility for diagnostic or management purposes (33).
- Maternal testing for gestational diabetes should be performed or repeated as indicated when the fetus is found to be LGA or macrosomic.

Treatment

Medical Management

- Among patients with diabetes, optimizing maternal glycemic control remains one of the cornerstones in prevention of macrosomia. Aggressive glycemic profiling and management with oral hypoglycemic agents or insulin is recommended.
- Maternal nutritional counseling may prevent excessive maternal weight gain, especially in the obese woman, and reduce the risk of macrosomia. However, studies evaluating this as a therapeutic option to prevent macrosomia are limited (26).

Fetal Surveillance

- The finding of fetal macrosomia alone is not necessarily an indication for antenatal fetal surveillance. However, comorbidities such as maternal diabetes, obesity, postterm pregnancy, and polyhydramnios often prompt initiation into an antenatal fetal surveillance program.

Delivery Management

- Induction of labor appears to increase the rate of cesarean delivery, without a reduction in neonatal morbidity (26,38). Therefore, early induction because of suspected macrosomia cannot be recommended.
- Although cesarean delivery may reduce the risk of shoulder dystocia and fetal morbidity from a traumatic vaginal delivery, this must be weighed against the increased maternal risks of cesarean delivery with both the current pregnancy and future pregnancies. There are no prospective trials that support reductions in fetal injury with altering mode of delivery among nondiabetic patients with suspected macrosomia.
- There are no specific recommendations for the weight at which elective cesarean section should be considered. In general, most experts consider cesarean delivery in diabetic women with estimations of fetal weight beyond 4250 to 4500. In nondiabetics, it is likely that benefits to elective cesarean section are only seen if estimations of fetal weight beyond 5000 g are used to recommend cesarean delivery.
- When fetal macrosomia is suspected, it is recommended to avoid operative vaginal deliveries as this may increase the risk of shoulder dystocia and traumatic delivery.

Prognosis

- Macrosomic fetuses have higher rates of many morbidities and even mortality. In women with diabetes, a birth weight over 4000 g has been shown to increase risks of hypoglycemia, respiratory distress syndrome, shoulder dystocia, and Erb palsy (29). The risk of brachial plexus injury is directly related to fetal weight and has been found to be 2.86% in fetuses weighing over 5000 g (31).

Prevention

- Optimization of maternal health prior to conception may reduce both prepregnancy weight and occurrence of diabetes and therefore decrease risk of complications from macrosomia.
- Strict glycemic control in women found to be diabetic early in pregnancy before the development of fetal macrosomia is likely to reduce complications from fetal macrosomia.

REFERENCES

1. Dessi A, Ottonello G, Fanos V. Physiopathology of intrauterine growth retardation: from classic data to metabolomics. *J Matern Fetal Neonatal Med.* 2012;25(S5):13–18.
2. ACOG Practice Bulletin Number 134. Intrauterine growth restriction. *Obstet Gynecol.* 2013;121(5):1122–1133.
3. Tyson RW, Staat BC. The intrauterine growth-restricted fetus and placental evaluation. *Semin Perinatol.* 2008;32(3):166–171.
4. Resnik R. Intrauterine Growth Restriction. *Obstet Gynecol.* 2002;99(3):490–496.
5. Guidetti DA, Divon MY, Braverman JJ, et al. Sonographic estimates of fetal weight in the intrauterine growth retardation population. *Am J Perinatol.* 1990;7:5–7.

6. Tuuli MG, Cahill A, Stamilio D, et al. Comparative efficacy of measures of early fetal growth restriction for predicting adverse perinatal outcomes. *Obstet Gynecol.* 2011;117(6):1331–1340.

7. Mongelli M, Gardosi J. Reduction of false-positive diagnosis of fetal growth restriction by application of customized fetal growth standards. *Obstet Gynecol.* 1996;88(5): 844–848.

8. Bukowski R, Uchida T, Smith GSC, et al. Individualized norms of optimal fetal growth: fetal growth potential. *Obstet Gynecol.* 2008;111(5):1065–1076.

9. Facco F, You W, Grobman W. Genetic thrombophilias and intrauterine growth restriction: a meta-analysis. *Obstet Gynecol.* 2009;113(6):1206–1209.

10. Committee on Practice Bulletins—Obstetrics, American College of Obstetricians and Gynecologists. ACOG Practice Bulletin No. 132. Antiphospholipid Syndrome. *Obstet Gynecol.* 2012;120(6):1514–1521.

11. Berkley E, Chauhan SP, Abuhamad A; Society for Maternal-Fetal Medicine Publications Committee. Doppler assessment of the fetus with intrauterine growth restriction. *Am J Obstet Gynecol.* 2012;206(4):300.

12. Alfirevic Z, Stampalija T, Gyte GM. Fetal and umbilical Doppler ultrasound in high-risk pregnancies. *Cochrane Database Syst Rev.* 2010;(1):CD007529.

13. Thompson JL, Kuller JA, Rhee EH. Antenatal surveillance of fetal growth restriction. *Obstet Gynecol Surv.* 2012;67(9):554–565.

14. Thornton JG, Hornbuckle J, Vail A, et al.; GRIT study group. Infant well-being at 2 years of age in the Growth Restriction Intervention Trial (GRIT): multicentered randomized controlled trial. *Lancet.* 2004;364(9433):513–520.

15. Duley L, Henderson-Smart DJ, Meher S, et al. Antiplatelet agents for preventing pre-eclampsia and its complications. *Cochrane Database Syst Rev.* 2007;98:253.

16. The GRIT Study Group. A randomized trial of timed delivery for the compromised preterm fetus: short term outcomes and Bayesian interpretation. *BJOG.* 2003;110:27–32.

17. The DIGITAT Study Group. Induction versus expectant monitoring for intrauterine growth restriction at term: randomized equivalence trial (DIGITAT). *BMJ.* 2010;341:c7087.

18. Morrison I, Olsen J. Weight-specific stillbirths and associated causes of death: an analysis of 765 stillbirths. *Am J Obstet Gynecol.* 1985;152:975–980.

19. Pilliod RA, Cheng YW, Snowden JM, et al. The risk of intrauterine fetal death in the small-for-gestational-age fetus. *Am J Obstet Gynecol.* 2012;207(4):318.

20. Bergella V. Prevention of recurrent fetal growth restriction. *Obstet Gynecol.* 2007;110(4): 904–912.

21. McIntire DD, Bloom SL, Casey BM, et al. Birth weight in relation to morbidity and mortality among newborn infants. *N Engl J Med.* 1999;340:1234–1238.

22. Abalos E, Duley L, Steyn DW, et al. Antihypertensive drug therapy for mild to moderate hypertension during pregnancy. *Cochrane Database Syst Rev.* 2007;(1):CD002252.

23. Mostello D, Jen Chang J, Allen J, et al. Recurrent preeclampsia: the effect of weight change between pregnancies. *Obstet Gynecol.* 2010;116:677.

24. Maggard MA, Yermilov I, Li Z, et al. Pregnancy and fertility following bariatric surgery: a systematic review. *JAMA.* 2008;300:2286.

25. Bujold E, Roberge S, Lacasse Y, et al. Prevention of preeclampsia and intrauterine growth restriction with aspirin started early in pregnancy: a meta-analysis. *Obstet Gynecol.* 2010;116(2):402–413.

26. American College of Obstetricians and Gynecologists. ACOG Practice Bulletin 22. Fetal Macrosomia. *Obstet Gynecol.* 2000;96(5):1–12.

27. Ju H, Chadha Y, Donovan T, et al. Fetal macrosomia and pregnancy outcomes. *Aust N Z J Obstet Gynaecol.* 2009;49(5):504–672.

28. King JR, Korst LM, Miller DA, et al. Increased composite maternal and neonatal morbidity associated with ultrasonographically suspected fetal macrosomia. *J Matern Fetal Neonatal Med.* 2012;25(10):1953–1959.

29. Esakoff TF, Cheng YW, Sparks TN, et al. The association between birthweight 4000 gm or greater and perinatal outcomes in patients with and without gestational diabetes mellitus. *Am J Obstet Gynecol.* 2009;200(6):672.

30. Bjorstad AR, Irgens-Hansen K, Daltveit AK, et al. Macrosomia: mode of delivery and pregnancy outcome. *Acta Obstet Gynecol Scand.* 2010;89(5):664–669.

31. Raio L, Ghezzi F, Di Naro E, et al. Perinatal outcome of fetuses with a birthweight greater than 4500 gm; an analysis of 3356 cases. *Eur J Obstet Gynecol Reprod Biol.* 2003;109(2):160–165.

32. Gross SJ, West DJ, Scardo JA, et al. Antepartum detection of macrosomic fetus: clinical versus sonographic, including soft-tissue measurements. *Obstet Gynecol.* 2000;95:639–642.

33. HAPO Study Cooperative Research Group. Hyperglycemia and adverse pregnancy outcome. *N Engl J Med.* 2008;358:1991–2992.

34. Okun N, Verma A, Mitchell BF, et al. Relative importance of maternal constitutional factors and glucose intolerance of pregnancy in the development of newborn macrosomia. *J Matern Fetal Med.* 1997;6:285–290.

35. Parker JD, Abrams S. Prenatal weight gain advice: an examination of the recent weight gain recommendations of the Institute of Medicine. *Obstet Gynecol.* 1992;79:664–669.

36. Bianco AT, Smilen SW, Davis Y, et al. Pregnancy outcome and weight gain recommendations for the morbidly obese woman. *Obstet Gynecol.* 1998;91:97–102.

37. Chauhan SP, West DJ, Scardo JA, et al. Antepartum detection of macrosomic fetus: clinical versus sonographic, including soft-tissue measurements. *Obstet Gynecol.* 2000;95:639.

38. Gonan O, Rosen DJ, Dolfin Z, et al. Induction of labor versus expectant management in macrosomia: a randomized study. *Obstet Gynecol.* 1997;89:913–917.

Multiple Gestations
John D. Yeast

KEY POINTS
- Prematurity is the greatest risk factor for multiple-gestation pregnancies.
- Monochorionic placentation creates additional risk for either fetus and requires careful surveillance.
- Higher-order multiple gestations also pose significant medical risks for maternal morbidity.

BACKGROUND
Definition
- Incidence with spontaneous ovulation
  - Twin gestation occurs in 15 out of 1000 pregnancies.
    - Monozygotic twin gestation is constant at 3 to 5 in 1000 births.
    - Dizygotic twin incidence varies by population group.
  - Triplet gestation occurs in 3.7 out of 10,000 pregnancies.
    - The frequency of triplets is influenced by the same factors as is that of twins.
  - Higher-order multiple gestation:
    - Incidence is less than 5 out of 1,000,000 pregnancies.
    - Live birth rate is significantly lower.
- Incidence in United States
  - Vital statistics data often do accurately differentiate spontaneous conceptions from assisted reproductive technology (ART).
  - Twin gestation:
    - Thirty-three out of 1000 births are twins (1).
    - There has been a 76% increase in incidence since 1980 (1,2).
    - Thirty-three percent of twins result from fertility therapies (2,3).
  - Triplet gestation and higher-order multiples (triplets/+):
    - Triplets and higher-order multiples accounted for 13.8 out of 10,000 pregnancies in 2010.
    - During the 1980s, the incidence rose greater than 400%. However, since 1995, the incidence has dropped nearly 30% (1,4).
    - Only 7% to 18% of triplets occur spontaneously.
    - Less than 7% of higher-order multiples result from spontaneous ovulation (5).
  - The gradual increase in maternal age over the past 20 years also has had some minor effect on the frequency of multiple-gestation birth.

Pathophysiology
- Zygosity and placentation
  - The outcome of multiple gestations, especially twins, correlates well with placentation and, to a lesser extent, zygosity.
  - The outcome for triplets and higher-order multiples is more influenced by the degree of prematurity.
  - Patterns of placental relationships remain important to siblings in triplets and higher-order multiples due to the possible combinations of zygosity.

- Zygosity
  - Monozygotic twins
    - There is a fixed incidence of 30% of monozygosity in spontaneous twins.
    - Monozygosity can occur in ART twins, especially after intracytoplasmic sperm injection.
  - Dizygotic twins
    - The rate of dizygotic twins is influenced by
      - Maternal age
      - Parity
      - Race and ethnicity
    - There is a 70% incidence of dizygosity in spontaneous twins.
    - There is a greater than 95% incidence of dizygosity in ART twins and higher-order multiples.
- Placentation
  - Monochorionic placenta
    - Derived from single embryo, identical
    - Monochorionic/diamniotic
      - There is a 68% incidence of monochorionic/diamniotic placentation in monozygotic twins.
      - Excess preterm birth and perinatal mortality are observed with a single placenta.
      - The perinatal fetal death rate is as high as 25% (6).
    - Monochorionic/monoamniotic
      - In monozygotic twins, the incidence of monochorionic/monoamniotic placentation is less than 2%.
      - Up to 50% perinatal mortality is reported due to cord entanglement.
  - Dichorionic/diamniotic placenta
    - Dichorionic placentation may occur in either monozygotic or dizygotic twins and higher-order multiples.
    - Dichorionic placentation occurs in monozygotic twins that divide earlier than 3 days after fertilization.
    - There is lower perinatal risk than with monochorionic placentation.
  - Evaluation of the placenta may help determine if same-sex twins are identical.
    - Placentation should always be documented
      - During ultrasound studies
      - In the delivery room
      - In the lab, if necessary
    - Same-sex twins with separate placentas have a monozygotic/dizygotic risk of 1:5 (Table 34-1).

Table 34-1	The Frequency of Placentation in Twin Pregnancies	
Placentation type	**Frequency**
Diamnionic/dichorionic, fused[a]	34.0%
Diamnionic/dichorionic, separate[a]	35.2%
Diamnionic/monochorionic[b]	29.6%
Monoamnionic/monochorionic[b]	1.2%

[a]May be mono- or dizygotic.
[b]Monozygotic only.
Source: Hollenbach KA, Hickok DE. Epidemiology and diagnosis of twin gestation. *Clin Obstet Gynecol*. 1990;33:3–9.

Table 34-2	Perinatal Outcome for Multiple-Gestation Pregnancy		
	Gestation		
Outcome	Singleton	Twins	Triplets
Percent delivering at <37 wk	9.4	50.7	91.0
Percent delivering at <32 wk	1.7	13.9	41.2
Percent SGA	9.4	35.6	36.6
Percent perinatal mortality	0.6	2.6	6.1

SGA, small for gestational age.
Source: Keith LG, Cervantes A, Mazela J, et al. Multiple births and preterm delivery. *Prenat Neonat Med.* 1998;3:125–129; Mathews MS, MacDorman MF. Infant mortality statistics from the 2009 period linked birth/infant death data set. *National Vital Statistics Reports.* 2013;61(8).

Epidemiology
- Of all live births, 3.3% are from multiple gestations.
- Just more than 58% of multiples are also low birth weight.
- Thirteen percent of all preterm births are multiples.
- Over 5% of all infants less than 1500 g are multiples (1).
- The average cost for twin pregnancy and delivery is almost $40,000.
- The average cost for triplets and higher-order multiple pregnancy and delivery exceeds $100,000 per pregnancy (4,7).
- Prematurity is the greatest risk for multiple-gestation pregnancies (Table 34-2). There is a significant increase (vs. singletons) in
  - Neonatal intensive care unit admissions
  - Low birth weight deliveries (8)
  - Perinatal deaths (8)

EVALUATION
Ultrasound Surveillance
Chorionicity
- Chorionicity is best determined by ultrasound in the first trimester or early second trimester (Fig. 34-1).

Monochorionicity
- Single placental bed
- Thin amniotic membrane
- At insertion of amnion into chorion, no increase in thickness

Dichorionicity
- Two separate placental beds or fused placentas with thickened amnion.
- Chorion separates leaves of amnion at insertion in placental bed (twin peak sign).

Fetal Growth
- Multiple-gestation fetuses have a high rate of growth restriction.
- Serial sonographic estimated fetal weights (EFW) are the only method to assure that fetal growth is within normal limits. Ultrasound references for expected twin growth are available.
- Ultrasound studies should be done every 3 to 6 weeks.
- EFW with less than 25% differences are concordant.
- EFW with greater than 25% difference are discordant and warrant more careful attention.

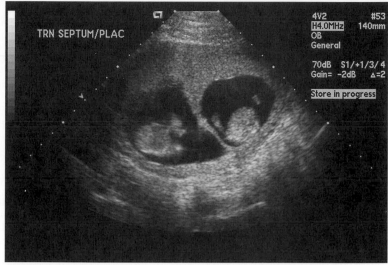

A

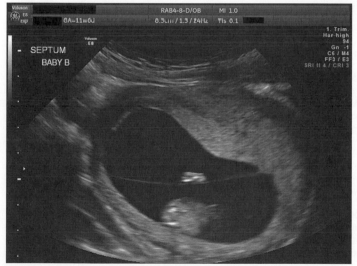

B

Figure 34-1. A: Dichorionic, diamniotic placenta. Note chorion present between leaves of amnion at placenta insertion. **B:** Monochorionic, diamniotic placenta. Note amnion appears thin at insertion without chorion present.

Cervical Length
- Endovaginal ultrasound measurement of the cervix at 22 to 28 weeks may aid in selecting patients at high risk of preterm delivery (9–11).
- Normal cervix with length greater than 3.5 cm is very reassuring.
- Cervical length less than 2.5 cm in an asymptomatic patient may indicate increased risk of spontaneous preterm birth and warrant careful surveillance.
- Cervical length less than 2.5 cm and abnormal examination or symptoms of preterm labor mandate immediate evaluation.

Amniotic Fluid Volume
- The amniotic fluid index (AFI) is the standard method of measuring amniotic fluid volume in singleton pregnancies.
- Reduced AFI may represent chronic placental dysfunction.
- The amniotic fluid volume in twins may be assessed by two different methods:
  - General assessment can be done using the same method as a singleton pregnancy (12).
  - A subjective assessment of fluid volume of each pregnancy can be made with a minimal objective measurement of a 2-cm vertical pocket in each gestational sac beyond 20 weeks' gestational age.
  - Amniotic fluid volume assessment should be performed at every ultrasound study and is recommended every 2 weeks beyond 32 weeks' gestational age.

DIAGNOSIS
Antepartum Surveillance
- In at-risk singleton gestations, antepartum surveillance reduces the risk of stillbirth (13).
- Some centers routinely perform antepartum testing in all multiple gestations.
- An alternative option is to perform antepartum testing in twins only if discordance or other risk factors exist.
- All higher-order multiples require some form of fetal surveillance.

Methods of Surveillance for Fetal Well-Being
- Nonstress tests (NSTs) are most the common tests used. NST is usually recommended twice weekly.
- Biophysical profiles (BPPs) may be used but are more costly and time-consuming than are NSTs. BPPs may be used as the primary antepartum surveillance methodology or may be used as a backup test following nonreactive or technically unsatisfactory NSTs.
- Fetal arterial and venous Doppler studies are a supplemental form of surveillance.
- Amniotic fluid volume should be assessed frequently as a measure of chronic placental function.

Initiation of Surveillance for Fetal Well-Being
- If testing is offered to uncomplicated twin pregnancies, begin at or near 32 weeks' gestational age.
- If additional risk factors are present in a twin gestation, testing may need to be initiated earlier.
- For triplets and higher-order multiple gestations, surveillance should start at 28 weeks' gestational age. Interpretation must take into account gestational age.

Techniques of Surveillance
- Obtaining satisfactory tests in multiple gestations requires staff experienced in such procedures.
- For NST, a combination of ultrasound localization and fetal heart rate monitoring is necessary to assure that all fetuses are correctly identified and tested.
- Interpretation of tests may be modified based on gestational age.

Fetal Movement
- Fetal movement or kick counts are reliable forms of surveillance in singletons.
- Mothers of twins may be able to distinctly differentiate and report movements of each fetus.
- Fetal movement in triplets and beyond cannot be considered a reliable assessment of fetal well-being.

TREATMENT
Antepartum Care
Frequency of Visits
- Frequent second-trimester visits may detect early signs of preterm labor.
  - Establish baseline blood pressure.
  - Establish baseline cervical findings.
  - Teach prematurity prevention skills.
  - Prepare the patient for reduction of activity.
- Twins and triplets.
  - Visits at least every 3 weeks in second trimester
  - Visits weekly by 24 to 26 weeks' gestational age
- Higher-order multiples may require more frequent visits and/or inpatient management.

Diet and Nutrition
- 2700 kcal per day for twin gestation
- 200 to 300 kcal per day for each additional fetus (14)
- Folate supplementation, 1 mg per day
- Iron supplementation, 30 mg per day elemental iron for twins
  - Additional 30 mg per day for triplets and higher-order multiples.
  - High doses iron may necessitate stool softeners.

Maternal Serum Screens for Aneuploidy
- Serum screening programs now have established norms for twin gestation.
- The twin pregnancy can be screened and results compared with normal values.
- Triplets and higher-order multiples cannot reliably be screened with serum programs.
- Targeted fetal DNA aneuploidy screening through maternal blood sampling may be utilized for twin gestations with increased risk of trisomies 21, 18, and 13. This new technology may have lower test accuracy than in singletons, is not currently marketed for higher-order multiple gestations, and does not provide a full karyotype evaluation.
- Patients with multiple gestation and traditional indications for invasive prenatal cytogenetic studies benefit from genetic counseling.
- Risks and benefits of amniocentesis and chorionic villus sampling must be carefully weighed in multiple-gestation pregnancy.

Prematurity Prevention Education
- Education late in the first and early in the second trimester regarding signs and symptoms of preterm labor can be beneficial.
- Instruction in promptly reporting important symptoms can allow early evaluation and treatment of preterm labor. Symptoms include
  - Vaginal spotting of blood
  - Change in vaginal discharge
  - Persistent contractions
- Early education empowers the patient to actively participate in her care.

Physical Activity
- No studies demonstrate a benefit for prophylactic bed rest (15).
- Limiting physical work, hours of ambulation, and environmental stress may be of some value.
- Women pregnant with triplets or higher-order multiples should limit physical activity by 24 to 26 weeks' gestational age and perhaps earlier.

Cervical Evaluation
- Changes in cervical dilation and length are sensitive markers for preterm delivery risk.
- Cervical assessment should begin early in the second trimester and continue at each visit beyond 18 to 20 weeks' gestational age.
- Ultrasound assessment of cervical length may be substituted for digital examination and may be more sensitive.

Screening for Preeclampsia
- Twin gestation carries 3.5 times the risk of preeclampsia versus singleton gestation.
- The risk of preeclampsia in a nulliparous patient with twins is 14 times that of a singleton gestation (16).
- Patients with triplets and higher-order multiples have an extremely high risk of preeclampsia.
- Race and chronic hypertension may further increase these risks.
- Surveillance should be conducted for signs and symptoms of preeclampsia as part of prenatal care.

Excess Maternal Morbidity
- Twin gestations
  - Additive risk of preeclampsia
  - Increased risks associated with tocolysis compared to singletons
- Triplets and higher-order multiple gestations
  - Ninety-eight percent of patients experience at least one maternal complication (17):
    o Preterm labor, 76%
    o Preeclampsia, 27%
      - HELLP syndrome, 9%
      - Eclampsia, 2%
    o Postpartum endometritis, 25%

Intrapartum Care

Twin Gestation
- Vertex/vertex twins (Table 34-3) with reassuring fetal status can be allowed a trial of labor and possible vaginal delivery.
- Nonvertex presentation of the first twin should prompt cesarean delivery as safest mode.
- Vertex/nonvertex twins may be candidates for vaginal delivery if an experienced operator is present (18). Options for delivery of second twin are
- Breech extraction of second twin
- External cephalic version second twin
- Cesarean delivery if operator not experienced in either procedure or per patient preference

Table 34-3	Presentation of Twin Gestation Near Term
Presentation	**Incidence (%)**
Vertex–vertex	40
Vertex–breech	26
Breech–vertex	10
Breech–breech	10
Vertex–transverse	8
Miscellaneous	6

Source: Boggess KA, Chisholm CA. Delivery of the nonvertex second twin: a review of the literature. *Obstet Gynecol Surv.* 1997;52:728–734.

Triplets and Higher-order Multiples
- Inability to monitor all fetuses during labor
- Cesarean safest mode of delivery

Operative Risks with Multiple Gestation
- Anticipate increased blood loss due to uterine distention and increased frequency of uterine atony.
- Blood should be screened and readily available for transfusion in cesarean delivery of multiple-gestation patients in the event of hemorrhage.

COMPLICATIONS
Preterm Delivery
- Twin gestations
  - Fifty percent deliver at less than 37 weeks' gestational age.
  - Fourteen percent deliver at less than 32 weeks' gestational age.
- Higher-order multiples
  - Triplets: 90% deliver at less than 37 weeks' gestational age
  - Quadruplets: 50% deliver at less than 32 weeks' gestational age (19)
- Management of preterm labor (see Chapter 8)
- Multifetal pregnancy reduction
  - Late first-trimester reduction of number of fetuses for triplets and higher-order multiples reduces risk of preterm delivery (19–22).
  - Women with quadruplets and higher order should be offered this option early during counseling.
  - The perinatal benefit of reduction for uncomplicated triplets is controversial.
  - There is no perinatal benefit of reduction for twin gestation.
  - The reduction procedure must be performed by an experienced operator.
- Bed rest
  - The value of bed rest in preventing preterm labor has not been proven.
  - However, bed rest is commonly utilized therapeutic option for
    ○ Management of preterm labor
    ○ Preterm, premature rupture of membranes
    ○ Early cervical dilation
  - Risks include
    ○ Weight loss
    ○ Bone density loss
    ○ Venous thrombosis
    ○ Pulmonary embolus
  - Prolonged bed rest should include
    ○ Dietary supplementation
    ○ Physical therapy
    ○ Antiembolic therapy
- Home health care
  - Home health care may be valuable for assessing maternal and fetal well-being.
  - No clear benefit has been demonstrated for home uterine activity monitoring in preventing preterm delivery (23,24).
  - For higher-order multiples, home monitors should be considered experimental therapy.
- Cerclage
  - Prophylactic cerclage in multiple gestation has not been shown to reduce prematurity rate.
  - Ultrasound indicated cerclage for asymptomatic cervical shortening in twins is not beneficial, may increase the risk of preterm birth, and should be avoided.

- Emergent (or "exam-indicated") cerclage in the second trimester with early cervical dilation may be of benefit.
- Controlled studies assessing the risk and benefits of cerclage in multiple gestations are lacking.
- Fetal fibronectin (fFN)
  - fFN has been shown to help identify patients at high risk of premature delivery (25).
  - It is most useful in patients with contractions with a closed or slightly dilated cervix.
  - Some nonrandomized studies suggest that screening multiple gestations with fFN may help identify patients who require more careful assessment (26,27).
  - The high negative predictive value of fFN test helps to select patients in whom interventions such as tocolysis and bed rest may be avoided.

Monochorionic Twin Gestation
- Monochorionic placentation places fetus at increased risk of morbidity and mortality.
- Twin–twin transfusion syndrome (TTTS; see also Chapter 37, Fetal Therapy)
  - Present in 8% to 10% monochorionic twins.
  - Diagnosis depends upon
    ○ Confirmed monochorionic, diamniotic twins
    ○ Oligohydramnios (less than 2 cm deepest vertical pocket of amniotic fluid [AF]) in one twin
    ○ Polyhydramnios (greater than 8 cm deepest vertical pocket of AF) in second twin
  - Mild cases may resolve without treatment.
  - Overall twin survival 15% to 70% (28).
  - Etiology is unbalanced vascular anastomoses in monochorionic placenta (29).
  - Treatment options for moderate–severe cases include
    ○ Serial amnioreduction (therapeutic amniocentesis) (30–32)
      − Early, aggressive use may reduce risk of fetal loss.
      − Reduces amniotic fluid pressure and may restore balanced vascular flow.
      − Consider when TTTS presents with preterm labor or when AF in larger sac exceeds 15 cm in depth.
    ○ Laser ablation of placental surface anastomoses (28)
      − Complex treatment performed in small number of centers
      − Secondary risks of preterm labor, rupture of membranes, and fetal death
  - Randomized studies have mixed results in regard to optimal treatment; morbidity and mortality remain high with or without treatment. Perinatal consultation recommended (28–34).
- Monochorionic twin gestation should have serial ultrasounds (every 2 weeks) starting at 16 to 18 weeks' gestation to allow early diagnosis of TTTS.
  - Twin reversed arterial perfusion sequence (TRAP)
    ○ Results from proximal arterial–arterial anastomosis.
    ○ Failure of development of perfused twin's heart and upper body.
    ○ Mortality of normal twin exceeds 50%.
    ○ Presumed TRAP diagnosis mandates referral to perinatal center.
    ○ Treatment options include
      − Ligation or coil occlusion of cord flow in acardiac twin
      − Hysterotomy and removal of acardiac twin
  - Monoamniotic twins
    ○ Rare: Occurs in less than 2% of monozygotic twins
    ○ Mortality reported as 50%, although may be less (35)
    ○ Risk of cord entanglement and sudden death of one or both twins
    ○ Intensive fetal surveillance not always successful in preventing loss
    ○ Delivery warranted as soon as combined perinatal–neonatal team feels comfortable with extrauterine outcome

Isolated Fetal Death
- Risk to surviving fetus varies widely based on clinical setting.
  - If monochorionic gestation, determine if findings point to TTS:
    - May require early delivery
    - Intense perinatal surveillance necessary
  - If dichorionic gestation, risk is minimal to surviving twin, especially in first and second trimester (36).
  - Fetal surveillance warranted using ultrasound and electronic fetal monitoring, especially proximate to fetal death.
- In monochorionic gestation, there is a 20% risk of subsequent death to the surviving twin and a 25% risk of central nervous system damage from vascular anastomosis.

PATIENT EDUCATION
- Prematurity prevention skills must be emphasized early in prenatal care
  - Lifestyle changes are necessary as pregnancy progresses.
  - The patient should be aware of signs and symptoms of preterm labor.
  - Patients should be encouraged to call clinicians with concerns and early symptoms.
- If the pregnancy is monochorionic, the physician must emphasize the importance of frequent office visits and frequent ultrasound surveillance.
- Patients should be prepared for likely cesarean delivery and educated and familiarized with the procedure and its risks and benefits.
- In higher-order multiples, the patient must understand maternal risks as well as significant risks of prematurity.
- Consider neonatal consultation and neonatal care unit tours to lessen anxiety over premature delivery.

REFERENCES
1. Martin JA, Hamilton BE, Ventura SJ, et al. Births: final data for 2010. National Vital Statistics Reports. vol 61, no 1. Hyattsville, MD: National Center for Health Statistics, 2012.
2. Corchia C, Mastrioiacovo P, Lanni R, et al. What proportion of multiple births are due to ovulation induction? A register-based study in Italy. *Am J Public Health.* 1996;86:851–854.
3. Kurinczuk JJ, Pemberton R, Binns S, et al. Singleton and twin confinements associated with infertility treatments. *Aust NZ J Obstet Gynaecol.* 1995;35:27–31.
4. Keith LG, Cervantes A, Mazela J, et al. Multiple births and preterm delivery. *Prenat Neonat Med.* 1998;3:125–129.
5. Lipitz S, Seidman DS, Alcalay M, et al. The effect of fertility drugs and in vitro methods on the outcome of 106 triplet pregnancies. *Fertil Steril.* 1993;60:1031–1034.
6. Hollenbach KA, Hickok DE. Epidemiology and diagnosis of twin gestation. *Clin Obstet Gynecol.* 1990;33:3–9.
7. Johnson TJ, Patel AL, Jegier BJ, et al. Cost of morbidities in very low birth weight infants. *J Peds.* 2013;162:243–249.
8. Mathews TJ, MacDorman MF. Infant mortality statistics from the 2009 period linked birth/infant death data set. *National Vital Statistics Reports.* 2013;61(8).
9. Imseis HM, Albert TA, Iams JD. Identifying twin gestations at low risk for preterm birth with a transvaginal ultrasonographic cervical measurement at 24 to 26 weeks' gestation. *Am J Obstet Gynecol.* 1997;177:1149–1155.
10. Crane JM, Van Den Hof M, Armson BA, et al. Transvaginal ultrasound in the prediction of preterm delivery: singleton and twin gestations. *Obstet Gynecol.* 1997;90:357–363.
11. Fuchs I, Tsoi E, Henrich W, et al. Sonographic measurement of cervical length in twin pregnancies in threatened preterm labor. *Ultrasound Obstet Gynecol.* 2004;23:42–45.
12. Porter TF, Dildy GA, Blanchard JR, et al. Normal values for amniotic fluid index during uncomplicated twin pregnancy. *Obstet Gynecol.* 1996;87:699–702.

13. Clark SL, Sabey P, Jolley K. Nonstress testing with acoustic stimulation and amniotic fluid volume assessment: 5973 tests without unexpected fetal death. *Am J Obstet Gynecol.* 1986;155:131–134.

14. Yeast JD. Maternal physiologic adaptation to twin gestation. *Clin Obstet Gynecol.* 1990;33: 3–9.

15. Goldenberg RL, Cliver SP, Bronstein J, et al. Bed rest in pregnancy. *Obstet Gynecol.* 1994;84:131–136.

16. Coonrod DV, Hickok DL, Zhu K, et al. Risk factors for preeclampsia in twin pregnancies: a population-based cohort study. *Obstet Gynecol.* 1995;85:645–650.

17. Malone FD, Kaufman GE, Chelmow D, et al. Maternal morbidity associated with triplet pregnancy. *Am J Perinatol.* 1998;15:73–77.

18. Boggess KA, Chisholm CA. Delivery of the nonvertex second twin: a review of the literature. *Obstet Gynecol Surv.* 1997;52:728–734.

19. Berkowitz RL, Lynch L, Stone J, et al. The current status of multifetal pregnancy reduction. *Am J Obstet Gynecol.* 1996;174:1265–1272.

20. Smith-Levitin M, Kowalik A, Birnholz J, et al. Selective reduction of multifetal pregnancies to twins improves outcome over nonreduced triplet gestations. *Am J Obstet Gynecol.* 1996;175(4PT.1):878–882.

21. Souter I, Goodwin TM. Decision making in multifetal pregnancy reduction for triplets. *Am J Perinatol.* 1998;15:63–71.

22. Blickstein I, Keith LG. The decreased rates of triplet births: temporal trends and biologic speculations. *Am J Obstet Gynecol.* 2005;193:327–331.

23. Dyson DC, Danbe KH, Bamber JA, et al. Monitoring women at risk for preterm labor. *N Engl J Med.* 1998;338:15–29.

24. Colton T, Kayne HL, Zhang Y, et al. A meta-analysis of home uterine activity monitoring. *Am J Obstet Gynecol.* 1995;173:1499–1505.

25. Ascarelli MH, Morrison JC. Use of fetal fibronectin in clinical practice. *Obstet Gynecol Surv.* 1997;52:S1–S12.

26. Goldenberg RL, Mercer BM, Meis PJ, et al. The preterm prediction study: fetal fibronectin testing and spontaneous preterm birth. *Obstet Gynecol.* 1996;87:643–648.

27. McMahon KS, Neerhof MG, Haney EI, et al. Prematurity in multiple gestations: identification of patients who are at low risk. *Am J Obstet Gynecol.* 2002;186:1137–1141.

28. Simpson LI; Society of Maternal Fetal Medicine. Twin-twin transfusion syndrome. *Am J Obstet Gynecol.* 2013;203:3–18.

29. Lewi L, Deprest J, Hecher K. The vascular anastomoses in monochorionic twin pregnancies and their clinical consequences. *Am J Obstet Gynecol.* 2013;208:9–30.

30. Elliott JP, Urig, MA, Clewell WH. Aggressive therapeutic amniocentesis for treatment of twin-twin transfusion syndrome. *Obstet Gynecol.* 1991;77:537–540.

31. Trespidi L, Boschetto C, Caravelli E, et al. Serial amniocentesis in the management of twin-twin transfusion syndrome: when is it valuable? *Fetal Diagn Ther.* 1997;12:15–20.

32. Moise KJ, Dorman K, Lamvu G, et al. A randomized trial of amnioreduction versus septostomy in the treatment of twin-twin transfusion syndrome. *Am J Obstet Gynecol.* 2005;193:701–707.

33. Robyr R, Quarello E, Ville Y. Management of fetofetal transfusion syndrome. *Prenat Diagn.* 2005;25:786–795.

34. Fox C, Kilby M, Khan K. Contemporary treatments for twin-twin transfusion syndrome. *Obstet Gynecol.* 2005;105:1469–1477.

35. Tessen JA, Zlatnik FJ. Monoamniotic twins: a retrospective controlled study. *Obstet Gynecol.* 1991;77:832–834.

36. Carlson NJ, Towers CV. Multiple gestation complicated by the death of one fetus. *Obstet Gynecol.* 1989;73:685–689.

Isoimmunization
James T. Christmas

KEY POINTS
- Rh isoimmunization is the primary cause of hemolytic disease of the newborn, although other "irregular" antigens can also be causative.
- All pregnant women must be screened for the presence of circulating antibodies that can cause fetal hemolysis and neonatal hemolytic disease.
- Pregnancies complicated by isoimmunization require assessment by specialists with the clinical experience and ultrasound skills necessary to manage the disease.
- For women who are Rh negative and not sensitized, Rh immunoglobulin can prevent isoimmunization in most situations.

BACKGROUND
Definition
- Isoimmunization, or maternal blood group immunization, is the development of circulating antibodies by the mother directed against an antigen of fetal origin. Isoimmunization is also referred to as maternal sensitization.
- Isoimmunization in pregnancy primarily involves the Rh system of red blood cell antigens, but it can also involve other, "irregular" antigens.
  - It is a disease of genetic predisposition, as these antigens are inherited.
  - The identification of the rhesus antigen and its relation to hemolytic disease of the newborn was described more than 60 years ago by Landsteiner and Weiner (1) and Levine et al. (2). Their classic works are at the cornerstone of modern immunohematology.
- The evolution of our understanding of the complexities of the Rh blood group system, combined with the development of sensitive screening tests for blood group antibodies, has given us the ability to diagnose and treat this unique disease of pregnancy. Indeed, we now have the capability to both treat and prevent this historically difficult problem.

Pathophysiology
- The pathophysiology of isoimmunization involves the following sequence:
  - Maternal sensitization against a fetal blood group antigen
  - Maternal production of IgG antibodies
  - Transplacental antibody passage to the fetus
  - Antibody-mediated hemolysis in the fetal circulation, resulting in fetal anemia
D Antigen
- In the Fischer-Race nomenclature system, the Rh complex contains three pairs of antigenic determinants (Dd, Cc, Ee). The d allele has never been immunologically identified (there is no specific antiserum).
- The presence of the D antigen determines that the individual is Rh positive. The Rh-positive individual is homozygous for D (i.e., DD) approximately 45% of the time. This results from having inherited a D-containing set of alleles from both parents. The remainder of Rh-positive individuals will be heterozygous for the D allele (Dd). A homozygous partner of an Rh-negative woman can produce only Rh-positive offspring; a heterozygous partner can produce either Rh-positive or Rh-negative offspring with equal

frequency in each pregnancy. Because the *d* allele cannot be identified, zygosity at the *D* locus cannot be known with certainty. However, the *Cc*, *Dd*, and *Ee* alleles are closely linked on chromosome 1, and the statistical likelihood of homo- or heterozygosity can be estimated based on the alleles identified at the *Cc* and *Ee* loci.

- Rh isoimmunization can occur only in the pregnancy with an Rh-positive fetus, and only that fetus or subsequent Rh-positive fetuses will be affected by the maternally produced Rh antibody.
- Although the allelic combination at the *Cc* and *Ee* loci can be used to predict the statistical likelihood of an Rh-positive fetus, recent advances in DNA testing have allowed direct fetal antigen determination for Rh and other blood group antigens from cultured amniocytes or from chorionic villus sampling.
- More recently, evaluation of circulating cell-free DNA in maternal plasma early in pregnancy has been demonstrated to accurately predict fetal RhD antigen status and is now commercially available (3). Accurate identification of fetal antigen status for other antigens still requires DNA testing from cultured amniocytes or chorionic villus sampling.

Atypical Antibodies

- Antibodies directed against antigens c and E, and less commonly against e and C, are associated with the risk of hemolytic disease and are considered "atypical" antibodies. A number of other red blood cell antigens that are not part of the Rh antigen complex are capable of stimulating isoimmunization as well (Table 35-1) and are also considered atypical antigens. Because of the efficacy with which Rh immunoglobulin prophylaxis programs prevent Rh D isoimmunization, hemolytic disease caused by these atypical antigens has become relatively more important.
- The general principles of management of sensitization with atypical antibodies are similar to those applied in the evaluation and treatment of Rh D isoimmunization. In the past, many have felt that atypical antibody titers did not reliably predict the severity of hemolytic disease; more recent studies suggest that management decisions should be made using the same protocol as for Rh D disease (4). As with all isoimmunized patients, referral to a high-risk center for evaluation and management is prudent.

Epidemiology

- The absence of the Rh antigen (Rh negativity) is predominantly a trait of Caucasians, with 15% to 16% of the Caucasian population identified as Rh negative. However, the distribution is not homogeneous. The Basque population of Spain has an incidence of 30% to 32% Rh negativity.
- The frequency of Rh negativity in Asian, Native American, and African populations is low. Approximately 8% of African Americans are Rh negative.
- These population statistics argue that Rh negativity was originally confined to the Basque population and that initially all of the races were Rh positive.

Etiology

- Blood group isoimmunization generally arises from one of two pathogenic incidents:
  - Incompatible blood transfusion
  - Fetal–maternal hemorrhage

Incompatible Blood Transfusion

- Transfusion isoimmunization, although uncommon, is generally related to development of atypical blood group antibodies.
- The majority of atypical antibodies are of little clinical consequence; however, severe hemolytic disease of the fetus and newborn can be related to a few atypical antibodies (Table 35-1).

Table 35-1	Atypical Maternal Blood Group Antibodies and Associated Risk of Fetal–Neonatal Hemolytic Disease
Antibody	**Relative hemolytic disease risk**
C	Common
Kell	Common
E	Common
Fyd	Common
e	Uncommon
C	Uncommon
Ce	Uncommon
Kpa	Uncommon
Kpb	Uncommon
CE	Uncommon
k	Uncommon
s	Uncommon
S	Very rare
U	Very rare
M	Very rare
Fyb	Very rare
N	Very rare
Doa	Very rare
Caa	Very rare
Dia	Very rare
Dib	Very rare
Lua	Very rare
Yta	Very rare
Jka	Very rare
Jkb	Very rare
Lea	None
Leb	None
P	None

Fetal–Maternal Hemorrhage
- Fetal–maternal bleeding is a much more common cause of Rh D isoimmunization than is incompatible blood transfusion, and it is a significant cause of atypical antibody development as well.
- As demonstrated in 1986 by Bowman et al. (5), 75% of pregnancies have some evidence of transplacental hemorrhage during gestation or at delivery. As measured by the sensitive tests developed by Kleihauer et al. (6) in 1957, the amount of fetal blood in the maternal circulation is most frequently less than 0.1 mL.
- Antepartum hemorrhage, gestational hypertension, manual removal of the placenta, cesarean delivery, and external cephalic version are all associated with larger volumes of blood loss and transplacental hemorrhage. Amniocentesis, for genetic or other indications, has also been associated with increased risk of maternal sensitization, particularly if the placenta is traversed during amniocentesis. A 5% to 25% incidence of fetal–maternal hemorrhage has been identified after abortion, both spontaneous and therapeutic.
- Maternal response to the introduction of Rh-positive fetal cells into maternal circulation is a two-step phenomenon.
  - The first, primary Rh immune response is frequently slow and weak in its development. This may be related to the relatively compromised immune response seen in the pregnant patient.

- ○ Immunoglobulin M (IgM) anti-D is often not identified before 8 to 9 weeks after exposure, and as many as 6 months may elapse before this primary response is seen.
- ○ The pregnant patient then frequently switches rapidly to the production of IgG anti-D, which does cross the placenta.
  - ▪ After the establishment of the primary response, a second exposure with a very small inoculum generally produces a rapid and profound increase in IgG anti-D.

Incidence

- Although the likelihood of Rh immunization appears to be dose dependent, a small inoculum may be sufficient to generate immunization. Zipursky and Israels (7) and Woodrow (8) have reported data indicating that 50% of patients would become immunized with an inoculum of 50 to 75 mL of Rh-positive cells.
- The secondary response, after initial immunization has occurred, can be provoked by as little as 0.1 mL of red blood cells.

ABO Incompatibility

- It appears that the risk of Rh immunization is approximately 16% when an Rh-negative woman has her first pregnancy with an ABO-compatible Rh-positive fetus.
  - If the mother is not immunized by the first pregnancy, the risk appears approximately the same for the second pregnancy.
  - Although subsequent pregnancy risks for nonresponding patients decrease, a patient undergoing five Rh-positive ABO-compatible pregnancies has a 50% likelihood of becoming Rh immunized.
- An ancillary consideration is the impact of fetal ABO incompatibility, which confers partial protection, thereby decreasing immunization risks markedly. Woodrow (8) calculated that the risk of Rh immunization after an ABO-incompatible Rh-positive pregnancy is approximately 2%.
- Although fetal–maternal hemorrhage sufficient to cause immunization can occur throughout the pregnancy and delivery process, as many as 2% of Rh-negative women become Rh immunized during otherwise uncomplicated pregnancies between 28 weeks of gestation and delivery (9):
  - This represents 12% of all Rh-negative women who would become Rh immunized as a result of Rh-positive pregnancies.
  - This has led to the recommendation for the administration of Rh immunoglobulin to all unsensitized Rh-negative pregnant women at 28 weeks of gestation.

Risk Factors

- Although the numbers are equivocal, it appears that approximately 2% of women having spontaneous or therapeutic abortions are at risk of becoming Rh immunized.
  - It is suggested that early abortion (6 to 8 weeks) carries a much lower risk than later abortion.
  - This risk increases to 5% after 20 weeks of gestation.
- The diagnosis and management of the Rh-immunized pregnancy depend on the early initial evaluation and identification of patients at risk.
  - A blood sample should be taken from every woman at her first antenatal visit for blood type, Rh blood grouping, and antibody screening.
  - This test should be universal and carried out independent of reported results of prior screening tests.

Paternal Antigen Status

- The Rh status and ABO group of the father of the baby should be determined when the mother is Rh negative. If he is Rh negative, the conceptus should be Rh negative, and the mother should not be at risk for Rh immunization, presuming that he is the biologic father of the baby (Table 35-2).

Table 35-2	Approximate Risk of Rh Isoimmunization	
Partner	**Fetus**	**Risk (%)**
D (−)	D positive	0
D positive, homozygous, ABO compatible	D positive	16
D positive, homozygous, ABO incompatible	D positive, ABO incompatible	2
D positive, heterozygous, ABO compatible	Rh unknown	8
D positive, heterozygous, ABO incompatible	ABO, Rh unknown	3.5

- For atypical antibodies, the patient's history should be reviewed to determine the likely etiology of the immunization (transfusion vs. prior fetal–maternal bleeding). Paternal antigen testing should be performed, and if the father is antigen negative, there is no risk of fetal hemolytic disease, no matter what the maternal antibody titer.
- In the case of uncertain paternity, patients should be made aware of the potential for catastrophic complications should the wrong male be tested as the father of the baby. If there is any uncertainty about paternity, the pregnancy should be treated as having unknown paternal antigen status with presumption of risk for Rh immunization or fetal disease to occur.

Evaluation
- All patients should be evaluated for prior sensitization.
- It is incumbent on the practitioner to follow sensitized pregnancies closely with both maternal and fetal surveillance.

Antibody Titers
- Serial antibody titers are the mainstay of maternal assessment. After it is determined that there is maternal sensitization and the possibility of fetal antigen positivity, additional antibody titer determinations should be performed as the pregnancy progresses.
- A second maternal antibody titer is performed at 18 to 20 weeks of gestation and then repeated monthly for the rest of the pregnancy.
- Rarely does significant hemolytic disease in the fetus occur before 20 weeks of gestation.

Fetal Assessment
- Fetal antigen status can be inferred from information gained from antigen testing of the father. When necessary, fetal antigen status can be determined directly using cell-free DNA testing (for RhD isoimmunization) or, for other antigens, by cord blood sampling or from fetal cells obtained by amniocentesis.
- Fetal anemia can be diagnosed from fetal blood obtained from cord blood sampling.
- Ultrasound is the primary tool for fetal surveillance throughout the pregnancy. It can provide several types of information, all of which are critical to successful management:
  - Fetal growth
  - Fetal well-being by biophysical profile scoring
  - Presence of ascites or hydrops as indicators of fetal anemia
  - Assessment of middle cerebral artery (MCA) blood flow by Doppler technology as a direct assessment of fetal anemia and risk of intrauterine death
- Antepartum fetal testing is used to monitor the development of fetal hypoxia due to fetal anemia.

MANAGEMENT
Documented Sensitization
- Those patients who have a positive antibody screen for the Dd antigen, or for one of the atypical antigens that are capable of causing significant hemolytic disease of the newborn, need close follow-up.

- Should amniocentesis or chorionic villus sampling be performed for genetic or other indications earlier in the pregnancy, fetal antigen typing can be performed on the cultured cells.
- As noted above, serial antibody titers need to be performed at least monthly from 18 to 20 weeks through the duration of the pregnancy.
  - Severe hemolytic disease of the newborn rarely occurs when the Coombs titer is 1:16 or less. Therefore, patients whose antibody titers are below this level can be managed expectantly and delivered at term with little change in routine obstetric care.
  - Patients whose antibody titer in the current or any previous pregnancy has exceeded 1:16 and who are carrying a potentially antigen-positive fetus must be considered at risk for severe hemolytic disease of the newborn.
- In general, in a first affected pregnancy, hydrops fetalis is unlikely before 26 to 28 weeks, and therefore, procedures to assess for fetal anemia can usually be delayed until that time. In patients who have previously had a severely affected fetus, fetal surveillance is usually started at 18 to 20 weeks' gestation.
- Traditionally, amniocentesis with analysis of amniotic fluid for breakdown products of hemoglobin has been used to identify fetuses likely to be severely anemic. In addition, fetal blood sampling can be used to assess the fetal antigen status and degree of anemia in affected pregnancies.
- Ultrasound evaluation of the fetus is a noninvasive method of evaluating the fetus at risk for significant anemia and hydrops. Hydrops is relatively easy to identify by ultrasound: Increased amniotic fluid volume, placental thickening, and hepatosplenomegaly are ultrasound signs of early hydrops.
- Noninvasive Doppler sonographic evaluation of blood flow in the fetal MCA Doppler has largely replaced serial amniocentesis for bilirubin concentration and/or fetal blood sampling as the primary method of surveillance for patients whose history or current antibody titer places them at risk for severe fetal anemia. Numerous studies have demonstrated that the degree of fetal anemia can be accurately predicted by Doppler studies of blood flow in the fetal MCA. MCA Doppler has replaced the other more traditional methods of fetal assessment because it is noninvasive, widely available, easy to repeat regularly, and well accepted by the mothers (10–12).
- Animal and human studies have demonstrated that blood flow in the brain is increased in fetuses with anemia because of an increase in cardiac output and decrease in blood viscosity (13,14).
- In pregnancies at risk for fetal anemia, Doppler ultrasound of blood flow in the MCA can be used to accurately identify the severely anemic fetus. The MCA is identified using color flow Doppler ultrasound, and duplex Doppler is then used to estimate the peak systolic velocity (Fig. 35-1). Normal values for peak systolic velocity in the MCA have been established for fetuses between 18 and 36 weeks of gestation (Table 35-3).
  - Fetuses with peak systolic velocity less than 1.5 multiples of the median are at low risk for significant anemia (11).
  - Fetuses with MCA Doppler estimated velocity greater than 1.5 multiples of the median are considered at risk for severe anemia and/or further investigated by either fetal blood sampling or amniotic fluid bilirubin studies.
- If gestational age is less than 36 weeks and fetal blood sampling reveals significant anemia (hematocrit less than 30%), intrauterine transfusion is performed.
- At or beyond 36 weeks' gestation, delivery is recommended for the anemic fetus (15).

Progressive Involvement with Successive Pregnancies
- Classically, significant fetal anemia and hydrops is not a complication of the first sensitized pregnancy; rather, it occurs in subsequent pregnancies. Each succeeding pregnancy will then demonstrate an earlier and more severe onset of anemia and hydrops.

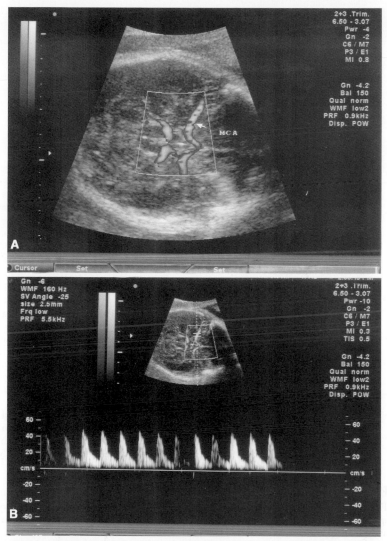

Figure 35-1. Ultrasound images of the fetal head demonstrating measurement of blood velocity in the MCA. **A:** The circle of Willis and its major branches are identified using color flow Doppler ultrasound. **B:** A pulsed Doppler gate has been placed over the proximal MCA, and the peak velocity is estimated (in this case, ~50 cm per second).

- The risk of hydrops in the first sensitized pregnancy is approximately 10%.
- Unfortunately, there is no way to predict when, during a subsequent pregnancy, a fetus may become hydropic. However, given the likelihood of similar or increased antibody levels in subsequent pregnancies, most physicians would recommend noninvasive assessment beginning at 18 to 20 weeks' gestation.

Table 35-3	Peak Systolic Velocity in the MCA as a Predictor of Moderate or Severe Fetal Anemia	
Gestational age (weeks)	PSV, cm/s (median)	PSV, cm/s (1.5 MOM)
20	25.5	34.8
22	27.9	41.9
24	30.7	46.0
26	33.6	50.4
28	36.9	55.4
30	40.5	60.7
32	44.4	66.6
34	48.7	73.1
36	53.5	80.2

Only fetuses with MCA PSV ≥ 1.5 MOM are at risk for moderate or severe fetal anemia. PSV, peak systolic velocity; MOM, multiples of the median; MCA, middle cerebral artery.
Adapted from Mari G, for the Collaborative Group for Doppler Assessment of the Blood Velocity in Anemic Fetuses. Non-invasive diagnosis by Doppler ultrasonography of fetal anemia due to maternal red-cell alloimmunization. *N Engl J Med.* 2000;342: 9–14, with permission.

Prognosis
- Fifty percent of all isoimmunized fetuses are mildly affected. The fetal anemia is mild at birth, and bilirubin levels do not rise to dangerous levels.
- Twenty-five percent to thirty percent of isoimmunized fetuses have moderate disease. In these cases, hematopoiesis is sufficient to keep up with the rate of hemolysis. Hepatic function is not compromised. In utero, the placenta is able to clear the breakdown products of hemolysis. After delivery, neonatal bilirubin levels rise rapidly. Exchange transfusion is needed to prevent neonatal death or severe neurologic impairment from kernicterus.
- In the remaining 20% to 25% of affected fetuses, severe anemia leads to extramedullary hematopoiesis, particularly in the liver. Liver obstruction and decreased hepatic synthetic activity lead to portal and umbilical hypertension, ascites, hydrops, and fetal death. Without either intrauterine transfusion or delivery, only a small proportion of severely affected fetuses can be expected to survive.

TREATMENT
The management of isoimmunization requires balancing the risks of preterm delivery against the uncertainties of the fetus remaining in utero and the potential risks of intrauterine therapy.
- For fetuses who are severely affected before 34 weeks of gestation, prematurity represents a formidable risk, and neonatal morbidity and mortality rates are elevated, making intrauterine transfusion the first therapeutic choice.
- For fetuses beyond 34 to 36 weeks, delivery with management in the NICU is the first choice in response to the diagnosis of severe hemolytic disease.

Transfusion
- The original intrauterine transfusion used the intraperitoneal transfusion technique and was first described by Liley (16) in 1963. Intraperitoneal transfusion involves the transfusion of packed antigen-negative red blood cells into the peritoneal cavity of the fetus. The cells enter the fetal bloodstream by way of the subdiaphragmatic lymphatic system.

Intraperitoneal transfusion may still be warranted for the severely affected fetus at very early gestational ages or if intravascular transfusion is technically not feasible (15).

- With increasing sonographic sophistication, intravascular transfusion, which provides more immediate diagnostic and therapeutic approaches, was described by Rodeck et al. (17) in 1981 (via fetoscope) and by Bang et al. (18) (via needle) in 1982. Numerous studies have demonstrated the efficacy of intravascular intrauterine transfusion with survival rates in severely affected pregnancies of 80% to 90%. Frigoletto et al. (19) and Hamilton (20) have summarized the value of intrauterine transfusion.

- Using continuous real-time ultrasound guidance, a 20-gauge needle is directed percutaneously into the umbilical vein, and condensed (hematocrit 70% to 80%) antigen-negative blood cross-matched to the mother is slowly infused until the fetal hematocrit is greater than 40%. Transfusions frequently need to be repeated every 1 to 3 weeks as the transfused cells have a finite life span and fetal growth results in a gradual increase in blood volume.

- Intravascular intrauterine transfusion results in survival rates of greater than 90%, even of severely affected fetuses. A recent large trial demonstrated normal neurologic outcome in 94% of those survivors (21).

- Other treatment modalities (promethazine, plasmapheresis, intravenous immune serum globulin) have not been shown to be of benefit in management of this disease.

Prevention

- Rh immunoglobulin is administered to pregnant women who are Rh negative and not sensitized. Its purpose is to prevent the maternal immunologic response to Rh-positive fetal cells that gain access to the maternal circulation and stimulate the formation of antibodies against the fetal Rh antigen.

- The exact mechanism by which Rh immunoglobulin accomplishes this is not well understood.

Antepartum Rh Immunoglobulin

- Rh immunoglobulin should be administered for prophylaxis at 28 weeks of gestation to those Rh-negative women in whom sensitization has not already occurred. A blood sample should be drawn to document a negative maternal antibody titer before administering Rh immunoglobulin.

- If such a patient undergoes amniocentesis or chorion villus sampling for any reason, Rh immunoglobulin should be administered if the father is Rh positive or his status is unknown.

- If a significant bleeding episode occurs during an Rh-negative unsensitized pregnancy, the Rh immunoglobulin should be administered.

- There are no risks or adverse side effects from giving Rh immunoglobulin, so the directive is to give it if the situation appears to have risk for fetal–maternal hemorrhage and subsequent isoimmunization.

Postpartum Rh Immunoglobulin

- Rh immunoglobulin should be administered to the mother as soon after delivery as cord blood findings indicate that the baby is Rh positive and that the mother is at risk.

- Adherence to the dictum that it is preferable to treat a woman with Rh immunoglobulin unnecessarily rather than fail to treat a woman who then becomes Rh sensitized is sensible.
  - A woman at risk who is inadvertently not given Rh immunoglobulin within 72 hours after delivery should still receive prophylaxis at least up to 2 weeks after delivery.
  - If prophylaxis is delayed, it may be ineffective.

- Current recommendations (22) are that all Rh-negative patients who have delivered an Rh-positive fetus be screened for excessive fetomaternal hemorrhage using a qualitative rosette test.

- A negative test indicates minimal fetomaternal bleeding, and a single vial of Rh immunoglobulin is administered.
- If positive, a quantitative Kleihauer-Betke stain is used to estimate the volume of fetomaternal hemorrhage.
- A vial of Rh immunoglobulin is administered for every 30 mL (or portion thereof) of calculated fetomaternal hemorrhage volume.

PATIENT EDUCATION

- Women of reproductive age should be informed of their blood type and Rh status.
- Women who are Rh negative should be informed about the risks and management issues of an Rh-negative pregnancy before becoming pregnant. Ideally, this should take place during an annual gynecologic checkup early in their reproductive life.
- Rh-negative women should understand the importance of Rh immunoglobulin in preventing Rh sensitization, so that they can be certain that they receive it in appropriate situations when they are pregnant.
- Couples contemplating pregnancy, in which the woman is Rh negative, should be counseled and offered the option of paternal testing if the man's Rh status is unknown.
- If a women becomes Rh sensitized, she should receive specific counseling before further pregnancies to explain the risks, management issues, and any additional evaluation that may be necessary.

REFERENCES

1. Landsteiner K, Weiner AS. An agglutinable factor in human blood recognized by immune sera for rhesus blood. *Proc Soc Exp Biol Med.* 1940;43:223.
2. Levine P, Katzin EM, Burnham L. Isoimmunization in pregnancy: its possible bearing on the etiology of erythroblastosis fetalis. *JAMA.* 1941;116:825.
3. Bombard AT, Akolekar R, Farkas DH, et al. Fetal RHD genotype detection from circulating cell-free fetal DNA in maternal plasma in non-sensitized RhD negative women. *Prenat Diagn.* 2011;31:802–808.
4. Bowman J. Hemolytic disease (erythroblastosis fetalis). In: Creasy R, Resnik R, eds. *Maternal fetal medicine principles and practice.* Philadelphia: W.B. Saunders, 1994:739.
5. Bowman JM, Pollock JM, Penston LE. Fetomaternal transplacental hemorrhage during pregnancy and after delivery. *Vox Sang.* 1986;51:117.
6. Kleihauer E, Braun H, Betke K. Demonstration von Fetalem Haemoglobin in den Erythrozyten eines Blutasstriches. *Klin Wochenschr.* 1957;35:637.
7. Zipursky A, Israels LG. The pathogenesis and prevention of Rh immunization. *Can Med Assoc J.* 1978;18:625.
8. Woodrow JC. *Rh immunization and its prevention.* In: *Series hematologia.* Vol 3. Copenhagen: Munksgaard, 1970.
9. Bowman JM, Pollock JM. Antenatal Rh prophylaxis: 28 week gestation service program. *Can Med Assoc J.* 1978;18:627.
10. Mari G, Adrignolo A, Abuhamad AZ, et al. Diagnosis of fetal anemia with Doppler ultrasound in the pregnancy complicated by maternal blood group immunization. *Ultrasound Obstet Gynecol.* 1995;6:400–405.
11. Mari G; for the Collaborative Group for Doppler Assessment of the Blood Velocity in Anemic Fetuses. Non-invasive diagnosis by Doppler ultrasonography of fetal anemia due to maternal red-cell alloimmunization. *N Engl J Med.* 2000;342:9–14.
12. McLean LK, Hedriana HL, Lanouette JM, et al. A retrospective review of isoimmunized pregnancies managed by middle cerebral artery peak systolic velocity. *Am J Obstet Gynecol.* 2004;190:1732–1738.
13. Fan FC, Chen RY, Schuessler GB, et al. Effects of hematocrit variations on regional hemodynamics and oxygen transport in the dog. *Am J Physiol.* 1980;238:H545–H552.
14. Moise KJ Jr, Mari G, Fisher DJ, et al. Acute fetal hemodynamic alterations after intrauterine transfusion for treatment of severe red blood cell count will immunization. *Am J Obstet Gynecol.* 1990;163:776–784.

15. Moise KJ, Argoti PS. Management and prevention of red cell alloimmunization in pregnancy: a systematic review. *Obstet Gynecol.* 2012;5:1132.

16. Liley A. Intrauterine transfusion of fetus in hemolytic disease. *Br Med J.* 1963;2:1107.

17. Rodeck CH, Kemp JR, Holman CA, et al. Direct intravascular fetal blood transfusion by fetoscopy in severe rhesus isoimmunization. *Lancet.* 1981;1:625–627.

18. Bang J, Bock JE, Trolle D. Ultra-sound guided fetal intravenous transfusion for severe rhesus haemolytic disease. *Br Med J.* 1982;284:373.

19. Frigoletto FD, Umansky I, Birnholz J, et al. Intrauterine fetal transfusion in 365 fetuses during fifteen years. *Am J Obstet Gynecol.* 1981;139:781–790.

20. Hamilton ET. Intrauterine transfusion. Safeguard or peril. *Obstet Gynecol.* 1977;50:255.

21. Lindenburg IT, Smits-Wintjens VE, et al. Long-term neurodevelopmental outcome after intrauterine transfusion for hemolytic disease of the fetus/newborn: the LOTUS study. *Am J Obstet Gynecol.* 2012;206:141.e1–141.e8.

22. Roback JD, Grossman BJ, Harris T, et al., eds. *Technical manual.* 17th ed. Bethesda: AABB, 2011.

Disease of the Placenta
Raymond W. Redline

KEY POINTS
- Placental pathology is determined by the dominant physiologic processes of pregnancy, vascular biology, immunology, and development.
- Adverse outcomes and recurrence risks can be explained and subclassified according to the underlying placental pathology.

BACKGROUND
Structure: The placenta is an invasive fetal organ that absorbs nutrients from a reservoir of maternal blood accumulating within its confines in the uterus (1,2):
- *Maternal–trophoblastic placenta*: Trophoblasts are the only fetally derived cells in direct contact with the mother. Trophoblast is separated into two main types:
  - *Villous trophoblast*: covers the placental villi and mediates gas exchange and transport of nutrients from maternal blood in the intervillous space
  - *Extravillous trophoblast*: infiltrates the uterus and its blood vessels attaching the placenta to the mother (basal plate), allowing maternal blood to enter the intervillous space, and separating the amniotic fluid from the uterus
- *Fetal stromal–vascular placenta*: Vascularized fetal connective tissue that transmits fetal blood to and from the placenta via the umbilical cord, chorionic plate, and villous trees.
- *Placental membranes*: Portion of the nonvascularized placenta lying outside the perimeter of the disc, which contains the amniotic fluid.
- *Umbilical cord*: Tubular structure composed of the major arteries and veins that connect the fetus to the placenta, a surrounding protective extracellular matrix (Wharton jelly), and covered by a surrounding simple squamous epithelium.

Development (3–5)
- Basal plate
  - *Uterine implantation*: Extravillous trophoblast from the periphery of the blastocyst invades the inner one-third of the uterus and secretes a fibrinoid extracellular matrix that forms the floor of the placenta (known as the basal plate).
  - *Maternal arterial remodeling*: Extravillous trophoblast first migrates upstream within the lumina of maternal spiral arteries, forming plugs that prevent uteroplacental blood flow in early pregnancy. Later, this extravillous trophoblast invades and remodels the spiral artery walls, enhancing perfusion of the placental intervillous space.
- Chorionic plate and villous trees
  - *Vasculogenesis/angiogenesis*: Fetoplacental blood vessels are induced within the extraembryonic endo-/mesoderm by angiogenic factors primarily produced by villous trophoblast. This network of vessels later develops connections with large fetal blood vessels entering the placenta through the body stalk/umbilical cord. Several generations of vascular branching create the roof of the placenta (known as the chorionic plate) and the villous trees, which project downward into the intervillous space. The "trunks and large branches" of the villous tree are known as proximal villi, while the "twigs" are termed distal villi.
  - *Vasculosyncytial membranes*: Specialized areas of close apposition between villous capillaries and trophoblast that form in the early third trimester at the tips of the distal villous tree (terminal villi) facilitating optimal uptake of nutrients.

- Membrane formation
  - *Regression of peripheral chorion*: The placenta is initially spherical, not discoid. When uteroplacental blood flow is initiated by maternal spiral artery remodeling, areas with inadequate perfusion become atrophic (chorion regression), losing their fetal and maternal blood vessels and forming a thin membrane composed of connective tissue (former chorionic plate), chorion laevae trophoblast (remnants of the basal plate and villous tree), and decidua capsularis (underlying endometrium). The remainder of the placenta (chorion frondosum) forms the mature placental disc.
  - *Amniochorionic fusion*: Amnion fuses with the membranous choriodecidual portion of the membranes at about 11 to 12 weeks' gestation.
  - *Apposition and fusion with the opposing endometrium*: Decidua capsularis fuses with the endometrial lining on the opposite side of the uterus (decidua vera) at about 18 to 19 weeks' gestation to complete the definitive placental membrane unit.
- Body stalk/umbilical cord
  - *Vascular remodeling*: Two fetal structures enter the primitive body stalk, the allantoic duct projecting from the dome of the bladder and the vitelline duct/yolk sac projecting from the midileum. Each is accompanied by paired veins and arteries. Only the allantoic vessels (one vein and two arteries) persist after embryogenesis in the human placenta.
  - *Umbilical cord formation*: The body stalk becomes sheathed by a skin-like ectodermal covering as the embryo undergoes rostral, caudal, and lateral folding.
  - *Wharton jelly*: A hydrated glycoprotein matrix accumulates around the large vessels in the body stalk/umbilical cord following enclosure by ectoderm.

GUIDELINES FOR SUBMISSION OF PLACENTA FOR PATHOLOGIC EVALUATION

Indications for Submission: College of American Pathologists Practice Guideline (6)

- Developed by a task force of pathologists, obstetricians, and neonatologists.
- Relatively liberal guidelines resulting in submission rate of 40% to 50% in a high-risk setting.
- Yield of significant placental findings with full compliance to guidelines = 64%.
- Indications are separated into three groups as listed below.

Maternal
- Delivery at less than 37 weeks or more than 42 weeks (accepted alternative is less than 34 weeks)
- Systemic disorders with concern for mother or infant (hypertension, diabetes, others)
- Peripartum fever or infection
- Unexplained or excessive third-trimester bleeding
- Unexplained or recurrent pregnancy complications
- Invasive procedures with suspected placental injury
- Thick or viscid meconium
- Severe oligohydramnios/polyhydramnios

Fetal/Neonatal
- Stillbirth or neonatal death
- NICU admission
- Small for gestational age (SGA)/large for gestational age (LGA) (less than 10th or greater than 90th percentile for gestational age)
- Birth depression/pH less than 7.0/Apgar less than 7 at 5 minutes/assisted ventilation greater than 10 min/hematocrit less than 35
- Neonatal seizures

- Suspected infection or sepsis
- Hydrops fetalis
- Multiple pregnancy (accepted alternative is all fused placentas, same sex twins, or discordant fetal growth)

Significant Gross Placental Abnormalities
- Structural abnormalities of the placental disc or membranes
- Suspected abnormal size or weight for gestational age
- Umbilical cord abnormalities (e.g., long/short/hypercoiled/abnormal insertion/single artery)

Placental storage for later submission: Infants may occasionally develop problems within the first few days after leaving the delivery suite. Storing all placentas (fresh refrigerated) for 1 week has been recommended by some to insure that all specimens from pregnancies with adverse outcome are examined.

Ancillary studies: Ancillary studies of placental tissue such as microbiologic culture, karyotype, molecular testing, and electron microscopy are rarely used for placental evaluation. A maternal blood sample for Kleihauer-Betke testing or flow cytometric fetal hemoglobin determination has been recommended in all cases of unexpected adverse outcome.

PLACENTAL PATHOLOGY IN SINGLETON PREGNANCIES (3,4)

Clinical information: The pathologist requires some basic clinical data to properly interpret placental findings. These include the indication(s) for submission, gestational age, maternal gravidity and parity, fetal weight, Apgar scores, and any more specific question that the submitting physician may have.

Gross examination: Placentas can be examined fresh either following refrigeration or after formalin fixation. Abnormalities of color, shape, and umbilical cord insertion site are documented along with any deformations, disruptions, or adherent clots. The trimmed placental disc is weighed and measured, and both the weight and fetoplacental weight ratio are compared with expected values for gestational age. Between three and five histologic sections are usually submitted for histologic analysis including samples of the umbilical cord, membranes and adjacent peripheral placenta, a full-thickness section of parenchyma at the umbilical cord insertion site, and sections of any pathologic lesion with adjacent normal parenchyma.

Selected Gross Abnormalities (See Subsequent Sections for Additional Detail)
- Abnormal shape: reflects reduced maternal perfusion and/or abnormal early fetal vascular branching
  - Accessory ("succenturiate") lobe (placental tissue completely separates from the main disc); bridging vessels can be torn (Fig. 36-1).
  - Bilobate/multilobate and over 50% indentation (relatively benign).
  - Thick: seen with severe maternal malperfusion and hydrops fetalis.
  - Thin: placental atrophy (seen with chronically decreased intervillous perfusion).
  - Decreased width ("short chorion"): associated with early marginal hypoxia.
- Abnormal color
  - Green: meconium, severe chorioamnionitis, and chronic hemorrhage (biliverdin)
  - Brown: chronic hemorrhage (hemosiderin) and stillbirth
- Abnormal weight for gestational age (see Kraus et al. (3) reference for table)
  - Decreased: seen with maternal malperfusion, villitis of unknown etiology (VUE), and small fetus
  - Increased: seen with diabetic mother, hydrops, and large fetus

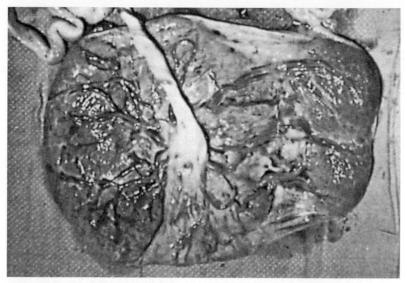

Figure 36-1. Accessory ("succenturiate") lobe: Fetal vessels bridge membranes separating an island of placental tissue on the right from the main placental disc on the left.

- Abnormal cord length (see Kraus et al. (3) reference for table)
  - Increased (greater than 70 cm): increased fetal movement and risk of entanglements
  - Reduced: decreased fetal movements
  - Excessive coiling: increased risk of vascular compromise
- Abnormal cord insertion: can cause acute or chronic fetal perfusion abnormalities
  - Membranous: Cord inserts in membranes (risk of torsion/rupture) (Fig. 36-2).
  - Furcate: Vessels separate from cord prior to insertion into disc (risk of torsion/rupture).
  - Chorionic plate vessel anomalously traveling in membranes (risk of rupture).
  - Tethered: Cord covered by a "hood" of amnion (risk of obstructed flow).
  - Marginal/peripheral ("battledore"): Cord inserts less than 3 cm from margin (relatively benign).
- Placental mass
  - Infarct: obstructed spiral artery (Fig. 36-3)
  - Chorangioma: fetal capillary vascular tumor in large stem villus (Fig. 36-4)
  - Perivillous fibrin plaque: localized increase in intervillous fibrin (relatively benign)
  - Others: entrapped uterine tumors (leiomyoma, stromal nodule)
- Placental hematoma/blood clot
  - Retroplacental and central with indentation: abruptio placenta
  - Retroplacental and marginal/retromembranous: acute or chronic marginal abruption
  - Intraplacental: fetomaternal hemorrhage with surrounding maternal clot
  - Large fetal/umbilical vessel: ruptured vasa previa
- Cystic villi
  - Septal cysts: intraplacental trophoblastic inclusion cyst (relatively benign)
  - Mesenchymal dysplasia: molar villi without trophoblast hyperplasia
  - Twin hydatidiform mole: high risk of persistent gestational trophoblastic disease (GTD)
  - Partial mole: low risk of persistent GTD
  - Trisomy 16: confined placental mosaicism (risk of occult fetal mosaicism)

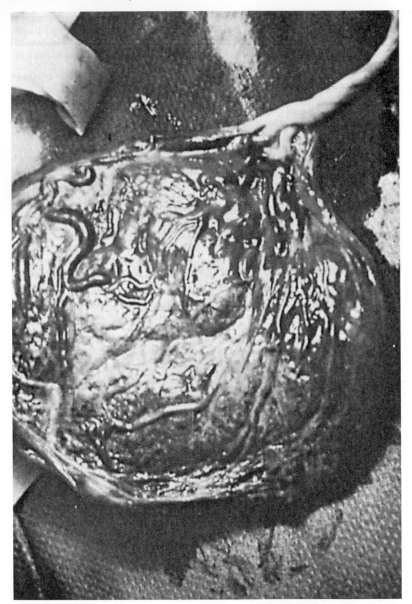

Figure 36-2. Membranous insertion of the umbilical cord: Umbilical vessels separate from the umbilical cord before inserting into the membranes near the placental margin.

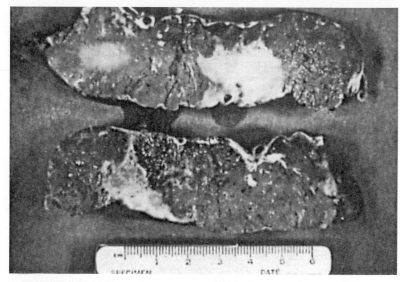

Figure 36-3. Villous infarcts: Firm, pale, granular lesions with their broadest base abutting the maternal surface are seen on cut section of the placenta.

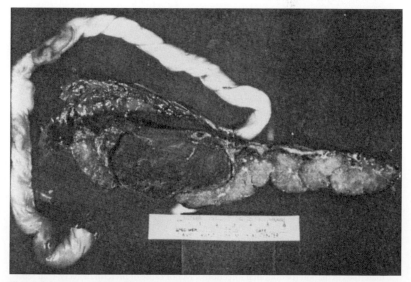

Figure 36-4. Chorangioma: Dark, rounded, smooth lesion incorporating a large chorionic vessel near the fetal surface is seen on cut section of the placenta.

Histologic Lesions (See Figs. 36-5 and 36-6) (2,7)

- Maternal–*trophoblastic*: Lesions in this category relate to abnormal trophoblast function in the early stages of pregnancy resulting in superficial implantation and damage to maternal arteries that can lead to vascular obstruction and/or rupture. They are most frequent with severe preeclampsia but may also be seen with idiopathic fetal growth restriction (FGR), preterm delivery, maternal obesity, essential hypertension, insulin-dependent diabetes, renal disease, thrombophilia, and collagen vascular diseases:
  - Developmental abnormalities involving extravillous trophoblast
    - *Inadequate arterial remodeling*: persistent smooth muscle in basal plate arteries
    - *Superficial uterine invasion*: increased placental site giant cells
    - *Excessive intraplacental extravillous trophoblast*: chorionic cysts
  - Maternal vascular malperfusion
    - *Complete/segmental occlusion and spiral arteries*: villous infarcts
    - *Partial/intermittent flow abnormalities and uterine arteries*: increased syncytial knots and *intervillous* fibrin, villous agglutination, and distal villous hypoplasia
  - Loss of maternal vascular integrity
    - *Abruptio placenta*
    - *Marginal abruption, recent or chronic*
  - Secondary/extrinsic lesions
    - *Decidual arteriopathy* (acute atherosis, mural hypertrophy)
- Fetal *stromal–vascular*: Lesions in this category reflect primary or secondary abnormalities affecting connective tissue and/or fetal vessels in the membranes, chorionic plate, or villous stroma. They are commonly seen with umbilical cord obstruction, diabetes, chromosomal abnormalities, and hydrops fetalis and may be associated with stillbirth, macrosomia, placentomegaly, neonatal encephalopathy, idiopathic FGR, and preterm delivery:
  - Developmental abnormalities involving villous stroma
    - *Distal villous immaturity (maturation defect): increased villous stroma and decreased vasculosyncytial membranes*
    - *Villous capillary proliferation: chorangiosis*
  - Fetal vascular malperfusion
    - *Complete/segmental occlusion, chorionic plate, or stem villous vessels (fetal thrombotic vasculopathy/FTV): large to intermediate sized foci of hyalinized avascular villi and chorionic or proximal villous occlusive thrombi*
    - *Partial/intermittent flow abnormalities and umbilical vessels: dilation or intimal fibrin cushions in large fetoplacental veins, scattered small foci of avascular villi, and patchy distal villous edema and immaturity*
  - Loss of fetal vascular integrity
    - *Small-vessel (fetomaternal) hemorrhage: intervillous thrombi*
    - *Large-vessel (vaginal bleeding with + fetal blood) hemorrhage: ruptured vasa previa*
  - Secondary/extrinsic lesions
    - *Prolonged meconium exposure: abundant pigment-laden macrophages in chorionic plate, green-stained umbilical cord, and meconium vascular necrosis*
    - *Increased circulating nucleated red blood cells (NRBC): indicative of subacute/chronic fetal hypoxemia*
    - *Hydrops fetalis: diffuse villous edema and increased villous cytotrophoblast*
- Inflammatory/*infectious*: Lesions in this category develop as a result of microbial infection of the placenta and/or its membranes:
  - *Acute chorioamnionitis*: Bacterial/fungal infections primarily localized to the placental membranes. Organisms ascend from cervicovaginal tract or lodge in the membranes from maternal circulation (periodontal infections). Major cause of preterm delivery, fetal sepsis, and fetal end-organ damage related to the fetal inflammatory response (FIR) syndrome.
    - Maternal inflammatory response

Categories of Placental Pathology

1. Maternal uterine/trophoblastic
Maldevelopment:
    defective arterial remodelling
    shallow implantation
    excessive intraplacental trophoblast
Malperfusion
    partial global: increased syncytial knots
    complete segmental: villous infarct
Loss of Integrity:
    abruptio placenta
    marginal abruption, acute or chronic
Secondary/extrinsic:
    decidual arteriopathy

2. Fetal stromal-vascular
Maldevelopment:
    distal villous immaturity
    chorangioma, chorangiosis
Malperfusion:
    partial global: umbilical cord compromise
    complete segmental:
        fetal thrombotic vasculopathy/FTV
Loss of integrity:
    small vessel hemorrhage
    large vessel hemorrhage
Secondary/extrinsic:
    meconium effects
    increased nucleated red cells (NRBC)
    hydrops fetalis

3. Inflammatory, infectious
Acute:
    chorioamnionitis
    villitis
    intervillositis
Chronic:
    villitis
    intervillositis
    deciduitis

4. Inflammatory, idiopathic
Villitis/VUE
Chorioamnionitis, lymphocytic
Fetal vasculitis, eosinophilic T cell
Intervillositis, histiocytic

5. Pathogenesis incompletely understood
Perivillous fibrin(oid) deposition, diffuse or localized
Intraplacental (thrombo) hematomas, atypical
Deciduitis, lymphoplasmacytic
Dysmorphic villi, nonspecific

6. Other
Malformations/deformations/disruptions
Benign tumors and heterotopias
Malignant/premalignant tumors
Genetic/chromosomal abnormalities

Figure 36-5. Placental classification scheme: outline of patterns of placental injury capable of causing adverse perinatal outcomes.

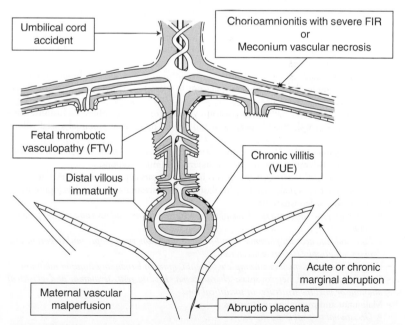

Figure 36-6. Diagram illustrating the site of action for specific patterns of injury: schematic diagram of the placenta showing from top to bottom; umbilical cord, chorionic plate, proximal villi, distal villi, peripheral draining maternal veins, and central supplying maternal artery. (FIR, fetal inflammatory response; FTV, fetal thrombotic vasculopathy; VUE, villitis of unknown etiology).

- Grade: mild-moderate versus severe
- Stage: 1. subchorionitis, 2. chorioamnionitis, and 3. necrotizing chorioamnionitis
  ○ FIR
    - Grade: mild-moderate versus severe
    - Stage: 1. umbilical/chorionic vein(s), 2. umbilical artery(s), and 3. Wharton jelly (funisitis)
- *Chronic placentitis*: Hematogenous infections by organisms of the so-called TORCH group (*T*oxoplasma, *r*ubella, *C*MV, *H*SV; *o*thers: syphilis, Varicella Zoster, miscellaneous other viruses, protozoans, and parasites). Inflammation primarily localizes to the villi and chorionic plate. Important causes of stillbirth, FGR, and severe neonatal morbidity.
  ○ Organisms/inclusions
  ○ Lymphohistiocytic villitis/chorionitis
  ○ Villous plasma cells, hemosiderin, and/or calcifications
- Inflammatory/*idiopathic*: Lesions in this category represent maternal immune responses occurring within the fetal compartment of the placenta (putative "graft versus host"–type reactions). They are important causes of FGR, preterm delivery, and recurrent pregnancy loss:
  - *Chronic villitis (villitis of unknown etiology [VUE])*
    ○ Low grade: small foci of less than 10 contiguous villi
    ○ High grade: foci of 10 or more contiguous villi and/or fetal vasculitis/obliterative fetal vasculopathy
  - *Chronic histiocytic intervillositis*: diffuse infiltration of the intervillous space by maternal monocyte/macrophages
  - Other: *chronic chorioamnionitis* and *eosinophilic T-cell fetal vasculitis*
- Pathogenesis *uncertain*: Lesions in this category are distinct and often associated with adverse outcomes, but their underlying pathogenesis is either unknown or controversial:
  - *Massive perivillous fibrin(oid) deposition ("maternal floor infarction")*: distal villi surrounded by fibrin, fibrinoid matrix, and extravillous trophoblast that obliterates the intervillous space
  - *Atypical intervillous thrombohematomas*: accumulations of clotted blood not completely surrounded by normal villi (adjacent to infarcted tissue, basal plate, or chorionic plate)
  - *Dysmorphic villi*: irregular villous contour, villous stromal trophoblast inclusions, nonspecific villous trophoblast hyperplasia, and altered patterns of proximal–distal villous branching
  - *Decidual plasma cells*: chronic endometritis seen with persistent microbial infections and/or other B-lymphocyte–mediated maternal immune responses
- *Other developmental abnormalities*: Lesions in this category represent structural anomalies not directly related to maternal–trophoblastic or fetal stromal–vascular development:
  - Malformations/deformations
    ○ *Umbilical cord: single artery, abnormalities of length, coiling, and insertion site (see previous section)*
    ○ *Placental disc accreta, placenta membranacea, and abnormal shape: multilobation and marginal atrophy (see previous section)*
  - Disruptions: *fragmented or incomplete placenta, amnion bands, and amnion nodosum*
  - Benign tumors and heterotopias: *chorangioma, hepatic rests, teratoma, and persistent allantoic or vitelline structures in umbilical cord*
  - Malignant and premalignant tumors
    ○ *Gestational trophoblastic disease*
      - Villous trophoblast: *partial mole (triploid), complete mole (diandry),* and *choriocarcinoma*
      - Extravillous trophoblast: *placental site trophoblastic tumor and epithelioid trophoblastic tumor*

- ○ *Metastatic tumors*
  - − Fetal: neuroblastoma, lymphoma/leukemia, and Langerhans cell histiocytosis
  - − Maternal: breast, GI malignancy, and melanoma most common
- Genetic/chromosomal disorders
  - ○ Fetoplacental: *trisomies, monosomy X, metabolic storage diseases, and fetoplacental overgrowth disorders (e.g., Beckwith-Wiedemann syndrome)*
  - ○ Placental: *mesenchymal dysplasia and confined placental mosaicism*

PLACENTAL PATHOLOGY IN MULTIPLE PREGNANCIES (1,3,8)

Dichorionic placentas (two separate or fused discs): Dichorionic placentas represent two chorionic sacs, which may be separate or contiguous (fused) within the uterus. By definition, they always have two amnions and lack vascular anastomoses. However, they may be seen with either dizygotic or monozygotic twins:

- *Pathologic diagnosis of chorionicity*: Assessment of chorionicity distinguishes two fused dichorionic placentas from a single monochorionic placenta. This is accomplished by examining the membrane that divides the two amnionic sacs. If two amnions and an intervening fused chorion are found at gross examination and confirmed histologically, the placenta is dichorionic and the various complications of monochorionic twin pregnancy (listed below) need not be further considered.
- *Early loss, vanishing twins/fetus papyraceous–compressus*: Spontaneous abortion affecting one or more of the gestations in a multiple pregnancy results in collapse of the affected chorionic sac and involution of the embryo or fetus. These abortions are often detected as firm plaques of yellow-brown tissue within the membranes of the viable twin and are confirmed histologically by identifying structural elements of the involuting fetus and chorionic sac.
- *Discordant growth*: Discordant growth in dichorionic twins may be due to genetic disparities in the conceptuses, disadvantageous implantation of one of the twin placentas, or acquired placental lesions such as those described above for singleton placentas. The most commonly identified placental lesions in the smaller twin are peripheral umbilical cord insertion, avascular villi suggestive of fetal vascular occlusion, and changes of maternal malperfusion.

Monochorionic placentas (one disc): A monochorionic placenta develops when a single fertilized zygote splits into two embryos after formation of the trophectoderm. Earlier separation of a single fertilized zygote will result in a dichorionic placenta. Very rarely, two separate blastocysts when cultured together in vitro may fuse to form a single placenta.

Monochorionic monoamnionic placentas: These placentas form following a very late split of the inner cell mass after formation of the amnion resulting in both embryos being contained within a single amnionic sac. Monoamnionic pregnancies always have vascular anastomoses (see next section), but these are almost always balanced, and transfusion syndrome is rare:

- *Umbilical cord entanglements*: Entanglement and obstructed flow in one or both umbilical cords is associated with death of one or both twins in up to 50% of monoamnionic twins. The cause of death may be either complete umbilical cord obstruction or acute fetofetal hemorrhage across large-caliber anastomoses triggered by asymmetric umbilical cord compression.
- *Conjoined pregnancy*: Partial attachment of the two fetuses, considered to represent secondary fusion of exposed germ layers prior to complete embryonic folding and closure rather than primary failure of the embryos to fully separate.
- *Twin reversed arterial perfusion sequence (TRAP), acardiac twin*: Closely opposed large-caliber artery–artery anastomoses can lead to reversal of arterial blood flow with subsequent perfusion of the affected twin by deoxygenated blood that largely bypasses the upper body before returning to the placenta. This leads to deficient development of the head, heart, and upper limbs and a so-called acardiac fetus. TRAP sequence is most

frequent in monoamnionic twins, but may also occur in monochorionic diamnionic placentas.

Monochorionic Diamnionic Placentas

- *Vascular anastomoses (surface, deep)*: Vascular anastomoses are observed in 80% of monochorionic diamnionic twin placentas. These may be separated into three groups: bidirectional surface artery–artery and vein–vein anastomoses and unidirectional deep arteriovenous anastomoses.
- *Twin–twin transfusion syndrome (TTTS)*: TTTS occurs in approximately 10% of monochorionic twins, usually between 16 and 26 weeks. Defined clinically by the combination of donor oligohydramnios and recipient polyhydramnios. It is usually characterized pathologically by unidirectional deep anastomoses in the absence of balancing bidirectional surface anastomoses. TTTS may be confirmed by placental injection studies, which are also useful in evaluating the efficacy of antenatal laser coagulation therapy used to obliterate deep anastomoses.
- *Twin anemia–polycythemia syndrome (TAPS)*: TAPS is defined by discrepancies in the hemoglobin concentrations (greater than 8 g/dL) and reticulocyte counts of the two fetuses/neonates. TAPS occurs in approximately 5% of previously uncomplicated monochorionic twin pregnancies, usually at a later stage than TTTS (TAPS may also develop secondarily following incomplete laser ablation in TTTS). TAPS is characterized pathologically by very small unidirectional deep vascular anastomoses.
- *Death of cotwin*: A catastrophic complication of monochorionic twin pregnancies leading to profound circulatory shifts resulting in death (15%) or neurodevelopmental abnormalities (25%) in the viable twin and preterm delivery in 68% of cases. Autopsy often documents ischemic lesions in the initially viable cotwin.
- *Discordant growth:* Discordant growth in monochorionic twins is most commonly correlated with unequal sharing of the placental chorionic surface and peripheral insertion of one or both umbilical cords.

UTILITY OF PLACENTAL EXAMINATION (2)

Current Pregnancy

- *Identify immediately treatable processes*: Prompt examination of the placenta can uncover processes not suspected by other clinical and laboratory modalities:
  - Mother: specific infections, retained placenta, GTD, and other maternal malignancies
  - Infant: elevated risk of neonatal sepsis (histologic chorioamnionitis with FIR), specific infections (CMV, *Candida*, syphilis, *Listeria*), metabolic storage disease, and fetal malignancy
- *Identify potential underlying influences of adverse outcomes*: Clinical outcomes as listed below are the result of diverse underlying processes that can be subgrouped by placental pathology:
  - Preterm delivery
  - Fetal growth restriction
  - Stillbirth
  - Central nervous system (CNS) injury
- *Quality assurance and risk management*: Information regarding the underlying cause of adverse outcomes provides useful feedback for healthcare providers and timely explanations for grieving parents that can sometimes preempt medicolegal action:
  - Distinguishing "perceived" from actual causes in specific clinical situations (e.g., chorioamnionitis and abruption)
  - Uncovering subacute and chronic disorders predisposing to birth asphyxia, neonatal encephalopathy, seizures, stroke, or cerebral palsy

Future Management

- *Estimate recurrence risks*: Some placental lesions have significant recurrence risks as listed below. Risk of perinatal morbidity and mortality in subsequent pregnancies may be an indication for high-risk referral:
  1. *Chronic histiocytic intervillositis/massive intervillositis* (75% to 90%)
  2. *Massive perivillous fibrin(oid) deposition/maternal floor infarction* (30% to 60%)
  3. *Chronic villitis/VUE* (25% to 50%)
  4. *Placenta accreta* (10% to 25%)
  5. Preeclampsia with *severe maternal malperfusion* (10% to 25%)
  6. Preterm *acute chorioamnionitis* (10% to 25%)
- *Clinical correlations of placental pathologic findings*: Some placental findings may be indicative of underlying maternal medical disease. Further evaluation could be considered depending on the patient's medical history and clinical index of suspicion for these conditions:
  - *Severe maternal malperfusion*: may be associated with maternal thrombophilia, glucose intolerance, renal insufficiency, autoimmune disease, or significant underlying cardiovascular disease
  - *Acute chorioamnionitis*: may be associated with underlying periodontal disease or chronic endometritis
  - *Recurrent thromboinflammatory syndromes (1 to 3 above)*: may be associated with maternal autoimmune diseases and risk of poor fetal growth
  - *Fetal thrombotic vasculopathy*: may be associated with maternal thrombophilia or diabetes
  - *Distal villous immaturity (maturation defect)*: may be associated with maternal diabetes or risk of poor fetal growth
  - *Placenta accreta*: associated with high risk of recurrent placental attachment abnormality, subsequent Caesarian section, or hysterectomy
  - *Placental hydrops*: may be associated with maternal RBC alloimmunization, fetal genetic aberration, or perinatal infection

Advances in Perinatal Biology and Therapeutics

- Continuing advances in the molecular characterization and potential treatment of pregnancy disorders require accurate phenotyping, which is provided in a comprehensive and cost-effective manner by placental pathology.

ANTENATAL EVALUATION OF PLACENTAL STRUCTURE AND FUNCTION

Ultrasound (9,10)

- Multiple pregnancies
  - First-trimester assessment of dividing membrane, one versus two sacs: twin peak sign (lambda sign) and intertwin membrane diameter greater than 1.5 to 2.0 mm indicative of dichorionicity.
  - Second trimester: Oligohydramnios (deepest vertical pocket less than or equal to 2 cm)/polyhydramnios (deepest vertical pocket greater than 8 cm) could be indicative of TTTS in monochorionic gestations.
- Singleton pregnancies
  - Amniotic fluid volume
    - Oligohydramnios: associated pathology *and maternal malperfusion/placental insufficiency* (FGR); membrane rupture should be excluded.
    - Polyhydramnios: associated pathology—*fetal genetic abnormalities, congenital infections or birth defects, and others.*
  - Periplacental hemorrhages
    - Preplacental (associated pathology: *marginal abruption*)

- ° Retroplacental (associated pathology: *abruptio placenta*)
- ° Subchorionic (associated pathology: *chronic abruption*)
- Placenta previa or low-lying placenta: distance from internal cervical os at time of delivery—1 to 10 mm (Cesarean delivery recommended), 10 to 20 mm (trial of labor could be considered), and greater than 20 mm (routine clinical management)
  - ° Often resolves before delivery (overall prevalence: 3% in second trimester, 0.6% at 32 weeks)
  - ° Associated pathology: *chronic abruption, peripheral umbilical cord insertion, and mild maternal malperfusion*
- Placenta accreta (occurs more frequently with previous Cesarean delivery and low anterior placenta): loss of anechoic uteroplacental separation zone, irregular anechoic regions, and loss of uterovesical delineation
  - ° *Accreta*: villi in contact with the myometrium without intervening decidual stromal cells.
  - ° *Increta/percreta*: villi invading into or through myometrial wall.
  - ° *Caesarian section scar pregnancy*: Placenta grows within a space created by dehiscence of a previous lower uterine segment incision.
- Placental diameter: chorion regression (less than 11.5 cm), secondary to early marginal hypoxia
  - ° Associated pathology: *maternal malperfusion*
- Placental thickness
  - ° Greater than 3 cm (and/or "jelly-like" placenta): thickened placenta with patchy, decreased echogenicity, and "wobbly" appearance upon abdominal pressure (associated pathology: *severe maternal malperfusion with distal villous hypoplasia, maternal floor infarction*)
  - ° Greater than 4 cm at umbilical cord insertion: may be associated with *placental hydrops*
- Placental lakes/anechoic areas (poorly reproducible)
  - ° Associated pathology: *intervillous thrombus, chorionic cysts, placental infarcts, placental fibrin deposits, and intercotyledonary distal villous hypoplasia*
- Placental grading (mostly of historic interest)
  - ° Associated pathology: *maternal malperfusion and calcified intervillous fibrin*

Doppler Blood Flow Studies
- Umbilical artery Doppler, ductus venosus Doppler, and middle cerebral artery (MCA) Doppler (cerebroplacental ratio): prediction of adverse outcome in FGR
  - Associated pathology: *distal villous hypoplasia (reduced villous branching) and maternal malperfusion*
- Uterine artery Doppler: when performed in early pregnancy, may have some predictive value for subsequent development of preeclampsia (65% positive predictive value with 10% false negative rate)
- Associated pathology: *decidual arteriopathy and superficial implantation*
- MCA Doppler: prediction of fetal anemia in cases of red blood cell alloimmunization
- For evaluation of placental mass lesions:
  - *Chorangioma* (fetal vascular flow)
  - *Intraplacental leiomyoma* (maternal vascular flow)
  - *Infarcts/intervillous thrombi/perivillous fibrin(oid)* (no flow)

Biochemical Markers in Early Pregnancy (11)
- Down syndrome screening: HCG, AFP, E3, inhibin, and PAPP-A
  - Associated pathology: *maternal malperfusion* (elevated AFP: *chronic villitis/VUE*)
- Preeclampsia screening: s-flt-1, s-Eng, PlGF, PAPP-A, ADAM-12, and PP13
  - Has modest predictive value (sensitivity 55% and 80% specificity) for preeclampsia in a low-risk population of nulliparous women (may perform better as predictor of pre-eclampsia associated with pathologic changes of severe *maternal vascular malperfusion*)

REFERENCES

1. Benirschke K, Burton G, et al., eds. *Pathology of the human placenta*. New York: Springer, 2012.
2. Redline RW. Placental pathology. In: Martin R, Walsh M, eds. *Fanaroff and Martin's neonatal-perinatal medicine*. St. Louis: Elsevier-Mosby, 2014.
3. Kraus FT, Redline R, et al. *Placental pathology*. Washington: American Registry of Pathology, 2004.
4. Redline RW. The placenta. In: Stocker T, Dehner L, Hussain A, eds. *Stocker and Dehner's Pediatric Pathology*. Philadelphia: LWW, 2014.
5. Brosens I, Pijnenborg, R, et al. The "Great Obstetrical Syndromes" are associated with disorders of deep placentation. *Am J Obstet Gynecol*. 2010;204(3):193–201.
6. Langston C, Kaplan C, et al. Practice guideline for examination of the placenta. *Arch Pathol Lab Med*. 1997;121:449–476.
7. Redline RW. Placental pathology: a systematic approach with clinical correlations. *Placenta*. 2008;29(suppl A):S86–S91.
8. Lewi L, Deprest J, et al. The vascular anastomoses in monochorionic twin pregnancies and their clinical consequences. *Am J Obstet Gynecol*. 2013;208(1):19–30.
9. Costantini D, Walker M, et al. Pathologic basis of improving the screening utility of 2-dimensional placental morphology ultrasound. *Placenta*. 2012;33(10):845–849.
10. Sebire NJ, Sepulveda W. Correlation of placental pathology with prenatal ultrasound findings. *J Clin Pathol*. 2008;61(12):1276–1284.
11. Myatt L, Clifton RG, et al. First-trimester prediction of preeclampsia in nulliparous women at low risk. *Obstet Gynecol*. 2012;119(6):1234–1242.

Fetal Therapy
Alan M. Coleman and Foong-Yen Lim

KEY POINTS
- Fetal therapy consists of prenatal interventions that are performed to maintain the well-being of the fetus while minimizing maternal complications.
- Improvements in prenatal imaging have led to earlier diagnosis of abnormalities at a time when interventions are still an option for improving fetal outcomes. They have assisted in risk stratification as well as operative planning.
- Referral to centers with experience in fetal intervention can be made when prenatal intervention may be needed or high-risk delivery is anticipated.
- Interventions can range from medical therapy administered to the mother to surgical interventions performed on the fetus, with trends now toward minimally invasive approaches and treatment of nonlethal conditions.
- Maternal safety and well-being are of paramount priority.

BACKGROUND
Central Nervous System
- **Myelomeningocele (MMC) (1)**
  - Open spinal cord defect due to the failure of the neural tube to fuse during embryogenesis.
  - One in 3000 live births but greatly depends on ethnic and geographic factors; also higher with anticonvulsants, obesity, diabetes, and low socioeconomic status (2).
  - In an MMC, a portion of the spinal cord and surrounding nerves protrude through the spinal defect. It is thought that exposure of the spinal cord to the amniotic fluid results in progressive neurologic damage, while loss of cerebrospinal fluid (CSF) through the defect causes hindbrain herniation and a Chiari type 2 malformation.
  - Fifteen percent of patients die within the 1st year of life but dependent on severity of defect, hindbrain herniation, and complications. Long-term prognosis is related to location of the defect.
  - Long-term complications may include ventriculomegaly/hydrocephalus, paralysis, breathing and feeding difficulties, learning disabilities, mental retardation, problems with bowel and bladder control, and sexual dysfunction.

Head and Neck
- **Cervical teratoma**
  - Neoplasm composed of all three germ layers located in the region of the neck; 1 in 20,000 to 40,000 live births and 3% to 6% of all teratomas (3).
  - Mortality is 80% to 100% in untreated infants, regardless of size.
    - Forty percent to forty-five percent of mortality secondary to airway obstruction, respiratory compromise related to pulmonary hypoplasia, retention of secretions, pneumonia, and acute hemorrhage of the tumor (4)
    - Increased risk of intrauterine fetal demise (IUFD), polyhydramnios, and preterm labor
  - Complications (2).
    - Laryngotracheomalacia, mandibular hypoplasia, and nerve compression (mandibular nerve, hypoglossal nerve, and recurrent laryngeal nerve) as a result of mass effect.

- ○ Transient or permanent hypoparathyroidism and hypothyroidism due to partial resection of glands or complete replacement by the tumor.
- ○ Developmental delay and mental retardation secondary to asphyxia and anoxia at birth.
- ○ Pulmonary hypoplasia (up to 30% of cases) as a result of hyperextension of the neck, pulling the trachea cephalad and the lungs into the apices of the thoracic cavities (4).
- ○ Rarely, the tumor may extend intracranially with increased morbidity and mortality.
- ○ The rate of malignant transformation is unknown.
- **Epignathus**
  - Teratoma usually originates from the palate or pharynx (Rathke pouch) (3); less than 1% of all teratomas (5); 10% have associated anomalies.
  - High risks of polyhydramnios, preterm labor and delivery, and significant prematurity.
  - High mortality rate secondary to airway obstruction.
- **Lymphangioma (2)**
  - Benign vascular malformation characterized by dilated cystic lymphatics more commonly located in the neck (cystic hygroma), axilla, thorax, and lower extremities; 1 in 1000 to 12,000 pregnancies, depending on inclusion of all perinatal deaths.
  - More than 60% of cases are associated with syndromes or genetic abnormalities.
  - High mortality when associated with nonimmune hydrops.
- **Micrognathia**
  - Malformation characterized by mandibular hypoplasia affecting 1 in 1600 fetuses.
  - Mandibular hypoplasia with posterior displacement of the tongue (glossoptosis) may obstruct the upper airway and predispose the patient to polyhydramnios and preterm labor.
  - Agnathia or otocephaly (total absence of the mandible) is the lethal form.
  - High frequency of associated anomalies and syndromes, including Pierre Robin syndrome (micrognathia, upper airway obstruction, and cleft palate) (2).
  - Poor prognosis is secondary to congenital anomalies.
  - Infants are at risk for aspiration, feeding difficulty, and airway obstruction.
- **Congenital high airway obstruction syndrome (CHAOS)**
  - CHAOS entails complete obstruction of the fetal airway resulting in a constellation of pathognomonic signs (see "Diagnosis" section).
  - Most common cause is laryngeal atresia. Other causes include subglottic stenosis or atresia, laryngeal or tracheal webs, tracheal atresia or agenesis, and laryngeal cyst (6).
  - True incidence is unknown as many of these fetuses die in utero or are stillborn.
  - May be associated with Fraser syndrome: autosomal recessive disorder characterized by laryngeal atresia, cryptophthalmos, syndactyly, and urogenital defects (6).
  - Mortality approaches 100% if no intervention takes place:
    - ○ A relatively better prognosis is seen if a decompressive fistula develops spontaneously in utero with resolution of hydrops and in those without other anomalies (6).
  - The postnatal course of the survivors may be complicated by bronchopulmonary dysplasia, diaphragmatic dysfunction, laryngotracheomalacia, long-term ventilator dependence, profound capillary leak, and liver and intestinal dysfunction.

Cardiothoracic
- **Hypoplastic left heart syndrome (HLHS) with intact or restrictive atrial septum (I/RAS)**
  - Condition of obstructed left ventricular (LV) outflow caused by abnormal development of left-sided cardiac structures including a hypoplastic left ventricle, an atretic or stenotic mitral valve, and a hypoplastic aorta and arch.
  - Constitutes 0.016% to 0.036% of all live births and 1% to 3.8% of all congenital cardiac anomalies (7).
  - HLHS with I/RAS manifests as profound hypoxia and pulmonary venous thickening as a result of in utero pulmonary hypertension and parenchymal damage.

- **Pericardial, cardiac, and mediastinal teratomas (5)**
  - Pericardial teratomas originate from within the pericardium, while the more rare cardiac teratomas originate from the myocardium. Together, these account for 7.5% of teratomas.
  - Mediastinal teratomas are also located in the anterior mediastinum but are noncardiac in origin, accounting for 2% to 3% of teratomas.
  - Pericardial effusion may lead to atriocaval compression and tamponade with subsequent hydrops. Increased risks of IUFD can also be observed with large tumors that cause significant mass effects or hydrops.
  - Survival is 75% for pericardial/cardiac and 69% mediastinal depending on whether pericardial effusions are controlled and surgical resection can be performed (5).
- **Congenital pulmonary airway malformation (CPAM), aka congenital cystic adenomatoid malformation (CCAM)**
  - Multicystic or "solid" mass of pulmonary tissue that can have a minute communication with the tracheobronchial tree and a pulmonary blood supply.
    - Etiology is failure of bronchiolar structure maturation at the fifth to sixth week of gestation versus focal pulmonary dysplasia.
    - Related to a spectrum of lesions as a result of airway obstruction or bronchial atresia (8).
  - One in 25,000 to 35,000 live births with no genetic or recurrence association (2).
  - Predominately a unilobar disease; less than 2% are bilobar.
  - Stocker classification (a histologic classification initially described in 1977 and revised in 2002).
    - Type 0 (formerly acinar dysplasia): Tracheobronchial; 1% to 3% of cases; a lethal, diffuse malformation of the entire lung
    - Type I: Bronchial/bronchiolar; 60% to 70% of cases; single or multiple large cysts
    - Type II: Bronchiolar; 15% to 20% of cases; numerous small diameter (less than 1 cm) cysts; high frequency of associated anomalies
    - Type III: Bronchiolar/alveolar duct; 5% to 10% of cases; large homogenous microcystic masses; cardiac compromise and hydrops more likely
    - Type IV: Distal acinar; 10% of cases; poorly differentiated large cysts (up to 10 cm), and associated with pleuropulmonary blastoma
  - Spontaneous regression is reported, but this may actually be an inability to detect lesions by ultrasound as they become isoechogenic to the surrounding lung or are "outgrown" relative to the fetus (2).
  - Prognosis is related to the size of the lesion and its growth. Mass growth can plateau in relationship to the fetus between 26 and 28 weeks' gestation, decreasing the risk of developing hydrops.
  - Large lesions causing mediastinal shift are at high risk for polyhydramnios, hydrops, and fetal demise. Mortality is 2% to 30% without hydrops but greatly increased when persistent.
  - Long-term complications are malignant transformation (4% risk) and recurrent infection.
- **Bronchopulmonary sequestrations (BPS)**
  - A nonfunctional mass of lung tissue not in communication with the bronchial tree and supplied by an anomalous systemic vessel (usually from the descending aorta) rather than the pulmonary circulation.
  - Intralobar (same pleural cover as normal lung, 75% of cases) versus extralobar (separate pleural cover, intrathoracic or subdiaphragmatic) (2).
  - Hybrid lesions (coexisting CCAM and BPS) have a systemic blood supply.
- **Congenital diaphragmatic hernia (CDH)**
  - Diaphragm defect arising from the failure of the pleuroperitoneal canal to close by 9 to 10 weeks leading to herniation of abdominal contents into the thoracic cavity with resultant pulmonary hypoplasia and pulmonary hypertensive vasculopathy (9).

- One in 3000 to 5000 live births but 1 in 2200 births if all cases of prenatally diagnosed CDH are included (i.e., intrauterine demise and neonatal deaths prior to transfer to tertiary care facility).
- Eighty-five percent to ninety percent are left sided, 10% to 15% are right, and the remaining approximately 2% are bilateral (2).
- Sixty percent are isolated, and forty percent are associated with major anomalies or genetic syndromes such as Cornelia de Lange and Fryns (9).
- Mortality rates in population studies range from 60% to 70% compared to various institution studies with mortality rates less than 30%; this discrepancy, termed "the hidden mortality," refers to a selection bias of not reporting terminations, stillbirths, or those that die before transfer to tertiary centers (10).
- Long-term complications (11).
  - Developmental delay and seizures (related to hypoxic events in neonatal period, extracorporeal membrane oxygenation [ECMO] use) and sensorineural hearing loss (related to prolonged antibiotic and furosemide use)
  - Prolonged ventilatory support, reactive airway disease
  - Failure to thrive, gastroesophageal reflux disease
  - Scoliosis, pectus deformities
- **Fetal hydrothorax**
  - Pleural effusion that is primary (chylous leak) or secondary (associated with immune or nonimmune hydrops) and can be unilateral or bilateral.
  - One in 15,000 pregnancies; the true incidence of primary hydrothorax is unknown due to underdiagnosis, spontaneous resolution, abortion, or death (12).
  - Associated with CDH (20% of cases), congenital heart disease (5%), and chromosomal abnormalities (5%).
  - Mortality for prenatally diagnosed chylothorax is up to 53% (12); improved prognosis when unilateral, tension-free, or spontaneously resolves. Mortality of secondary hydrothorax is related to associated anomalies and/or syndromes.

Abdominal–Pelvic
- **Sacrococcygeal teratoma (SCT)**
  - Teratoma located in the sacrum/coccyx; 1 in 23,000 to 40,000 live births (2).
  - The American Academy of Pediatrics Surgical Section (AAPSS) classification is based on the extent of external and presacral tumor (13):
    - Relates to the ability to make the diagnosis prenatally, ease of resection, and malignant potential secondary to a delay in diagnosis
  - Coexisting anomalies are seen in 11% to 38% of cases, with many related to the development and mass effect of the tumor itself (14).
  - Mortality in neonates with diagnosis made postnatally is 5%. With prenatal diagnosis, the mortality can be greater than 50% (14,15):
    - Postnatal mortality is related to tumor hemorrhages, difficulty of resection, and malignant degeneration.
    - Prenatal mortality is related to high-output cardiac failure (arteriovenous shunting or tumor hemorrhage/anemia), polyhydramnios and premature labor, and dystocia with tumor rupture.
  - Long-term complications.
    - Neurogenic bowel, neurogenic bladder, and renal dysplasia are related to mass effect and obstruction in utero or complications from resection (16).
    - Recurrence rate is 11%. Malignant potential is 5% to 10% if the diagnosis is made prior to 2 months of age or excision performed before 4 months of age. This risk increases to 50% to 90% if the diagnosis is delayed after this (2).
      - Malignant elements are histologically present in 7% to 30% of tumors, but this does not signify malignancy.

Genitourinary Tract
- **Bladder outlet obstruction (BOO)**
  - Also known as lower urinary tract obstruction (LUTO).
  - Posterior urethral valves (PUV) are the most common cause in males (1 in 4000 live births) and account for 10% of all urologic anomalies. Urethral atresia is the most common cause of BOO in females (2). Other causes include urogenital sinus, cloaca, and anterior urethral valves.
  - Presentation can range from normal amniotic fluid to oligohydramnios and anhydramnios, renal dysplasia, and pulmonary hypoplasia when complete obstruction is present.

Multiple Gestations
- **Twin–twin transfusion syndrome (TTTS)**
  - Complication of monochorionic twins resulting from unbalanced blood flow through vascular communications in the placenta (17).
  - TTTS occurs in 5% to 15% of monochorionic twins:
    - Recipient: usually larger, hypervolemic with polyhydramnios; increased vascular preload results in right ventricular (RV) congestive heart failure
    - Donor: usually smaller, growth restricted with oligohydramnios related to poor renal perfusion from hypovolemia and vasoconstriction
  - Quintero TTTS staging (18).
    - I: oligohydramnios in donor twin (deepest vertical pocket [DVP] less than 2 cm) and polyhydramnios in recipient twin (DVP greater than 8 cm)
    - II: nonvisualized bladder in donor
    - III: abnormal Doppler findings in one or both twins
    - IV: hydrops in one or both twins
    - V: death of one or both twins
  - Cincinnati TTTS staging stratifies TTTS into three groups based on severity of cardiomyopathy in the recipient twin (A = mild, B = moderate, C = severe), defined using atrioventricular (AV) regurgitation, RV/LV thickness, and Tei index (17).
  - Other staging systems exist (cardiovascular profile score [CVPS] and Children's Hospital of Philadelphia [CHOP] system) with severity based on points assigned on echocardiographic and Doppler findings (17).
  - Perinatal mortality is 60% to 100% for both twins if untreated (2).
  - Long-term complications include health problems related to prematurity, central nervous system (CNS) sequelae ranging from mild disability or developmental delay to cerebral palsy, mental retardation, cardiomyopathy, and renal failure.
- **Twin reversed arterial perfusion (TRAP) sequence**
  - Anomaly of monochorionic gestation characterized by one twin (acardiac twin) having an absent, rudimentary, or nonfunctioning heart (2).
    - "Pump" twin: the twin with a usually structurally normal heart perfusing the acardiac twin with deoxygenated blood along the umbilical artery, hence, reversed arterial perfusion.
    - Acardiac twin: the twin with rudimentary to no cardiac structure; most common form is absence of the head (anencephalic) with variable development of trunk and limbs (60% to 75% of cases) and hydrops.
  - 1% of monozygotic twins (1 in 35,000 to 50,000 births), but this does not account for early pregnancy losses (2).
  - The risk of aneuploidy is about 9%.
  - When the ratio of the acardiac twin's total body volume to the pump twin's estimated fetal weight exceeds 0.7, the risk of adverse pregnancy outcome is greater than 90% (2,19).
  - Complications are IUFD, polyhydramnios (~50%), preterm labor (~75%), and CNS sequelae.

Other Conditions
- **Amniotic band syndrome (ABS)**
  - A constellation of defects (see "Diagnosis" section) occurring as a result of entrapment of fetal body parts by constrictive tissue bands causing a tourniquet-like effect or disruption of development; 1 in 1200 to 15,000 live births (2).
    - Results from amnion rupture, either spontaneously or secondary to instrumentation.
    - Alternatively, ABS may occur from vascular disruptions.
  - 10% of cases involve the umbilical cord with very high risk of fetal demise without intervention.
- **Chorioangioma**
  - A vascular tumor of placental origin. It is the most common placental tumor, occurring in 0.6% to 1% of placentas, and is benign in histologic presentation.
  - Large tumors (greater than 4 cm) occur 1 in 3500 to 9000 placentas.
  - Etiology is unknown, but it is associated with increased maternal age, diabetes, hypertension, and multiple gestation (20).
  - Complications are polyhydramnios, abruptio placentae, and preterm labor.
  - Fetal risks are anemia, consumptive coagulopathy, growth restriction, prematurity, cardiac failure, and hydrops.
  - Perinatal mortality is 18% to 40% (20).

EVALUATION
History and Physical Exam
- The history should focus on the current obstetric history, past medical history, family history of related abnormalities, and current medical conditions that may affect management strategies, delivery modalities, and possible prenatal interventions.
- Surgical history should be reviewed, particularly if fetoscopic or open fetal procedures are being considered. All procedures that have previously been attempted (e.g., amnioreductions and thoracenteses) should also be reviewed.
- Physical exam should be thorough and include all maternal systems in addition to an evaluation of the fetus.

Laboratory Tests
- Physiologic changes typical of pregnancy should be acknowledged but still recognized as a possible derangement related to the fetal complication.
- Testing should include urinalysis for proteinuria, the presence of which can signify a preeclamptic condition known as maternal mirror syndrome.
- Amniocentesis for karyotype is performed to evaluate for possible chromosome abnormality before subjecting the mother to more invasive procedures.

Fetal Imaging (See "Diagnosis" Section for Specific Findings)
- Ultrasonography, fetal echocardiography, and fetal magnetic resonance imaging (MRI)

DIAGNOSIS
Central Nervous System
- **Myelomeningocele (2)**
  - Maternal serum markers for open neural tube defects include alpha-fetoprotein (from CSF leakage into the amniotic fluid) and acetylcholinesterase.
  - Ultrasonography can identify intracranial findings suspicious for a spinal abnormality earlier (12 to 16 weeks) than visualization of a developed vertebra (21). Vertebral defect level needs to be diagnosed for intervention candidacy.
    - Intracranial findings include small biparietal diameter or head circumference, absent or diminished cerebellum, cerebral ventriculomegaly or hydrocephalus, and lemon (frontal bone scalloping) and banana (compressed cerebellum) signs.

- ○ Arnold-Chiari type 2 malformation characterized by beaking of the tectum, hindbrain herniation, elongation and kinking of the medulla, and obliteration of the cisterna magna.
  - ○ Spinal findings can be better visualized by 16 weeks' gestation and include splaying or widening of the ossification centers, scoliosis or kyphosis, and cystic meningeal sac.
- MRI provides superior visualization of intracranial findings and may serve a role in assessment in situations where evaluations are hindered by maternal body habitus, oligohydramnios, low fetal head position, or posterior position of fetal spine (22).

Head and Neck
- **Cervical teratoma**
  - Ultrasonography defines tumor features, growth, and physiologic effects:
    - ○ Multiloculated, irregular masses with solid and cystic components that are typically well demarcated and unilateral.
      - – Differentiated from cystic hygroma (typically septated cystic masses with poorly defined borders in the posterior neck) and vascular malformations (relatively more vascular lesions usually without calcifications)
    - ○ Evaluate for signs of hydrops and tracheal/esophageal obstruction including a small or empty stomach, hyperextension of the neck (flying fetus sign), and polyhydramnios (seen in 20% to 40% of cases) (2).
  - Echocardiography to diagnose high-output cardiac failure or cardiac compromise.
  - MRI is useful in distinguishing cervical teratomas from lymphangiomas and other diagnoses, as well as intracranial and airway involvement (3).
- **Epignathus**
  - Diagnosis is by ultrasound, which is also used to follow tumor growth similar to a cervical teratoma.
  - MRI is useful in determining intracranial extension of the mass and evaluating the airway (3).
- **Lymphangioma**
  - It usually appears as a septated cystic mass lacking solid components on ultrasonography:
    - ○ Anterior neck location increases the risk of airway obstruction.
    - ○ Posterior neck location has a worse prognosis related to the high incidence of associated anomalies (2).
  - MRI is useful in differentiating from cervical teratomas or diagnosing lymphangiomas in locations other than the neck.
- **Micrognathia**
  - Diagnosis is by ultrasound. It is also important to evaluate the patient for associated anomalies and airway management (23).
    - ○ Jaw index: anterior–posterior mandibular diameter/biparietal diameter × 100; index below fifth percentile has a high risk for an obstructed airway.
    - ○ Polyhydramnios is concerning for airway obstruction.
- **CHAOS (24)**
  - Ultrasound demonstrates pathognomonic signs of large distended and echogenic lungs, an inverted diaphragm, compressed mediastinal structures, a dilated tracheobronchial tree leading to the level of obstruction, and hydrops.
  - Echocardiography is used to evaluate cardiac anatomy and function.
  - MRI allows differentiation of highly echogenic lungs from solid organs and lung lesions such as type III CPAMs. It also provides a larger field of view that may add to or change the initial ultrasound diagnosis, thereby affecting counseling and surgical management.

Cardiothoracic
- **HLHS and I/RAS**
  - Ultrasonography allows initial diagnosis of structurally abnormal heart as well as identification of any other congenital abnormality.

- Echocardiography confirms the diagnosis and evaluates the extent of the structural disease. Size of the interatrial communication, AV valve function, and size of the ascending aorta should be assessed (7).
- **Pericardial, cardiac, and mediastinal teratomas (5)**
  - Ultrasonography demonstrates a cystic and solid mass in the mediastinum, adjacent to the heart, or protruding into a chamber.
  - Echocardiography delineates location of the mass. It also allows assessment of cardiac function and evaluation for cardiac tamponade from a large pericardial effusion.
  - Serial ultrasounds are necessary to monitor for hydrops that can occur as a result of tamponade from a large pericardial effusion or mass effect from an anterior mediastinal mass.
- **CPAM**
  - A solid or cystic lung tumor with the absence of systemic vascular supply.
  - Ultrasonography allows characterization of lung lesion into microcystic (less than 5 mm) versus macrocystic (greater than 5 mm with echolucency) (25).
    - Type 3 (microcystic) lesions appear as a large hyperechogenic mass and have an increased risk of developing hydrops. These lesions can become isoechogenic with surrounding normal lung between 30 and 34 weeks.
    - Doppler can demonstrate lack of systemic vascular flow to possibly rule out bronchopulmonary sequestration or hybrid lesions.
    - CPAM or CCAM volume ratio (CVR) = CPAM or CCAM volume calculated as an ellipse [0.52 × product of all three dimensions of the lung mass] divided by the head circumference (26).
      - CVR greater than 1.6 has greater than 75% chance of developing hydrops.
      - Growth of lesion usually plateaus at 26 weeks, while the fetus continues to grow; risk for developing hydrops is alleviated once the lesion's growth plateaus.
      - However, there is still an underlying risk for pulmonary hypoplasia.
    - Evaluate for associated anomalies such as renal dysgenesis, cardiac abnormalities, jejunal atresia, hydrocephalus, and skeletal anomalies.
  - Echocardiography assessment for cardiac anomalies (e.g., truncus arteriosus and tetralogy of Fallot) and impaired cardiac function secondary to mediastinal shift and ventricular compression.
  - MRI can better delineate these lesions from normal lung tissue and confirm other anatomical findings.
- **BPS**
  - Sonographic diagnosis established by an echodense triangular area of lung tissue with a systemic feeding vessel as noted on Doppler evaluation (25).
    - Polyhydramnios can indicate esophageal obstruction.
    - Pleural effusions and hydrops can be secondary to venous obstruction by compression or torsion of its vascular pedicle.
  - MRI will assist in identifying whether the lesion is intralobar, extralobar, or subdiaphragmatic. It also helps differentiate the lesion (higher T2 signal intensity) from normal lung and other diagnoses, such as foregut duplication.
- **CDH**
  - Ultrasonography requires 3-plane inspection of the chest, noting abnormal location of abdominal viscera or shift of the mediastinum (27).
    - Lung to head ratio (LHR) = 2-dimensional measurement of the lung, at the level of the four-chamber heart, contralateral to the hernia divided by head circumference.
      - LHR less than 1 has increased risk of mortality.
      - Observed to expected LHR (O:E LHR) = LHR divided by normative LHR at a given gestational age. More accurate late gestation. O:E LHR less than 25% is classified as severe with increased mortality.

- ○ Liver herniation can be discerned with Doppler view of "kinked" hepatoportal vessels. Liver herniation into the hemithorax ("liver-up" position) is associated with 57% mortality.
- Echocardiography for structural defects and function.
  - ○ Modified McGoon Index = combined diameters of the pulmonary arteries divided by the diameter of the descending aorta. Ratio of less than 1 correlates to reduced survival and higher incidence of postnatal pulmonary hypertension (28).
- MRI for confirmation of diagnosis, detailed anatomic survey, and lung volumes (27).
  - ○ Total lung volumes (TLV) = lung volume of both lungs measured by trace method or 3D reconstruction software.
  - ○ Percent predicted lung volumes (PPLV) = TLV divided by predicted lung volume (total thoracic volume – mediastinal volume). PPLV less than 15% has 60% mortality, while PPLV greater than 20% has a 100% survival.
- **Fetal hydrothorax**
- Ultrasonography will demonstrate a peripherally located anechoic space surrounding compressed lungs (2).
  - ○ The presence of septations or solid components suggests alternative diagnoses (e.g., CDH, CPAM, and BPS). Also evaluate for other anatomic anomalies.
  - ○ Signs of tension such as mediastinal shift away from the effusion, diaphragmatic flattening or eversion, or polyhydramnios can result in lung hypoplasia, cardiac failure, and hydrops.
- Echocardiography is used to assess for structural defects and signs of cardiac dysfunction.

Abdominal–Pelvic
- **SCT**
  - Alpha-fetoprotein may be elevated prenatally. It is most useful in evaluating for postnatal recurrence following resection.
  - Ultrasound will demonstrate a sacral mass and document tumor growth (29). Note that SCT type IV has no exophytic component, sometimes resulting in the diagnosis being delayed until childhood when it becomes symptomatic.
    - ○ Types/classification is based on the extent of external and presacral tumor (AAPSS) (13).
    - ○ Purely cystic tumors have favorable outcomes compared to solid tumors.
    - ○ Doppler is necessary to monitor for umbilical artery flow reversals and elevated middle cerebral artery velocities indicating possible high-output states.
      - − Hydrops, placentomegaly, hepatomegaly, and polyhydramnios
  - Echocardiography can further evaluate for high-output cardiac failure as noted by a dilated IVC, increased descending aorta flow velocities, increased combined cardiac output, and increased cardiac to thoracic ratios (2).
  - MRI delineates tumor composition and important anatomic relationships, particularly in the setting of pelvic extension where bony shadowing can impact staging and tumor measurements, and also assists in operative planning (30).

Genitourinary Tract
- **BOO**
  - Ultrasonography can diagnose the marked and persistent dilation of the bladder with a thickened wall (greater than 2 mm). A typical "keyhole" appearance of the proximal urethra can be seen with PUV (31).
    - ○ Poor prognostic signs include the presence of subcortical renal cysts, increased echogenicity of the kidneys (i.e., renal dysplasia), and other anatomic anomalies. All of these can be indicative of renal damage, which may exclude the patient from intervention since renal damage may be irreversible.

- ○ The finding of oligohydramnios with the presence of ascites indicates possible rupture of the urinary tract.
- Fetal urine electrolytes are used to follow renal function but are only valid at 20 weeks' gestation or later (31).
  - ○ Sodium less than 100, chloride less than 90, osmolarity less than 210, and β_2-microglobulin less than 6 indicate preserved renal function and favorable prognosis.
- MRI may be more sensitive in defining subcortical cysts and defining pelvic anatomy especially early in gestation.

Multiple Gestations
- **TTTS**
  - Ultrasonography provides data to properly stage TTTS based on amniotic fluid status of both twins, visibility of the bladder, abnormal Doppler finding, and presence of hydrops fetalis. Abnormal Doppler findings (usually in the donor twin) include (2)
    - ○ Absent or reversed end-diastolic velocity in the umbilical artery
    - ○ Reversed flow in the ductus venosus
    - ○ Pulsatile flow in the umbilical vein
  - Echocardiography to evaluate
    - ○ The degree of cardiomyopathy (particularly in the recipient twin) by presence of AV valvular incompetence, ventricular wall thickening, and ventricular function (assessed by Tei index)
    - ○ Risk for congenital hearts defects that present in 7% of all monochorionic/diamniotic twin gestations with a higher incidence in those with TTTS (17)
  - MRI is useful for evaluation of CNS injury (ischemia, hemorrhage, or dilated venous sinuses), which is present in up to 8% of TTTS infants (32).
- **TRAP syndrome**
  - Ultrasonography demonstrates in one twin the absence of normal cardiac structure and movement with possible anencephaly or holoprosencephaly. Other useful findings that may predict increased adverse outcomes include the following:
    - ○ Ratio of estimated fetal weight of acardiac twin (this can be difficult since biometric parameters may be absent or inaccurate) to pump twin is predictive of outcomes. When the ratio exceeds 0.5, adverse pregnancy outcome is approximately 65%, while the risk increases to greater than 90% if the ratio is greater than 0.7 (2,19).
    - ○ Doppler studies can demonstrate reversal of flow in the umbilical artery of the acardiac twin with 67% having a single umbilical artery.
    - ○ Evaluation of structural abnormalities of pump twin.
  - Echocardiography may identify congestive heart failure in the pump twin (AV enlargement, pericardial effusion, tricuspid regurgitation).

Other
- **ABS (33)**
  - Sonographic diagnosis is based on a constellation of abnormalities rather than visualization of actual bands. A band in the absence of defects is not ABS. Defects typical of ABS include
    - ○ Absent digits or limbs or swelling of extremities
    - ○ Craniofacial deformities, encephaloceles, or anencephaly
    - ○ Abdominal wall defects
    - ○ Spinal deformities
    - ○ Limb–body wall complex (anterolateral body wall defect with herniation of abdominal and/or thoracic organs, spinal deformity, limb abnormalities, and craniofacial defects)
  - Echocardiography is useful to evaluate for structural cardiac defects.
  - MRI may better define anatomy and visualization of bands.

- **Chorioangioma (34)**
  - Ultrasonography diagnosis demonstrates a well-circumscribed placental mass with different echogenicity, while Doppler demonstrates presence of blood flow within the mass or feeding vessels.
  - Monitor by serial ultrasound exams for polyhydramnios, appropriate fetal growth and blood flow, and hydrops.
  - Serial fetal echocardiography to monitor for cardiac compromise and high cardiac output states.

TREATMENT (2,35)
Decision for Intervention During Pregnancy
- Consideration for interventions is made when the fetus would otherwise have a high associated morbidity or mortality given the natural history of the fetal condition.
- Deterioration of maternal health is generally a contraindication to fetal intervention. In such situations, emergent delivery is usually the most judicious option.

Anesthesia Considerations (35)
- Conscious sedation and local anesthetics with or without regional anesthesia are usually adequate for percutaneous shunting procedures and straightforward fetoscopic interventions.
- The addition of epidural anesthesia to local anesthetics and intravenous sedatives provides further maternal comfort when the fetoscopic intervention is expected to be more extensive or if more than one port for fetoscopic instruments is needed. This is usually adequate even if conversion to laparotomy is necessary.
- For open fetal surgeries and ex utero intrapartum therapy (EXIT) procedures, anesthesia consists of high concentrations of volatile anesthetic agents to provide optimal uterine relaxation, thereby preserving uterine–placental circulation.
  - Potential anesthesia complications include maternal hypotension and direct fetal cardiac depression, which can be minimized by using supplemented intravenous anesthesia (SIVA) or total intravenous anesthesia (TIVA) after epidural placement and induction until uterine relaxation is needed. At that point, the volatile anesthetic agents are gradually increased to achieve the desired uterine relaxation while decreasing SIVA/TIVA infusion.
  - Maternal blood pressure is maintained using phenylephrine, ephedrine, and prudent use of intravenous fluid boluses.
- A cocktail of fentanyl (5 to 20 mg/kg), atropine (20 mg/kg), and vecuronium (0.2 mg/kg) is administered intramuscularly into the fetus after the fetus is exposed following hysterotomy.
- Maternal monitoring should include electrocardiography, pulse oximetry, blood pressure by cuff and/or arterial catheter, and urine output by Foley catheter.
- Fetal monitoring with open procedures includes pulse oximetry, intraoperative fetal echocardiography, and occasional fetal blood gases if indicated.
- Postoperative pain management following open fetal surgery is usually by epidural.
- Tocolytic options after open fetal surgery are magnesium sulfate, indomethacin (risk for oligohydramnios and fetal ductal constriction), intravenous nitroglycerin, and terbutaline.

Percutaneous Procedures
- Thoracentesis
  - Large fetal hydrothorax with significant lung compression or mediastinal shift
    o Needle aspiration of pleural fluid is performed under ultrasound guidance to determine characteristics of the effusion as well as to decompress the thoracic cavity to allow the lungs to expand/develop (12).

- ○ Differentiate between primary (chylothorax identified by greater than 80% lymphocytes on cell count) and secondary effusion. Pursue further evaluation with viral testing, cultures, and karyotype analysis.
    - ○ A single aspiration may be therapeutic. Repeat thoracentesis may be considered for recurrences. Thoracoamniotic shunting is recommended for large, recurrent pleural effusions nonresponsive to thoracentesis.
- Pericardiocentesis
    - Pericardial effusion resulting in tamponade with cardiac dysfunction or pulmonary hypoplasia. This occurs frequently with mediastinal and pericardial teratomas.
- Thoracoamniotic shunts
    - Indications.
        - ○ Fetal hydrothorax confirmed as primary with recurrence (usually after a second thoracentesis has been performed; note that only 5% to 22% resolve spontaneously) causing mediastinal shift or hydrops. This is associated with greater than 65% survival (12).
        - ○ BPS with mediastinal shift, polyhydramnios, and hydrops secondary to the pleural effusion may be corrected with shunting.
        - ○ CPAM with a single large dominant cyst or several large cysts (see "Unique Therapy" section below).
    - The procedure involves placement of a pigtail catheter (Harrison double-pigtail or Rocket shunt) under local or regional anesthesia, with or without conscious sedation, into the fetal chest with ultrasound guidance, leaving one end of the catheter in the pleural cavity (for pleural effusions) or in the predominant lung cyst and the other end positioned in the amniotic cavity.
    - Potential complications include laceration of the intercostal artery (which can be lethal), shunt failure, or shunt migration. If the shunt is not visible in the baby's chest at delivery, retained shunt in the mother or internalization of the shunt into the baby should be ruled out. The shunt should be removed after birth and an occlusive dressing applied to avoid pneumothorax. Postnatal chest radiograph is performed shortly after birth to guide further therapy.
- Vesicoamniotic shunts (see BOO in the "Unique Therapy" section below)

OPEN FETAL SURGERY

- General considerations (2,35)
    - Intraoperative ultrasound is used to locate the placenta and plan the hysterotomy.
    - Hysterotomy is performed using an absorbable uterine stapling device to minimize bleeding.
    - Maintenance of uterine volume by leaving as much of the fetus in the uterine cavity as possible along with constant or intermittent infusion of warmed lactated Ringer solution into the uterine cavity (to minimize the risk of cord compression).
    - Once the fetus is exposed, vascular access is obtained preferably using a peripheral IV line. This is then used to administer fluid, blood, and medications.
    - Infusion of warmed lactated Ringer solution (to restore fluid volume) and administration of intraamniotic antibiotics prior to completion hysterotomy closure.
    - Aggressive tocolytic regimens are required postoperatively.
    - Potential complications associated with open fetal surgery include hemorrhage, chorioamniotic separation, leakage of amniotic fluid, preterm premature rupture of membrane (PPROM), preterm labor, hysterotomy dehiscence or uterine rupture, and need for repeat cesarean section for delivery.
- **MMC**
    - Goal of prenatal MMC repair is to prevent secondary injury to nerves from amniotic fluid exposure, direct trauma, or hydrostatic pressure and thereby improve neurologic outcomes (1).

- Management of MMC study (MOMS) trial (36).
  - ○ Randomized, prospective trial started in 2003 and concluded in 2011 evaluating outcomes of prenatal versus postnatal repair of MMC.
  - ○ Inclusion criteria: maternal age greater than 18 years of age, 19 to 25 6/7 weeks' gestation, normal karyotype, upper boundary of MMC between T1 and S1, and Arnold-Chiari II malformation.
  - ○ Refer to the cited article for complete exclusion criteria.
  - ○ Results demonstrated that 40% of the prenatally repaired group required ventriculoperitoneal shunting compared to 82% of postnatally repaired group. Improved hindbrain herniation, mental development, and motor function were also observed.
  - ○ However, prenatal repair was associated with increased risks of spontaneous ruptured membranes (46%), oligohydramnios (21%), preterm delivery (79%), and various hysterotomy dehiscences (10%).
- After laparotomy/hysterotomy, the MMC defect is closed primarily or with a prosthetic patch; the skin is then closed over the dura primarily or, if tension was present, with the use of relaxing incisions or a biologic patch. Refer to MOMS trial publication for complete surgical details (36).
- **SCT**
- Goal of open fetal surgery for SCT is to debulk the tumor by removing the exophytic portion of the SCT to reverse the high cardiac output state.
- Indications for surgical consideration include signs of cardiac failure or early hydrops and usually less than 27 weeks' gestation (gestational age too early to deliver secondary to mortality/morbidity of prematurity) (14,15).
- The procedure involves delivery of the tumor through a hysterotomy while the fetal head, torso, and upper extremities remain in the uterus. The tumor is dissected free of the perineal structures, the anus, and the rectum. The tumor base is usually transected using a thick tissue stapling device, and the skin is reapproximated. The fetus is then returned into the amniotic cavity, the hysterotomy closed, and the maternal laparotomy repaired.

Fetoscopic Surgery
- General considerations
  - Intraoperative ultrasound is used to plan the approach after fetal position, placental edges, and placental cord insertion are mapped out.
  - Potential complications are similar to open approaches but less prevalent because of the minimally invasive approach. The smaller fetoscopic incisions have very low risk of uterine dehiscence and do not mandate cesarean delivery. Therefore, they may allow future vaginal deliveries unless obstetrically contraindicated.
- **Selective fetoscopic laser photocoagulation**
  - TTTS
    - ○ Goal of selective fetoscopic laser photocoagulation (SFLP) is to coagulate all superficial placental connecting vessels between the fetuses to interrupt their vascular communication.
    - ○ Several studies have shown SFLP to be the preferred therapy over serial amnioreductions when available, demonstrating improved overall survival greater than 80%, survival of at least one of the paired twins greater than 90%, and better neurologic outcomes (37,38).
    - ○ Adjunctive maternal therapy with nifedipine to treat the hypertensive cardiomyopathy in the recipient twin 24 to 48 hours prior to laser therapy has been reported to improve survival in recipient twins. The patient is maintained on nifedipine (20 mg po every 6 hours) after laser therapy until complete resolution of twin cardiomyopathy (39).
- Fetoscopic devascularization of chorioangioma

- ° Indications include high cardiac output state related to the chorioangioma, hydrops fetalis, or evidence of imminent fetal demise; lesions greater than 4 to 5 cm are high risk (20,40).
- ° Techniques used to devascularize the tumor include
  - ‐ Bipolar cauterization
  - ‐ Laser photocoagulation
  - ‐ Vascular clip
  - ‐ Or any combination of these techniques to stop the blood supply to the tumor
- ° Other reported techniques include ultrasound-guided interstitial laser therapy, in utero endoscopic suture ligation, and microcoil embolization. Although injection of absolute alcohol had been reported, theoretically, there is an increased risk of fetal injury from dissemination of alcohol into fetal circulation.
- • Fetoscopic release of amniotic bands
  - ° Indications include cord involvement at risk for fetal demise and threatened limbs or body parts as indicated by visualization of a constricting band, edema, and abnormal Doppler flow related to the amniotic band (41).
  - ° The bands may be cut and lysed using microsciscors or laser.
  - ° Patients are at risk for preterm labor and PPROM.
  - ° Despite band lysis, limbs may have secondary lymphedema or fail to grow.
  - ° Postnatal orthopedic or plastic surgeries may be necessary for extremity or facial deformities. Abdominal defects, if present, are usually repaired after birth following lysis of abdominal bands.
- • **Radiofrequency ablation (RFA)**
  - • TRAP sequence
    - ° The goal of therapy is to completely interrupt the umbilical circulation to the acardiac twin.
    - ° The technique uses thermal energy created by high-frequency radio waves to coagulate the umbilical cord of the acardiac twin. The tines of the RFA device are deployed intrafetally to minimize thermal injury to the pump twin.
    - ° Use of sclerosing agents, coils, fetoscopic cord ligation, photocoagulation, and thermocoagulation has been reported with varying degrees of success (42).
    - ° Eighty percent to ninety-five percent survival rate of pump twin reported (19).
  - • Tumors
    - ° RFA of tumors such as SCT and lung lesions has been reported but with increased risk of thermal injury and destruction of surrounding tissues.
- • **Fetoscopic endotracheal occlusion (FETO) (43,44)**
  - • CDH
    - ° Goal of fetoscopic intervention is to place a detachable balloon in the fetal trachea between 26 and 28 weeks' gestation (this may broaden to 24 to 30 weeks) under direct fetoscopic view to block the normal egress of lung fluid, increasing airway pressure, thereby accelerating lung growth. The tracheal occlusion is usually reversed around 34 weeks' gestation by ultrasound-guided puncture or fetoscopic retrieval.
    - ° European FETO consortium provided data in a prospective nonrandomized trial demonstrating improved survival in patients with O:E LHR less than 25% to 49%.
    - ° Pitfalls included PPROM (25% prior to 34 weeks) and airway management difficulties due to delivery prior to balloon removal.
    - ° Evaluation through a multicenter, prospective randomized study is currently under way to assess outcomes compared to current management strategies.
- • **Fetoscopic decompression of atretic airway or CHAOS (45)**
  - • The goal is to convert a completely obstructed airway to a partial obstruction with resolution of hydrops. Further studies are required to decide on the utility of this therapy.
- • **Fetoscopic release of BOO (see "Unique Therapy" section)**

Ex Utero Intrapartum Therapy (46,47)
- General considerations
  - Allows time and a controlled environment for indicated procedures to be performed on the high-risk fetus right before delivery. The uteroplacental blood flow and fetal gas exchange are maintained by optimizing uterine relaxation through the use of inhalation anesthetic agents.
  - Maternal risks.
    - Patients are at risk of uterine atony following delivery that may result in severe maternal hemorrhage requiring hysterectomy. Bleeding risk is minimized by allowing the uterine tone to return prior to umbilical cord ligation and delivery of the baby following discontinuation of volatile anesthetic agents and administration of oxytocin. Blood loss is further decreased with the use of a uterine stapling device for the hysterotomy.
    - Possibility of immediate delivery prior to completion of fetal intervention in the setting of maternal complications, abruption, increased uterine tone, or loss of uteroplacental gas exchange.
    - If a low transverse hysterotomy cannot be utilized for the EXIT procedure, the patient will need to be managed like a patient with a history of classical cesarean for future pregnancies.
  - Other pitfalls can include (2)
    - Failure to maintain adequate uterine volume and relaxation
    - Failure to monitor mother and fetus adequately and recognize decompensation
    - Failure to recognize fetal and maternal indications for terminating the EXIT procedure
- Indications
  - **EXIT to airway**
    - CHAOS
    - Cervical teratomas
    - Epignathus
    - Large cystic hygroma or lymphatic malformations with airway involvement
    - Carefully selected patients with severe micrognathia (jaw index of less than fifth percentile without lethal anomalies)
    - Other forms of internal or external airway obstruction
  - **EXIT to resection of high-risk tumors**
    - Large intrathoracic mass (CPAM, BPS, complete unilateral bronchial atresia, mediastinal teratoma, pericardial teratoma) with significant mediastinal shift and airway deviation/compression, and the baby is expected to have significant risk of cardiopulmonary compromise shortly after birth.
    - SCT with same indications for open fetal resection but greater than 27 weeks' gestation (15).
  - **EXIT to ECMO or cesarean section delivery with ECMO standby**
    - Severe CDH (LHR less than 1, O:E LHR less than 25%, liver up, TLV less than 18 mL, PPLV less than 15%)
    - Severe cardiac disease: HLHS with I/RAS or aortic stenosis with I/RAS
    - Other conditions where immediate cardiopulmonary collapse or instability is expected once separation from the placenta (i.e., delivery) occurs
  - EXIT for separation of conjoined twins

Unique Therapy Options for Specific Diagnoses
- **HLHS with I/RAS or aortic stenosis with HLHS**
  - Cesarean delivery of HLHS with I/RAS patients in a hybrid cardiac catheterization laboratory is advocated to facilitate potential cardiac intervention while decreasing morbidity/mortality associated with transport and logistics (48).

- Percutaneous balloon valvuloplasty (49) for aortic stenosis with evolving HLHS.
  - Up to 40% of these fetuses develop moderate to severe aortic regurgitation, with a majority of infants still requiring a repeat valvuloplasty or intervention postnatally.
- Percutaneous balloon atrial septostomy (49) for HLHS with I/RAS.
  - Surgical survival has only been 58%, but fetal intervention leaving an atrial septal defect greater than 3 mm (by ballooning alone or stent placement) has resulted in higher oxygen saturation at birth and less urgency to perform decompression.
- **CPAM**
  - Percutaneous thoracoamniotic shunting of a dominant cyst should be considered at the earliest sign of hydrops.
  - Maternal steroids (betamethasone 12.5 mg intramuscularly q24 hours × 2 doses) should be considered in cases complicated by hydrops fetalis or cases with CVR greater than 1.6 (where the risk of developing hydrops is ~75%) (50–52).
    - If the growth of the solid component of the lesion slows down following steroid administration, resolution of the hydrops may occur. Survival improves to greater than 85% if hydrops resolves.
    - A repeat course of maternal steroids may be necessary, but results are variable (50–52).
  - Open fetal surgery should be considered for CPAM with persistent hydrops refractory to steroids or large cystic lesions not responsive to shunting procedures (35).
    - The goal is to resect the lung lesion, eliminating mass effect and mediastinal shift while preserving as much normal lung as possible.
    - The procedure involves exposure of the chest ipsilateral to the lesion. A thoracotomy is performed with lobectomy, although resection of multiple lobes or pneumonectomy may be required depending on the extent of the lesion.
  - EXIT procedure should be considered if the fetus is expected to have high risk of cardiorespiratory compromise with conventional therapy after birth. In such situations, EXIT allows resection of the lung lesion, decompression of the airway, and placement on ECMO if indicated while on placental support.
- **BOO (2,30,35)**
  - Vesicoamniotic (VA) shunting can be used to bypass the BOO, albeit not completely decompressing the urinary tract:
    - VA shunt can become obstructed or displaced. Functional shunt failure occurs in 40% to 50% of cases following successful placement.
    - Survival following shunting ranges from 40% to 85%.
    - Despite restoring amniotic fluid with good pulmonary outcomes, 50% of patients develop renal failure secondary to ongoing dysplastic changes in the kidney from significant intravesical pressure.
  - Fetoscopic release of BOO is a potential option for those with PUV, severe oligohydramnios or anhydramnios, and a favorable urinalysis results and preserved renal parenchyma.
    - A fetoscope is placed in the uterus through small incisions and used to inspect and pass instruments into the fetal bladder and urethra. Fetal cystoscopy is used to disrupt the valves by hydroablation, guide wire passage, or laser ablation.
    - Long-term outcomes still need to be shown compared to other therapies.
  - Open vesicostomy should be considered in patients with PUV, oligohydramnios, and a favorable prognosis. However, this approach still needs to be proven more effective than shunting or fetoscopic intervention to justify increased risks to mother and fetus.
    - The procedure requires amnioinfusion prior to hysterotomy because of oligohydramnios. The fetal bladder is exposed and marsupialized to the skin through an incision below the umbilical cord, with complete urinary diversion and pressure resolution.
    - Benefits from definitive decompression and protection of bladder and kidneys. Complications are similar to other open fetal procedures.

686 | Part V • Fetal Complications

- Amnioport placement for serial amnioinfusion may be used as an adjunct therapy for patients with severe oligohydramnios to achieve better pulmonary outcome. Its potential benefits when compared to serial needle amnioinfusion include decreased risk of membrane rupture, infection, maternal discomfort, and maternal and fetal injuries. Its impact on outcome is currently being evaluated.

PATIENT EDUCATION

More information about fetal therapy and patient support can be found at the following locations:
- North American Fetal Therapy Network (NAFTnet): http://www.naftnet.org/
- Society for Maternal-Fetal Medicine (SMFM): www.smfm.org
- Fetology: Diagnosis and management of the fetal patient (textbook-reference below) (53)

REFERENCES

1. Adzick NS. Fetal surgery for spina bifida: past, present, future. *Semin Pediatr Surg.* 2013; 22(1):10–17.
2. Bianchi DW, et al. *Fetology : diagnosis and management of the fetal patient.* 2nd ed. New York: McGraw-Hill Medical Pub, Division. xix, 2010:1004.
3. Tonni G, et al. Cervical and oral teratoma in the fetus: a systematic review of etiology, pathology, diagnosis, treatment and prognosis. *Arch Gynecol Obstet.* 2010;282(4):355–361.
4. Wolfe K, et al. Fetal cervical teratoma: what is the role of fetal MRI in predicting pulmonary hypoplasia? *Fetal Diagn Ther.* 2013;33(4):252–256.
5. Isaacs H, Jr. Perinatal (fetal and neonatal) germ cell tumors. *J Pediatr Surg.* 2004;39(7): 1003–1013.
6. Roybal JL, et al. Predicting the severity of congenital high airway obstruction syndrome. *J Pediatr Surg.* 2010;45(8):1633–1639.
7. Connor JA, Thiagarajan R. Hypoplastic left heart syndrome. *Orphanet J Rare Dis.* 2007;2:23.
8. Kunisaki SM, et al. Bronchial atresia: the hidden pathology within a spectrum of prenatally diagnosed lung masses. *J Pediatr Surg.* 2006;41(1):61–65; discussion 61–65.
9. Pober BR. Genetic aspects of human congenital diaphragmatic hernia. *Clin Genet.* 2008;74(1):1–15.
10. Mah VK, et al. Are we making a real difference? Update on 'hidden mortality' in the management of congenital diaphragmatic hernia. *Fetal Diagn Ther.* 2011;29(1):40–45.
11. Peetsold MG, et al. The long-term follow-up of patients with a congenital diaphragmatic hernia: a broad spectrum of morbidity. *Pediatr Surg Int.* 2009;25(1):1–17.
12. Deurloo KL, et al. Isolated fetal hydrothorax with hydrops: a systematic review of prenatal treatment options. *Prenat Diagn.* 2007;27(10):893–899.
13. Altman RP, et al. Sacrococcygeal teratoma: American Academy of Pediatrics Surgical Section Survey-1973. *J Pediatr Surg.* 1974;9(3):389–398.
14. Wilson RD, et al. Sacrococcygeal teratomas: prenatal surveillance, growth and pregnancy outcome. *Fetal Diagn Ther.* 2009;25(1):15–20.
15. Roybal JL, et al. Early delivery as an alternative management strategy for selected high-risk fetal sacrococcygeal teratomas. *J Pediatr Surg.* 2011;46(7):1325–1332.
16. Le LD, et al. Prenatal and postnatal urologic complications of sacrococcygeal teratomas. *J Pediatr Surg.* 2011;46(6):1186–1190.
17. Habli M, et al. Twin-to-twin transfusion syndrome: a comprehensive update. *Clin Perinatol.* 2009;36(2):391–416, x.
18. Quintero RA, et al. Staging of twin-twin transfusion syndrome. *J Perinatol.* 1999;19(8 Pt 1): 550–555.
19. Livingston JC, et al. Intrafetal radiofrequency ablation for twin reversed arterial perfusion (TRAP): a single-center experience. *Am J Obstet Gynecol.* 2007;197(4):399.e1–399.e3.
20. Zanardini C, et al. Giant placental chorioangioma: natural history and pregnancy outcome. *Ultrasound Obstet Gynecol.* 2010;35(3):332–336.

21. Blumenfeld Z, et al. The early diagnosis of neural tube defects. *Prenat Diagn.* 1993;13(9): 863–871.

22. Glenn OA, Barkovich J. Magnetic resonance imaging of the fetal brain and spine: an increasingly important tool in prenatal diagnosis: part 2. *AJNR Am J Neuroradiol.* 2006;27(9):1807–1814.

23. Lee W, et al. Three-dimensional ultrasonographic presentation of micrognathia. *J Ultrasound Med.* 2002;21(7):775–781.

24. Mong A, et al. Congenital high airway obstruction syndrome: MR/US findings, effect on management, and outcome. *Pediatr Radiol.* 2008;38(11):1171–1179.

25. Cavoretto P, et al. Prenatal diagnosis and outcome of echogenic fetal lung lesions. *Ultrasound Obstet Gynecol.* 2008;32(6):769–783.

26. Crombleholme TM, et al. Cystic adenomatoid malformation volume ratio predicts outcome in prenatally diagnosed cystic adenomatoid malformation of the lung. *J Pediatr Surg.* 2002;37(3):331–338.

27. Kline-Fath BM. Current advances in prenatal imaging of congenital diaphragmatic [corrected] hernia. *Pediatr Radiol.* 2012;42(suppl 1):S74–S90.

28. Vuletin JF, et al. Prenatal pulmonary hypertension index: novel predictor of severe postnatal pulmonary artery hypertension in antenatally diagnosed congenital diaphragmatic hernia. *J Pediatr Surg.* 2010;45(4):703–708.

29. Neubert S, et al. Sonographic prognostic factors in prenatal diagnosis of SCT. *Fetal Diagn Ther.* 2004;19(4):319–326.

30. Danzer E, et al. Diagnosis and characterization of fetal sacrococcygeal teratoma with prenatal MRI. *AJR Am J Roentgenol.* 2006;187(4):W350–W356.

31. Ruano R. Fetal surgery for severe lower urinary tract obstruction. *Prenat Diagn.* 2011; 31(7):667–674.

32. Kline-Fath BM, et al. Twin-twin transfusion syndrome: cerebral ischemia is not the only fetal MR imaging finding. *Pediatr Radiol.* 2007;37(1):47–56.

33. Neuman J, et al. Prenatal imaging of amniotic band sequence: utility and role of fetal MRI as an adjunct to prenatal US. *Pediatr Radiol.* 2012;42(5):544–551.

34. Zalel Y, et al. Role of color Doppler imaging in diagnosing and managing pregnancies complicated by placental chorioangioma. *J Clin Ultrasound.* 2002;30(5):264–269.

35. Mattei P. *Fundamentals of pediatric surgery,* xxviii. New York: Springer, 2011:921.

36. Adzick NS, et al. A randomized trial of prenatal versus postnatal repair of myelomeningocele. *N Engl J Med.* 2011;364(11):993–1004.

37. Crombleholme TM, et al. A prospective, randomized, multicenter trial of amnioreduction vs selective fetoscopic laser photocoagulation for the treatment of severe twin-twin transfusion syndrome. *Am J Obstet Gynecol.* 2007;197(4): 96.e1–96.e9.

38. Rossi AC, D'Addario V. Laser therapy and serial amnioreduction as treatment for twin-twin transfusion syndrome: a metaanalysis and review of literature. *Am J Obstet Gynecol.* 2008; 198(2):147–152.

39. Crombleholme TM, et al. Improved recipient survival with maternal nifedipine in twin-twin transfusion syndrome complicated by TTTS cardiomyopathy undergoing selective fetoscopic laser photocoagulation. *Am J Obstet Gynecol.* 2010;203(4): 397.e1–397.e9.

40. Jones K, et al. Fetoscopic laser photocoagulation of feeding vessels to a large placental chorioangioma following fetal deterioration after amnioreduction. *Fetal Diagn Ther.* 2012; 31(3):191–195.

41. Keswani SG, et al. In utero limb salvage: fetoscopic release of amniotic bands for threatened limb amputation. *J Pediatr Surg.* 2003;38(6):848–851.

42. Tan TY, Sepulveda W. Acardiac twin: a systematic review of minimally invasive treatment modalities. *Ultrasound Obstet Gynecol.* 2003;22(4):409–419.

43. DeKoninck P, et al. Results of the fetal endoscopic tracheal occlusion for congenital diaphragmatic hernia and the set up of the randomized controlled TOTAL trial. *Early Hum Dev.* 201187(9):619–624.

44. Deprest JA, et al. Fetal surgery for congenital diaphragmatic hernia is back from never gone. *Fetal Diagn Ther.* 2011;29(1):6–17.

45. Saadai P, et al. Long-term outcomes after fetal therapy for congenital high airway obstructive syndrome. *J Pediatr Surg.* 2012;47(6):1095–1100.
46. Moldenhauer JS. Ex utero intrapartum therapy. *Semin Pediatr Surg.* 2013;22(1):44–49.
47. Morris LM, et al. Ex utero intrapartum treatment procedure: a peripartum management strategy in particularly challenging cases. *J Pediatr.* 2009;154(1):126.e3–131.e3.
48. Michelfelder E, et al. Hypoplastic left heart syndrome with intact atrial septum: Utilization of a hybrid catheterization facility for cesarean section delivery and prompt neonatal intervention. *Catheter Cardiovasc Interv.* 2008;72(7):983–987.
49. McElhinney DB, et al. Current status of fetal cardiac intervention. *Circulation.* 2010;121(10):1256–1263.
50. Curran PF, et al. Prenatal steroids for microcystic congenital cystic adenomatoid malformations. *J Pediatr Surg.* 2010;45(1):145–150.
51. Morris LM, et al. High-risk fetal congenital pulmonary airway malformations have a variable response to steroids. *J Pediatr Surg.* 2009;44(1):60–65.
52. Peranteau WH, et al. Effect of maternal betamethasone administration on prenatal congenital cystic adenomatoid malformation growth and fetal survival. *Fetal Diagn Ther.* 2007;22(5):365–371.

Neonatal Resuscitation

Brett H. Siegfried, Kenneth F. Tiffany and Glen A. Green

KEY POINTS

- At least one person qualified to perform neonatal resuscitation should be in attendance at every delivery.
- Anticipation and preparation are critical for a smooth, successful resuscitation.
- The key characteristics for determining the need for further resuscitation after the initial steps of stabilization are respirations and heart rate.
- The most important and effective action in neonatal resuscitation is to ventilate the infant's lungs with blended air.
- The steps of evaluation, decision, and action outlined in the algorithm of resuscitation of the newborn infant should be followed to ensure optimal neonatal resuscitation.
- Not initiating or discontinuing neonatal resuscitation may be appropriate in certain circumstances.

BACKGROUND

Definition

Hypoxic ischemic encephalopathy (HIE) usually involves a complex combination of hypoxemia, hypercapnia, and circulatory insufficiency that may be induced by a variety of perinatal events.

Pathophysiology

Physiologic Changes During Hypoxia

- The events that occur during hypoxia in the human newborn probably are analogous to those that occur in the fetal primate model described by Dawes (1) (Fig. 38-1):
  - The initial brief response to hypoxia is one of hypertension and hypercapnia.
  - A period of primary apnea then occurs, followed by gasping in an effort to establish respirations.
  - If there is no reversal of the hypoxia, the fetus enters a phase of secondary apnea, bradycardia, and shock.
  - At this point, central nervous system and multisystem organ damage begins to occur. If resuscitative measures are not initiated, the infant will die.
  - Decreased central nervous system blood flow and hypoxemia may lead to cerebral edema and hypoxic ischemic encephalopathy. Further neurologic injury also may occur as the result of hemorrhage in ischemic and damaged portions of the brain.

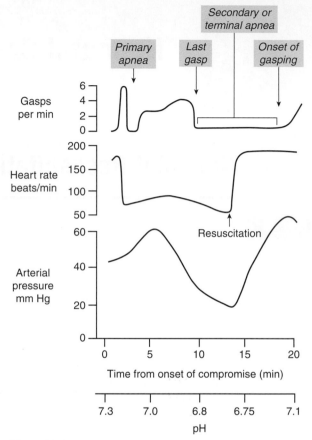

Figure 38-1. Sequence of physiologic events in animal models from multiple species involving complete total asphyxia. Note the prompt increase in heart rate as soon as resuscitation has begun. (Used with permission of the American Academy of Pediatrics. *Textbook of neonatal resuscitation.* 6th ed. American Academy of Pediatrics and American Heart Association, 2011.)

• Primary and secondary apnea cannot be easily distinguished in the clinical setting. Therefore, any apnea at birth is assumed to be secondary apnea, and neonatal resuscitation should be initiated as taught in the American Heart Association–American Academy of Pediatrics Neonatal Resuscitation Program (NRP) (2).

Etiology

Although the causes of neonatal cardiopulmonary depression and hypoxia are often unknown, many causes have been identified, including drugs, trauma, hemorrhage, developmental anomalies, infection, and iatrogenic causes. Some of the common causes of neonatal hypoxia ischemia are summarized in Table 38-1.

Table 38-1	Causes of Neonatal Cardiorespiratory Depression and Hypoxia	
Etiology	**Example**	**Major effect**
Maternal drugs	Anesthetics, narcotics, alcohol, magnesium sulfate, sedatives	Respiratory depression
Physical/mechanical trauma	Prolapsed cord, abruptio placentae ruptured umbilical cord, forceps, breech delivery	Interruption of blood supply, hypovolemia, shock
Maternal illness	Infant of diabetic mother, maternal group B *Streptococcus* infection, toxemia, Rh disease	Cardiopulmonary insufficiency, polycythemia, hypoglycemia, anemia
Development	Congenital heart disease, diaphragmatic hernia, choanal atresia, Intrauterine infection	Cardiac and pulmonary insufficiency
Environmental	Delivery in cool environment, lack of heat source	Hypothermia
Postmaturity	Meconium aspiration syndrome, persistent pulmonary hypertension	Pneumonia, pulmonary hypertension
Iatrogenic	Pulmonary air leak resulting from excessive inflation pressure with resuscitation	Pulmonary and cardiac dysfunction

Epidemiology

Many newborn infants may experience some degree of cardiorespiratory depression, characterized by a heart rate less than 100 beats/min (bpm), some degree of hypotension, and hypoventilation and/or apnea in the delivery room. However, true intrapartum hypoxia occurs in approximately 1.5 per 1000 term live births (3). HIE has a worldwide mortality of 10% to 60% of affected infants, and approximately 25% of survivors have long-term neurodevelopmental delay (4).

TREATMENT

Goal of Resuscitation

- The aim of a successful resuscitation should be the immediate reversal of hypoxemia, hypercapnia, and circulatory insufficiency to prevent permanent damage to the central nervous system or other organs. This can be accomplished by means that are directed at
  - Reducing oxygen consumption by drying the infant and conducting the resuscitation on a radiant warmer
  - Clearing the airway of secretions, meconium, and other material
  - Performing effective positive-pressure ventilation (PPV)
  - Maintaining adequate perfusion to the vital organs

Procedures

The following discussion is a summary of the guidelines of the American Heart Association–American Academy of Pediatrics NRP based on the *Textbook of Neonatal Resuscitation*, sixth edition (2).

Principles of Successful Resuscitation

- Anticipation.
  - Good communication between the care providers for the mother and the neonatal resuscitation team is critical:

- Pertinent information in the perinatal history that may affect the infant should be disclosed.
- A review of the mother's medical chart and medication record is recommended before delivery if possible.
- A successful resuscitation depends on
  - Anticipating a clinical situation likely to require neonatal resuscitation
  - Having a skilled team available to respond to a compromised infant
- Personnel.
  - At least one person demonstrating competence at neonatal resuscitation, preferably with NRP certification, should be present at every delivery.
  - If the newborn is severely depressed, there should be at least two people at the resuscitation:
    - One person to ventilate and intubate if necessary
    - A second person to monitor the heart rate and perform chest compressions if needed
  - If prolonged resuscitation is required, a team of three or more people is recommended.
  - The resuscitation team members must not only know what tasks to perform but must be able to perform these tasks efficiently and effectively.
- Equipment and preparation.
  - Appropriate resuscitation equipment and medications must be immediately available, and equipment must be in working order (Table 38-2).
  - If there is enough time before delivery, the resuscitation team should
    - Check the equipment to make sure it is functioning properly.
    - Ensure blended oxygen and suction are available.
    - Ensure ample heat (radiant warmer) is available.
    - Draw up medications if appropriate.
    - Introduce themselves to the parents, and explain the procedures to be completed and the difficulties that may be expected.
  - Universal precautions should be followed because blood and other body fluid exposures are possible in the delivery room.
- The ABCs of resuscitation should be followed.
  - Airway
    - Establish an open airway by positioning the infant to maximize the airway.
    - Suction the mouth, nose, and, in some cases, the trachea to ensure an open airway.
    - Endotracheal tube (ETT) intubation may be necessary to ensure a patent airway in some situations.
  - Breathing
    - Breathing can be stimulated by tactile stimulation (optional).
    - If necessary, PPV may be administered via a bag and mask, a T-piece device, or an ETT.
  - Circulation
    - Stimulate and maintain circulation of blood with chest compressions, fluids, or drugs when indicated.

Initial Steps in Resuscitation
- Initial evaluation.
  - Within a few seconds of life, the initial assessment of the newborn should be performed and the need for routine care or further neonatal resuscitation determined.
  - The algorithm (Fig. 38-2) shows the steps of evaluation, decision, and action.
  - The resuscitator should rely on respiratory effort, heart rate, and color to evaluate the infant's condition. If, as a result of assessing these signs, the infant is determined to be in distress, the resuscitator should initiate measures long before the 1-minute Apgar score is assigned.

Table 38-2   Neonatal Resuscitation Supplies and Equipment

Suction equipment
  Bulb syringe
  Mechanical suction and tubing
  Suction catheters, 5F or 6F, 8F, and 10F, 12F, or 14F
  8-F feeding tube and 20-mL syringe
  Meconium aspiration device
Bag and mask equipment
  Device for delivering positive-pressure ventilation, capable of delivering 90%–100% oxygen
  Face masks, newborn and premature sizes (cushioned rim masks preferred)
  Oxygen source
  Compressed air source
  Oxygen blender to mix oxygen and compressed air with flowmeter (flow rate up to 10 L/min) and tubing
  Pulse oximeter and oximeter probe
Intubation equipment
  Laryngoscope with straight blades, No. 0 (preterm) and No. 1 (term)
  Extra bulbs and batteries for laryngoscope
  Tracheal tubes, 2.5-, 3.0-, 3.5-, and 4.0-mm internal diameter (ID)
  Stylet (optional)
  Scissors
  Tape or securing device for tracheal tube
  Alcohol sponges
  CO_2 detector or capnograph
  Laryngeal mask airway
Medications
  Epinephrine 1:10,000 (0.1 mg/mL)—3-mL or 10-mL ampules
  Isotonic crystalloid (normal saline or Ringer lactate) for volume expansion—100 or 250 mL
  Dextrose 10%, 250 mL
  Normal saline for flushes
Umbilical vessel catheterization supplies
  Umbilical catheters, 3.5F, 5F
  Three-way stopcock
  Syringes, 1, 3, 5, 10, 20, and 50 mL
  Needles, 25-, 21-, and 18-gauge or puncture device for needleless system
Miscellaneous
  Gloves and appropriate personal protection
  Radiant warmer or other heat source
  Firm, padded resuscitation surface
  Clock with second hand (timer optional)
  Warmed linens
  Stethoscope (with neonatal head)
  Tape, ½ or ¾ inch
  Cardiac monitor and electrodes or pulse oximeter with probe (optional for delivery room)
  Oropharyngeal airways (0, 00, and 000 sizes or 30-, 40-, and 50-mm lengths)
For very preterm babies
  Size 00 laryngoscope blade (optional)
  Reclosable, food grade plastic bag (1-gallon size) or plastic wrap
  Chemically activated warming pad (optional)
  Transport incubator to maintain baby's temperature during move to the nursery

Used with permission of the American Academy of Pediatrics, *Textbook of Neonatal Resuscitation*, 6th edition, copyright American Academy of Pediatrics and American Heart Association, 2011.

Newborn Resuscitation

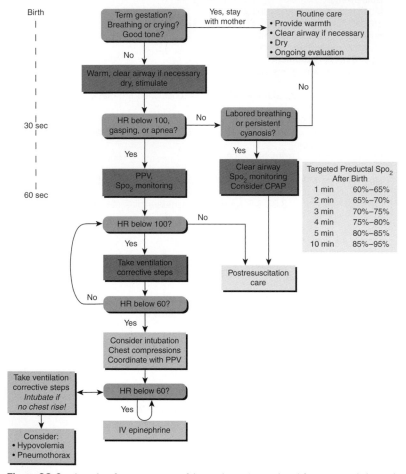

Figure 38-2. Algorithm for resuscitation of the newborn. (Reproduced from Kattwinkel J, et al. Part 15: neonatal resuscitation: 2010 American Heart Association Guidelines for cardiopulmonary resuscitation and emergency cardiovascular care. *Circulation.* 2010;122:S909–S919, with permission.)

- The Apgar scores (Table 38-3) should be obtained at 1 minute and 5 minutes after birth:
  - The Apgar score is *not* used to determine when to initiate resuscitation or to determine what course of action to take during resuscitation.
  - When the 5-minute Apgar is less than 7, Apgar scores should be assigned every 5 minutes for up to 20 minutes or until the score is ≥7.
  - The Apgar score at 5 and 10 minutes is a useful component in predicting acute multisystem organ dysfunction.

Table 38-3	Apgar Score		
	Score		
Sign	**0**	**1**	**2**
Heart rate	Absent	<100 beats/min	≥100 beats/min
Respirations	Absent	Weak cry; hypoventilation	Good, strong cry
Muscle tone	Limp	Some flexion	Active motion
Reflex irritability	No response	Grimace	Cough or sneeze
Color	Blue or pale	Body pink, extremities blue	Completely pink

- Initial steps of the resuscitation process should take no more than a few seconds to accomplish and include the following:
- Warmth.
  - Place the infant on an overhead radiant heater.
  - Dry the infant thoroughly with preheated towels or blankets.
  - Remove the wet towels to prevent heat loss.
  - Perinatal hyperthermia (greater than 36.5°C–37°C) should be avoided.
  - Therapeutic hypothermia is currently recommended for neonates ≥36 weeks with evidence of moderate/severe HIE (5).
- Position the infant and clear the airway:
  - Place the infant on the back or side with the head slightly extended in the neutral position ("sniffing" position).
  - Suction the mouth and nose to clear the airway.
  - The mouth should be suctioned first with a bulb syringe to decrease the risk of aspiration, and then the nose is subsequently suctioned.
  - A shoulder roll consisting of a rolled towel or blanket may be used to elevate the shoulders slightly.
  - If large amounts of secretions are coming from the mouth, the infant's head may be turned to the side to facilitate removal of these secretions.
- Initiation of breathing.
  - The infant may be stimulated by both drying and suctioning.
  - However, if the infant does not breathe immediately, slapping or flicking the soles of the feet or rubbing the infant's back with a warm blanket is an optional method to stimulate breathing. Other methods of infant stimulation are not recommended and may be harmful.
  - If there is no response to tactile stimulation within a few seconds, PPV should begin.
- Continued assessment is the next step in the resuscitative process and involves evaluating the infant's respiratory efforts, heart rate, and color to determine further action:
  - If the infant is apneic or gasping, PPV should be initiated with bag and mask and blended oxygen. If there is adequate respiratory effort, the infant's heart rate should be evaluated.
  - If the heart rate is greater than 100 bpm, the infant's color should be evaluated. If the heart rate is less than 100 bpm, PPV must be initiated. Continued monitoring of the heart rate will determine whether chest compressions or medication is indicated.
  - If central cyanosis is persistent despite blended oxygen, PPV should be initiated.
- In summary, if the infant is apneic, is gasping, or has inadequate respirations or the heart rate is less than 100 bpm, PPV must be initiated immediately to ensure adequate oxygenation.
- The administration of blended oxygen alone or persistent efforts to provide tactile stimulation to a nonbreathing infant or one whose heart rate is less than 100 bpm is of no value, delays appropriate management, and increases the risk of central nervous system and other organ damage.

Positive-Pressure Ventilation
• Adequate ventilation *must* be established for neonatal resuscitation to be successful.
• The equipment required for PPV should be available in the delivery room at all times and includes
  • A resuscitation bag or T-piece resuscitator capable of delivering blended oxygen
  • Neonatal masks of various sizes
  • An oxygen source
  • A flowmeter and blender
  • Pulse oximetry
  • Suction equipment (bulb, mechanical suction)
  • Appropriate-sized suction catheters
  • A syringe and orogastric catheter
  • Oral airways
• Resuscitation devices.
  • Size should be less than 750 mL.
  • Self-inflating bags (Fig. 38-3).
    ○ Refill independently of gas flow because of elastic recoil of the bag.
    ○ An oxygen reservoir attached to the air inlet is necessary to deliver high oxygen concentration because air is pulled in during reinflation of the bag.
    ○ If a pressure release valve is present, the pressure limit should be approximately 30 to 35 cm H_2O, and an override feature should be included to allow delivery of higher pressure if necessary to provide good chest expansion.
    ○ Blow-by oxygen should not be delivered through the mask because the flow of oxygen is unreliable unless the bag is being squeezed.
  • Flow-inflating bags (Fig. 38-4).
    ○ Bag inflation requires compressed gas flowing into it and requires the patient outlet to be at least partially occluded.
    ○ Adjustment of the gas flowing into the bag and adjustment of the gas flowing out through the flow-control valve are required for proper use.
    ○ A manometer should be used due to the possible high pressures that could be delivered.

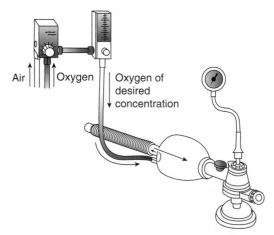

Air | Oxygen | Oxygen of desired concentration

Figure 38-3. Self-inflating bag. (Used with permission of the, American Academy of Pediatrics. *Textbook of neonatal resuscitation.* 6th ed. American Academy of Pediatrics and American Heart Association, 2011.)

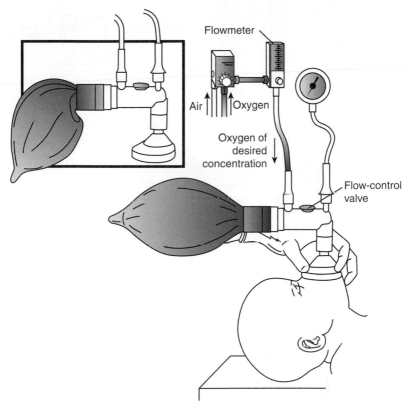

Figure 38-4. Flow-inflating bag. Flow-inflating bag inflates only with a compressed gas source and with mask sealed on face; otherwise, the bag remains deflated (inset). (Used with permission of the American Academy of Pediatrics. *Textbook of neonatal resuscitation.* 6th ed. American Academy of Pediatrics and American Heart Association, 2011.)

- ○ Blow-by oxygen can be delivered through the mask with a flow-inflating bag.
- ○ More experience and training are necessary to safely and effectively use a flow-inflating bag than to use a self-inflating bag. Therefore, it is generally recommended that a self-inflating bag be used in the delivery room.
- T-piece resuscitator (Fig. 38-5).
  - ○ The T-piece resuscitator requires gas flow from a compressed gas source.
  - ○ It requires a tight mask-to-face seal to deliver a breath and can deliver up to 100% free-flow oxygen.
  - ○ Advantages include consistent pressure, reliable control of peak inspiratory pressure, and positive end-expiratory pressure.
  - ○ Disadvantages include the following: requirement of compressed gas supply, pressure should be set prior to use, and a risk of administering prolonged inspiratory time.
- The resuscitation bag or T-piece resuscitator connected to an oxygen source with a mask of appropriate size should be immediately available and checked for proper functioning.

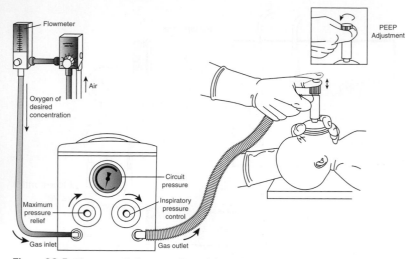

Figure 38-5. Flow-controlled, pressure-limited device (T-piece resuscitator). Pressures are preset by adjusting controls on the device and are delivered by occluding and opening the aperture in the PEEP cap. (Used with permission of the American Academy of Pediatrics. *Textbook of neonatal resuscitation.* 6th ed. American Academy of Pediatrics and American Heart Association, 2011.)

- PPV should be initiated when
  - The infant is apneic or gasping.
  - Respirations are unable to sustain a heart rate greater than 100 bpm.
  - Saturation remains below target values (Fig. 38-6) despite increasing to 100% free-flow oxygen.
- Before the initiation of PPV, the infant should be placed in position with the head slightly extended to provide an open airway.
- The mask should be applied over the nose and mouth and the seal checked by ventilating the infant two to three times.
- The chest should be observed for appropriate excursion. If the chest does not rise, the following actions should be performed:
  - Reapply the mask, and ensure a tight seal is present.

Targeted Productal Spo$_2$ After Birth

1 min	60%–65%
2 min	65%–70%
3 min	70%–75%
4 min	75%–80%
5 min	80%–85%
10 min	85%–95%

Figure 38-6. SpO$_2$ targets during neonatal resuscitation. Pulse oximetry probe should be on the right wrist to obtain preductal values. Used with permission of Wolters Kluwer.

- Reposition the head.
- Check for secretions, and, if present, suction.
- Ventilate with the mouth slightly open.
- Increase inflation pressure.
- If the chest still does not rise, then immediately intubate the trachea to secure the airway.
- After PPV has been performed for 30 seconds while increasing the oxygen to maintain oxygen saturations in the targeted range, the heart rate should be counted for 6 seconds and multiplied by 10:
  - If the heart rate is greater than 100 bpm and spontaneous breathing is present, PPV can be gradually discontinued.
  - If the heart rate is greater than 100 bpm and spontaneous breathing is absent or ineffective, then continue PPV.
  - If the heart rate is less than 60 bpm, continue PPV, initiate chest compressions, and consider endotracheal intubation.
- Resuscitation with blended oxygen is recommended. However, if oxygen is not available and PPV is indicated, use room air.
- The laryngeal mask airway, a mask designed to fit over the laryngeal inlet, is an alternative method of establishing an airway in neonatal resuscitation in infants with a birth weight greater than 1500 g (Figs. 38-7 and 38-8).

Endotracheal Intubation
- Endotracheal intubation is required in the following situations:
  - When prolonged PPV is needed
  - When PPV with appropriate inflation pressures is ineffective
  - When meconium must be suctioned from the trachea
  - When chest compressions are performed
  - When tracheal administration of medications is desired
  - When diaphragmatic hernia is suspected and PPV is needed

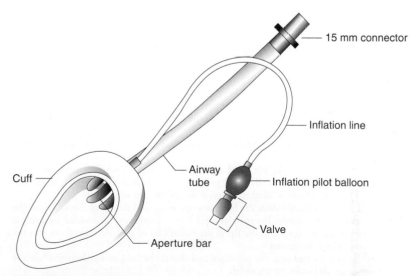

Figure 38-7. Laryngeal mask airway.

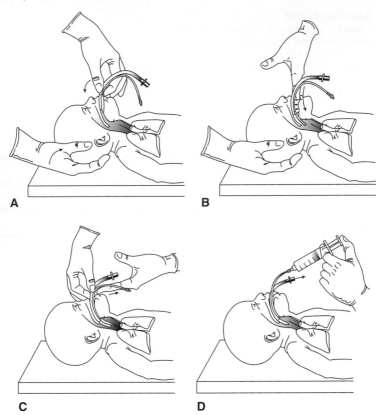

Figure 38-8. A–D: Inserting the laryngeal mask airway. The cuff should be inserted while deflated and then be inflated after insertion.

- The following steps should be taken for endotracheal intubation (Fig. 38-9):
  - Select the appropriate size ETT on the basis of the estimated fetal weight (Table 38-4) (2). A stylet may be inserted as an aid to intubation but should not extend beyond the tip of the tube.
  - The infant should be properly positioned under a radiant warmer with the neck slightly extended.
  - With a laryngoscope in the left hand and the head stabilized with the right hand, the blade of the laryngoscope is advanced to just past the base of the tongue into the val-lecula. The blade is gently lifted to visualize the glottis and vocal cords.
  - The ETT is introduced beside the laryngoscope blade and the tip of the tube into the glottis between the cords. Inserting the ETT too deeply can be avoided by using a length from tip of the tube to the tip of the infant's lip of no more than 6 cm plus the infant's weight in kilograms.
  - With the tube in position, the proximal end should be held and stabilized while the laryngoscope and stylet are removed.
  - The ETT is connected to the resuscitation bag, and ventilation is initiated.

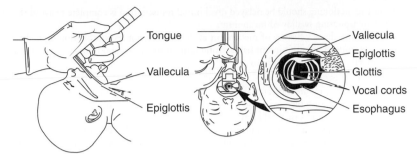

Figure 38-9. Identification of landmarks before placing ETT through glottis. (Used with permission of the American Academy of Pediatrics. *Textbook of neonatal resuscitation.* 6th ed. American Academy of Pediatrics and American Heart Association, 2011.)

- The tube should be stabilized while an assistant assesses the effects of the endotracheal intubation by
  - Observing symmetric chest wall movement
  - Auscultating equal bilateral breath sounds
  - Confirming the stomach is not being inflated
  - Observing a fog of moisture in the tube during exhalation
  - Noting improvement in the infant's heart rate, color, and activity
- The tube should be taped and secured.
- The primary method for confirming a successful endotracheal intubation is demonstrating an increasing heart rate and detecting CO_2 by an exhaled CO_2 detector (colorimetric devices and capnographs).
- If the infant is to remain intubated, confirmation by chest X-ray should be done to ensure that the tip of the tube is in the appropriate position.
- If the newborn has had a history of meconium in the amniotic fluid, then
  - Direct laryngoscopy should be performed immediately after birth with suctioning of residual meconium from the hypopharynx and intubation/suction of the trachea **if**
    - Respirations are absent or depressed.
    - The heart rate is less than 100 bpm.
    - The infant's muscle tone is decreased.
  - If the infant develops apnea or respiratory depression after being initially vigorous, tracheal suctioning should be performed before PPV is given.

Table 38-4	Endotracheal Tube Sizes for Infants of Various Weights and Gestations		
Tube size (mm, inside diameter)	Weight (g)	Gestational age (wk)	Depth of ETT insertion (cm) at lip[a]
2.5	<1000	<28	7
3.0	1000–2000	28–34	8
3.5	2000–3000	34–38	9
3.5–4.0	>3000	>38	9–10

[a]In infants less than 750 g, the ETT may need to be secured at 6 cm at the lip.

- Gastric suctioning should be delayed until initial resuscitation is complete to avoid the risk of aspirating swallowed meconium.
- Infants that have a history of meconium at delivery do not require suctioning if they are vigorous. A vigorous infant has a strong respiratory effort, good muscle tone, and a heart rate greater than 100 bpm.

Chest Compressions
- Chest compressions are indicated if
  - Effective PPV with blended oxygen has been given for a period of 30 seconds.
  - The heart rate is less than 60 bpm.
- Chest compressions must be administered in conjunction with PPV with 100% oxygen **AND** the thumb method (Fig. 38-10A–D) is the preferred technique for performing chest compressions (6):
  - Both thumbs are placed on the lower third of the sternum just below an imaginary line passing between the nipples, and the fingers encircle the chest to support the back.
  - If the resuscitator's hands are too small to encircle the chest, then two-finger compression should be performed, with the other hand supporting the back (Fig. 38-10E).

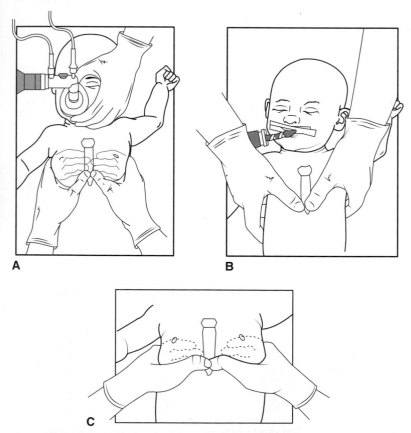

Figure 38-10. A–C: Thumb technique of chest compressions administered from the bottom (**A**), from the top (**B**), and for small chests, with thumbs overlapped (**C**).

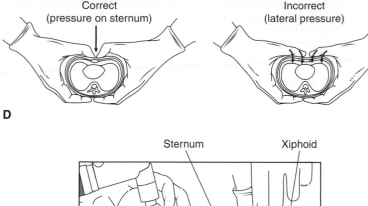

Figure 38-10 *(Continued)*. D: Correct and incorrect application of pressure with thumb technique of chest compressions. **E:** Correct finger position for two finger technique. (Used with permission of the American Academy of Pediatrics. *Textbook of neonatal resuscitation.* 6th ed. American Academy of Pediatrics and American Heart Association, 2011.)

- The sternum should be compressed at the rate of 90 times per minute to a depth of approximately one-third of the anterior–posterior diameter of the chest. The depth of compressions should be adequate enough to produce a palpable pulse.
- Ventilation should continue at 30 breaths/min.
- Chest compressions should be interposed in a 3:1 ratio with ventilation.
- The "compressor" should count aloud so that the "ventilator" knows when to insert the ventilation. The cadence should be "one-and-two-and-three-and-breathe-and...."
- The heart rate should be checked approximately every 30 seconds. If the heart rate is less than 60 bpm, compressions should be continued in conjunction with ventilation. If the heart rate is greater than 60 bpm, compressions may be discontinued but PPV maintained at a more rapid rate of 40 to 60 bpm.
- Once the heart rate is greater than 100 bpm and the baby is breathing spontaneously, PPV should be slowly withdrawn.

Medications
- Volume expanders and medications may be required during resuscitation to stimulate the heart, improve tissue perfusion, or correct anemia.

- Typically, volume expanders and cardiotonic drugs are administered to newborns who do not respond to effective ventilation, blended oxygen, and chest compressions.
- Routes of administration include
  - The preferred route of drug administration is the umbilical vein because it can be rapidly identified and catheterized:
    - A 3.5- to 5-French catheter can be emergently inserted into the umbilical vein 2 to 4 cm below the skin and just deep enough to get a free flow of blood return.
    - If the catheter tip is too deep and in the liver, infusions of hyperosmolar and vasoactive drugs may damage the liver.
  - Epinephrine may be administered through the ETT.
  - Intraosseous access may be an alternative route for administration of medications and volume expanders if umbilical or other venous access is not available.
  - The rate of administration of medications must be carefully considered, especially in the preterm infant, because the brain vasculature is vulnerable to rapid changes in vascular pressure and osmolarity.
- Initial pharmacologic therapy is administered to improve myocardial function and enhance tissue perfusion.
- **Epinephrine**.
  - Epinephrine should be given if
    - There is no heart rate at birth in an infant who had signs of life shortly before delivery.
    - The heart rate is less than 60 bpm after 30 seconds of effective chest compressions and ventilation with blended oxygen.
  - The intravenous dose of epinephrine is 0.01 to 0.03 mg/kg (0.1 to 0.3 mL/kg of 1:10,000 solution drawn in a 1-mL syringe) and may be repeated every 3 to 5 minutes if necessary.
  - In emergency situations, while intravenous access is being attempted, epinephrine may be administered through the ETT. The endotracheal dose of epinephrine is 0.05 to 0.1 mg/kg (0.5 to 1 mL/kg of 1:10,000 solution drawn in a 3-mL or 5-mL syringe). However, endotracheal epinephrine may be erratically absorbed (7), and intravenous access should be obtained as soon as possible, especially if the response is poor.
  - The use of high-dose intravenous epinephrine in neonatal resuscitation is not recommended.
  - Reassessment of heart rate and perfusion should be performed 30 to 60 seconds after a dose of epinephrine is given.
- **Volume expanders**.
  - Volume expanders are given to correct hypovolemia and increase vascular volume, subsequently improving tissue perfusion.
  - Acute bleeding may not be evident because many times fetal–maternal hemorrhage occurs through the placenta before delivery.
  - Hypovolemia should be suspected any time the infant
    - Is not responding to resuscitative efforts
    - Has poor perfusion
    - Has a weak pulse
  - The preferred volume expander is an isotonic crystalloid solution and includes
    - Normal saline (0.9% NaCl)
    - Ringer's lactate
  - If the infant has had a large amount of blood loss, O negative packed red blood cells may be indicated for volume replacement.
  - The usual dose is 10 mL/kg given intravenously over 5 minutes (term infants) or over 10 minutes (preterm infants).
  - Sodium bicarbonate is no longer recommended in neonatal resuscitation (8).

Postresuscitation Care
- Admission to a special or intensive care unit
  - If an infant has required prolonged resuscitation, then the infant should be admitted to a special or intensive care unit for close observation and monitoring for at least 24 hours. Monitoring for postresuscitation complications is necessary. Baseline laboratory studies, including a blood gas (either from an umbilical sample or from the baby) to assess the infant's pH and base deficit, may be useful to determine the infant's risk for HIE.
  - Useful laboratory tests include serum glucose, calcium (ideally ionized), arterial blood gas, complete blood count, and chest radiograph.
- Hypotension
  - Hypotension should be treated with volume expanders or vasopressors.
  - Dopamine.
    - ○ Continuous dopamine infusion may improve peripheral perfusion and increase blood pressure.
    - ○ Infants receiving dopamine should be continuously monitored and frequently assessed for heart rate and blood pressure.
    - ○ Dopamine infusion generally begins at 5 mcg/kg/min and may be increased gradually to a maximum of 20 mcg/kg/min.
  - Preterm infants are unlikely to be hypovolemic in the absence of obvious blood loss, and hypoperfusion in the preterm infant is best treated with a vasopressor.
- Acute renal failure
  - Acute renal failure is common in infants with severe HIE.
  - Close monitoring of urine output, serum electrolytes, and creatinine is necessary.
  - Renal failure is often nonoliguric and, therefore, may be missed if serum creatinine is not measured daily (9).
- Hypoglycemia
  - Hypoglycemia is common in the postresuscitation period and may require boluses of 2 mL/kg of 10% dextrose in water (200 mg/kg) as well as a continuous glucose infusion at a rate of 6 to 8 mg/kg/min.
- Hypocalcemia
  - Hypocalcemia, as measured in an ionized sample, frequently occurs 24 to 48 hours after resuscitation and may require IV calcium supplementation.
- Metabolic acidosis
  - Metabolic acidosis is typically a reflection of tissue hypoperfusion and anaerobic metabolism. Recognizing and treating the cause of the acidosis are the primary recommended interventions (8).
- Central nervous system sequelae
  - Central nervous system sequelae may include
    - ○ Cerebral edema
    - ○ Cerebral hemorrhage
    - ○ Seizures
    - ○ Development of the syndrome of inappropriate antidiuretic hormone secretion
  - Initial management should consider fluid restriction to 50 to 60 mL/kg/day.
  - Further management and evaluation depends on the individual symptoms and clinical course.
- Therapeutic hypothermia
  - Cooling infants to 33.5°C to 34.5°C has been shown to improve neurodevelopmental outcomes in infants with moderate to severe hypoxic–ischemic encephalopathy (HIE).
  - Criteria include
    - ○ Gestational age ≥36 weeks
    - ○ Evidence of an acute perinatal hypoxic–ischemic event
    - ○ Ability to start hypothermia within 6 hours after birth

- Once the decision is made to proceed with hypothermia therapy, the care team should ensure the child does not become hyperthermic (temperature greater than 36.5°C–37°C) (10).
- Persistent pulmonary hypertension
  - Persistent pulmonary hypertension may occur with pulmonary vasospasm, causing right-to-left shunting of blood and subsequent hypoxia and acidosis.
  - Expedient and aggressive ventilatory support with blended oxygen is required, and in some situations, inhaled nitric oxide therapy and/or extracorporeal membrane oxygenation may be necessary.
- Documentation
  - All observations and actions taken during resuscitation should be documented in the medical record and, ideally, on a delivery room resuscitation record.

Outcome
- Cerebral palsy
  - Fewer than 10% of children with cerebral palsy have a history of HIE (11,12).
  - Mental retardation and epilepsy in the absence of cerebral palsy are not associated with HIE.
  - Only a severe or prolonged hypoxic ischemic insult will cause brain injury that results in motor and intellectual impairment.
  - Full-term infants with permanent brain damage from HIE show neurologic dysfunction soon after birth. A newborn with severe HIE should demonstrate all of the findings that include (12)
    - Apgar scores of 0 to 3 for greater than 5 minutes
    - Neurologic manifestations such as seizures, hypotonia, or coma
    - Profound metabolic acidosis or mixed acidemia (pH less than 7.0) on an umbilical cord arterial blood gas assessment or a pH <7.1 with significant base excess (>−12) on an arterial blood gas obtained on the infant in the first 30–60 minutes of life.
    - Multisystem organ dysfunction (e.g., cardiovascular, gastrointestinal, hematologic, pulmonary, or renal system)
  - Unfortunately, the incidence of cerebral palsy in term infants has remained unchanged in the last 20 to 30 years despite technologic advances in obstetrics and neonatology.

COMPLICATIONS: WITHHOLDING AND DISCONTINUING RESUSCITATION
- Withholding resuscitation
  - The resuscitation of certain types of newly born infants is unlikely to result in survival or survival without severe disabilities.
  - The 2011 NRP considers withholding resuscitation in the delivery room appropriate for infants with
    - Confirmed gestation of less than 23 weeks or birth weight of less than 400 g
    - Anencephaly
    - Confirmed lethal genetic disorder or malformation (2)
  - Attitudes toward the resuscitation of, and medical care given to, a child with trisomy 13 or 18 are evolving, and more of these children are surviving both the neonatal period and the first year of life (13).
  - In uncertain cases where antenatal information is incomplete or unreliable, initiation of resuscitation may be done, and after assessment of the infant, resuscitation and/or further support may be continued or discontinued.
  - Not initiating support and later withdrawing support are generally considered to be ethically equivalent. Later withdrawal of support does, however, allow further time to obtain more complete clinical information and to provide counseling to the family.
  - In general, there is no advantage to delayed or partial support, and if the infant survives, the outcome may be worsened as a result of performing delayed or partial resuscitation.

- Discontinuation of resuscitation
  - Prolonged resuscitation that results in only delayed death or in the survival of a severely disabled infant is undesirable, and it is reasonable to want to avoid this outcome.
  - Resuscitation of newborns after 10 minutes of asystole is likely to result in only delayed death or survival of a severely disabled infant (14).
  - Discontinuation of resuscitation of infants with severe HIE is addressed by the 2011 NRP textbook. Discontinuation of resuscitation may be appropriate if no signs of life (no heart rate and no respiratory effort) are present after 10 minutes of adequate resuscitative efforts (2).

PATIENT EDUCATION

- Parent and family care
  - Ideally, the resuscitation team should introduce themselves to the family before the delivery, and the probable plan of care should be discussed and any questions addressed.
  - After delivery, the family should be informed of any resuscitation and/or procedures that were needed and why they were indicated.
  - Great effort should be made to allow the parents contact with their newborn infant as soon as possible.
  - Admission plans for the infant, particularly if the infant will not be staying with the parents, should be explained to the parents and family.

REFERENCES

1. Dawes G. *Fetal and neonatal physiology.* Chicago: Year Book Medical Publishers, 1968.
2. Kattwinkel J. *Textbook of neonatal resuscitation: American Heart Association and American Academy of Pediatrics.* 6th ed. Elk Grove Village. American Academy of Pediatrics, 2011.
3. Kurinczuk JJ, White-Koning M, Badawi N. Epidemiology of neonatal encephalopathy and hypoxic-ischaemic encephalopathy. *Early Hum Dev.* 2010;86:329–338.
4. Vannucci RC. Current and potentially new management strategies for perinatal hypoxic-ischemic encephalopathy. *Pediatrics.* 1990;85:961–968.
5. Jacobs SE, et al. Cooling for newborns with hypoxic ischaemic encephalopathy. *Cochrane Database Syst Rev.* 2013;1:CD003311.
6. David R. Closed chest cardiac massage in the newborn infant. *Pediatrics.* 1988;81:552–554.
7. Orlowski JP, Gallager JM, Porembka DT. Endotracheal epinephrine is unreliable. *Resuscitation.* 1990;19:103–113.
8. Poland RL. Dogma disputed: why intravenous sodium bicarbonate doesn't work. *NeoRev.* 2009;10:e558–e563.
9. Karlowicz MG, Adelman RD. Nonoliguric and oliguric acute renal failure in asphyxiated term neonates. *Pediatr Nephrol.* 1995;9:718–722.
10. Shankaran S, et al. Whole-body hypothermia for neonates with hypoxic-ischemic encephalopathy. *N Engl J Med.* 2005;3535:1574–1584.
11. Blair E, Stanley FJ. Intrapartum asphyxia: a rare cause of cerebral palsy. *J Pediatr.* 1988;112:515–519.
12. American College of Obstetricians and Gynecologists' Task Force on Neonatal Encephalopathy and Cerebral Palsy, American College of Obstetricians and Gynecologists, American Academy of Pediatrics. Neonatal encephalopathy and cerebral palsy: Defining the pathogenesis and pathophysiology. Washington: American College of Obstetricians and Gynecologists, 2003.
13. Carey JC. Perspectives on the care and management of infants with trisomy 18 and trisomy 13: striving for balance. *Curr Opin Pediatr.* 2012;24:672–678.
14. Kattwinkel J, et al. Part 15: neonatal resuscitation: 2010 American Heart Association Guidelines for cardiopulmonary resuscitation and emergency cardiovascular care. *Circulation.* 2010;122:S909–S919.

Neonatal Complications
Tushar A. Shah and Jamil H. Khan

RESUSCITATION OF THE NEWBORN: SPECIAL CIRCUMSTANCES
Key Points
- Certain conditions require specific resuscitative measures.
- Antenatal diagnosis can help optimize preparation and management.
- Communication with the family before and after delivery can ease the shock of significant neonatal abnormalities.

Background
In a number of circumstances and diagnoses, independent of neonatal asphyxia, specific resuscitative measures should be undertaken for the newborn infant that fall outside of the usual neonatal resuscitation guidelines and may require additional equipment and technical skills. Given the ever-increasing accuracy of antenatal diagnosis, many of these problems may be anticipated in advance; thus, attention to the management of many uncommon problems is appropriate. This chapter reviews some of these special circumstances and outlines specific treatment recommendations.

Meconium-Stained Amniotic Fluid
Background
- Meconium is a viscous substance from the fetal intestinal tract consisting of water, lanugo, desquamated fetal intestinal cells, skin cells, vernix, amniotic fluid, pancreatic enzymes, and bile pigment.
- It is present in the amniotic fluid in 10% of all pregnancies and in 30% to 40% of postterm infants at delivery.

Epidemiology
- Meconium staining of amniotic fluid (MSAF) occurs in approximately 8% to 25% of all births, primarily in situations of advanced fetal maturity or fetal stress (1).
- Risk factors for MSAF include postmaturity (gestational age beyond 41 weeks), small for gestational age (SGA), fetal distress, and compromised in utero conditions including placental insufficiency and cord compression (2).
- Meconium aspiration syndrome (MAS) is defined as respiratory distress in an infant born through MSAF whose symptoms cannot be otherwise explained. It occurs in 5% of patients born through MSAF (3).
- An estimated 25,000 to 30,000 cases and 1000 deaths related to MAS occur annually in the United States with many more cases in developing countries (1). The incidence of MAS had decreased recently secondary to a decrease in number of deliveries beyond 41 weeks' gestation in developed countries (4).
- Previously, differentiating thin versus thick meconium was used to guide management decisions, but current Neonatal Resuscitation Program guidelines do not differentiate between the two consistencies (5).

Pathophysiology
- Meconium aspiration causes injury to lung tissues through a variety of mechanisms including complete or partial obstruction of airways, sepsis, inflammation, complement activation and cytokine production, inhibition of surfactant synthesis and function, apoptosis of epithelial cells, and increased pulmonary vascular resistance (3).

- Controversy exists as to whether meconium-stained amniotic fluid always indicates some degree of asphyxia. Meconium-stained fluid alone generally does not indicate asphyxia; however, in the presence of other indications of fetal compromise, its presence is a marker of fetal distress (6).
- MAS may be fatal and often requires aggressive neonatal care, including treatment with extracorporeal membrane oxygenation (ECMO).

Prevention
- Obstetric: The usual methods of assessing fetal well-being should be used to determine the optimal timing and method of delivery.
  - Amnioinfusion: In clinical settings with standard peripartum surveillance, the evidence does not support the use of amnioinfusion for MSAF. In settings with limited peripartum surveillance (developing countries), where complications of MSAF are common, amnioinfusion appears to reduce the risk of MAS (7).
  - Antepartum suctioning: Suctioning of the oropharynx upon delivery of the head and before delivery of the shoulders is used commonly in obstetric practices to decrease the possibility of meconium aspiration with the first breath. A multicenter, randomized, prospective study concluded that antepartum suctioning does not decrease the incidence of MAS even in high-risk infants. On the contrary, it may lead to complications including bradycardia, desaturations, and increased incidence of pneumothorax (8).
- Neonatal
  - If the infant has respiratory depression, a heart rate less than 100 beats per minute (bpm), or hypotonia, the infant should be rapidly intubated to clear the airway of meconium (5).
  - Gregory et al. (9) found that 9% of infants who had no meconium in the pharynx after obstetrical suctioning had meconium below the vocal cords in the trachea; therefore, visualization of the cords without intubation is insufficient
- The procedure for intubation is as follows:
  - The infant is placed on a radiant warmer.
  - Before any other resuscitative measures are begun, the infant is intubated under direct visualization using a laryngoscope (No. 0 or 1 blade) with the largest appropriate endotracheal tube (usually, a 3.5 or 4.0 tube for a term infant).
  - Suctioning of the pharynx during this procedure with a large suction catheter may be needed to visualize the airway.
  - Once the infant is intubated, a suction device is quickly attached directly to the hub of the endotracheal tube, suction is applied, and the tube is slowly removed, clearing meconium from the trachea.
  - If meconium is obtained from below the vocal cords, this intubation and suctioning procedure should be repeated until no further meconium is obtained.
  - To decrease the possibility of hypoxia while intubating and suctioning, blow-by oxygen should be administered at the patient's mouth.
- Duration of tracheal suctioning:
  - If repetitive intubation is difficult or if multiple intubations continue to yield meconium, one reaches a point at which continual depression of the newborn becomes a greater concern than does complete removal of meconium.
  - Clinical judgment, especially the presence of bradycardia, can guide the timing of initiation of manual ventilation.
  - Usually, after 2 to 5 minutes of intubation and suctioning, or if sustained bradycardia less than 60 bpm occurs, standard resuscitative measures should be considered.
- When not to intubate:
  - Randomized controlled trials do not support routine use of endotracheal intubation at birth in vigorous meconium-stained babies to reduce mortality or MAS (1,10).
  - If a vigorous infant with thick meconium is not initially intubated but later becomes distressed, intubation and removal of meconium from the airway may be necessary.

- Gastric suctioning:
  - Although many clinicians routinely suction out the stomach contents when meconium is noted in the amniotic fluid, there is no evidence to support this practice (11).

Management
- The respiratory manifestations include increased work of breathing, tachypnea, and cyanosis.
- Fifteen to twenty percent of infants with the MAS develop persistent pulmonary hypertension of the newborn (PPHN). Pneumothorax and pneumomediastinum are common complications in infants with severe MAS.
- Management consists mainly of supportive respiratory and cardiovascular care with options for oxygen therapy, conventional or high-frequency mechanical ventilation, vasopressors, inhaled nitric oxide, surfactant therapy, and ECMO.
- No specific long-term deficits in pulmonary function have been attributed to MAS. The ultimate prognosis depends not so much on the pulmonary disease as on the accompanying asphyxial insult and treatment required (3).

Pneumothorax
Background
Definition
- Pneumothorax is a collection of free gas in the thorax between the visceral and parietal pleura, which may compromise respiratory function.
- A pneumothorax can progressively increase in volume, leading to a shift of the mediastinal structures, known as a tension pneumothorax.

Pathophysiology
- Uneven ventilation in the lung and partial airway obstruction, especially when coupled with positive-pressure ventilation, can lead to overdistention and rupture of alveoli, with leakage of air into the pleural space and accumulation of gas.
- As gas accumulates under pressure, collapse of the lung, a shift in mediastinal structures, and decreased cardiac output resulting from decreased venous return can lead to acute deterioration.

Epidemiology
- Pneumothorax is estimated to occur in 1% to 2% of all term births, usually without symptoms (3).
- It is seen more frequently in infants with pulmonary disease and transient tachypnea of the newborn (10%), respiratory distress syndrome (5% to 20%), and MAS (20% to 50%).

Associations
- Pneumothorax is often seen with pulmonary disease, especially if positive-pressure ventilation with high pressures is used.
- Other air leaks (pneumomediastinum, pneumopericardium, subcutaneous emphysema, even pneumoperitoneum) may be seen in patients with pneumothorax.
- Pneumothorax is very common in patients with pulmonary hypoplasia (discussed later in this chapter).

Evaluation
History and Physical
- The infant may be asymptomatic.
- Often, a sudden deterioration, with cyanosis, bradycardia, and hypotension, is seen.
- A shift in cardiac sounds or change in breath sounds may occur.

Laboratory Tests
- Diagnosis may be made by transillumination, which reveals increased light transmission through the affected hemithorax.
- Usually, a chest radiograph will definitively diagnose a pneumothorax, but if the patient is deteriorating, treatment should be started based on a positive transillumination, without delay.

Treatment
- If asymptomatic, no treatment is needed. Careful observation is usually sufficient, and the pneumothorax will likely resorb.
- Mildly symptomatic pneumothorax with only modest oxygen requirements, tachypnea, and normal blood gases should be followed closely.
- Nitrogen washout: Placing the infant in 100% oxygen may facilitate resorption of a pneumothorax, but this management strategy has not been studied in infants. Considering the risks of oxygen toxicity and absorption atelectasis, this intervention is best avoided in all infants. It should be especially avoided in premature infants because of the association of hyperoxia with retinopathy of prematurity.
- Symptomatic pneumothorax may be treated emergently by tapping the pleural space anteriorly using a needle, aspiration kit, or Angiocath catheter.
  - It is usually necessary to place a chest tube after this procedure.
  - Insertion of a polyvinyl chloride chest tube, usually 10 or 12 French, in the fourth intercostal space in the anterior axillary line and aimed anteriorly, is the preferable method for treating symptomatic pneumothorax.

Complications
- Prognosis is generally good but depends on the underlying pulmonary disease.
- Pneumothorax is associated with an increased incidence of intraventricular hemorrhage in premature infants.

Congenital Diaphragmatic Hernia
Background
Definition
- The presence of normally intra-abdominal organs in the thorax via a defect in the diaphragm.
- The diagnosis of congenital diaphragmatic hernia may be known from antenatal ultrasonography or may be suspected clinically.

Etiology
- Failure of the Bochdalek foramen to close at 8 to 10 weeks of gestation allows the bowel to migrate into the thoracic cavity.

Pathophysiology
- The presence of the intestines and other organs in the chest can impair lung growth in utero. This leads to pulmonary insufficiency and PPHN secondary to pulmonary hypoplasia, lower number of alveoli, and airway and vascular muscular hypertrophy (3).

Epidemiology
- Incidence is 1 in 2500 to 1 in 4000, with 90% on the left; 56% of cases are prenatally diagnosed (12).
- Over the last 10 to 15 years, average survival for Congenital Diaphragmatic Hernia (CDH) has improved from 50% to 70% to 80% and as high as 90% in some institutions (13). Poor outcomes are associated with large defects, presence of liver in the chest, earlier displacement of abdominal contents into the chest, and lung area to head circumference ratio (LHR) less than 1—all indicators of the severity of the pulmonary hypoplasia.

Evaluation
History and Physical
- Clinical findings that may be present include
  - Scaphoid abdomen
  - Shift in heart sounds to the right
  - Unequal breath sounds
  - Respiratory distress
- Note that commonly there may be no symptoms other than respiratory distress.

Laboratory Tests
- A chest radiograph showing abdominal organs in the thorax confirms the diagnosis.

Treatment

Initial Management

- If the diagnosis is suspected prenatally, the mother should be counseled about the potential need for ECMO and offered delivery in a tertiary center with that capability (12).
- Avoid bag and mask ventilation and immediately intubate and begin manual ventilation because face mask ventilation may lead to gaseous distension of the intestines, further compressing the lungs. An orogastric tube should be placed to evacuate the stomach.
- The infant should be transferred to a tertiary neonatal intensive care unit (NICU) for further management.

NICU and Surgical Management

- Standardized, multidisciplinary treatment guidelines that include input from neonatology, pediatric surgery, ECMO specialists, and respiratory therapy are critical to successful management (14).
- Use of strategies aimed at minimizing lung injury (gentle ventilation or permissive hypercapnia), tolerance of postductal acidosis and hypoxemia, and adhering to center-specific criteria for ECMO are strategies most consistently reported by successful centers (12).
- Surgical repair with reduction of the intestines into the peritoneal cavity and repair of the diaphragmatic defect is the definitive treatment.
- Mean age for repair is variable across centers because timing of surgery is dependent on the patient's clinical condition. Though some studies have revealed no differences in outcomes of infants undergoing early versus delayed repair (15), others show that early repair in the face of unstable cardiorespiratory status may have worse outcomes, and delayed repair may improve survival in patients with borderline prognosis (16). There is no evidence that timing of surgery influences survival (17). Currently, repair is delayed at most centers until the patient's cardiovascular status is stabilized, and the risk of PPHN is lessened.

Complications

- Factors associated with mortality in CDH are severity of pulmonary hypertension, birth weight, associated defects/anomalies, gestational age at birth, inborn status, and need for ECMO (13).
- ECMO is used in approximately 30% of cases and is associated with a 51% survival. The sickest infants likely require ECMO, and though the overall outcomes are worse, ECMO likely improves survival in these patients (13).
- Infants born with CDH are at higher risk of morbidities such as pulmonary vascular abnormalities causing pulmonary hypertension, obstructive airway disease, gastroesophageal reflux disease requiring surgery, neurodevelopmental delay, chest wall deformities, and scoliosis (3).
- Although fetal surgical interventions such as tracheal occlusion have not been successful so far, minimally invasive techniques such as percutaneous fetoscopic endoluminal tracheal occlusion have shown promise and are currently being investigated in randomized clinical trials (18).

Associations

- CDH is commonly associated with multiple congenital anomalies including cardiac, urogenital, chromosomal, syndromic, and musculoskeletal. The reported incidence of associated malformations varies between 20% and 60% (19).

GASTROINTESTINAL MALFORMATIONS

Omphalocele

Background

Definition

- An omphalocele is a congenital defect in the formation of the umbilical and supraumbilical portions of the abdominal wall.
- Giant omphalocele is defined as an abdominal wall defect larger than 4 cm with the liver partly extruded in the defect (20).

Etiology
• Before 10 weeks of gestation, there is an embryologically normal defect in the anterior abdominal wall.
• If this defect fails to close, a saclike herniation of the peritoneum and abdominal contents through the abdominal wall remains.

Epidemiology
• Omphalocele occurs in 1 in 4000 to 1 in 10,000 births.

Evaluation
History and Physical
• Omphaloceles have the appearance of a transparent sac containing bowel protruding from the anterior abdominal wall.
• Omphaloceles have a large base with the umbilical cord implanted on the sac.
• Rupture of the sac can occur before delivery.

Treatment
Initial Management
• Most studies have concluded that there is no advantage to cesarean delivery for patients with abdominal wall defects (21).
• After delivery, the infant must be immediately placed on the radiant warmer, basic resuscitation performed, and then the defect gently wrapped in warm saline-soaked sterile gauze.
• The entire lower half of the infant should be placed in a sterile "bowel bag." This minimizes heat and water loss from the bowel and protects the exposed abdominal organs.
• Emergent transfer to a tertiary NICU is necessary for pediatric surgical repair.

Surgical Repair
• For most defects, a primary repair with the bowel being reduced into the peritoneal cavity is the procedure of choice.
• For larger defects, a staged repair, involving suspension of either the native sac or a synthetic silo above the patient, with gradual reduction of the contents, may be employed.
• For giant omphaloceles, a "skin-only" closure leaving a larger ventral hernia that may be repaired later may be needed.
• If the defect is too large for even a skin-only closure, then the sac may be treated with topical antimicrobials and allowed to epithelialize.

Complications
• Prognosis generally depends on the associated anomalies.
• Survival is 70% or better with isolated omphalocele, and recent reviews suggest even greater survival in patients with normal karyotype (22), but omphalocele with accompanying serious cardiac disease has been associated with a mortality of up to 80%.

Associations
• Up to two-thirds of patients with omphaloceles have associated anomalies, including trisomies (30%), cardiac lesions (20%), other gastrointestinal anomalies, and other midline defects such as bladder exstrophy.

Gastroschisis
Background
Definition
• Gastroschisis is the herniation of abdominal contents through an abdominal wall defect without a covering membrane of peritoneum or amnion from the umbilical cord.
• These defects occur on the right side of the umbilicus.

Etiology
• The cause is controversial: rupture of a hernia of the umbilical cord at the site of involution of the right umbilical vein versus interruption of the omphalomesenteric artery.

Epidemiology
- The incidence of gastroschisis varies from 1 to 5 per 10,000 live births and is similar in male and female fetuses. Worldwide, the prevalence of gastroschisis has increased two- to threefold in the past three decades (23,24).
  - Risk factors for gastroschisis include young maternal age, lower socioeconomic status, and exposure to external agents such as vasoconstricting decongestants, nonsteroidal anti-inflammatory agents, cocaine, and possibly pesticides/herbicides (3).

Evaluation
History and Physical
- The abdominal defect is usually small, but it may have a large amount of abdominal contents present outside of the peritoneal cavity, with the potential for vascular occlusion.
- No covering membrane is present, although a fibrous material adherent to the intestines may be seen.

Treatment
- Management is the same as for omphalocele, but repair is more urgent.

Complications
- Gastroschisis has a mortality rate of 10% to 30%.
- Establishment of enteral feedings is usually a slow process. Exclusive human milk feeding after gastroschisis repair has been shown to decrease time to achieve full enteral feeds and time to discharge (25).
- Some patients have a significant shortening of the intestine and may suffer long-term, life-threatening consequences of "short gut."

Associations
- About 50% of gastroschisis infants are born prematurely.
- There are associated anomalies in 5% to 25% of gastroschisis cases with the majority being intestinal atresias (3).
- A recent report suggests a 4% incidence of congenital heart disease in patients with gastroschisis (26).

Intestinal Atresias
Background
Definition
- Intestinal atresias are complete obstructions of the bowel lumen.

Pathophysiology
- The cause may be failure of recanalization of the intestine or an early vascular accident.

Epidemiology
- The most common site of intestinal atresia is the small intestine. The incidence of jejunal and ileal atresia ranges from 1:1500 to 12,000 births (27). Atresia of the colon is a relatively rare, with an incidence of 1:40,000 to 60,000 live births (28).

Evaluation
History and Physical
- Proximal obstructions (duodenal, jejunal) are often present with polyhydramnios, bile-stained amniotic fluid, and distended bowel loops on antenatal ultrasonography.
  - Duodenal atresia classically presents with the "double bubble" sign of dilated stomach and proximal duodenum, with no fluid distally on antenatal ultrasound.
- The abdomen is distended at birth.
- Distal obstructions (distal ileum or colon) may yield unremarkable antenatal ultrasound findings and may present in the neonatal period with vomiting or minimal if any passage of stool.

Laboratory Tests
- Plain radiographs reveal intestinal dilation distal to the obstruction.
- Contrast studies may help locate the atresia as well as rule out obstruction due to other causes, such as malrotation with midgut volvulus.

Treatment
Initial Management
- Continuous nasogastric suction with a Replogle tube is used to prevent vomiting.
- Intravenous fluid therapy is started, and the infant should be transferred to a tertiary NICU for surgical repair.
- Midgut malrotation with volvulus, which requires emergent surgery, must be ruled out.
- Surgical management involves exploratory laparotomy, excision of the stenotic area with reanastamosis, and a search for multiple atresias.

Complications
Prognosis
- Survival is greater than 90%, with most mortality caused by associated malformations.

Associations
- Duodenal atresia is associated with Down syndrome (30%), annular pancreas (20%), and other anomalies.
- Prematurity may occur in relation to the presence of polyhydramnios.

Tracheoesophageal Fistula and Esophageal Atresia
Background
Definitions
- Esophageal atresia (EA) describes a congenital failure of development of the complete lumen of the esophagus.
- A tracheoesophageal fistula (TEF) is an abnormal communication between the trachea and the esophagus.
- EA occurs in 95% of TEF cases.
- Most commonly, there is a fistula between the trachea and the distal portion of the esophagus.

Pathophysiology
- Initial theory of disruption in tracheoesophageal septation is now controversial.
- Specific absences of certain fibroblast growth factor elements allow the nonbranching development of the fistulous tract from the foregut, which then establishes continuity with the developing stomach (29). Sonic hedgehog–signaled apoptosis in the developing foregut can lead to EA (30).

Epidemiology
- EA occurs in 1 in 3000 to 1 in 5000 live births (31).

Evaluation
History and Physical
- Antenatal
  - One-third of patients have polyhydramnios.
  - Poor swallowing and small fetal stomach volume may be seen.
- Postnatal
  - The infant appears to have excessive secretions despite frequent suctioning.
  - Coughing, respiratory distress, and cyanosis.
  - In patients with a distal fistula, the stomach may dilate with air, leading to the reflux of gastric secretions back into the lungs, leading to reactive bronchoconstriction and chemical pneumonitis (3).

Laboratory Tests
- Inability to pass a nasogastric tube into the stomach suggests the diagnosis.

- An x-ray with a coiled tube in the esophagus confirms the diagnosis.
- Injection of a small amount of air into the tube at the time of an x-ray may highlight the distal pouch before the atresia.

Treatment

Initial Management

- Prevention of aspiration is critical.
- The infant should be positioned with the head elevated and low, continuous suction applied to the upper esophageal pouch.
- The infant should be transferred to a tertiary NICU for repair.

Surgical Repair

- Primary surgical repair with ligation of the TEF and anastomosis of proximal and distal parts of the esophagus is performed, when possible.
- If there is a long gap between the proximal and distal esophagus, other procedures are necessary.

Complications

Prognosis

- Survival is greater than 95% in term infants without associated anomalies or respiratory problems.
- Significant lung disease, prematurity, and associated anomalies reduce survival.
- Problems with swallowing and gastroesophageal reflux should be expected.

Associations

- Thirty percent to forty percent have other anomalies, particularly VATER/VACTERL (vertebral defects, anal atresia, cardiac defects, TEF with EA, and radial, renal, and limb anomalies).
- The affected organ systems most commonly associated with EA/TEF are cardiovascular (35% to 45%), gastrointestinal (25%), genitourinary (25%), skeletal (15%), and neurologic (10%) (3).

AIRWAY MALFORMATIONS

Choanal Atresia or Stenosis

Background

Definition

- Choanal atresia is a complete blockage or severe narrowing of the nasal airway at the posterior nares.

Pathophysiology

- The vast majority of affected newborns are obligate nose breathers. The entire length of the neonate's tongue is in close proximity to the hard and soft palate, which creates a vacuum and resultant respiratory distress when nasal obstruction is present (3).

Etiology

- Atresia may occur from failure of canalization of the nasal choanae.
- Stenosis may be congenital and is often exacerbated by aggressive nasal suctioning (12).

Epidemiology

- Choanal atresia occurs in 1 in 2500 to 1 in 10,000 live births.

Evaluation

History and Physical

- Apnea and cyanosis that improve with crying.
- Failure to pass a nasal catheter into the nasopharynx suggests choanal atresia.

Laboratory Tests

- Computed tomography scans may help differentiate bony atresia from mucosal swelling.
- Nasal endoscopy may also be useful.

Treatment
Initial Management
- Ensure adequate airway. Use of an oral airway requires close observation.
- Endotracheal intubation, if necessary, provides the optimal airway until definitive surgical repair can be made.
- Stenosis with edema may be treated with topical vasoconstrictors and steroids.
- Definitive surgical repair usually endoscopic through the transnasal route.

Complications
Prognosis
- Outcome is good, depending on associated anomalies. Repeated dilations may be necessary during the first year of life to maintain choanal patency (3).

Associations
- About 50% of patients with choanal atresia have craniofacial syndromes (Treacher Collins, Apert, etc.) and CHARGE association (coloboma of eyes, heart defects, atresia choanae, retarded growth and development, genital anomalies, ear anomaly/deafness).

Congenital Defects Involving the Tongue and Mandible
Background
Definition
- A variety of defects in the upper airway may cause respiratory distress from blockage of the airway.
- Upper airway obstruction may be seen in a variety of conditions, including
  - Pierre Robin sequence (1 in 2000 live births) consists of micrognathia with a 60% incidence of cleft palate.
  - Macroglossia often is part of Beckwith-Wiedemann syndrome (macroglossia, macrosomia, omphalocele).

Treatment
Management
- Airway compromise may occur, and ventilation with bag and mask may be difficult.
- Careful attention to positioning, such as positioning on the side or prone, may allow the infant to breathe on her or his own.
- An appropriate-size oral airway may be useful.
- Intubation may be extremely difficult, and in rare cases, emergent cricothyrotomy may be necessary.
- Lower airway obstruction is rare.
  - It may be seen with large goiter or intrinsic laryngeal or tracheal stenoses or atresias.
  - Frank airway atresias have a dismal prognosis.
  - Stenoses may be stabilized clinically with positive-pressure ventilation if needed, before definitive repair.

Pulmonary Hypoplasia
Background
Definition
- Pulmonary hypoplasia is characterized by a decrease in the number and size of both airways and alveoli.

Pathophysiology
- Inadequate lung size leads to rapid respiratory failure.

Etiology
- Pulmonary hypoplasia most commonly results from oligohydramnios caused by either
  - Prolonged rupture of the membranes without reaccumulation of amniotic fluid or
  - Inadequate production of amniotic fluid by the fetus

- It is thought that constraint of fetal breathing movements and a lack of intra-amniotic fluid exerting pressure against the flow of fetal lung fluid out of the trachea may cause hypoplasia.

Epidemiology
- The incidence of pulmonary hypoplasia is variable. It is commonly seen in association with severe renal insufficiency or long-standing oligohydramnios.

Evaluation
History and Physical
- Antenatal ultrasound may raise suspicion for pulmonary hypoplasia based on other diagnoses that are commonly associated with it (see below).
- Both fetal lung ultrasound and magnetic resonance imaging may help quantitate the degree of pulmonary hypoplasia (32), but results from these tests are not definitive.
- Babies born with significant pulmonary hypoplasia exhibit severe cyanosis and respiratory failure characterized by gasping respirations almost immediately after delivery.
- Limb contractures and dysmorphic facies secondary to in utero compression may be present.

Laboratory Tests
- Chest x-rays reveal small lungs.
- Postmortem lung weights and histology may lead to a definitive diagnosis.
- Renal ultrasound should be obtained, especially if Potter syndrome is suspected (see below).

Treatment
Initial Management
- Usually, infants with pulmonary hypoplasia require immediate intubation, aggressive ventilatory support to prevent respiratory failure, and transfer to a NICU.
- There is a high risk for pneumothorax.
- High-frequency ventilation and surfactant therapy may be beneficial.
- Some infants who present with early severe respiratory failure consistent with pulmonary hypoplasia may benefit from inhaled nitric oxide (33).
- ECMO may be helpful but is reserved for those patients with less severe degrees of hypoplasia.

Complications
Prognosis
- The outcome is generally poor.
- Pulmonary hypoplasia associated with bilateral renal agenesis (Potter syndrome) is uniformly lethal and should be managed accordingly.

Associations
- Pulmonary hypoplasia is associated with
  - Congenital diaphragmatic hernia
  - Renal disease leading to severe oligohydramnios or anhydramnios (Potter syndrome, bladder outlet obstruction, etc.)
  - Prolonged premature rupture of membranes without reaccumulation of amniotic fluid

CONGENITAL CARDIAC DISEASE
Background
Definition
- Any anatomic or physiologic congenital abnormality of the heart

Etiology
- Anatomic congenital heart disease is caused by abnormalities in the formation of the heart.
- Abnormalities in cardiac rhythm or function may be caused by viral infections, maternal disease, or inherited metabolic diseases and are often sporadic and idiopathic.

Evaluation
- Antenatal diagnosis of congenital heart disease allows the physician to anticipate physiologic abnormalities, which may need no special treatment if the patient is not in distress.
- All of these conditions should be evaluated by a pediatric cardiologist for definitive management.
- In patients with significant mixing of oxygenated and deoxygenated blood in the heart, some degree of cyanosis may be apparent in the delivery room. If the infant is otherwise well, the usual response to cyanosis (oxygen administration followed by positive-pressure ventilation) is not necessary.

Ductal-Dependent Lesions
- Ductal-dependent lesions are congenital heart defects in which either the pulmonary or systemic circulation is dependent on flow of blood through the ductus arteriosus.
- Although the ductus does not close immediately after delivery, one should be prepared to begin continuous infusion of prostaglandin E_1 soon after delivery.

Congenital Heart Block
Background
Definition
- Complete congenital heart block is a total failure of atrial impulses to be conducted to the ventricles.

Pathophysiology
- Low heart rate due to absent conduction of atrial electric impulses to the ventricle, with the resultant heart rate being a ventricular rate

Etiology
- Complete congenital heart block can originate in either a structural interruption in or a degeneration of the cardiac conduction tissue.

Epidemiology
- Complete congenital heart block occurs in about 1 in 15,000 pregnancies (34).

Evaluation
History and Physical
- The heart rate is 50 to 90 bpm and is usually detected antenatally.
- Diagnosis during labor may lead to emergent delivery for bradycardia.
- Congestive failure may develop with heart rates lower than 50 bpm.

Treatment
- If the diagnosis is established and the newborn is not in distress, careful observation is often sufficient without the usual intervention for delivery room bradycardia.
- Acute symptomatic bradycardia can be treated with chronotropic agents such as isoproterenol and cardiac pacing if necessary.

Complications
Prognosis
- About 10% of fetuses with congenital heart block are born with hydrops fetalis and congestive heart failure, and their prognosis is poor.
- Neonatal mortality rate in infants born with a congenital heart block ranges from 20% to 30% (3).

- Structural heart disease occurs in 40% of infants with congenital heart block.
- Most of the remaining affected infants have mothers with connective tissue disease, particularly lupus, or serologic markers for these diseases without clinical symptoms.

NEUROLOGIC DISEASES AND NEURAL TUBE DEFECTS
Myelomeningocele
Background
Definition
- Myelomeningocele (MMC) is a protrusion of the membranes (*meningo-*) and neural elements (*myelo-*) outside the spinal canal.
- It is usually visible as a midline cystic structure on the back.

Etiology
- Disorder of primary neurulation, from either failure of closure of the neural tube during the 3rd and 4th weeks of gestation or disordered midline axial integration during gastrulation (35).
- Low levels of folic acid have been associated with neural tube defects (NTD), and treatment with folic acid before conception is a critical public health measure to reduce the incidence of NTDs (36).

Epidemiology
- Incidence of NTDs has steadily declined over the past three to four decades. It is estimated that ≥2500 infants with NTDs are born annually in the United States (36).

Evaluation
History and Physical
- A cystic structure that may be intact or ruptured, in the midline of the back, most commonly in the lumbosacral area
- Often seen on antenatal ultrasound

Laboratory Tests
- Elevated maternal serum α-fetoprotein (AFP) is usually seen.

Treatment
- Cesarean section delivery is preferred to avoid damage to the nerves and to avoid rupture of the sac.
- Neonatal management:
  - Care should be taken to protect the sac and its contents and to avoid rupture of an intact sac.
  - The infant should be placed prone or on the side with the lesion protected with warm, saline-soaked gauze.
  - Antibiotic administration should be initiated.
  - Because of the potential for developing severe latex allergy later in life, latex-free gloves and supplies must be used when caring for these patients.
  - Surgery should be undertaken within the first 72 hours after birth to prevent further deterioration of the spinal cord and nerve roots and to prevent infection (3).
  - In utero repair of this condition is still considered investigational (37). Fetal surgery of MMC before 26 weeks of gestation may preserve neuromotor function, reverse hindbrain herniation, and reduce the need for ventriculoperitoneal shunting (38).

Complications
Prognosis
- Varying degrees of paresis of the legs and sphincter dysfunction are seen. The degree of neuromotor impairment depends mostly on the level of the lesion and may change after surgery.
- About 80% will have a normal IQ.

- These infant require long-term neurosurgical, orthopedic, and urologic follow-up.
- Past efforts to establish criteria for nontreatment have, in general, been abandoned. Currently, most infants are offered palliative surgical care to correct the defect (3).

Associations
- Other central nervous system abnormalities are common; 90% have the Arnold-Chiari type II malformation, which often leads to hydrocephalus and the need for a ventriculo-peritoneal shunt (39).

Encephalocele
Background
Definition
- An encephalocele is a protrusion of the membranes and brain tissue from the cranium that is closed or covered by skin.
- It is less common than MMC but has a similar etiology and embryology.
- Encephalocele is seen in chromosomal disorders such as trisomies 13 and 18 and conditions such as Walker-Warburg, Meckel-Gruber, and Dandy-Walker syndromes (3).
- Treatment is surgical, but if large amounts of neural tissue are in the lesion, conservative management may be used.
- Overall, the prognosis is poor, but more favorable if only membranes are involved (cranial meningocele).

Hydrops Fetalis
Background
Definition
- Fetal hydrops is defined as the finding of serous fluid accumulation in two or more body cavities, which may include ascites, pleural or pericardial effusions, or skin or trunk edema (40).

Pathophysiology
- Fetal hydrops develops due to an imbalance between interstitial fluid collection and lymphatic removal. Fluid accumulation in the fetus can be due to (a) congestive heart failure, (b) obstructed lymphatic flow, or (c) decreased plasma osmotic pressure (3).

Etiology
- *Immune hydrops fetalis* results in severe hemolytic disease in the fetus (erythroblastosis fetalis), usually resulting from the D antigen in the Rh group.
  - Immune hydrops fetalis is now uncommon because of the use of anti-D immunoglobulin (RhoGAM) (41), but immune hydrops due to minor blood groups can occur.
- *Nonimmune hydrops fetalis* can result from a variety of nonimmunologic causes, including congenital heart disease (structural, supraventricular tachycardia), chromosomal anomalies (Turner syndrome, trisomies), infections (parvovirus B19, cytomegalovirus, syphilis, others), and chorioangioma of the placenta.
  - Many are idiopathic.

Epidemiology
- There is a wide range of estimates, from 1 in 100 to 1 in 14,000 pregnancies.

Evaluation
History and Physical
- Antenatal ultrasound reveals abnormal amounts of pleural, peritoneal, and pericardial fluid, with marked skin edema.
- The infant may be extremely edematous, with rapid, severe respiratory compromise.

Treatment
Fetal Intervention
- Fetal intervention may improve outcomes in select circumstances (40,42).

Initial Management
- The management team must be prepared to perform a complete resuscitation and to intubate rapidly.
- If the newborn fails to respond to these measures, then thoracentesis or paracentesis may be required to allow adequate air entry, particularly if the abdomen is tight or if large pleural effusions are present (43).
- These procedures involve inserting a large (16 or 18 gauge) intravenous catheter into the pleural space (usually at the fourth intercostal space in the anterior axillary line) or the peritoneal cavity (on the side of the abdomen, taking care to avoid the liver and spleen), removing the needle, and aspirating back using a large (25 to 50 mL) syringe attached to a stopcock, until no more fluid can be obtained.
- Additional personnel may be needed so multiple body cavities can be tapped rapidly if necessary.
- Pericardiocentesis is best performed by someone with experience in the procedure.

Complications
- Prognosis remains poor, with only 20% to 33% survival.

LETHAL ANOMALIES

Background
- The ever-increasing use and accuracy of obstetrical ultrasound has made the antenatal diagnosis of lethal anomalies increasingly more frequent.
- Antenatal diagnosis of a lethal anomaly should lead to caring and open discussion with the family well in advance of delivery to give them a full understanding of the anomaly and the reason for its lethality.
- Explicit communication at the time of delivery to reiterate the diagnosis, answer any questions, and review the management plan is essential.

Treatment
- At delivery, the infant should be wiped dry, wrapped in a warm blanket, and given to the family to hold unless they expressly refuse.
- An explanation of visible abnormalities and relating them to antenatal findings is often useful.
- Contacting a chaplain (and arranging for baptism if the family so desires), a bereavement counselor, a social worker, and other support personnel is of great benefit.
- The infant should undergo a thorough examination at some point to confirm the diagnosis and to search for findings that may not have been seen antenatally.
- Chromosome studies may be appropriate if they have not already been performed.
- Permission for complete autopsy should always be sought.

Aftercare
- A follow-up meeting with the parents, a few weeks or months after the delivery, may help them with the grieving process and may resolve unanswered questions.
- Results of an autopsy, if performed, can also be reviewed at this time.
- Referral for genetic counseling before contemplating another pregnancy should be offered.

EXTREME PREMATURITY AND THE LIMIT OF VIABILITY
Background
- Viability refers to the gestational age when a fetus reaches an anatomical threshold when critical organs can sustain life. A more practical definition states that viability is the age at which the infant has a 50% chance of long-term survival (44).

- The Neonatal Resuscitation Program (NRP) states "where gestation, birth weight, and/or congenital anomalies are associated with almost certain early death, and unacceptably high morbidity among the rare survivors, resuscitation is not indicated" and states this may apply when the gestational age is less than 23 weeks, birth weight is less than 400 g, anencephaly is present, or with a confirmed diagnosis of trisomy 13 or 18 (5). Some parents of patients with trisomy 13 or 18 or at 22 weeks' gestation have opted for full care for their babies and would advocate for at least offering this care. The NRP also states that parents have a primary role in determining goals of care, stressing the importance of a fully informed decision.
- In a survey of New England neonatologists, most agreed that resuscitation is clearly indicated at 25 weeks of gestation. Between 24 and 25 weeks' gestation, 40% thought that resuscitation is clearly beneficial, and none surveyed believed it to be futile. Although few physicians believe that resuscitation is clearly beneficial between 23 and 24 weeks' gestation, only about 5% thought resuscitation was clearly futile. Between 22 and 23 weeks' gestation, more than 80% thought resuscitation was futile (45).
- In spite of improved survival at early gestational ages, the incidence of significant morbidity such as chronic lung disease, impaired vision, mental retardation, and cerebral palsy remains a matter of concern for the families and those in the medical profession responsible for the care of these infants.
- Survival to 3 years for babies admitted for intensive care increased from 39% in 1995 (EPICure) to 52% in 2006 (EPICure2). A higher proportion of infants survived without disability during the same period (6% vs. 16%). Survival increased from 9% to 23% at 25 weeks (survival without disability 6% vs. 24%) and from 5% to 20% at 24 weeks (survival without disability 0.5% vs. 20%). There was no improvement in survival or survival without disability at 23 weeks (46).
- In a study of Very Low Birthweight (VLBW) infants born in Neonatal Research Network Centers between 2003 and 2007, rates of survival were 6% at 22 weeks, 26% at 23 weeks, 55% at 24 weeks, and 72% at 25 weeks. Rates of survival without morbidity increased from 0% at 22 weeks to 8% at 23 weeks, 9% at 24 weeks, and 20% at 25 weeks (47). A web-based tool derived from these data using gestational age and four other variables (estimated weight, gender, single vs. multiple fetuses, maternal steroid administration) is available to help estimate prognosis and counsel families.
- In a multicenter study including 3065 ELBW babies born in Japan in 2005, Itabashi et al. (48) report survival to discharge at 22 and 23 weeks of 34% and 54%, respectively.
- Seri et al. (44) conclude that infants born at less than 23 weeks' gestation and less than 500 g are too immature to survive and provision of care for these patients is unreasonable. On the other hand, infants who are born at greater than or equal to 25 weeks' gestation and with a birth weight of greater than or equal to 600 g are mature enough and warrant initiation of intensive care. For infants born with gestational age and birth weight between these two groups, medical decision-making should be based on gestational age, birth weight, clinical condition upon delivery, and parental wishes.

Management
- Communication among the family, obstetrician, and pediatrician/neonatologist to discuss the situation and make a tentative delivery room plan is optimal.
- It is always advisable to check current outcome statistics, hospital policies, and local regulations (if any) concerning care in this situation, as these factors continue to evolve. Potential treatment plans include
  - Full intervention in delivery room
  - Immediate assessment of viability and resuscitation if the newborn is deemed potentially viable
    - Factors that may help decide if a newborn is viable include
      - Fetal foot length less than 40 mm
      - Translucent gelatinous skin with bruising
      - No activity and minimal response to resuscitative efforts

- No resuscitation based on historical information
  - If the delivering obstetrician and the family desire no intervention, then not calling a pediatrician to the delivery is an option, as, once present, the pediatrician may feel obligated to exercise professional judgment and act on behalf of the neonatal patient.
  - Once the decision has been made not to resuscitate the newborn, a belated resuscitation delayed by more than a few minutes should not be offered, as the expected outcome is very poor (49).
- When significant uncertainty about viability exists (such as at 23 to 24 weeks' gestation), many professionals advocate beginning resuscitation and intensive care but stating overtly to the family that if it becomes clear that survival is unlikely, intensive care should be withdrawn.
  - This approach may be ethically superior, in that one gains the knowledge of whether the patient will respond to treatment.
  - Emotionally, however, families may find it more difficult to stop treatments that have already begun.

MULTIPLE BIRTHS

- Multiple gestation pregnancies are more likely to result in premature birth, cesarean delivery, and depressed infants.
- The usual resuscitative measures should be used, but there should be separate resuscitation teams, infant warmers, and equipment for each infant.

UNSUSPECTED MAJOR MALFORMATIONS

- When unexpected major malformations are discovered at the time of delivery, appropriate communication with the family is of utmost importance.
  - In addition to any special care related to the specific condition, a caring, honest, and sensitive approach should be taken with the family.
  - Initially, a brief description of the anomaly, coupled with whatever reassurance is appropriate, should be given to the parents, and they should be allowed to see the infant and, if stable, hold him or her.
  - Because of the shock inherent in this situation, parents are unlikely to absorb the initial information and will need additional communication.
- Parents also go through a grieving process for the loss of the hoped-for normal child and will need to reattach to their child.
  - There is often a tendency for parents, especially the mother, to feel guilt for the anomaly.
  - Mothers should be reassured they are not to blame for the anomaly, unless there is clear evidence that the diagnosis does relate to a known teratogen, such as in the case of anomalies associated with the fetal alcohol syndrome:
    - This should be discussed in an open and sensitive manner.
- The infant should be referred for any further evaluation and treatment as needed.
- Appropriate follow-up counseling and support services should be provided.

PATIENT EDUCATION
Antenatal Diagnoses of Major Malformations
- Present findings to parents in a timely manner, including
  - Appropriate private setting
  - Father or support people present, if possible
  - Adequate time to discuss diagnosis
  - Provision of written information, Internet and other sources, and so on
  - Offering a full range of options in a nonjudgmental (unbiased) manner, which may include
    - Termination of pregnancy if appropriate
    - Nonintervention if appropriate

- Informing parents of support groups for parents who have babies with the same diagnosis, if available and if the parents so desire
- Scheduling a second meeting to make decisions and answer questions
- Consultation with appropriate medical and/or surgical specialists who would be involved in the care of the baby
- Consultation with neonatology if the condition is likely to result in need for NICU care
- Plan for delivery at a regional high-risk perinatal center to facilitate optimal care, keeping baby near mother, if treatment in neonatal period expected

Lethal Abnormalities
- Present findings to parents in a timely manner (as noted above).
- Consider consultation with appropriate medical and/or surgical specialists if parents desire.
- Formulate delivery room plan.
- Consider a neonatology consult if the neonatologist will be present at delivery.
  - A consultation may be especially useful if uncertainty exists about the lethality of conditions.
- Anticipate needs for bereavement support.

Threatened Preterm Delivery at the Threshold of Viability
- Schedule a neonatology consult as soon as feasible.
- Review current statistics and expected outcomes.
- Consider pertinent hospital policies and local regulations (if any).
- Formulate delivery room options/plan in advance (details in "Extreme Prematurity and the Limit of Viability," above).
  - Important that plan is conveyed to the on-call team who may end up caring for the mother and baby
  - Important to regularly revisit the plan, as expected outcomes change rapidly at the threshold of viability

REFERENCES

1. Fanaroff AA. Meconium aspiration syndrome: historical aspects. *J Perinatol.* 2008;28 (suppl 3):S3–S7.
2. Martin RJ, Fanaroff AA, Walsh MC. *Fanaroff and Martin's neonatal-perinatal medicine: diseases of the fetus and infant.* St. Louis: Mosby/Elsevier, 2011.
3. Dargaville PA, Copnell B; Australian and New Zealand Neonatal Network. The epidemiology of meconium aspiration syndrome: incidence, risk factors, therapies, and outcome. *Pediatrics.* 2006;117:1712–1721.
4. Yoder BA, Kirsch EA, Barth WH, et al. Changing obstetric practices associated with decreasing incidence of meconium aspiration syndrome. *Obstet Gynecol.* 2002;99:731–739.
5. Zaichkin J, Kattwinkel J, McGowan J; American Heart Association, American Academy of Pediatrics. *Textbook of neonatal resuscitation.* Elk Grove Village: American Heart Association, American Academy of Pediatrics, 2011: pp 1 online resource (xiii, 328 p.).
6. Balchin I, Whittaker JC, Lamont RF, et al. Maternal and fetal characteristics associated with meconium-stained amniotic fluid. *Obstet Gynecol.* 2011;117:828–835.
7. Xu H, Hofmeyr J, Roy C, et al. Intrapartum amnioinfusion for meconium-stained amniotic fluid: a systematic review of randomised controlled trials. *BJOG.* 2007;114:383–390.
8. Vain NE, Szyld EG, Prudent LM, et al. Oropharyngeal and nasopharyngeal suctioning of meconium-stained neonates before delivery of their shoulders: multicentre, randomised controlled trial. *Lancet.* 2004;364:597–602.
9. Gregory GA, Gooding CA, Phibbs RH, et al. Meconium aspiration in infants—a prospective study. *J Pediatr.* 1974;85:848–852.
10. Halliday HL. Endotracheal intubation at birth for preventing morbidity and mortality in vigorous, meconium-stained infants born at term. *Cochrane Database Syst Rev.* 2001;(1):CD000500.

11. Wiswell TE. Delivery room management of the meconium-stained newborn. *J Perinatol.* 2008;28(suppl 3):S19–S26.
12. Logan JW, Rice HE, Goldberg RN, et al. Congenital diaphragmatic hernia: a systematic review and summary of best-evidence practice strategies. *J Perinatol.* 2007;27:535–549.
13. Wynn J, Krishnan U, Aspelund G, et al. Outcomes of congenital diaphragmatic hernia in the modern era of management. *J Pediatr.* 2013;163(1):114–119.
14. Finer NN, Tierney A, Etches PC, et al. Congenital diaphragmatic hernia: developing a protocolized approach. *J Pediatr Surg.* 1998;33:1331–1337.
15. Moyer V, Moya F, Tibboel R, et al. Late versus early surgical correction for congenital diaphragmatic hernia in newborn infants. *Cochrane Database Syst Rev.* 2002;(3):CD001695.
16. Langer JC, Filler RM, Bohn DJ, et al. Timing of surgery for congenital diaphragmatic hernia: is emergency operation necessary? *J Pediatr Surg.* 1988;23:731–734.
17. Rozmiarek AJ, Qureshi FG, Cassidy L, et al. Factors influencing survival in newborns with congenital diaphragmatic hernia: the relative role of timing of surgery. *J Pediatr Surg.* 2004;39:821–824; discussion 821–824.
18. Deprest JA, Nicolaides K, Gratacos E. Fetal surgery for congenital diaphragmatic hernia is back from never gone. *Fetal Diagn Ther.* 2011;29:6–17.
19. Lally KP, Lally PA, Lasky RE, et al.; Group CDHS. Defect size determines survival in infants with congenital diaphragmatic hernia. *Pediatrics.* 2007;120:e651–e657.
20. van Eijck FC, Klein WM, Boetes C, et al. Has the liver and other visceral organs migrated to its normal position in children with giant omphalocele? A follow-up study with ultrasonography. *Eur J Pediatr.* 2010;169:563–567.
21. Anteby EY, Yagel S. Route of delivery of fetuses with structural anomalies. *Eur J Obstet Gynecol Reprod Biol.* 2003;106:5–9.
22. Heider AL, Strauss RA, Kuller JA. Omphalocele: clinical outcomes in cases with normal karyotypes. *Am J Obstet Gynecol.* 2004;190:135–141.
23. Vu LT, Nobuhara KK, Laurent C, et al. Increasing prevalence of gastroschisis: population-based study in California. *J Pediatr.* 2008;152:807–811.
24. Loane M, Dolk H, Bradbury I; EUROCAT Working Group. Increasing prevalence of gastroschisis in Europe 1980–2002: a phenomenon restricted to younger mothers? *Paediatr Perinat Epidemiol.* 2007;21:363–369.
25. Kohler JA Sr, Perkins AM, Bass WT. Human milk versus formula after gastroschisis repair: effects on time to full feeds and time to discharge. *J Perinatol.* 2013;33(8):627–630.
26. Kunz LH, Gilbert WM, Towner DR. Increased incidence of cardiac anomalies in pregnancies complicated by gastroschisis. *Am J Obstet Gynecol.* 2005;193:1248–1252.
27. Best KE, Tennant PW, Addor MC, et al. Epidemiology of small intestinal atresia in Europe: a register-based study. *Arch Dis Child Fetal Neonatal Ed.* 2012;97:F353–F358.
28. Ashcraft KW, Holcomb GW, Murphy JP, et al. *Ashcraft's pediatric surgery.* Philadelphia: Saunders/Elsevier, 2010: xxi, 1101.
29. Spilde TL, Bhatia AM, Miller KA, et al. Thyroid transcription factor-1 expression in the human neonatal tracheoesophageal fistula. *J Pediatr Surg.* 2002;37:1065–1067.
30. van den Brink GR Hedgehog signaling in development and homeostasis of the gastrointestinal tract. *Physiol Rev.* 2007;87:1343–1375.
31. Pedersen RN, Calzolari E, Husby S, et al.; EUROCAT Working group. Oesophageal atresia: prevalence, prenatal diagnosis and associated anomalies in 23 European regions. *Arch Dis Child.* 2012;97:227–232.
32. Tanigaki S, Miyakoshi K, Tanaka M, et al. Pulmonary hypoplasia: prediction with use of ratio of MR imaging-measured fetal lung volume to US-estimated fetal body weight. *Radiology.* 2004;232:767–772.
33. Chock VY, Van Meurs KP, Hintz SR, et al.; NICHD Neonatal Research Network. Inhaled nitric oxide for preterm premature rupture of membranes, oligohydramnios, and pulmonary hypoplasia. *Am J Perinatol.* 2009;26:317–322.
34. Glatz AC, Gaynor JW, Rhodes LA, et al. Outcome of high-risk neonates with congenital complete heart block paced in the first 24 hours after birth. *J Thorac Cardiovasc Surg* 2008;136:767–773.

35. Dias MS, Partington M. Embryology of myelomeningocele and anencephaly. *Neurosurg Focus*. 2004;16:E1.
36. Pitkin RM. Folate and neural tube defects. *Am J Clin Nutr*. 2007;85:285S–288S.
37. Arca MJ, Teich S. Current controversies in perinatal care: fetal versus neonatal surgery. *Clin Perinatol*. 2004;31:629–648.
38. Danzer E, Johnson MP, Adzick NS. Fetal surgery for myelomeningocele: progress and perspectives. *Dev Med Child Neurol*. 2012;54:8–14.
39. Talamonti G, D'Aliberti G, Collice M. Myelomeningocele: long-term neurosurgical treatment and follow-up in 202 patients. *J Neurosurg*. 2007;107:368–386.
40. Cass DL, Olutoye OO, Ayres NA, et al. Defining hydrops and indications for open fetal surgery for fetuses with lung masses and vascular tumors. *J Pediatr Surg*. 2012;47:40–45.
41. Ismail KM, Martin WL, Ghosh S, et al. Etiology and outcome of hydrops fetalis. *J Matern Fetal Med*. 2001;10:175–181.
42. Grethel EJ, Wagner AJ, Clifton MS, et al. Fetal intervention for mass lesions and hydrops improves outcome: a 15-year experience. *J Pediatr Surg*. 2007;42:117–123.
43. Carlton DP, McGillivray BC, Schreiber MD. Nonimmune hydrops fetalis: a multidisciplinary approach. *Clin Perinatol*. 1989;16.839–851.
44. Seri I, Evans J. Limits of viability: definition of the gray zone. *J Perinatol*. 2008;28(suppl 1): S4–S8.
45. Peerzada JM, Richardson DK, Burns JP. Delivery room decision-making at the threshold of viability. *J Pediatr*. 2004;145:492–498.
46. Moore T, Hennessy EM, Myles J, et al. Neurological and developmental outcome in extremely preterm children born in England in 1995 and 2006: the EPICure studies. *BMJ*. 2012;345:e7961.
47. Stoll BJ, Hansen NI, Bell EF, et al.; Eunice Kennedy Shriver National Institute of Child Health and Human Development Neonatal Research Network. Neonatal outcomes of extremely preterm infants from the NICHD Neonatal Research Network. *Pediatrics*. 2010;126:443–456.
48. Itabashi K, Horiuchi T, Kusuda S, et al. Mortality rates for extremely low birth weight infants born in Japan in 2005. *Pediatrics*. 2009;123(2):445–450.
49. Paris JJ, Goldsmith JP, Cimperman M. Resuscitation of a micropreemie: the case of MacDonald v Milleville. *J Perinatol*. 1998;18:302–305.

Index

Note: Page numbers in *italics* indicate figures; those followed by "t" indicate tables.